How Synthetic Drugs W

Insights into Molecular Pharmacology of Classic an

Pharmaceuticals

How Synthetic Drugs Work

Insights into Molecular Pharmacology of Classic and New Pharmaceuticals

Edited by

Imran Kazmi
Department of Biochemistry, Faculty of Science, King Abdulaziz University, Jeddah, Saudi Arabia

Sanmoy Karmakar
Department of Pharmaceutical Technology, Jadavpur University, Kolkata, West Bengal, India

Md. Adil Shaharyar
Department of Pharmaceutical Technology, Jadavpur University, Kolkata, West Bengal, India

Muhammad Afzal
Department of Pharmacology, College of Pharmacy, Jouf University, Sakaka, Aljouf, Saudi Arabia

Fahad A. Al-Abbasi
Department of Biochemistry, Faculty of Science, King Abdulaziz University, Jeddah, Saudi Arabia

ELSEVIER

ACADEMIC PRESS
An imprint of Elsevier

Academic Press is an imprint of Elsevier
125 London Wall, London EC2Y 5AS, United Kingdom
525 B Street, Suite 1650, San Diego, CA 92101, United States
50 Hampshire Street, 5th Floor, Cambridge, MA 02139, United States
The Boulevard, Langford Lane, Kidlington, Oxford OX5 1GB, United Kingdom

ISBN: 978-0-323-99855-0

For Information on all Academic Press publications
visit our website at https://www.elsevier.com/books-and-journals

Publisher: Mica H. Haley
Acquisitions Editor: Andre G. Wolff
Editorial Project Manager: Samantha Allard
Production Project Manager: Omer Mukthar
Cover Designer: Miles Hitchen

Typeset by MPS Limited, Chennai, India

Contents

List of contributors xxi

1. **Introduction to molecular pharmacology: basic concepts** 1

Muhammad Afzal, Imran Kazmi, Rupinder Kaur, Salman Bakr I. Hosawi, Mohammed Kaleem, Sami I. Alzarea and Muhammad Masood Ahmad

Pharmacology 1
Drugs 1
Brief history of pharmacology 1
Routes of drug administration 2
Enteral routes 2
Parenteral routes of drug administration 3
Local routes of drug administration 4
Pharmacokinetics 4
Passive diffusion 4
Filtration 5
Specialized transport 5
Carrier transport 5
Pinocytosis 6
Absorption 6
Factors affecting absorption of drugs 6
Physical factors 6
Drug distribution 7
Volume of distribution 7
Water compartments in the body 7
Plasma compartment 7
Extracellular fluid 7
Total body water 7
Other sites 8
Apparent volume of distribution 8
Plasma protein binding of the drugs 8
Drug metabolism 8
Kinetics of metabolism 8
Phase I reactions 9
Phase II reactions 9
Drug excretion 9

Pharmacodynamics: drug receptor interactions or mechanism of drug effects 10
Principles of drug action 10
Mechanism of drug actions 11
Physical action 11
Chemical action 12
Through enzymes 12
Through receptors 12
Some important definitions[75] 12
Agonists 12
Inverse agonist 12
Antagonist 12
Partial agonist 12
Ligand 13
Nature of receptors 13
Transducer mechanisms 13
G protein–coupled receptors 13
Receptors with intrinsic ion channels 16
Enzymatic receptors 17
Nuclear receptors 19
Reference 20

2 Mechanism of action of cholinergic drugs 27
Khandekar Hussan Reza, Partha Pratim Das, Chowdhury Mobaswar Hossain, Md. Adil Shaharyar, Soupayan Pal, Sk Zeeshan Ali and Imran Kazmi

Introduction 27
Chemistry of autonomic neurotransmitters 29
Biochemistry of acetylcholine 29
Signal transduction mechanisms involved in drug response 30
Nicotinic receptor 31
Muscarinic receptors 32
Inhibition of adenylyl cyclase 34
Conclusion 44
References 44
Further reading 46

3 Mechanism of action of adrenergic drugs and recent updates 47
Raisur Rahman, Shakir Saleem and Ruqaiyah Khan

Background 47
The Nervous System 47
Peripheral Nervous System 47
Adrenergic Drugs 48
Pharmacological Actions 49

Adrenergic Nerve Receptors 49
Molecular structure of G protein–coupled receptor 51
G-proteins 51
Difference between α and β receptors 52
Conclusion 59
References 59

4 Insight into the mechanism of steroidal and non-steroidal anti-inflammatory drugs 61
Kazi Asraf Ali, Arindam Maity, Sanhati Dutta Roy, Siddhartha Das Pramanik, Partha Pratim Das and Md. Adil Shaharyar

Introduction to inflammation and its role 61
Pathophysiology of inflammation and inflammatory pathway 63
Inflammatory mediators 65
Inflammatory diseases 65
Rheumatoid arthritis (RA) 66
Asthma 67
Chronic obstructive pulmonary disease 67
Inflammatory bowel disease (IBD) 68
Multiple sclerosis 69
Allergic rhinitis 69
Inflammatory disease and their treatments 69
Classification of non steroidal anti-inflammatory drugs and corticosteroids in broad category 69
Classification of NSAIDs 72
Classification of corticosteroids 73
Mechanism of action of corticosteroids and non steroidal anti-inflammatory drugs 74
Molecular mechanism of action of each class of NSAIDs 74
Anti-inflammatory mechanism of corticosteroids 82
Contraindications of corticosteroids 86
Contraindications of nonsteroidal anti-inflammatory drugs 86
Conclusion 86
References 87

5 Insight into the mechanism of action of anti-diabetic drugs 95
Gayatri Thapa, Amrita Kumari, Debankini Dasgupta, Shwetlana Bandyopadhy, Nilanjan Sarkar, Kalyan Roy, Gauthaman Karunakaran, Imran Kazmi, Samit Karmakar and Mainak Chakraborty

Introduction 95
Biochemical background of diabetes mellitus 95
Classification of diabetes 96

Type 1 diabetes mellitus 96
Pathophysiology of type-1 diabetes 96
Type 2 diabetes mellitus 96
Other specific types of diabetes[14] 97
Genetic defects in insulin action 97
Diseases of the exocrine pancreas 97
Endocrinopathies 98
Drug or chemical-induced 98
Infections 99
Uncommon forms of immune-mediated diabetes 99
Other genetic syndromes sometimes associated with diabetes 99
Etiology 99
Genetic component 99
Sulfonylureas 103
Effect of amaryl in adipose cells: regulation of key metabolic proteins/enzymes 105
Biguanides 105
Metformin 107
Metformin and organic cation transporters 107
K_{ATP} channel modulators (nonsulfonyl ureas): meglitinides 108
Repaglinide 108
α-Glucosidase inhibitors 108
Dipeptidyl peptidase-4 inhibitors 110
Mechanism of action 110
Dipeptidyl peptidase-4 inhibition in the gut 110
Thiazolidinediones 112
Mechanism of action 112
Bromocriptine 115
GLP-1 agonist 115
Liraglutide 116
Albiglutide 117
Other glucose-lowering agents 117
Pramlintide: amylin analog 117
References 118

6 Molecular mechanism of action of estrogens, progestins, and androgens 123
Muhammad Arshad Malik and Muhammad Shahid Nadeem

Introduction 123
Synthesis of endogenous estrogens, progesterone, and androgens 124
Mechanism of action of endogenous steroid sex hormones (estrogens, progesterone, and androgens) 127
Role of estrogen, progesterone, and androgen in diseases 127
Hormonal imbalance in females 127
Hormonal imbalance in males 129
Cancer 130

Synthetic estrogens, progestins, and androgens for treatment of hormone-related diseases 132
Hormonal therapy 132
Mechanism of action of synthetic estrogens 133
Mechanism of action of progestins 140
Mechanism of action of synthetic Androgens 148
References 157

7 Mechanism of action of sedatives, hypnotics, and antianxiety drugs 161
Muhammad Azhar Nisar and Muhammad Zubair Saleem

Introduction 161
Generalized mode of action of anxiolytics, sedatives/hypnotics 161
Anxiety and antianxiety medications 164
Novel molecules with diverse pharmacological targets 164
Sedatives and hypnotics 170
Benzodiazepines 170
Additional agents 171
Hypnotics are used to induce and maintain anesthesia 171
Sedatives/anesthetics administered intravenously 173
Closing remarks 174
References 174

8 Mechanism of action of antiepileptic drugs 177
Haider Ali, Naushad Ahmad Khan, Mirza Masroor Ali Beg, Mohammed Zahed Sarwar, Nurida Kemelbek Kyzy, Tilekeeva Ulankul Muktarovna, Kudaibergen Osmonaliev, Faez Iqbal Khan and Muhammed Burak Ay

Introduction 177
Pathophysiology and pathogenesis of epilepsy 178
Role of GABA 180
Role of glutamate 180
General treatment 182
Phenobarbital mechanism of action 183
Bromide (potassium bromide/sodium bromide) 183
Phenytoin mechanism of action 183
Benzodiazepines mechanism of action 184
Carbamazepine mechanism of action 184
Ethosuximide mechanism of action 184
Valproic acid mechanism of action 185
Gabapentin mechanism of action 185
Newer antiepileptic drugs 186
Mechanism of action of eslicarbazepine acetate 186
Levetiracetam 186
Brivaracetam 186

Lacosamide 186
Conclusion 187
References 187

9 **Mechanism of action of anti-Parkinson's drugs** 195
Muhammad Shahid Nadeem, Salman Bakr I. Hosawi, Bibi Nazia Murtaza and Imran Kazmi

Introduction to Parkinson's disease 195
Parkinson's disease symptoms, and its subtypes 196
Epidemiology and risk factors for Parkinson's disease 198
Substantia nigra and its association with neuronal components 199
Pathophysiology and pathoanatomy of Parkinson's disease 201
Anti-Parkinson's disease drugs 202
Levo-DOPA 202
Dopamine agonists 203
Catechol-o-methyltransferase 203
Catechol-O-methyltransferase inhibitors and Parkinson's disease 204
Monoamine oxidase 206
Monoamine oxidase-A and monoamine oxidase-B 206
Inhibitors of monoamine oxidase-A and monoamine oxidase-B 207
Monoamine oxidase-B inhibitor selegiline and Parkinson's disease 207
Monoamine oxidase-B inhibitor lazabemide in Parkinson's disease 207
Summary 208
References 210

10 **Mechanism of action of antipsychotics and antimanics** 215
Muhammad Shahid Nadeem, Muhammad Naeem Riaz, Salman Bakr I. Hosawi, Hisham N. Altayb, Aziz Ud-din and Tanzeela Fazal

Introduction 215
Psychological disorders at a glance 216
Behaviors represented by a psychological disorder 217
Definition of physiological disorders 217
Common symptoms of psychological disorders 218
Physical symptoms of psychological disorders 219
Some serious symptoms that might indicate a life-threatening condition 219
Causes psychological disorders 219
Risk factors for psychological disorders 219
Treatment of psychological disorders 220
Common treatments for psychological disorders 220
Ways to improve your psychological disorders 220
Potential complications of psychological disorders 221
Etiology of schizophrenia 221

Genetic factors 221
Neurotransmitters 222
Pregnancy and birth complications 222
Season of birth 222
Cannabis use 223
Genetic factors for psychological diseases 223
Genetics of schizophrenia 223
Familial clustering 223
Genetic changes 223
Environmental factors 228
Pollution 228
Pathophysiology of psychotic disease 230
Psychoses 230
Schizophrenia—split mind 231
Chlorpromazine 232
Mechanism of action of antipsychotics 239
Mechanisms of action of lithium 239
Assume 239
Unclear 243
Electrolytes, membrane transport, membrane potential 243
Monoaminergic signaling 244
Second messenger system 244
Transcription factors 245
Regulation of intracellular calcium 246
Glycogen synthase kinase 246
Carbamazepine 246
Valproic acid 247
Mechanism 247
Olanzapine 249
Risperidone 249
Lithium carbonate 251
Carbamazepine 252
Sodium valproate 252
Lamotrigine 253
References 253

11 Mechanism of action of antidepressants 255

Kuldeepak Sharma, Ankush Sundriyal, Aanchal Loshali, Mohit Agrawal, Chinnabonia Gopala Krishna and Yogendra Singh

Introduction 255
Pathophysiology of major depression 255
Monoamines and other neurotransmitters hypotheses 256
Neurotrophic hypotheses 257
Stress-responsive/HPA axis hypotheses 258
Dysbiosis/gut/brain axis hypotheses 259

Glutamate hypotheses 260
Assimilation of hypotheses on depression pathophysiology 260
Fundamental pharmacology of antidepressants 261
Selective serotonin reuptake inhibitors 261
Serotonin-norepinephrine reuptake inhibitors 262
5-Hydroxytryptamine receptor modulators 263
Monoamine oxidase inhibitors 264
Glutamate signaling antagonist 265
Adverse effect and interaction of antidepressant drugs 266
Conclusion 267
References 267

12 Mechanism on the action of drugs for heart failure 275
Waleed Hassan Almalki

Introduction 275
Classification of heart failure 275
Etiology 277
Pathophysiology 277
Changes in hemodynamics 277
Changes of neurohormones 279
Changes in the cell 279
Management of heart failure 281
Diuretics 281
Vasodilators 282
Digoxin 282
Positive ionotropic 282
Atrioventricular node inhibition 282
Angiotensin-converting enzyme inhibitors 283
Angiotensin-II blockers (AT1 antagonists) 283
Beta-blockers 283
Calcium channel blockers 284
Newer agents 284
Conclusion 285
References 285

13 Mechanism of action of antiarrhythmic drugs 289
Hindol Mazumdar, Rudranil Bhowmik, Md. Adil Shaharyar, Avishek Mandal, Kumar Anand, Susmita Patra, Reshma Kumari, Sandipan Jana, Pallab Kanti Haldar and Sanmoy Karmakar

Introduction 289
Signs and symptoms of cardiac arrhythmia 290
General approach 290
Palpitations 290
Syncope and presyncope 291
Sudden cardiac arrest and aborted sudden cardiac death 292

Physical findings 293
Genetics of cardiac arrhythmias 293
The QT-opathies 294
Long-QT syndrome 294
The other channelopathies 299
Catecholaminergic polymorphic ventricular tachycardia 299
Principles of electrophysiology 300
Descriptive physiology 300
Mechanisms of cardiac arrhythmias 302
Types of cardiac arrhythmias 305
Bradycardia 305
Supraventricular tachyarrhythmia 306
Atrioventricular nodal tachycardias 308
Ventricular tachyarrhythmia 309
Antiarrhythmic drugs 311
Classification of antiarrhythmic drugs 311
Class I antiarrhythmic drugs 311
Specific class IA drugs 313
Specific class IB drugs 314
Specific class IC drugs 314
Class II antiarrhythmic drugs 315
Class III antiarrhythmic drugs 316
Class IV antiarrhythmic drugs 318
Other antiarrhythmic drugs 319
New developments in antiarrhythmic therapy 320
Conclusion 320
References 321

14 Insights into the mode of action of antianginal and vasodilating agents 329

Susmita Patra, Pratibha Gupta, Reshma Kumari, Sandipan Jana, Pallab Kanti Haldar, Rudranil Bhowmik, Avishek Mandal, Md. Adil Shaharyar, Hindol Mazumdar, Kumar Anand and Sanmoy Karmakar

Pathophysiology associated with angina pectoris 329
USFDA classification of antianginal drugs 332
Mechanism of action of nitrates 333
Mechanism of action of beta-blockers 335
Mechanism of action of calcium channel blocker 337
Mechanism of action of potassium channel opener 338
Other drugs 339
Dipyridamole 339
Trimetazidine 340
Ranolazine 340
Fasudil 341

Ivabradine 342
Conclusion 343
References 344

15 Mechanism of action of drugs used in hypertension 349

Rudranil Bhowmik, Md. Adil Shaharyar, Kumar Anand, Hindol Mazumdar, Avishek Mandal, Pallab Mandal, Suparno Chakraborty, Parag Panday and Sanmoy Karmakar

Etiology of hypertension 350
Normal regulation of blood pressure 350
Control of renin secretion 352
Renin and prorenin receptor 353
Classification of antihypertensive drugs 354
Diuretics 355
Sympatholytic agents 356
Ca^{2+} channel blockers 358
Angiotensin-converting enzyme inhibitors 359
AngII receptor antagonist 360
Direct renin inhibitor 361
Vasodilators 361
D1 receptor agonist 362
Conclusion 362
References 362

16 Mechanism of action of diuretic and anti-diuretic drugs 369

Raja Chakraverty, Kalyan Samanta, Pallab Mandal and Samit Karmakar

Introduction 369
Brief anatomy and physiology of the nephron 369
Classification of diuretics (according to site of their action) 370
Normal physiology of different parts of nephron and related diuretics 371
Glomerulus and Bowman's capsule 371
Diuretic acting on glomerulus 371
Adenosine receptor antagonist: caffeine, theophylline, theobromine 371
Drugs acting on proximal convoluted tubule 373
Carbonic anhydrase inhibitors: acetazolamide, dorzolamide, ethoxzolamide, methazolamide, etc 373
Sodium-glucose cotransporter 2 inhibitors: dapagliflozin, canagliflozin, empagliflozin, etc 373
Diuretics acting on thick ascending limb 376
Loop diuretics: furosemide, torsemide, bumetanide and ethacrynic acid, etc 376
Mechanism of hypocalcaemia and hypomagnesemia 376

Mechanism of hypokalemia and metabolic alkalosis 377
Distal convoluted tubule 377
Diuretics acting on distal convoluted tubule 378
Thiazide diuretics: chlorothiazide, chlorthalidone, hydrochlorothiazide, indapamide, metolazone 378
Diuretics acting on tubule system 383
Aldosterone receptor antagonist or mineralocorticoid receptor antagonist (K + sparing diuretics): spironolactone, eplerenone 383
Inhibitors of renal epithelial Na + channel (K + sparing diuretics): triamterene, amiloride 383
Antidiuretic hormone receptor (vasopressin) antagonist: tolvaptan, conivaptan 384
Nonspecific cation channel inhibitor: natriuretic peptides: (1) atria natriuretic peptide, (2) brain natriuretic peptide, (3) C-type natriuretic peptide and urodilatin 385
Others 385
Osmotic diuretics: mannitol, urea, isosorbide, glycerol 385
Conclusion 386
References 387
Further reading 390

17 Mechanism of action of drugs used in gastrointestinal diseases 391

Himani Nautiyal, Imran Kazmi, Mohammed Kaleem, Muhammad Afzal, Muhammad Masood Ahmad, Ameeduzzafar Zafar and Rupinder Kaur

Overview 391
Introduction 391
Neuronal and hormonal control over gastrointestinal tract 392
Gastrointestinal acid regulation 392
Peripheral regulation of acid 392
Gastrin 393
Peptic ulcer 394
Potential causes of peptic ulcer 395
Drugs used for neutralizing and inhibiting acid release 396
Antacids 396
Histamine receptor antagonist 398
H^+/K^+ ATPase inhibitor/ Proton pump inhibitor (PPIs): Omeprazole, Lansoprazole, Rabeprazole, Pantoprazole, Esomeprazole Mechanism of Action 399
Antiemetics and emetics 401
Vomiting 401
Stimulants for vomiting 404
Classification of antiemetics 404
Antihistamines and anticholinergic 407
Cannabinoids 408

Glucocorticoids 408
Vitamin B6 409
Emetics 409
Ipecacuanha 409
Apomorphine 409
Laxatives, purgatives, and cathartics 409
Classification (laxatives, purgatives, and cathartics) 410
Antidiarrheal agents 410
Oral rehydration supplements 410
References 415

18 Mechanisms of action of antibacterial agents (AMA) 421

Raja Chakraverty, Kalyan Samanta, Pallab Mandal, Samit Karmakar and Sanmoy Karmakar

Introduction 421
Classification of β-lactams 421
Cell wall biosynthesis inhibitors[7–9] 422
Carbapenems 422
Cephalosporins 422
Protein synthesis inhibitors that bind the 30S subunit 422
Protein synthesis inhibitors that bind the 50S and 30S ribosomal subunits 423
Membrane function inhibitors 424
Inhibitors of nucleic acid synthesis 424
ATP synthase inhibitors 425
Conclusion 425
References 425

19 Mechanism of action of antifungal agents 431

Sandipan Jana, Srijon Gayen, Reshma Kumari, Susmita Patra, Pallab Kanti Haldar, Rudranil Bhowmik, Md. Adil Shaharyar, Avishek Mandal, Hindol Mazumdar and Sanmoy Karmakar

Introduction 431
Pathophysiology fungal diseases 432
Mechanism of antifungal agents 437
Black fungus and COVID-19 441
Source 441
Reasons for sudden development 441
Symptoms 442
Treatments 442
Conclusion 442
References 443
Further reading 445

20 Insights into the mechanism of action of antiviral drugs 447

Reshma Kumari, Sandipan Jana, Susmita Patra, Pallab Kanti Haldar, Rudranil Bhowmik, Avishek Mandal, Kumar Anand, Hindol Mazumdar, Md. Adil Shaharyar and Sanmoy Karmakar

Introduction 447
Virus life cycle and pathogenesis 447
Classification of drugs based on viral targets 448
Pathophysiology of viruses 450
Human immunodeficiency virus 450
Antihuman immunodeficiency virus drugs 453
Zidovudine 453
Stavudine 453
Lamivudine (3TC) and emtricitabine (FTC) 453
Abacavir 454
Nucleotide reverse transcriptase inhibitors 454
Protease inhibitors 455
Ritonavir 455
Saquinavir 455
Indinavir 456
Nelfinavir 456
Lopinavir 456
Atazanavir 456
Fosamprenavir 456
Tipranavir 456
Darunavir 457
Integrase inhibitors 457
Fusion peptide inhibitor 457
Adhesion inhibitor 458
CCR5 receptor inhibitor 458
Herpesvirus 458
Antiherpes drugs 459
Penciclovir and famciclovir 460
Idoxuridine 460
Trifluridine 460
Foscarnet 460
Docosanol 461
Influenza virus 461
Antiinfluenza drugs 462
Oseltamivir and zanamivir 462
Amantadine and rimantadine 463
Hepatitis virus 463
Antihepatitis B drugs 463
Antihepatitis C drugs 464
Varicella zoster virus 465
Antivaricella zoster virus drugs 467

Cytomegalovirus 467
Anticytomegalovirus drugs 467
Ganciclovir and valganciclovir 468
Antirespiratory syncytial virus drugs 468
Severe acute respiratory syndrome coronavirus 2 468
Anti-Covid drugs 468
Conclusion 469
References 470

21 Insight into the molecular mechanism of action of anticancer drugs 477

Monalisha Sengupta, Arijit Guha, Rudranil Bhowmik, Imran Kazmi, Salman Bakr I. Hosawi, Fahad Al-Abbasi and Mohammed Kaleem

Introduction 477
Pathophysiology 478
United States Food and Drug Administration 479
Newer United States Food and Drug Administration–approved drugs 479
Classification of anticancer drugs/therapies 483
Mechanism of action 486
Drugs acting on endothelium 486
Drugs acting on extracellular matrix 490
Drugs acting on Host Cell 491
Drugs acting on immune system 491
Drugs directed against tumor DNA 492
Conclusion 496
References 496

22 An insight into the agents used for immunomodulation and their mechanism of action 503

Avishek Mandal, Priti Das, Rudranil Bhowmik, Hindol Mazumdar, Md. Adil Shaharyar, Reshma Kumari, Sandipan Jana, Susmita Patra, Pallab Kanti Haldar and Sanmoy Karmakar

Introduction 503
Immunomodulators 504
Immunosuppressants 505
Glucocorticoid 505
Mechanism of action of classical immunomodulatory drugs 506
Prednisone 507
Hydrocortamate 507
Calcineurin inhibitors 509
Cyclosporine 509
Tacrolimus 509
Mammalian target of rapamycin inhibitors 510
Sirolimus 510

Everolimus 511
Antimetabolite 511
Leflunomide 511
6-Mercaptopurine pathology and treatment 511
Alkalyting agent 512
Steroid-free medications 512
Oral signs and symptoms 513
Cyclophosphamide 513
Definition of biologics 513
Biologics are divided into three groups based on their chemical composition 514
Mechanism of action of newer immunomodulators 514
Usage of biologics for clinical indications 514
Tumor necrosis factor-alpha Inhibitor 515
Categorization 515
Etanercept 516
Infliximab 516
Interleukin-1 inhibitors 518
Anakinra 518
Daclizumab 518
Polyclonal antibody 519
Antithymocyte immunoglobulin (ATG) 519
Monoclonal antibodies 520
Alemtuzumab 520
Vaccine 521
Bacillus Calmette-Guérin 521
Antihelminthics 521
Albendazole 521
Discussion 522
Conclusion 522
References 523

23 Mechanism of opioids action and their receptor-dependent signaling 529

Muhammad Zubair Saleem and Muhammad Azhar Nisar

Introduction 529
Opioid receptors 530
Opioid ligands 533
Molecular recognition of opioids 533
Classic mechanism 535
Ion channels 535
Adenylate cyclase 536
Mitogen-activated protein kinase signaling 536
Tolerance 538
Conclusion 539
References 539

24 Application of molecular pharmacology in research techniques and drug development 545

Mainak Chakraborty, Nilanjan Sarkar, Amrita Kumari, Kalyan Roy, Gauthaman Karunakaran, Priti Das, Jafar Abdulla Mohamed Usman and Samit Karmakar

Introduction 545
Molecular pharmacology methods and their application in drug discovery approaches 546
Molecular approaches based on network 547
Mechanism-based approach in drug discovery 548
Molecular biology method in human disease and drug discovery 549
Human disease networks and molecular pharmacology 549
Molecular pharmacology in treatment response prediction 549
Investigation of disease mechanisms by molecular pharmacology 550
Gene regulation and disease state 551
Molecular pharmacology approaches in drug discovery 551
Drug–target networks and molecular pharmacology 551
Predictions of drug–target interactions 552
Investigations of drug adverse effects by molecular pharmacology approaches 552
Drug repositioning and molecular pharmacology 553
Predictions of drug combination and molecular pharmacology approaches 553
Conclusion 553
References 554

Index 557

List of contributors

Muhammad Afzal Department of Pharmacology, College of Pharmacy, Jouf University, Sakaka, Aljouf, Saudi Arabia

Mohit Agrawal School of Medical & Allied Sciences, K.R. Mangalam University, Gurgaon, Haryana, India

Muhammad Masood Ahmad Department of Pharmaceutics, College of Pharmacy, Jouf University, Sakaka, Aljouf, Saudi Arabia

Fahad Al-Abbasi Department of Biochemistry, Faculty of Science, King Abdulaziz University, Jeddah, Saudi Arabia

Haider Ali Faculty of Medicine, Ala-Too International University, Bishkek, Kyrgyzstan

Kazi Asraf Ali Department of Pharmaceutical Technology, Maulana Abul Kalam Azad University of Technology, Haringhata, West Bengal, India

Sk Zeeshan Ali Bioeuivalence Study Centre, Department of Pharmaceutical Technology, Jadavpur University, Kolkata, West Bengal, India

Waleed Hassan Almalki Department of Pharmacology and Toxicology, College of Pharmacy, Umm Al-Qura University, Makkah, Saudi Arabia

Hisham N. Altayb Department of Biochemistry, Faculty of Science, King Abdulaziz University, Jeddah, Saudi Arabia

Sami I. Alzarea Department of Pharmacology, College of Pharmacy, Jouf University, Sakaka, Aljouf, Saudi Arabia

Kumar Anand Bioeuivalence Study Centre, Department of Pharmaceutical Technology, Jadavpur University, Kolkata, West Bengal, India

Muhammed Burak Ay Faculty of Medicine, Ala-Too International University, Bishkek, Kyrgyzstan

Shwetlana Bandyopadhy Department of Pharmaceutical Technology, NSHM Knowledge campus Kolkata, Group of Institutions, Kolkata, West Bengal, India

Mirza Masroor Ali Beg Faculty of Medicine, Ala-Too International University, Bishkek, Kyrgyzstan

Rudranil Bhowmik Bioeuivalence Study Centre, Department of Pharmaceutical Technology, Jadavpur University, Kolkata, West Bengal, India

Mainak Chakraborty Department of Pharmaceutical Technology, NSHM Knowledge campus Kolkata, Group of Institutions, Kolkata, West Bengal, India

Suparno Chakraborty TCG Life Sciences Pvt Ltd (formerly "Chembiotek Research International"), R&D Centre, Chemistry, Kolkata, West Bengal, India

Raja Chakraverty ICMR Research Scholar, Department of Pharmacology, IPGME&R-SSKM Hospital, Kolkata, West Bengal, India; ICMR Research Scholar, Department of Pharmacology, IPGMER-SSKM Hospital, Kolkata, West Bengal, India

Priti Das TCG Life Sciences Pvt Ltd (formerly "Chembiotek Research International"), Kolkata – R&D Centre, Chemistry, Kolkata, West Bengal, India

Siddhartha Das Pramanik Department of Pharmaceutical Technology, School of Medical Science, Adamas University, Barasat, West Bengal, India

Debankini Dasgupta Department of Pharmaceutical Technology, NSHM Knowledge campus Kolkata, Group of Institutions, Kolkata, West Bengal, India

Tanzeela Fazal Department of Chemistry, Abbottabad University of Science and Technology (AUST), Abbottabad, Pakistan

Srijon Gayen Bioeuivalence Study Centre, Department of Pharmaceutical Technology, Jadavpur University, Kolkata, West Bengal, India

Arijit Guha Bagda Rural Hospital, Mohanpur, West Bengal, India

Pratibha Gupta Department of Pharmaceutical Technology, Adamas University, Barasat, Kolkata, West Bengal, India

Pallab Kanti Haldar Bioeuivalence Study Centre, Department of Pharmaceutical Technology, Jadavpur University, Kolkata, West Bengal, India

Salman Bakr I. Hosawi Department of Biochemistry, Faculty of Science, King Abdulaziz University, Jeddah, Saudi Arabia

Chowdhury Mobaswar Hossain Department of Pharmaceutical Technology, Maulana Abul Kalam Azad University of Technology (MAKAUT), West Bengal, India; NH-12, Haringhata, Simhat, Nadia, West Bengal, India

Sandipan Jana Bioeuivalence Study Centre, Department of Pharmaceutical Technology, Jadavpur University, Kolkata, West Bengal, India

Mohammed Kaleem Department of Biochemistry, Faculty of Science, King Abdulaziz University, Jeddah, Saudi Arabia

Samit Karmakar Medical College Kolkata, Kolkata, West Bengal, India

Sanmoy Karmakar Bioeuivalence Study Centre, Department of Pharmaceutical Technology, Jadavpur University, Kolkata, West Bengal, India

Gauthaman Karunakaran Government Pharmacy College, Gangtok, Sikkim, India

Rupinder Kaur Chandigarh College of Pharmacy, Landran, Mohali, Punjab, India

Imran Kazmi Department of Biochemistry, Faculty of Science, King Abdulaziz University, Jeddah, Saudi Arabia

Nurida Kemelbek Kyzy Faculty of Medicine, Ala-Too International University, Bishkek, Kyrgyzstan

Faez Iqbal Khan Department of Biological Sciences, School of Science, Xi'an Jiaotong-Liverpool University, Suzhou, Jiangsu, China

Naushad Ahmad Khan Faculty of Medicine, Ala-Too International University, Bishkek, Kyrgyzstan

Ruqaiyah Khan Department of Pharmacology, College of Pharmacy, Princess Noura University, Riyadh, Saudi Arabia

Chinnabonia Gopala Krishna A.M. Reddy Memorial College of Pharmacy, Narasaraopet, Andhra Pradesh, India

Amrita Kumari Usha College of Pharmacy, Dhatkidih, Jamshedpur, Jharkhand, India; Ranchi College of Pharmacy and Research Centre, Ranchi, Jharkhand, India

Reshma Kumari Bioeuivalence Study Centre, Department of Pharmaceutical Technology, Jadavpur University, Kolkata, West Bengal, India

Aanchal Loshali Department of Pharmaceutical Sciences and Technology, Sardar Bhagwan Singh University, Dehradun, Uttarakhand, India

Arindam Maity Department of Pharmaceutical Technology, JIS University of Technology, Kolkata, West Bengal, India

Muhammad Arshad Malik Department of Biological Sciences, Faculty of Basic & Applied Sciences, International Islamic University Islamabad, Islamabad, Pakistan

Avishek Mandal Bioeuivalence Study Centre, Department of Pharmaceutical Technology, Jadavpur University, Kolkata, West Bengal, India

Pallab Mandal Bioeuivalence Study Centre, Department of Pharmaceutical Technology, Jadavpur University, Kolkata, West Bengal, India

Hindol Mazumdar Bioeuivalence Study Centre, Department of Pharmaceutical Technology, Jadavpur University, Kolkata, West Bengal, India

Tilekeeva Ulankul Muktarovna Department of Basic and Clinical Pharmacology, Kyrgyz State Medical Academy, Bishkek, Kyrgyzstan

Bibi Nazia Murtaza Department of Zoology, Abbottabad University of Science and Technology (AUST), Abbottabad, Pakistan

Muhammad Shahid Nadeem Department of Biochemistry, Faculty of Science, King Abdulaziz University, Jeddah, Saudi Arabia

Himani Nautiyal Siddhartha Institute of Pharmacy, Dehradun, Uttarakhand, India

Muhammad Azhar Nisar Department of Pathology and Laboratory Medicine, Tulane University School of Medicine, New Orleans, LA, United States

Kudaibergen Osmonaliev Faculty of Medicine, Ala-Too International University, Bishkek, Kyrgyzstan

Soupayan Pal Bioeuivalence Study Centre, Department of Pharmaceutical Technology, Jadavpur University, Kolkata, West Bengal, India

Parag Panday Infoclin Consultency, Kolkata, West Bengal, India

Susmita Patra Department of Pharmaceutical Technology, Adamas University, Barasat, Kolkata, West Bengal, India

Partha Pratim Das Department of Pharmaceutics, Bengal School of Technology, Chinsurah, Hooghly, West Bengal, India

Raisur Rahman Department of Paediatrics, University Hospitals Plymouth, Plymouth, United Kingdom

Khandekar Hussan Reza Department of Pharmaceutics, Bengal School of Technology, Chinsurah, Hooghly, West Bengal, India

Muhammad Naeem Riaz Department of Pharmacy, COMSATS University, Abbottabad, Pakistan

Kalyan Roy Government Pharmacy College, Gangtok, Sikkim, India

Sanhati Dutta Roy Department o Pharmaceutical Technology, NSHM Knowledge Campus, Kolkata, West Bengal, India

Muhammad Zubair Saleem Fujian Provincial Key Laboratory of Natural Medicine Pharmacology, Fujian Medical University, Fuzhou, P.R. China

Shakir Saleem Department of Public Health, College of Health Sciences, Saudi Electronic University, Riyadh, Saudi Arabia

Kalyan Samanta ICMR Research Scholar, Department of Pharmacology, IPGME&R-SSKM Hospital, Kolkata, West Bengal, India; MD-PGT, Department of Pharmacology, IPGMER-SSKM Hospital, Kolkata, West Bengal, India

Nilanjan Sarkar Department of Pharmaceutical Technology, NSHM Knowledge campus Kolkata, Group of Institutions, Kolkata, West Bengal, India

Mohammed Zahed Sarwar Faculty of Medicine, Ala-Too International University, Bishkek, Kyrgyzstan

Monalisha Sengupta Narayana Superspeciality Hospital, Howrah, West Bengal, India

Md. Adil Shaharyar Bioeuivalence Study Centre, Department of Pharmaceutical Technology, Jadavpur University, Kolkata, West Bengal, India

Kuldeepak Sharma Institute of Pharmacology and Toxicology, Faculty of Medicine, University of Ljubljana, Slovenia

Yogendra Singh Department of Pharmacology, Maharishi Arvind College of Pharmacy, Jaipur, Rajasthan, India

Ankush Sundriyal Department of Pharmaceutical Sciences and Technology, Sardar Bhagwan Singh University, Dehradun, Uttarakhand, India

Gayatri Thapa Himalayan Pharmacy Institute, Rangpo, Sikkim, India

Aziz Ud-din Department of Genetic Engineering and Biotechnology, Hazara University, Mansehra, Pakistan

Jafar Abdulla Mohamed Usman Prosthetic dentistry, Faculty of dentistry, MAHSA University, Jln SP2 Selangor, Malaysia

Ameeduzzafar Zafar Department of Pharmaceutics, College of Pharmacy, Jouf University, Sakaka, Aljouf, Saudi Arabia

Chapter 1

Introduction to molecular pharmacology: basic concepts

Muhammad Afzal[1], Imran Kazmi[2], Rupinder Kaur[3], Salman Bakr I. Hosawi[2], Mohammed Kaleem[2], Sami I. Alzarea[1] and Muhammad Masood Ahmad[4]

[1]Department of Pharmacology, College of Pharmacy, Jouf University, Sakaka, Aljouf, Saudi Arabia, [2]Department of Biochemistry, Faculty of Science, King Abdulaziz University, Jeddah, Saudi Arabia, [3]Chandigarh College of Pharmacy, Landran, Mohali, Punjab, India, [4]Department of Pharmaceutics, College of Pharmacy, Jouf University, Sakaka, Aljouf, Saudi Arabia

Pharmacology

Pharmacology is the branch of medical science that deals with study of drugs and their effects on biological systems.[1] The word "pharmacology" is derived from two Greek words *pharmacon* (meaning drugs) and *logos* (meaning the study or science).[2] Thus, pharmacology is the study of actions of drugs on living systems.[3] It encompasses all aspects of drug action on biological system including biochemical, physiological, its mechanism, therapeutic significances, and adverse effects of drugs.[4]

Drugs

Drugs refer to any chemical substance that affects the processes of living system.[5] They include chemical substances of known chemical structure that are used or intended to be used for diagnosis, prevention, cure, or mitigation of the diseases.[6] Drugs do nothing new with the living system but only changes the physiology of the cell.[7]

Brief history of pharmacology

The knowledge of drugs and their use in the treatment of illnesses are as old as the human civilization.[8] In the ancient times, people used natural substances in crude forms, observed the diseased states, and utilized their personal experiences after consuming plants and other herbs as remedies.[9] In middle ages, humans discovered that extracts from plants, animals, and minerals had

How Synthetic Drugs Work. DOI: https://doi.org/10.1016/B978-0-323-99855-0.00001-4

medicinal values and these information became the foundation of pharmacology.[10] Pharmacology in its present form is hardly 100 years old.[11]

Pharmacological studies are divided into two parts, namely, pharmacokinetics and pharmacodynamics Pharmacokinetics examines movement of drug through the body or what the body does with the drug after administration.[12] Pharmacodynamics examines the effect of the drug over a period of time on the body or what the drug does with the body[13] (Fig. 1.1).

Routes of drug administration

The path through which a drug or a chemical enter into the body comes under the routes of administration. On the basis of site of drug administration they are basically calssified into, enteral (oral), parenteral (injectional) and local route (topical).[14] Selection of routes of drug administration depends on its convenience, compliance, and also on the basis of physicochemical properties of the drug. Hence, it is very important to know the characteristics of different routes and techniques involved.[15] Numerous health professionals are engaged in the administration of drugs in patients.[16] Hence, before administering drugs, five "rights" must be considered carefully: right patient, right drug, right dose, right site, and right timing.[17] The patient must be explained about the drug, its route of administration, and the peculiarities of drug administration if any[18] (Fig. 1.2).

Enteral routes

1. Oral route is the easiest, most economic, and common route of drug administration.[19] The main site of drug absorption is small intestine, and the drug's ability to produce pharmacological effect is affected by fraction of administered drug absorbed across the intestinal epithelial membranes.[20] First-pass effect is another major influencer of oral drug bioavailability.[21] First-pass metabolism is the alteration of orally administered drug before it reaches the systemic circulation apparently in the way of portal to systemic circulation via liver.[22]

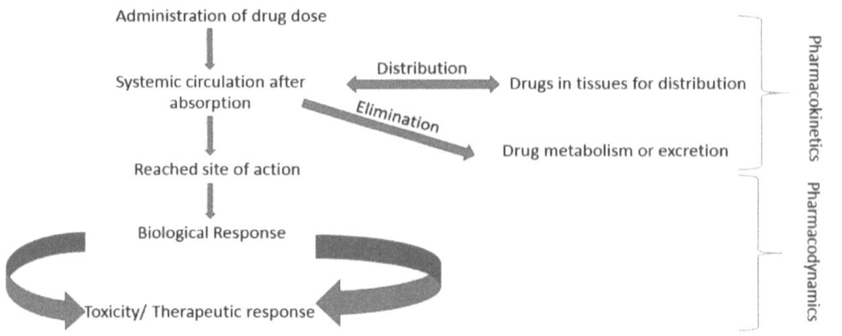

FIGURE 1.1 Illustration of pharmacokinetic and pharmacodynamic steps.

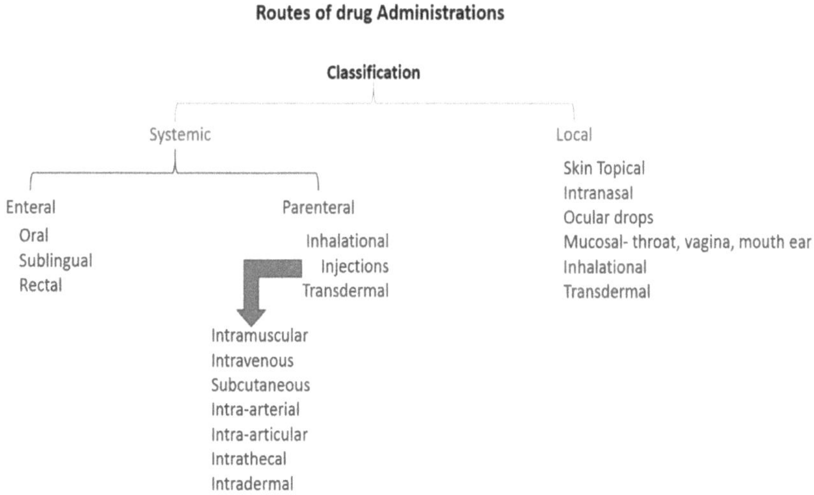

FIGURE 1.2 Different routes of drug administration.

2. Sublingual or buccal is another enteral route and is considered the second fastest route of drug administration. It offers advantage of liver bypass and diminished first-pass effect.[23] The drug is directly applied under the tongue (sublingually) or on the mucosal membranes of the cheeks (buccally). It is absorbed passively into venous blood, bypasses hepatic portal circulation, and is directly drained into superior vena cava. The passive absorption from buccal cavity is less and slow because the sublingual tissue is more permeable and has fast access to underlying blood capillaries.[24]
3. Rectal route offers fast and effective absorption of drugs through the massively vascularized mucosa. Rectally administered drugs undergo passive diffusion as in case of sublingual and buccal route and partially bypass liver.[25]

Parenteral routes of drug administration

1. Intravenous route is the most common among parental route of medication. It offers fastest drug absorption and does not have first-pass effect because the drug is directly poured into the venous circulation.[26] Because of superficial location on the skin, peripheral veins provides very fast and convenient access to systemic circulation and are often utilized in parental drug administration. The veins of upper extremity are preferred because of the lower chances of thrombophlebitis and thrombosis than lower limbs.[27] The cephalic or median basilic veins of the arms or metacarpal veins on the dorsum of hands are preferred. In the lower extremities, the dorsal venous plexuses of foot can also be considered in some situations.[28]
2. Intramuscular route can be considered if insufficient absorption, high first-pass effect, and patient's noncompliance are observed when oral route of medication

used. The drug is administered as a depot formulation intramuscularly, and it is slowly dissolved into circulation, which results in sustained actions. Haloperidol decanoate and vaccines are administered intramuscularly.

3. Subcutaneous route is taken into consideration when the molecular size of the drug particulates is large enough to cross the intestinal mucosal membranes.[29] The requirements of enhanced bioavailability and rapid absorption than oral route are the another factors to administer drug subcutaneously.[30] It is convenient and does not require assistance, and patients can administer themselves without any significant skill requirements, for example, insulin.[31]
4. Other routes include transdermal and inhalational routes of drug administration.[32]

Local routes of drug administration

1. Intranasal route of drug administration offers local actions as well as systemic absorption of the drugs. Nasal mucosa provides very large highly vascularized surface area.[33] Nasal decongestants are applied intranasally and utilized for the local actions. While some intranasal formulations for systemic effects are also available, calcitonin and desmopressin are delivered intranasally and produce systemic effects.[34]
2. Vaginal route of drug administration is less common inconvenient route but often used to deliver low, consistent concentrations of the drug for prolonged periods to achieve stable and sustained plasma concentrations.[35] The commonly administered formulations include tablets, ointments, creams, lotions, gels, and pessaries[36] (Fig. 1.2).

Pharmacokinetics

Pharmacokinetics is the quantitative estimation of the drug movement in, thorough, and out of the body.[35] The response intensity depends on concentration of the drug at site of action, which considerably depends on pharmacokinetic characteristics. Pharmacokinetics finally determine the dose, latency of onset, time to produce maximum effect, total duration of action, and dose frequencies.[37] Pharmacokinetic considerations mainly include absorption, distribution, metabolism, and excretion (ADME) of the drug. All pharmacokinetic processes involves transport of drug molecules across the cell membranes.[38] Drugs are basically transported across the plasma membrane via:

1. Passive diffusion and filtration
2. Specialized transport (Fig. 1.1).

Passive diffusion

In passive diffusion, drugs flow across biological membrane in the direction of concentration gradient. Mostly, the drugs cross biological membranes through this process where the membrane does not play any significant role. As the drug molecule are foreign substances, specialized mechanisms are only developed for normal metabolic products only.[39]

Lipid solubility affects diffusion considerably; highly lipid-soluble drugs dissolve in lipid bilayer of plasma membranes and diffuse quickly. Also, the higher the significant difference in concentration gradient across the cell membrane, faster the diffusion.[40]

Effect of pH:

$$pH = pK_a + \log[A-]/[HA] \ \{\text{where A} - \text{is ionized drug and HA is Unionized for a weak electrolyte}\}$$

If for a weak acid, the concentration of ionized drug is equal to concentration of unionized drug,

Then, $[A-]/[HA] = 1$
Since $\log 1 = 0$
Then, $pH = pK_a$

Thus, pK_a is numerically equal to pH when the drug is 50% ionized. Thus, weakly acidic drugs are ionized more at alkaline pH. Weakly basic drugs are more ionized at acidic pH. Lipid-soluble drugs readily cross biological membranes, and thus, their transport is pH independent.[41]

Filtration

Filtration refers to the phenomenon where drug molecules cross biological membranes through aqueous pores or throughout the paracellular spaces.[42] In glomeruli, lipid-insoluble drugs cross biological membranes if the molecular size of the drug molecule is lower than the pore size of the luminal membranes.[43]

Specialized transport

Carrier transport

Carrier transport is the way of drug transport across cell membrane where the drug combines with some components of the membrane, make the complexes, and then the complex translocates from one side to another.[44] The carriers for the polar molecules form lipophilic coating over hydrophilic groups and facilitate their passage through membranes.[45] They are of two kinds:

Active transport

Movement occurs from lower concentration to higher concentration, and it requires energy, resisted by metabolic poisons.[46]

Facilitated diffusion

It is more rapid than simple diffusion, does not require energy, transports even nondiffusible substances but from higher concentration to lower.[47]

Pinocytosis

Its operates rarely for absorption of drugs and transports particulates by forming some vesicles. It mainly operates for proteins and big molecules.[48]

Absorption

Absorption refers to the transfer of administered drug to blood stream from the site of administration.[49] Its rate and efficiency are mainly affected by the route of administration, that is, for intravenous route, 100% absorption is there, because the total amount of drug is directly poured into the blood vessel.[50] Drugs administered from other routes may have partial absorptions and lower bioavailability. Oral administration of the drug requires first to dissolve in gastrointestinal fluids and then penetrate the epithelial layers of intestine. The disease states and the presence of food can affect the process.[51]

Factors affecting absorption of drugs

Physical factors

Blood perfusion to the site of administration

The higher the perfusion rate, the higher the absorption of the site, that is, the intestine has greater blood perfusion than stomach, and thus, absorption is much higher from the intestine than stomach.[52]

Surface area available for absorption

The higher the surface area, the higher the absorption. The intestinal surface area because of microvilli is much greater (1000-fold) than stomach, and thus, more efficient absorption of drugs take place from the intestine.[53]

Retention time at the surface area

If the drugs move faster from the intestinal surface (e.g., in case of diarrhea), drug will not get absorbed well because of less contact time to the surface provided for the absorption. On the contrary, if anything delays movement of drug from stomach to intestine, it also delays the absorption of drugs.[54]

Drug distribution

It is the process in which drug apparently leaves bloodstream and enters the interstitial fluid or inside the cells of the tissues. It basically depends on the following factors.[55]

1. Blood perfusion
2. Permeability of capillaries
3. Degree of plasma protein binding of the drug
4. Lipid solubility of the drug.

Volume of distribution

Volume of distribution is the hypothetical volume of different water compartments in our body into which drugs are dispersed. It does not have any physiological basis.[56]

Water compartments in the body

Plasma compartment

If a drug has a very high molecular weight/size, has very high plasma protein binding capacity, or it cannot penetrate through the capillary membranes because of its size, it remains in the plasma, which is 6% of the total body weight (70 kg), about 4 L of total body fluids.[57]

Extracellular fluid

Drugs with low molecular weights are hydrophilic, but they can move from blood compartment to interstitial fluid through the slit junctions of the capillary epithelium. Because of hydrophilic nature, drug molecules cannot penetrate plasma membranes of the cells. Hence, the drugs remains in plasma and interstitial fluid only, which constitute about 20% of the total body weight (70 kg), that is, about 14 L. Amino glycosides are the example of this type of distribution.[58]

Total body water

Drugs with low molecular weights and hydrophobic nature can enter the interstitial fluid and are free to reach in cellular compartments (intracellular fluid). The drugs thus have acmes in plasma, extracellular fluid, and intracellular fluid, which is about the 70% of the total body weight (70 kg), that is, about 42 L. Ethanol and the drugs with high lipid solubility exhibit this type of distribution.[59]

Other sites

In special conditions, for example, in pregnancy, fetus can also take the drugs and increase the volume of distribution than the usual.

Apparent volume of distribution

A drug is not restricted to only one water compartment of the body, it distributes to several compartments and binds with different cellular components either to lipids, proteins, or nucleic acids. The volume into which the drugs distribute is called the apparent volume of distribution.[60]

Plasma protein binding of the drugs

Plasma protein binding affects the distribution of the drug and the biological activity. Drug molecules after absorption into systemic circulation may bind to plasma proteins and the bound drugs cannot cross biological membrane and are finally not available to elicit a pharmacological response. Only the free drugs (not bound to plasma proteins) are biologically active. There are two proteins that extensively bind with drug molecules: albumin and globulin. Acidic drugs bind to albumin, and basic drugs bind to globulin with higher affinities.[61]

Drug metabolism

The absorbed drugs after eliciting their pharmacological response are eliminated from biological system after biotransformation (a mechanism that transforms drug molecules into excretable forms). Biotransformation is the chemical alteration of drugs inside biological system, which is often called as metabolism of drugs. This process of drug metabolism converts lipophilic drugs into polar and excretable substances. Liver is the main site of metabolism of drugs, some drugs specifically metabolized at some other sites too, such as kidneys and intestines. Metabolism of drugs can inactivate the active drug or can lead to the activation of drug from its inactive form; biotransformation can also generate more active compounds from the administered drugs or partially reduce the biological activities of the parent compound.[62]

Kinetics of metabolism

1. First-order kinetics

   The rate of metabolism is proportional to the free amount of the drug in plasma, and it describes the constant fraction of drug metabolized per unit time.[63]

2. Zero-order kinetics

With fewer drugs when the doses are too large, the enzymes are saturated by the free amount of the drug, and the rate of metabolism becomes constant over a period. There are two different types of reactions of drug metabolism. The kidneys do not eliminate lipophilic drugs efficiently, as they can cross the biological membranes readily and are reabsorbed in the renal tubules. Hence, to be excreted, the drug molecules undergo two different sets of reactions in liver.[64]

Phase I reactions

Transform lipophilic drugs into polar compounds by introducing a polar functional group such as OH or NH_2 groups. Phase I reactions may either enhance, diminish, or not affect the drug's biological activity at all. The phase I reactions are carried out by microsomal CYTP450 system, also called mixed function oxidases.[65] The reactions involved are:

1. Oxidation
2. Reduction
3. Hydrolysis
4. Cyclization
5. Decyclization.

Phase II reactions

This phase includes conjugation reactions. The metabolites of phase I reactions that are sufficiently polarized can be excreted via kidneys. However, some metabolites are still lipophilic and reabsorbed in renal tubules, subsequent conjugation reaction make such substance completely inactive and excretable from the body.[66] These conjugation reactions include (Fig. 1.3):

- Glucuronide conjugation
- Acetylation
- Methylation
- Sulfate conjugation
- Glycine conjugation
- Glutathione conjugation
- Ribonucleoside/nucleotide synthesis.

Drug excretion

The passage to eliminate systemically absorbed drugs out of the body is excretion.[67] Drugs and transformed residues are eliminated in:

1. Urine: It is the most important route for drug elimination and takes place mainly through the kidneys;

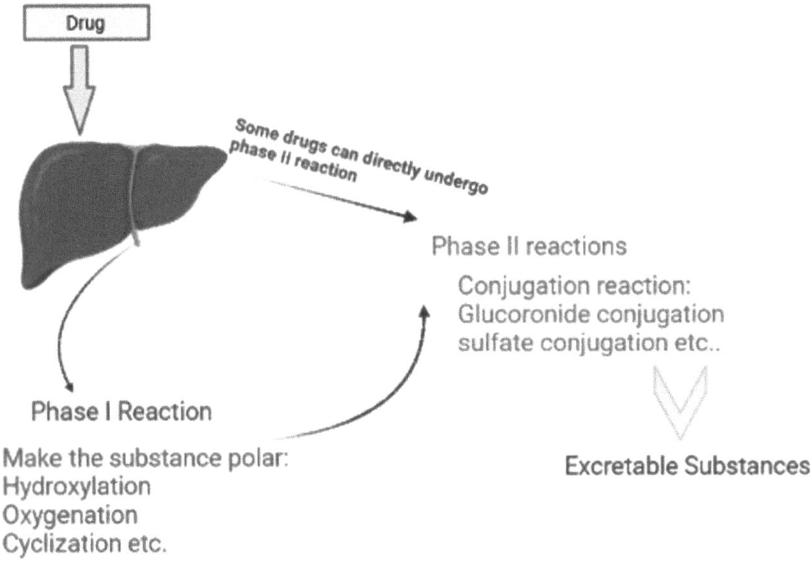

FIGURE 1.3 Drug metabolic reactions in liver.

2. Feces: Most of the drugs excreted via feces are derived from bile, except unabsorbed fractions;
3. Exhaled air: Gases and volatile liquids are excreted through exhaled air, alcohol, inhalation anesthetics;
4. Saliva and sweat: It is a minor route through which only a few substances are excreted, for example, lithium, rifampin, and heavy metals;
5. Milk: The excretion of drugs in milk is important for the infant; more lipid soluble and less protein bound drugs can enter easily into the breast milk.

Pharmacodynamics: drug receptor interactions or mechanism of drug effects

Pharmacodynamics is what the drug does to the body, that is, it is the study of drug effects. It is an attempt to elucidate the complete sequences from drug action to drug effect as well as the relationship of dose to drug effect, modifications of drug effect by another drug, and other influencers are also the part of pharmacodynamic studies.[68]

Principles of drug action

Drugs, except gene-targeted ones, do nothing new to biological system (cell, tissue, or organ). They just change the physiology of the cell, tissue, or organ they affect.[69] The fundamental drug action can be classified as:[70]

Stimulation

Selective enhancement of activities of specialized cells, for example, adrenaline has excitatory action on heart, pilocarpine has effect on salivary glands.

Depression

Certain drugs selectively diminish the activities of specialized cells, for example, quinidine suppresses heart.

Irritation

Irritation is a nonselective, mostly the noxious effect, especially to less specialized cells (epithelial, or to the cells of connective tissue). Milder irritation can possibly enhance ongoing pace of the activities, for example, bitters enhance gastrointestinal secretions; counterirritants increase blood flow to the applied area. However, strong irritation causes inflammation, cellular damage, and ultimately, it leads to loss of function.

Replacement

Replacement of natural metabolites or hormones in their deficiency states, dopamine precursor in Parkinsonism states, or growth hormones in its deficiency states.

Cytotoxic action

The invading microbes and cancer cells are selectively targeted without considerably affecting host cells. This is especially used to treat neoplasm and diseases created by microbes and parasites i.e., penicillins, albendazole, fluconazole, methotrexate etc.

Mechanism of drug actions

It is quite difficult to explain the mechanism of action of drugs on the basis of their physical and chemical actions. Only a few drugs act by these mechanisms, and most of the drugs act in a complex manner.[71] The basic mechanisms of drug action are broadly categorized into four types.[72]

Physical action

This is attributed to the physical property of the drug.

Mass of the drug	Laxatives
Adsorptive surface	Charcoal
Osmotic properties	Mannitol

Chemical action

The drugs react chemically with extracellular moieties.

Antacids	React with gastric acid
EDTA	Reacts with toxic materials

Through enzymes

Almost all the reactions in biological system are carried out via catalytic reaction mediated through enzymes.[73] Enzyme's activities can be modified via drug interruptions.

Enzyme's inhibition:

Acetylcholinesterase inhibitors enhance availability of acetylcholine to its receptors and potentiate cholinergic activities.

Enzyme's stimulation:

Sympathetic surge stimulates adenylyl cyclase activity in heart.

Through receptors

Sufficiently large number of drugs can mediate their effect via action on cellular macromolecules. These cellular macromolecules govern the number of physical and chemical reactions in the cells (e.g., enzymatic reaction, transmembrane permeability, morphology, and nuclear functions).[74] These specific macromolecules to which drugs bind and initiate the response but itself alone has no properties are termed as "receptors."

Some important definitions[75]

Agonists

A substance that binds with the receptor and has intrinsic activity.

Inverse agonist

A substance that produces an effect opposite to that of agonist.

Antagonist

A substance that binds with receptor with more affinity but does not have any intrinsic activity.

Partial agonist

A substance that binds with receptor but does not activate receptor fully (produces submaximal response only).

Ligand

Any endogenous or exogenous molecule that binds with receptor regardless of any functional change. Agonists and antagonists both act as a ligand for a particular type of receptor.

Nature of receptors

Receptors are mostly protein macromolecules, and sometimes, nucleic acids can also serve as receptors. Receptors have been studied extensively via radio ligand bindings studios and by gene cloning technology receptor proteins isolated. Their amino acid sequence has been studied very well. Molecular cloning further adds to it, and by utilizing this technology, the structure of different receptors studied and subclassifications could become possible. Receptors possess two important features: recognition of ligand and signal transduction, and thus, the receptor has ligand-binding site and an effector domain, and both of them undergo conformational changes.[76]

Transducer mechanisms

Significant progress has been made in the scientific field in terms of analytical techniques and their utilization in medical fields for the study of biological system and discoveries to reduce sufferings of humanity. Considerable developments have been made in understanding the mechanism of signal transduction, and mostly, it is found to be a highly complex multistep process that has evolved in amplification and integration of concurrently received intracellular and extracellular signals at each step.[77] On the basis of morphological and translation of signals into functional response mechanisms, receptors are classified into four major categories;

1. G protein–coupled receptors (GPCR) or Metabotropic receptor
2. Receptors linked to ion channels or Ionotropic receptor
3. Receptors linked to protein tyrosine kinases
4. Gene transcription regulatory receptor or Nuclear receptor.

G protein–coupled receptors

A GPCR is constituted by a single polypeptide of 1100 amino acid residues and has seven transmembrane helices (three extracellular and three intracellular loops), and these receptors are linked to G proteins, which possess three subunits, alpha which is bound to guanosine triphosphate (GTP) on activation, and beta–gamma subunit (Fig. 1.4). GPCR comprises an extracellular domain that binds with ligand and is the amino terminal of the chain. The intracellular terminal is the carboxylic acid group and is associated with G proteins (Gs, Gi, G0, Gq, G13, etc.).[78] Binding of a ligand with the

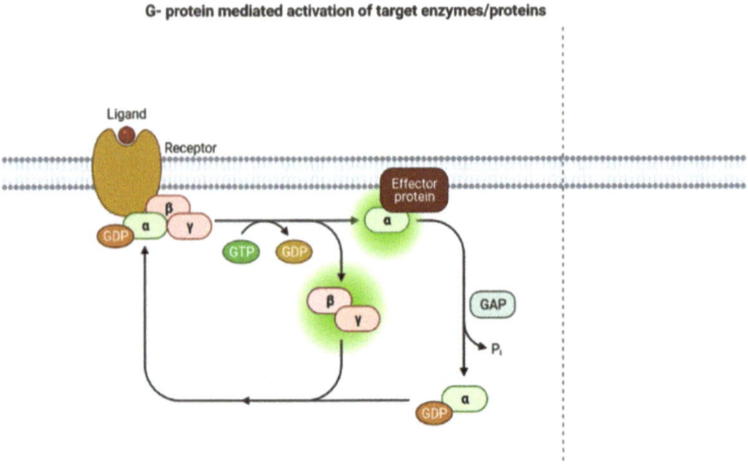

FIGURE 1.4 G protein–mediated activation of target protein.

extracellular domain of the receptors lead to conformational changes in the receptor that in turn activate the G protein. Activation of G protein leads to displacement of GDP with GTP from the alpha subunit. The active alpha subunit finally activates or inhibits the effectors.[79] The beta–gamma subunit is also found to modify certain effectors (Fig. 1.4).

There are three different pathways of G protein–coupled receptors to transduce their signal.

These are also called as signal-transduction mechanisms.

1. Cyclic adenosine monophosphate (cAMP) pathway;
2. Ionositol triphosphate/diacylglycerol (IP3/DAG) pathway;
3. GPCR linked to ion channels.

1. *cAMP Pathway*

   β-1 Receptors for norepinephrine are the classical examples for this pathway. Binding of ligand (norepinephrine) to the receptor brings about the conformational changes in receptor protein and G protein coupled to the receptor gets activated via guanosine triphosphate–guanosine diphosphate (GTP–GDP) exchange.[80] The activated alpha-GTP subunit activates intracellularly located membrane-bound adenylyl cyclase enzyme,[81] which leads to conversion of intracellular adenosine triphosphate (ATP) to cyclic adenosine monophosphate (cAMP) by hydrolytic reactions. cAMP phosphorylates and activates protein kinase A (PK_A), the activated PK_A causes phosphorylation and activation of numerous proteins including troponin and phospholamban (Heart). Activated troponin and phospholamban interact with Ca^{2+} and results in increased force of contraction, faster contraction (troponin action), and faster relaxation (phospholamban action). Ca^{2+} ions are made available via activation of membrane-bound Ca^{2+} channels by Gs and their phosphorylation by PK_A, and from the intracellular reservoirs.[82] The cAMP activation causes phosphorylation of many enzymes, structural proteins, ion channels, carrier proteins, and brings about the contraction, impulse generation (heart),[83] visceral smooth muscle (relaxation), glycogen breakdown in liver, lipolysis, suppression of secretions of mediators, junctional neurotransmission modulation, and hormone synthesis (Fig. 1.5).

2. *IP3/DAG Pathway*

   Histaminergic H-1 receptors are the example of receptors that transduce their signal via IP3-DAG pathway.[84]

Binding of ligand to the receptor causes activation of receptors and the coupled G protein (Gq) gets activated via GDP–GTP exchange. G protein gets dissociated in alpha-GTP subunit, and beta–gamma subunit.[85] The activated alpha-GTP subunit then activates a membrane bound nearly located phospholipase-C enzyme (intracellular, membrane-bound enzyme). Phospholipase-C (PLC) acts on membrane phospholipids phosphoionositol bisphosphate (PIP2) and hydrolyzes it into inositol triphosphate IP3 and diacylglycerol (DAG).[86] IP3 primarily releases Ca^{2+} from intracellular calcium ion depots, while DAG mobilizes Ca^{2+} as well as activates protein kinase C (PKC), and finally causes phosphorylation and activation of many other functional proteins. Ca^{+2} ions are veritable second messenger and activate numerous proteins via Ca^{2+} CAM-dependent and CAM-independent mechanisms [87] (Fig. 1.6).

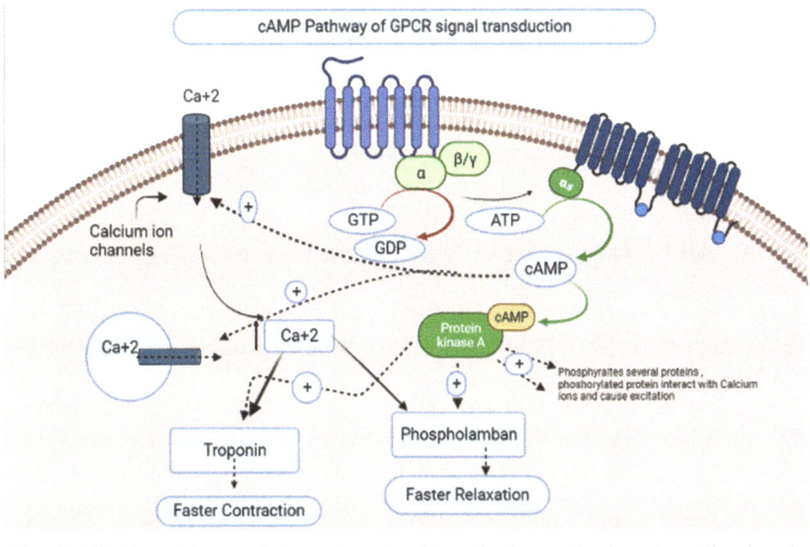

FIGURE 1.5 G protein–coupled receptors signal transduction mechanism via cyclic adenosine monophosphate pathway.

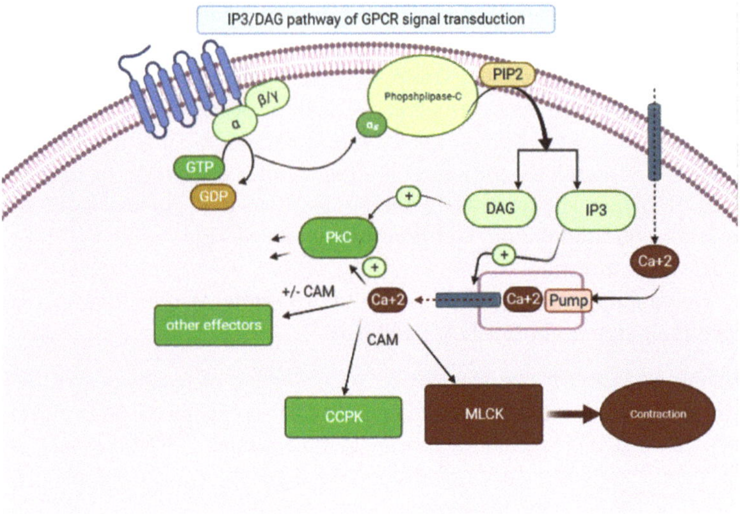

FIGURE 1.6 G protein–coupled receptors signal transduction mechanism via IP3/DAG pathway.

3. *G protein–coupled receptor linked to ion channels*
   G protein activation can also modulate the channels for Ca^{2+}, K^{+}, Na^{+} specifically and bring about depolarization and hyperpolarization or changes in cellular Ca^{2+} such as stimulation of Gs in cardiac and skeletal muscles opens Ca^{2+} channels and Gi/Go opens K^{+} channels and brings about the contraction and relaxation, respectively[88] (Fig. 1.7).

Receptors with intrinsic ion channels

$GABA_A$ (gamma amino butyric acid), nicotinic, and N-methyl- D- aspartate (NMDA) are the receptors with intrinsic ion channels.[89] These are cell surface receptors enclosing ion channels selective for (Na^{+}, K^{+}, Ca^{2+}, or Cl^{-}). Binding of the ligand opens the ion channels and allows the permeation of the respective ion in or out of the cell.[90] Flow of the ions inside or outside the cell brings about the depolarization and hyperpolarization in the cell, which depends on the intracellular ionic composition and the ion flowing through.

Ligand-gated ion channels are composed of five subunits (two alpha, one beta, one gamma, and one delta) of proteins.[91] All these subunits have large intra- and extracellular domains and four membrane-spanning domains in each of which the amino acid chains traverse through the width of the cell membrane. These subunits are arranged round the channels like a rosette and the alpha subunits bear the ligand-binding sites[92] (Fig. 1.5).

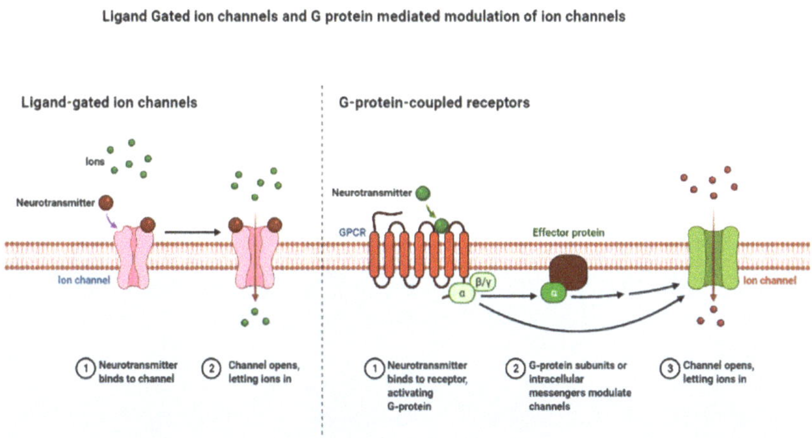

FIGURE 1.7 Ligand-gated ion channels and G protein–mediated modulation of ion channels.

Rho/Rho kinase

This pathway of signal transduction involves activation via some GPCRs (and also some non GPCR mechanism), involving $G_{12/13}$ type of G proteins.[93] The free subunit of G protein–activated guanosine nucleotide exchange factor and phosphorylates another GTPse (Rho) via GDP–GTP exchange, which in turn, activates the Rho kinase. Subsequently Rho kinase phosphorylates activate numerous target proteins and regulate a wide variety of cellular proteins.[94]

The mitogen activated protein kinases

The mitogen activated protein (MAP) kinases are activated by cytokines and growth factors as well as from GPCRs.

Enzymatic receptors

These receptors are also called as kinase-linked receptors. They are structurally and physiologically different than ion channels and GPCRs. Numerous proteins, growth factors, cytokines, and hormone's actions are transduced through these receptors. Because of their inherent enzymatic activities, they are also referred as receptor tyrosine kinases.[95]

The receptor tyrosine kinases have very large extracellular domain (ligand-binding site) and intracellular domain (effector domain), and contain about 400–700 residues in each. In case of insulin, extracellular domain is a separate polypeptide chain linked to rest of the receptor with disulfide bond; in case of growth factor receptor, tyrosine kinase is a single long chain of amino acid of about 1000 residues, while in case of cytokines, it is a dimeric chain.[96] However, in all cases these receptors trigger kinase cascade. Growth factors and insulin receptors process tyrosine kinase activity and involve the incorporation of ATP and sites of substrate binding.[97] Receptors for cytokine do not have tyrosine kinases at intracellular domain but possess some kinase activity after ligand binding, incorporates Janus kinases (JAK), which further activates kinase cascade.

There are two well defined pathways of signal transduction via receptor tyrosine kinases

1. Rat Sarcoma (RAS)/Rapidly Accelerated Fibrosarcoma (RAF) pathway
2. Janus kinases (JAK)/Signal Transducer and Activator of Transcription (STAT) pathway.

Rat Sarcoma (RAS)/Rapidly Accelerated Fibrosarcoma (RAF) pathway

The effects of numerous growth factors are mediated via this signal transduction mechanism. RAS (a proto-oncogene product), works like G protein and transduces its signal undergoing phosphorylation (GDP–GTP exchange), which is facilitated by SH2-domain protein Grb, which is phosphorylated by protein tyrosine kinase.[98] Activated RAS activates RAF, which is the first reaction of serine–threonine cascade, each of which phosphorylates and activates next in the line.[99] The last one of these are the MAP kinases, which finally phosphorylates the transcriptional factors, which ultimately causes gene expressions (Fig. 1.8).

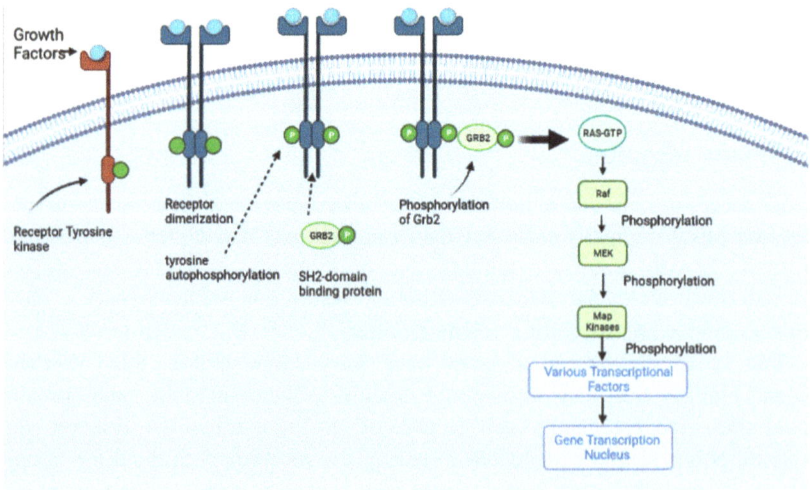

FIGURE 1.8 RAS/RAF pathway of signal-transduction mechanism.

Janus kinases (JAK)/Signal Transducer and Activator of Transcription (STAT) pathway

This pathway involves response to many cytokines. The receptor dimerization occurs after binding of the ligand to the receptor-binding site. After dimerization, the kinase unit JAK is attracted and associated with receptor dimer (JAK belongs to protein family), which has different specificity for different cytokine receptors.[100] From the JAK targets, STAT are family of transcriptional factors that are phosphorylated. STAT are the SH2-domain proteins associated to phosphorylated tyrosine groups on the receptors–JAK complex, phosphorylate themselves, get activated and finally this activated stat migrate to nucleus and results in gene expressions[101] (Fig. 1.9).

Nuclear receptors

Steroid and thyroid hormone receptors are the classical examples of these types of receptors.[102] The mechanisms of DNA transcription are totally different from these receptors as we discussed so far about the previous receptors.[103] Most of these receptors are located intranucleously, and their ligands are lipophilic compounds. They contain very highly specific regions of about 60 residues in its middle that makes DNA-binding domains. The receptors also possess two loops of about 15 residues, which are knotted together by four cysteine residues clustered around a zinc atom,[104] and these structures are present in variety of proteins involved in DNA transcription and fingers are believed to wrap around the DNA helix. The ligand-binding domain resides just below this central region, and upstream to this are the different regions that regulate gene transcriptions.[105]

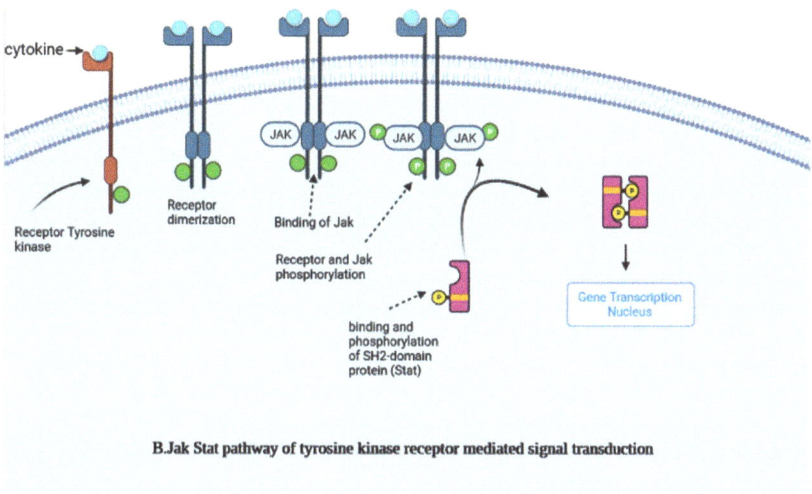

FIGURE 1.9 JAK/STAT pathway of signal-transduction mechanism.

Binding of ligand to the receptor molecule causes conformational changes, which facilitate receptor dimerization. Receptor dimers then bind to DNA-specific sequence hormone-responsive elements, which are at about 200 base pair upstream to the genes that are regulated, leading to DNA polymerase activity and expressions of specific mRNA finally translated to ribosomes for protein synthesis.[106,107]

Reference

1 Satoskar RS, Bhandarkar SD. *Pharmacology and Pharmacotherapeutics*. India: Elsevier; 2020.

2 Cassin B. *3. Logos-Pharmakon. Jacques the Sophist*. Fordham University Press; 2019:39–58.

3 Ritter J, Flower RJ, Henderson G, Kong Loke Y, MacEwan DJ, Rang HP. *Rang and Dale's Pharmacology*. Elsevier; 2019.

4 Maher TJ. *Systems pharmacology. Translational Systems Medicine and Oral Disease*. Elsevier; 2020:207–217.

5 Oglah MK, Mustafa YF, Bashir MK, Jasim MH, Mustafa YF. Curcumin and its derivatives: a review of their biological activities. *Syst Rev Pharm*. 2020;11(3):472.

6 Benek O, Korabecny J, Soukup O. A perspective on multi-target drugs for Alzheimer's disease. *Trends Pharmacol Sci*. 2020;41(7):434–445.

7 Billman GE. Homeostasis: the underappreciated and far too often ignored central organizing principle of physiology. *Front Physiol*. 2020;11:200.

8 Khan MSA, Ahmad I. *Herbal medicine: current trends and future prospects. New Look to Phytomedicine*. Elsevier; 2019:3–13.

9 Singh A, Banerjee P, Anas M, Singh N, Qamar I. Traditional nutritional and health practices targeting lifestyle behavioral changes in humans. *J Lifestyle Med*. 2020;10(2):67.

10 Inoue M, Hayashi S, Craker LE. *Role of medicinal and aromatic plants: past, present, and future. Pharmacognosy-Medicinal Plants*. IntechOpen; 2019.

11 Wiedemar N, Hauser DA, Mäser P. 100 Years of suramin. *Antimicrob Agents Chemother*. 2020;64(3):e01168-19.

12 Hashida M. Role of pharmacokinetic consideration for the development of drug delivery systems: a historical overview. *Adv Drug Deliv Rev*. 2020;157:71–82.

13 Cossart AR, Neil Cottrell W, Campbell SB, Isbel NM, Staatz CE. Characterizing the pharmacokinetics and pharmacodynamics of immunosuppressant medicines and patient outcomes in elderly renal transplant patients. *Transl Androl Urol*. 2019;8(Suppl. 2):S198.

14 Tran P, Pyo Y-C, Kim D-H, Lee S-E, Kim J-K, Park J-S. Overview of the manufacturing methods of solid dispersion technology for improving the solubility of poorly water-soluble drugs and application to anticancer drugs. *Pharmaceutics*. 2019;11(3):132.

15 Chenthamara D, Subramaniam S, Ramakrishnan SG, et al. Therapeutic efficacy of nanoparticles and routes of administration. *Biomat Res*. 2019;23(1):1–29.

16 Cascone S, Lamberti G. Hydrogel-based commercial products for biomedical applications: a review. *Int J Pharm*. 2020;573:118803.

17 Vallerand AH, Sanoski CA. *Davis's Canadian Drug Guide for Nurses*. FA Davis; 2020.

18 de Magalhães AMM, Kreling A, Brandão Chaves EH, Pasin SS, Castilho BM. Medication administration—nursing workload and patient safety in clinical wards. *Revista Brasileira de Enfermagem*. 2019;72:183–189.

19 Uddin MN, Allon A, Roni MA, Kouzi S. Overview and future potential of fast dissolving buccal films as drug delivery system for vaccines. *J Pharm Pharm Sci*. 2019;22:388–406.

20 Nikolić V, Ilić-Stojanović S, Petrović S, Tačić A, Nikolić L. *Administration routes for nano drugs and characterization of nano drug loading. Characterization and Biology of Nanomaterials for Drug Delivery*. Elsevier; 2019:587–625.

21 Lee JS, Kim SH. Dose-dependent pharmacokinetics of tofacitinib in rats: influence of hepatic and intestinal first-pass metabolism. *Pharmaceutics*. 2019;11(7):318.

22 Franco V, Gershkovich P, Perucca E, Bialer M. The interplay between liver first-pass effect and lymphatic absorption of cannabidiol and its implications for cannabidiol oral formulations. *Clin Pharmacokinet*. 2020;59(12):1493–1500.

23 Márquez Valls M, Labrador AM, Bellowa LH, et al. Biopharmaceutical study of triamcinolone acetonide semisolid formulations for sublingual and buccal administration. *Pharmaceutics*. 2021;13(7):1080.

24 Guo Y-g, Singh AP. Emerging strategies for enhancing buccal and sublingual administration of nutraceuticals and pharamaceuticals. *J Drug Deliv Sci Technol*. 2019;52:440–451.

25 Jain KK. An overview of drug delivery systems. *Drug Deliv Syst*. 2020;1–54.

26 Nolan JP, Deakin CD, Ji C, et al. Intraosseous versus intravenous administration of adrenaline in patients with out-of-hospital cardiac arrest: a secondary analysis of the PARAMEDIC2 placebo-controlled trial. *Intens Care Med*. 2020;46(5):954–962.

27 Zhang H-Y, Niu W, Olaleye OE, et al. Comparison of intramuscular and intravenous pharmacokinetics of ginsenosides in humans after dosing XueShuanTong, a lyophilized extract of panax notoginseng roots. *J Ethnopharmacol*. 2020;253:112658.

28 Granfeldt A, Avis SR, Lind PC, et al. Intravenous vs. intraosseous administration of drugs during cardiac arrest: a systematic review. *Resuscitation*. 2020;149:150–157.

29 Cook IF. Subcutaneous vaccine administration—an outmoded practice. *Human Vaccines Immunother*. 2021;17(5):1329–1341.

30 Papa P, Oricchio F, Ginés M, et al. Pharmacokinetics of subcutaneous levetiracetam in palliative care patients. *J Palliative Med*. 2021;24(2):248–251.

31 Rice BA, Saunders MA, Jagielo-Miller JE, Prendergast MA, Akins CK. Repeated subcutaneous administration of PT150 has dose-dependent effects on sign tracking in male Japanese quail. *Exp Clin Psychopharmacol*. 2019;27(6):515.

32 Keshavarz A, Kadry H, Alobaida A, Ahsan F. Newer approaches and novel drugs for inhalational therapy for pulmonary arterial hypertension. *Expert Opin Drug Deliv*. 2020;17(4):439–461.

33 Alshweiat A, Ambrus R, Csóka I. Intranasal nanoparticulate systems as alternative route of drug delivery. *Curr Med Chem*. 2019;26(35):6459–6492.

34 Islam SU, Shehzad A, Ahmed MB, Lee YS. Intranasal delivery of nanoformulations: a potential way of treatment for neurological disorders. *Molecules*. 2020;25(8):1929.

35 Jalalvandi E, Jafari H, Amorim CA, Freitas Siqueira Petri D, Nie L, Shavandi A. Vaginal administration of contraceptives. *Sci Pharm*. 2021;89(1):3.

36 Iqbal Z, Dilnawaz F. Nanocarriers for vaginal drug delivery. *Recent Pat Drug Deliv Formul*. 2019;13(1):3–15.

37 Lucas AJ, Sproston JL, Barton P, Riley RJ. Estimating human ADME properties, pharmacokinetic parameters and likely clinical dose in drug discovery. *Expert Opin Drug Discov*. 2019;14(12):1313–1327.

38 Glassman PM, Muzykantov VR. Pharmacokinetic and pharmacodynamic properties of drug delivery systems. *J Pharmacol Exp Ther*. 2019;370(3):570–580.

39 Alagga AA, Gupta V. *Drug Absorption*. StatPearls; 2021 [Internet].

40 Gopinath A, Wilson M. Factors affecting drug absorption and distribution. *Anaesth Intensive Care Med*. 2020;21(5):223–228.

41 Wanat K. Biological barriers, and the influence of protein binding on the passage of drugs across them. *Mol Biol Rep.* 2020;47(4):3221–3231.
42 Matyszewska D. The influence of charge and lipophilicity of daunorubicin and idarubicin on their penetration of model biological membranes–langmuir monolayer and electrochemical studies. *Biochim Biophy Acta (BBA)-Biomembranes.* 2020;1862(2):183104.
43 Lakey JH. Recent advances in neutron reflectivity studies of biological membranes. *Curr Opin Colloid Interface Sci.* 2019;42:33–40.
44 Zhang R, Qin X, Kong F, Chen P, Pan G. Improving cellular uptake of therapeutic entities through interaction with components of cell membrane. *Drug Deliv.* 2019;26 (1):328–342.
45 Vergalli J, Bodrenko IV, Masi M, et al. Porins and small-molecule translocation across the outer membrane of gram-negative bacteria. *Nat Rev Microbiol.* 2020;18(3):164–176.
46 Martinez MN, Greene J, Kenna L, Kissell L, Kuhn M. The impact of infection and inflammation on drug metabolism, active transport, and systemic drug concentrations in veterinary species. *Drug Metab Dispos.* 2020;48(8):631–644.
47 Koepsell H. Organic cation transporters in health and disease. *Pharmacol Rev.* 2020;72 (1):253–319.
48 Omran Z, Whitehouse C, Halwani M, Zamzami MA, Baothman OA, Rauch C. Pinocytosis as the biological mechanism that protects Pgp function in multidrug resistant cancer cells and in blood–brain barrier endothelial cells. *Symmetry.* 2020;12(8):1221.
49 Battaglia L, Panciani PP, Muntoni E, et al. Lipid nanoparticles for intranasal administration: application to nose-to-brain delivery. *Expert Opin Drug Deliv.* 2018;15(4):369–378.
50 Reinholz J, Landfester K, Mailänder V. The challenges of oral drug delivery via nanocarriers. *Drug Deliv.* 2018;25(1):1694–1705.
51 Kumar AR, Sreekar Aeila AS. Sustained release matrix type drug delivery system: an overview. *World J Pharma Pharm Sci.* 2019;8(12):470–480.
52 Currie GM. Pharmacology, Part 2: Introduction to pharmacokinetics. *J Nuclear Med Technol.* 2018;46(3):221–230.
53 Valluri S, Kawatra SK. Use of frothers to improve the absorption efficiency of dilute sodium carbonate slurry for post combustion CO_2 capture. *Fuel Process Technol.* 2021;212:106620.
54 Sofi HS, Abdal-Hay A, Ivanovski S, Zhang YS, Sheikh FA. Electrospun nanofibers for the delivery of active drugs through nasal, oral and vaginal mucosa: current status and future perspectives. *Mater Sci Eng: C.* 2020;111:110756.
55 Hu P, Guo C, Zhang Y, Lv J, Zhang Y, Xu J. Occurrence, distribution and risk assessment of abused drugs and their metabolites in a typical Urban River in North China. *Front Environ Sci Eng.* 2019;13(4):1–11.
56 Chan R, De Bruyn T, Wright M, Broccatelli F. Comparing mechanistic and preclinical predictions of volume of distribution on a large set of drugs. *Pharm Res.* 2018;35(4):1–11.
57 Zhang D, Hop CECA, Patilea-Vrana G, et al. Drug concentration asymmetry in tissues and plasma for small molecule–related therapeutic modalities. *Drug Metab Dispos.* 2019;47 (10):1122–1135.
58 He H, Yuan D, Wu Y, Cao Y. Pharmacokinetics and pharmacodynamics modeling and simulation systems to support the development and regulation of liposomal drugs. *Pharmaceutics.* 2019;11(3):110.
59 Heikenfeld J, Jajack A, Feldman B, et al. Accessing analytes in biofluids for peripheral biochemical monitoring. *Nat Biotechnol.* 2019;37(4):407–419.

60 Jung SY, Hwang S, Clarke JM, et al. Pharmacokinetic characteristics of vactosertib, a new activin receptor-like kinase 5 inhibitor, in patients with advanced solid tumors in a first-in-human phase 1 study. *Investig New Drugs*. 2020;38(3):812–820.

61 Kamble S, Loadman P, Abraham MH, Liu X. Structural properties governing drug-plasma protein binding determined by high-performance liquid chromatography method. *J Pharm Biomed Anal*. 2018;149:16–21.

62 Correia MA. Drug biotransformation. *Basic Clin Pharmacol*. 2018;4:48–59.

63 Saha N. *Clinical pharmacokinetics and drug interactions. Pharmaceutical Medicine and Translational Clinical Research*. Elsevier; 2018:81–106.

64 Bruck SD. *Pharmacological basis of controlled drug delivery. Controlled Drug Delivery*. CRC Press; 2019:1–14.

65 Coleman MD. *Human Drug Metabolism*. John Wiley & Sons; 2020.

66 He C, Wan H. Drug metabolism and metabolite safety assessment in drug discovery and development. *Expert Opin Drug Metab Toxicol*. 2018;14(10):1071–1085.

67 Routes AE. Drug Absorption, Distribution and Elimination; Pharmacokinetics; 2019.

68 van den Anker J, Reed MD, Allegaert K, Kearns GL. "Developmental changes in pharmacokinetics and pharmacodynamics. *J Clin Pharmacol*. 2018;58:S10–S25.

69 Miles R, Wanklyn S, Ross J. *Principles of drug therapy. Oxford Textbook of Palliative Medicine*. Oxford University Press; 2021:364.

70 Neal MJ. *Medical Pharmacology at a Glance*. John Wiley & Sons; 2020.

71 Cronstein BN, Aune TM. Methotrexate and its mechanisms of action in inflammatory arthritis. *Nat Rev Rheumatol*. 2020;16(3):145–154.

72 Wu T-H, Karim N, Moscow JA. Distinguishing mechanisms of adverse drug reactions from mechanisms of actions of drugs. *Oncotarget*. 2018;9(65):32404.

73 Guengerich FP. A history of the roles of cytochrome P450 enzymes in the toxicity of drugs. *Toxicol Res*. 2021;37(1):1–23.

74 Wootten D, Christopoulos A, Marti-Solano M, Babu MM, Sexton PM. Mechanisms of signalling and biased agonism in G protein-coupled receptors. *Nat Rev Mol Cell Biol*. 2018;19(10):638–653.

75 Müller CE, Baqi Y, Namasivayam V. *Agonists and antagonists for purinergic receptors. Purinergic Signaling*. Springer; 2020:45–64.

76 Zhou Q, Yang D, Wu M, et al. Common activation mechanism of class A GPCRs. *eLife*. 2019;8:e50279.

77 Byrne EFX, Luchetti G, Rohatgi R, Siebold C. "Multiple ligand binding sites regulate the hedgehog signal transducer smoothened in vertebrates. *Curr Opin Cell Biol*. 2018;51:81–88.

78 Zhao P, Furness SGB. The nature of efficacy at G protein-coupled receptors. *Biochem Pharmacol*. 2019;170:113647.

79 Muratspahić E, Freissmuth M, Gruber CW. Nature-derived peptides: a growing niche for GPCR ligand discovery. *Trends Pharmacol Sci*. 2019;40(5):309–326.

80 Xu X, Kaindl J, Clark MJ, et al. Binding pathway determines norepinephrine selectivity for the human β 1 AR over β 2 AR. *Cell Res*. 2021;31(5):569–579.

81 Qi C, Sorrentino S, Medalia O, Korkhov VM. The structure of a membrane adenylyl cyclase bound to an activated stimulatory G protein. *Science*. 2019;364(6438):389–394.

82 VerPlank JJS, Tyrkalska SD, Fleming A, Rubinsztein DC, Goldberg AL. CGMP via PKG activates 26S proteasomes and enhances degradation of proteins, including ones that cause neurodegenerative diseases. *Proc Natl Acad Sci*. 2020;117(25):14220–14230.

83 Iqbal SM, Lemmens-Gruber R. Phosphorylation of cardiac voltage-gated sodium channel: potential players with multiple dimensions. *Acta Physiol.* 2019;225(3):e13210.

84 Massari NA, Nicoud MB, Medina VA. Histamine receptors and cancer pharmacology: an update. *Br J Pharmacol.* 2020;177(3):516–538.

85 Vedel L, Nøhr AC, Gloriam DE, Bräuner-Osborne H. Pharmacology and function of the orphan GPR139 G protein-coupled receptor. *Basic Clin Pharmacol Toxicol.* 2020;126:35–46.

86 Katan M, Cockcroft S. "Phosphatidylinositol (4, 5) bisphosphate: diverse functions at the plasma membrane. *Essays Biochem.* 2020;64(3):513–531.

87 Singh N, Bhalla N. Moonlighting proteins. *Ann Rev Gene.* 2020;54:265–285.

88 Pivovarov AS, Calahorro F, Walker RJ. Na + /K + -pump and neurotransmitter membrane receptors. *Invert Neurosci.* 2019;19(1):1–16.

89 Alexander SPH, Mathie A, Peters JA, et al. The concise guide to pharmacology 2021/22: ion channels. *Br J Pharmacol.* 2021;178:S157–S245.

90 Cottone G, Chiodo L, Maragliano L. Thermodynamics and kinetics of ion permeation in wild-type and mutated open active conformation of the human A7 nicotinic receptor. *J Chem Inform Model.* 2020;60(10):5045–5056.

91 Phillips MB, Nigam A, Johnson JW. Interplay between gating and block of ligand-gated ion channels. *Brain Sci.* 2020;10(12):928.

92 Chowdhury L. *Handbook of Pharmacology for the Anaesthesiologist.* Jaypee Brothers Medical Publishers; 2019.

93 Seyedabadi M, Ghahremani MH, Albert PR. Biased signaling of G protein coupled receptors (GPCRs): molecular determinants of GPCR/transducer selectivity and therapeutic potential. *Pharmacol Ther.* 2019;200:148–178.

94 Choi E-K, Kim J-G, Kim H-J, et al. Regulation of RhoA GTPase and novel target proteins for ROCK. *Small GTPases.* 2020;11(2):95–102.

95 LeRoith D, Holly JMP, Forbes B. The insulin-like growth factors: ligands, binding proteins and receptors. *Mol Metab.* 2021;101245.

96 Karl K, Hristova K. Pondering the mechanism of receptor tyrosine kinase activation: the case for ligand-specific dimer microstate ensembles. *Curr Opin Struct Biol.* 2021;71:193–199.

97 Chen L, Marsiglia WM, Chen H, et al. Molecular basis for receptor tyrosine kinase A-loop tyrosine transphosphorylation. *Nat Chem Biol.* 2020;16(3):267–277.

98 Takács T, Kudlik G, Kurilla A, Szeder B, Buday L, Vas V. The effects of mutant ras proteins on the cell signalome. *Cancer Metastasis Rev.* 2020;39(4):1051–1065.

99 Terrell EM, Morrison DK. Ras-mediated activation of the raf family kinases. *Cold Spring Harb Perspect Med.* 2019;9(1):a033746.

100 Sperti M, Malavolta M, Ciniero G, et al. JAK inhibitors in immune-mediated rheumatic diseases: from a molecular perspective to clinical studies. *J Mol Graph Model.* 2021;104:107789.

101 Shouse G, Nikolaenko L. Targeting the JAK/STAT pathway in T cell lymphoproliferative disorders. *Curr Hematol Malig Rep.* 2019;14(6):570–576.

102 Handa RJ, Price RH, Wilson ME. *Steroid hormone receptors and the assessment of feedback sensitivity. Methods in Neuroendocrinology.* CRC Press; 2020:49–68.

103 Behr A-C, Plinsch C, Braeuning A, Buhrke T. Activation of human nuclear receptors by perfluoroalkylated substances (PFAS). *Toxicol In Vitro.* 2020;62:104700.

104 Qiu J, Wilkens C, Barrett K, Meyer AS. Microbial enzymes catalyzing keratin degradation: classification, structure, function. *Biotechnol Adv.* 2020;107607.

105 Song Y, Xuan A, Bu C, Ci D, Tian M, Zhang D. Osmotic stress-responsive promoter upstream transcripts (PROMPT s) act as carriers of MYB transcription factors to induce the expression of target genes in *Populus simonii*. *Plant Biotechnol J*. 2019;17(1): 164–177.

106 Venezia D, Nicole AV, Marcel V, Catez F, Diaz J-J. Emerging role of eukaryote ribosomes in translational control. *Int J Mol Sci*. 2019;20(5):1226.

107 Mathias CB, McAleer JP, Szollosi DE. *Pharmacology of Immunotherapeutic Drugs*. Springer; 2020.

Chapter 2

Mechanism of action of cholinergic drugs

Khandekar Hussan Reza[1], Partha Pratim Das[1], Chowdhury Mobaswar Hossain[3,4], Md. Adil Shaharyar[2], Soupayan Pal[2], Sk Zeeshan Ali[2] and Imran Kazmi[5]

[1]Department of Pharmaceutics, Bengal School of Technology, Chinsurah, Hooghly, West Bengal, India, [2]Bioeuivalence Study Centre, Department of Pharmaceutical Technology, Jadavpur University, Kolkata, West Bengal, India, [3]Department of Pharmaceutical Technology, Maulana Abul Kalam Azad University of Technology (MAKAUT), West Bengal, India, [4]NH-12, Haringhata, Simhat, Nadia, West Bengal, India, [5]Department of Biochemistry, Faculty of Science, King Abdulaziz University, Jeddah, Saudi Arabia

Introduction

The central nervous system (CNS; brain and spinal cord) and the peripheral nervous system (PNS; neuronal tissues outside the CNS) are the two parts of the nervous system. The nervous system's motor (efferent) part can be classified into two categories: autonomic and somatic. In the autonomic nervous system (ANS), functions are not under direct conscious control but are mostly autonomous.[1]

The ANS is further divided into two major divisions: sympathetic thoracolumbar (thoracic and lumbar spinal nerves) and parasympathetic craniosacral (especially the third, seventh, ninth, and tenth cranial nerves and the third and fourth sacral spinal nerve roots). Both have nuclei that start in the CNS (brain stem or spinal cord) and grow into preganglionic efferent fibers that end in the motor ganglia. The sympathetic preganglionic fibers are either short and end in the paravertebral ganglia, or they are slightly longer and end in the prevertebral ganglia. Postganglionic sympathetic fibers innervate the tissues via the ganglia, as illustrated in Fig. 2.1.[3] In general, parasympathetic preganglionic fibers terminate in ganglion cells, which get distributed diffusely or in networks on the walls of the innervated organs.

The primary transmitter molecules for ANS are acetylcholine (Ach) or norepinephrine (NE). Many peripheral ANS fibers produce ACh; hence, they are known as cholinergic fibers. Almost all of the efferent fibers that

How Synthetic Drugs Work. DOI: https://doi.org/10.1016/B978-0-323-99855-0.00002-6

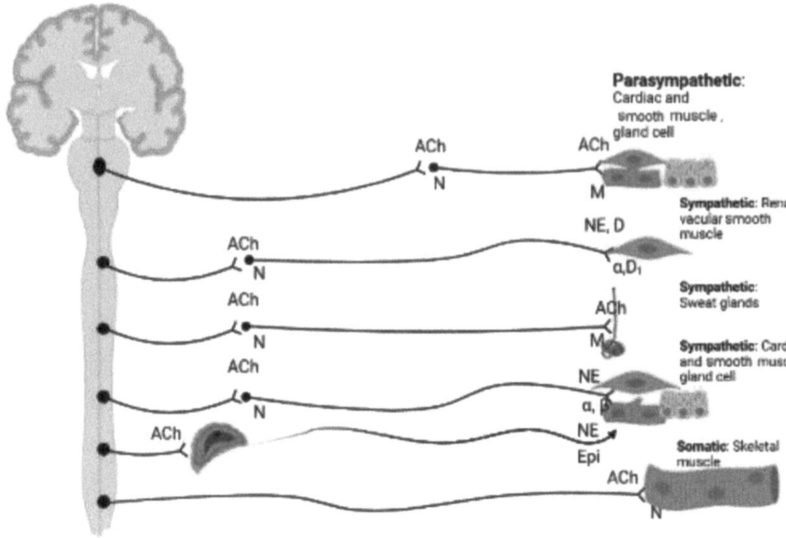

FIGURE 2.1 Somatic and autonomic nerve origin and distribution. ACh is released by somatic neurons in the brain and the spinal cord (CNS) to activate nicotinic receptors (N) on skeletal muscle.[2] *CNS*, Central nervous system.

leave the CNS are cholinergic. Furthermore, the majority of parasympathetic postganglionic fibers and a few sympathetic postganglionic fibers are cholinergic.

Most postganglionic sympathetic fibers secrete NE (also known as noradrenaline); they are noradrenergic (often referred to simply as "adrenergic") fibers, that is, they function by secreting NE (noradrenaline).[3,4] The release of neurotransmitter NE by sympathetic nervous system (SNS) results in an increase in overall activity and attention: the "fight or flight" response. The blood pressure and heart rate rise, glycogenolysis occurs, gastrointestinal peristalsis takes places, in addition to other reactions in the body.[4] The parasympathetic nervous system (PSNS) facilitates "rest and digest" processes by releasing ACh, which reduces heart rate and blood pressure, resets gastrointestinal peristalsis/digestion, and so on.[4,5] The PSNS solely innervates the brain, viscera, and external genitalia, keeping much of the musculoskeletal system and skin uninvolved, making it substantially smaller than the SNS.[6] Drugs acting on ANS (also termed as autonomic drugs) are used clinically to either imitate or inhibit the normal functions of the SNS and PSNS. Certain drugs mimic the function of the neurotransmitters at postsynaptic ends for SNS (sympathomimetics or adrenergic agonist) and PSNS (parasympathomimetics, cholinomimetic, or cholinergic).[1,2] On the other hand, some of the drugs produce an inhibitory effect by blocking the activity of neurotransmitters at the effector end of SNS (sympatholytics or antiadrenergic) and PSNS (parasympatholytic or anticholinergic).[1,7] In this chapter, we are going to discuss neurotransmitters, their synthesis, action, and degradation, as well as discuss the mechanism of how the neurotransmitters and drugs act at effectors end. We also emphasize the mechanism of actions produced by the neurotransmitters at the various receptor ends triggering various physiological outcomes. We will also overview the drug actions mediated via these receptors.

Preganglionic parasympathetic neurons originate from the brain and sacral spinal cord connecting with ganglia near or within smooth muscle and the heart. The release of ACh activates nicotinic receptors (N) on postganglionic neurons. It also activates muscarinic receptors (M) on target organs. These neurons also secret ACh, which activates muscarinic receptors (M) on target organs. Preganglionic sympathetic neurons exit the spinal cord at the thoracic and lumbar levels (thoracolumbar) and synapse with ganglia near the cord, releasing each to activate N_N receptors (type of nicotinic receptors) on postganglionic neurons. The majority of these are dispersed to smooth muscle and the heart, where they release NE to activate α and β receptors. The adrenal medulla is a postganglionic neuron that secrets primarily epinephrine (Epi) (80% Epi and 20% NE), which moves to the target tissue via circulation.

Chemistry of autonomic neurotransmitters

The major physiological action mediated by ANS involving SNS and PSNS involves the interaction of neurotransmitters with their respective receptors at the postsynaptic end of neurons.[1] Two major neurotransmitters play a central role in ANS activity. ACh mediates through ganglion and PSNS results in inhibitory "rest and digest activity."[5] On the other hand, NE mediates via SNS producing "fight or flight" response.[2] Herein, we discuss the biochemistry involving synthesis, storage, and degradation of ACh.

Biochemistry of acetylcholine

ACh is synthesized in the cytoplasm from acetyl-CoA (synthesized in mitochondria) and choline through the enzymatic action of the enzyme choline acetyltransferase. Choline is transported into the neuron terminal by a sodium-dependent choline transporter. ACh formed is transported into the vesicles by vesicular acetylcholine transporter (VAChT) driven by proton efflux. Most of the vesicular ACh is bound to negatively charged vesicular proteoglycan. Vesicles contain vesicle-associated membrane proteins (VAMPs), which align them to the inner neuronal cell membrane potentiating the release of transmitter. Inner surface of the nerve terminal membrane contains synaptosomal nerve–associated proteins (SNAPs) and docks the vesicle with VAMPs. VAMPs and SNAPs are together termed as "fusion proteins." The release of transmitter from the vesicles is a calcium-dependent process. The influx of calcium ions takes place via N-type calcium channels. Calcium's interaction with VAMPs results in the fusion of the vesicle membrane with the terminal membrane and opening of a pore into the synapse. The opening of the pore and influx of cations result in the release of the ACh from the proteoglycan and exocytotic expulsion into the synaptic cleft. This process is described in Fig. 2.2. Various drugs may also act as presynaptic end, which may modulate the function and release of each. Such modulated drug actions are briefed in Table 2.1.

Signal transduction mechanisms involved in drug response

Drugs generally interact with the receptors targeted to bind with basic neurotransmitters categorized under ANS. The list includes Epi, NE, ACh, and dopamine. The transmitters bind with the receptors, resulting in conformational change that results in a defined physiological outcome. Drugs generally modulate the binding of the receptors by enhancing, inhibiting, or moderating their activities. There are two sets of receptors that are linked to

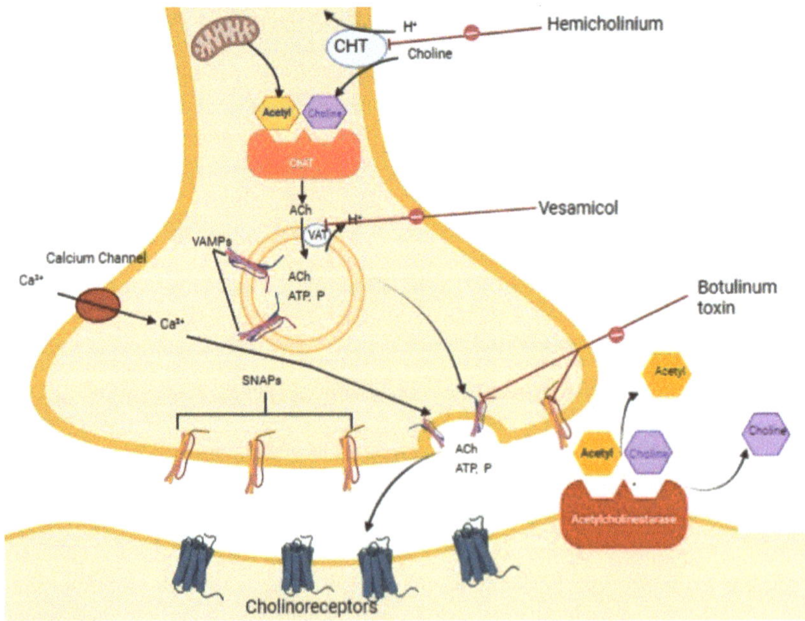

FIGURE 2.2 Synthesis, storage, and release of ACh at synaptic end a block diagram. *ACh*, Acetylcholine.

TABLE 2.1 List of drugs or chemicals inhibiting the synthesis or release of acetylcholine (ACh).

Name of drug	Category	Site of Action
Hemicholinium	Cholinergic antagonist	Inhibits the choline transporter preventing the entry of choline into the cell[8]
Vesamicol	Cholinergic antagonist	VAChT inhibitor preventing the entry of ACh in the vesicle[9]
Botulinum toxin	A neurotoxic protein from *Clostridium botulinum* and related species	Prevents the release of the neurotransmitter ACh from the axon endings by inhibiting SNAPs and VAMPs at the neuromuscular junction, thus causing flaccid paralysis[10]

SNAP, Synaptosomal nerve–associated protein; *VAMP*, vesicle-associated membrane protein; *VAT*, vesicle-associated transport.

the function of ANS: nicotinic and muscarinic. These receptors are named after the nerves that normally innervate them. The term "adrenoceptor" is commonly used to describe receptors that respond to catecholamines such as Epi or NE.[11] The general class of adrenoceptors can be further subdivided into α- and β-adrenoceptor types. Cholinoreceptors are the receptors (both nicotinic and muscarinic) that respond to ACh.[12]

Nicotinic receptor

The isolation of protein obtained from the muscle from the Torpedo electric organ by Jean-Pierre Changeux allowed the first reading of the corresponding amino acid sequence.[13] One such form of receptor is a pentamer comprising four polypeptide subunits (e.g., two α chains, one β, one γ, and one δ chain, within the molecular weights from 43,000 to 50,000), as shown in Fig. 2.3. The α subunits comprises the binding site, and the adjacent subunit to it provides the complementary site.[13] ACh binding to sites on the α subunits causes a conformational change resulting in the opening of a central ligand-gated sodium channel, with size ranging within 0.5 nm in diameter, through which sodium ions enters.[14]

Nicotinic receptors (see Fig. 2.3) are further classified into two types: N_N and N_M. The N_N type receptors are located at autonomic ganglia and are generally the pentamer of αβ subunits. They generally open for cations like sodium, potassium, and calcium. Drugs like hexamethonium and trimethaphan act as an agonist to the receptor. On the other hand, N_M type receptors are located at neuromuscular junctions. They are pentamers comprising two

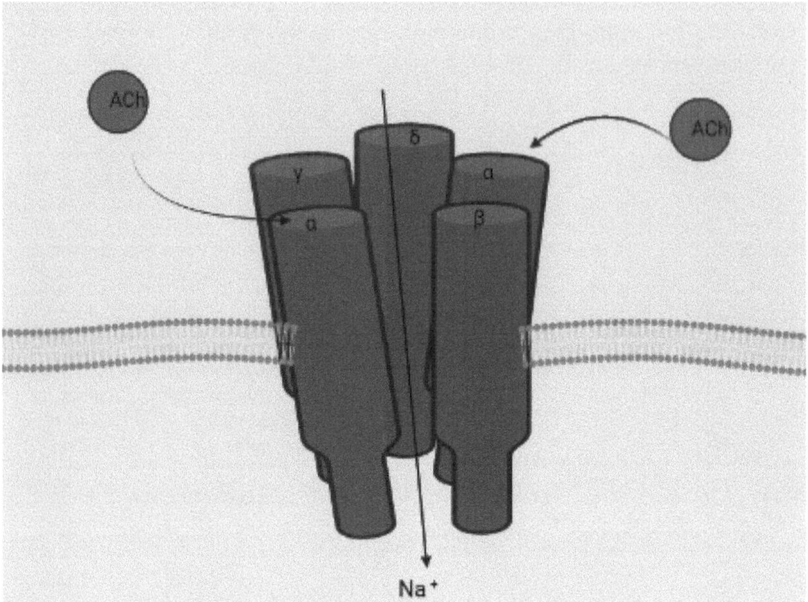

FIGURE 2.3 The nicotinic acetylcholine receptor.

α, one β, one γ, and one δ subunits and generally open for cations like sodium and potassium. Drugs like tubocurarine and α bungarotoxin are agonist to the receptor.[15]

Muscarinic receptors

It is the receptor subtype classified under G protein-coupled receptor family. The receptors are connected to the effectors (e.g., enzyme, channel, or effector protein) through GTP-activated proteins (G protein). Muscarinic receptors are found throughout the human body and mediate a variety of physiological functions. The precise location and functional role of all of these subtypes are yet to be fully elucidated into five types ($M_{1'}$ to M_5).[16]

They generally comprise seven α-helical trans-membrane amino acid segments with three extracellular and intracellular loops. The drugs generally bind between the helices extracellular. G protein comprises three subunits: α, β, and γ.[17] The α subunit interacts with effectors resulting in their activation or their deactivation. The classification of G proteins based on the α subunit is summarized in Table 2.2.

Muscarinic receptors ($M_{1'}$ to M_5) generally regulate mainly using G_i, G_o, and G_q subunits. Hence, they act via inhibition of adenylyl cyclase, opening of potassium channel, downregulation of calcium channel, and activation of phospholipase C (PLC).[18] The locations and functions are enumerated in Table 2.3.

TABLE 2.2 G protein classification based on the type of α subunit.

α Subunit type	Functions
G_s	Activation of adenylyl cyclase Opening of calcium channel
G_i	Inhibition of adenylyl cyclase Opening of potassium channel
G_o	Downregulation of calcium channel
G_q	Activation of phospholipase C
G_{13}	Sodium–potassium exchange

TABLE 2.3 Location and outcome of muscarinic receptor.

Name of receptor	Location	Type of G-protein	Affected effectors pathway	Physiological outcome
M_1	Nerves gastrin gland (GIT)	G_q	Activation of phospholipase C	Enhances acid secretion
M_2	Heart, nerves, smooth muscles	G_i	Inhibition of adenylyl cyclase Opening of potassium channel	Produces a negative chronotropic effect, reducing pacemaker rate and contractility strength, which in turn reduce the heart rate
M_3	Glands Smooth muscles Endothelium	G_q	Activation of phospholipase C	Increases gland secretion Smooths muscle contraction Releases EDRF[a] resulting vasodilatation
M_4	CNS	G_i	Inhibition of adenylyl cyclase	Inhibitory autoreceptor for ACh release
M_5	CNS	G_q	Activation of phospholipase C	Modulates the activity of ACh in CNS

ACh, Acetylcholine; CNS, central nervous system; *GIT*, gastro intestinal tract.
[a]*EDRF = Endothelial-derived relaxing factor.*

The signal transduction resulting in physiological outcome is controlled by three effector pathways explained below with the reference to Fig. 2.4.

Inhibition of adenylyl cyclase

ACh or other drug ligands binding to M_2 or M_4 receptors inhibit the activation of the adenylyl cyclase enzyme via G_i α subunit of G protein, which results in downregulation of phosphokinase A. This lowers the interaction of various proteins like troponin and phospholamban with calcium, thereby reducing the contractility of myocytes (mainly cardiac). *Activation of phospholipase C:*ACh or other drug ligands binding to M_1, M_3, or M_5 receptors activate PLC via G_q α subunit of G protein. The PLC hydrolyzes membrane phospholipid phosphatidylinositol 4,5-biphosphate (PIP_2) producing inositol 1,4,5-triphosphate (IP_3) and diacylglycerol (DAG). IP_3 promotes mobilization of calcium from intracellular organizer pools. DAG along with calcium activates protein kinase C which upon phosphorylation results in enhanced smooth muscle contraction and glandular secretion and acid secretion (gastric parietal cell). Cytosolic calcium interacts with calmodulin, activating myosin light chain kinase, which results in contraction.[19]

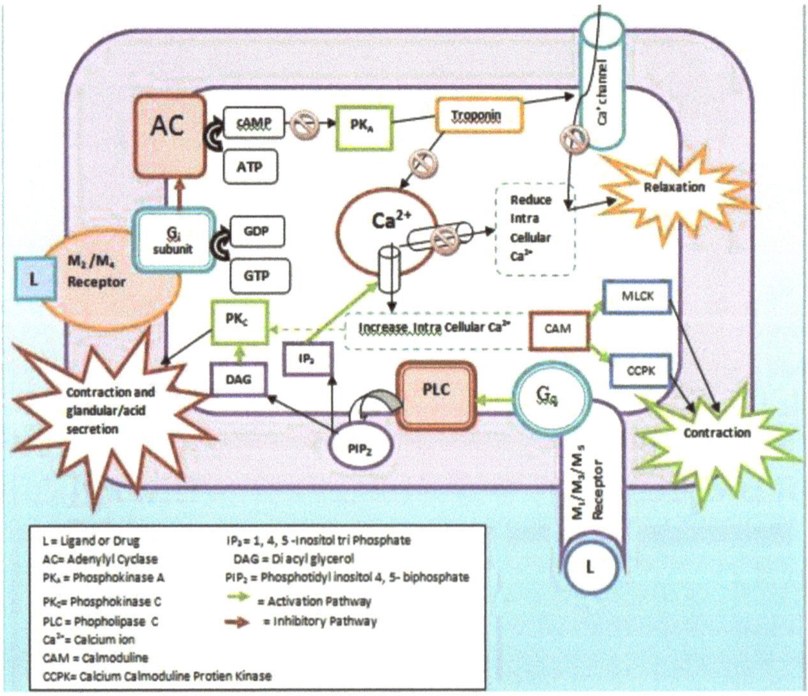

FIGURE 2.4 Signal transduction process for muscarinic receptors.

Cholinergic agonists

Cholinergic agonists are the drugs that interact with muscarinic and nicotinic receptors and produce effects that are similar to ACh. Muscarinic receptors are widely distributed and exhibit the activities on heart, blood vessels, smooth muscles, glands, and eyes, whereas nicotinic receptors help in interaction between the autonomic ganglia and skeletal muscles. Table 2.4 summarizes some cholinergic agonists.

Anticholinesterases

Anticholinesterase acts similar to cholinoreceptor stimulants. In the classification of anticholinesterase, all chemical agents act on different site of action with different intensity.

Physostigmine: Physostigmine is parasympathomimetic reversible cholinesterase, mainly used in glaucoma.
Neostigmine: Physostigmine is parasympathomimetic reversible cholinesterase, mainly used as myasthenia gravis.
Pyridostigmine: Pyridostigmine is parasympathomimetic reversible cholinesterase, mainly used as Myasthenia Gravis. It is used along with atropine.
Edrophonium: Edrophonium is a reversible anticholinesterase inhibitor used as a diagnostic agent in Myasthenia Gravis and postoperative decurarization.
Tacrine: Lipophilic tacrine can cross the blood–brain barrier and has a longer duration of action by increasing the ACh and is used for partial symptomatic improvement in Alzheimer's disease.
Rivastigmine and donepezil: Rivastigmine and donepezil both are acetylcholinesterase inhibitors and used in Alzheimer's disease.

The activities of various anticholinesterases are enumerated in Table 2.5.

Anticholinergic drugs

Anticholinergic agents block the effects of cholinergic agonists at autonomic effectors via muscarinic receptors. Anticholinergic prototype like atropine stimulates the CNS action on medullary centers like vagal, respiratory, and vasomotor. It depresses the vestibular excitation and has antimotion sickness property. By blocking the M_2 receptors on sino atrial (SA) nodes, it causes the tachycardia. It also causes the mydriasis as well as miosis. All smooth muscles are relaxed by M_3 receptors and decrease the lacrimation, salivation, gastric, and tracheobronchial secretion. Body temperature increases by the anticholinergic, and in particular, atropine has a mild anesthetic action on cornea. The mechanism of action and effects of various anticholinergics are summarized in Table 2.6.

TABLE 2.4 Cholinergic agonists.

Drug	Spectrum of action	Mechanism of action	Therapeutic effects	Clinical applications
Acetylcholine[20]	Both muscarinic and nicotinic	Cholinergic agonist	Produces stimulation of both sympathetic and parasympathetic ganglia	Miosis of the iris soon after delivery of the lens in cataract surgery, in penetrating keratoplasty, iridectomy, and other anterior segment surgery
Methacholine[21]	Muscarinic agonist	Stimulates the parasympathetic nervous system	A bronchoconstrictor agent, an epitope, a cholinergic agonist and a vasodilator agent	Clinically it is used in asthma
Carbachol[22]	Both Muscarinic and nicotinic	Parasympathomimetic	Intraocular administration results miosis decreasing intraocular pressure and increased aqueous humor outflow	Cardiac failure, bronchial asthma, peptic ulcer, hyperthyroidism, gastrointestinal spasm, urinary tract obstruction, and Parkinson's disease
Bethanechol[23]	Muscarinic (M3)	Bethanechol exerts its parasympathomimetic effects by a direct action on muscarinic (cholinergic) receptors	Stimulates the PSNS by binding to postganglionic muscarinic receptors	Leads to increased detrusor muscle tone to promote bladder emptying and increased smooth muscle tone, which restores gastrointestinal peristalsis and motility
Muscrine[24]	Muscarinic receptors	Mimicking parasympathetic nerve activity	Activates muscarinic receptors and drugs that enhance cholinergic activity, by slowing the breakdown of acetylcholine	Toxicological use

Pilocarpine[25]	Muscarinic	Increases secretion by the exocrine glands, and produces contraction of the iris sphincter muscle and ciliary muscle (when given topically to the eyes) by mainly stimulating muscarinic receptors	Increases secretion by the exocrine glands	Used in the eye to treat elevated intraocular pressure, various types of glaucoma, and to induce miosis
Arecholine[26]	Both muscarinic and nicotinic	Stimulates muscarinic receptor	Used in the form of various salts as a ganglionic stimulant, a parasympathomimetic, and a vermifuge	Used as a euphoriant

TABLE 2.5 Activities of various anticholinesterases.

Drug	Spectrum of action	Mechanism of action	Therapeutic effects	Clinical applications
Physostigmine[27]	Both nicotinic and muscarinic receptors	Inhibits acetylcholinesterase, the enzyme responsible for the breakdown of used acetylcholine.	Increase in availability of acetylcholine at the synapse	Applied topically to the conjunctiva and the treatment of severe anticholinergic toxicity.
Neostigmine[28]	Both nicotinic and muscarinic receptors	Inhibits acetylcholinesterase, the enzyme responsible for the breakdown of used acetylcholine.	Increase in availability of acetylcholine at the synapse	Treatment of myasthenia gravis and to reverse the effects of muscle relaxants.
Pyridostigmine[29]	Both nicotinic and muscarinic receptors	Reversible acetylcholinesterase inhibitor.	Increase in availability of acetylcholine at the synapse	Used for symptomatic treatment of myasthenia gravis and congenital myasthenic syndromes and to reverse neuromuscular blockade by nondepolarizing muscle relaxants.
Edrophonium[30]	Both nicotinic and muscarinic receptors	Inhibits the action of the enzyme acetylcholinesterase.	A rapid-onset, short-acting cholinesterase inhibitor used in cardiac arrhythmias and in the diagnosis of myasthenia gravis	Used to diagnose and evaluate myasthenia gravis.
Rivastigmine[31]		Increasing the concentration of acetylcholine through reversible inhibition of its hydrolysis by cholinesterase.	Increase in availability of acetylcholine at the synapse	Can treat mild to moderate dementia in Alzheimer's and Parkinson's.

Donepezil[32]		Selectively and reversibly inhibits the acetylcholinesterase enzyme.	Donepezil improves the cognitive and behavioral signs and symptoms of Alzheimer's disease	Used to treat the behavioral and cognitive effects of Alzheimer's disease and other types of dementia.
Galantamine[33]	Nicotinic acetylcholine receptors	Reversible, competitive inhibitor of the acetylcholinesterase by binding to the choline-binding site and acyl-binding pocket of the enzyme active site.	Enhances ACh levels in the synaptic cleft	Used to manage mild to moderate dementia associated with Alzheimer's disease.
Tacrine[34]		Reversibly binds with and inactivates cholinesterases.	Muscle relaxants, as a respiratory stimulant, and in the treatment of Alzheimer's disease and other CNS disorders	Used for the management of Alzheimer's disease symptoms.
Dyflos[35]		Irreversible inhibition of cholinesterase.	Powerful miotic	Used mainly in the treatment of glaucoma.
Echothiophate[36]		Long-acting cholinesterase inhibitor which enhances the effect of endogenously liberated acetylcholine in iris, ciliary muscle, and other parasympathetically innervated structures of the eye.	It depresses both plasma and erythrocyte cholinesterase levels in most patients after a few weeks of eye drop therapy	Used as a miotic in the treatment of glaucoma.
Malathion[37]		Nonsystemic, wide-spectrum organophosphate insecticide. It inhibits acetylcholinesterase activity of most eukaryotes.	Potent neurotoxins, causing muscle spasms and ultimately death	Used to control mosquitos and other flying insects. Pharmaceutically, malathion is used to eliminate head lice.

ACh, Acetylcholine. *CNS*, Central nervous system.

TABLE 2.6 Anticholinergic drugs.

Drug	Spectrum of action	Mechanism of action	Therapeutic effects	Clinical applications
Atropine[38]	Muscarinic antagonist	Atropine binds to and inhibits muscarinic acetylcholine receptors, producing a wide range of anticholinergic effects	Atropine in clinical doses counteracts the peripheral dilatation and abrupt decrease in blood pressure produced by choline esters	Excitatory CNS effects, potent on heart, bronchial muscles, and intestines
Homatropine[39]	Muscarinic receptor antagonist	Blocking muscarinic receptors and cholinergic signaling pathways.	Blocks the response of the iris sphincter muscle and causes the pupil to become unresponsive to light upon dilation or mydriasis	Used to dilate the pupil, treat inflammation of the uveal tract, and suppress a cough
Ipratropium bromide[40]	Anticholinergic	Inhibition of the parasympathetic nervous system in the airways and hence, inhibit their function	Generates bronchial secretions and constriction	Used in the control of symptoms related to bronchospasm in COPD
Tiotropium bromide[41]	Antimuscarinic	Antagonist of muscarinic receptors M_1 to M_5	Inhibition of the M_3 receptor in the smooth muscle of the lungs leads to relaxation of smooth muscle and bronchodilation	Used in the management of COPD
Cyclopentolate[42]	Anticholinergic	Blocks the muscarinic receptors	Produces dilatation of the pupil (mydriasis) and prevents the eye from accommodating for near vision (cycloplegia)	Used to cause mydriasis and cycloplegia for diagnostic testing

Tropicamide[43]	Muscarinic receptor antagonist	Nonselective muscarinic antagonist that binds to all subtypes of muscarinic receptors	Relaxes the pupillary sphincter muscle and causes pupil dilation; By blocking the muscarinic receptors of the ciliary body, tropicamide also prevents accommodation	Used to induce mydriasis and cycloplegia for diagnostic procedures
Propantheline[44]	Antimuscarinic	(1) A specific anticholinergic effect (antimuscarinic) at the acetylcholine-receptor sites, and (2) A direct effect upon smooth muscle (musculotropic)	A muscarinic antagonist used as an antispasmodic, in rhinitis, in urinary incontinence, and in the treatment of ulcers	Used to treat urinary incontinence, hyperhidrosis, as well as cramps and spasms of the stomach, intestines, and bladder
Oxiphenonium[45]	Anticholinergic	Action is achieved via a dual mechanism: (1) a specific anticholinergic effect (antimuscarinic) at the acetylcholine-receptor sites and (2) a direct effect upon smooth muscle (musculotropic)	Has a direct relaxing effect on smooth muscle. Used to treat or prevent spasm in the muscles of the gastrointestinal tract in the irritable bowel syndrome	Treatment of gastric and duodenal ulcer, and to relieve visceral spasms, eye drops for mydriatic effect
Clidinium[46]	Anticholinergic	Inhibits muscarinic actions of acetylcholine at postganglionic parasympathetic neuroeffector sites primarily by inhibiting the M1 muscarinic receptors	Has a pronounced antispasmodic and antisecretory effect on the gastrointestinal tract	Used to treat peptic ulcer disease, colicky abdominal pain, diverticulitis, and IBS
Pipenzolate methyl bromide[47]	Antimuscarinic agent	Inhibiting muscarinic (cholinergic) receptors on smooth muscles and prevents the effect of acetylcholine	Gastrointestinal motility disorders and arrhythmia	Relaxation of smooth muscles of the gastrointestinal tract and genitourinary tract and reduces the painful spasm and cramp

(*Continued*)

TABLE 2.6 (Continued)

Drug	Spectrum of action	Mechanism of action	Therapeutic effects	Clinical applications
Isopropamide[48]	Anticholinergic	Inhibit parasympathetic nerve impulses by selectively blocking the binding of the neurotransmitter acetylcholine to its receptor in nerve cells	Relieves symptoms of spastic and painful symptoms of gastrointestinal conditions and symptoms of flu, colds, and related conditions	Used in the treatment of peptic ulcer and other gastrointestinal disorders marked by hyperacidity and hypermotility
Dicyclomine[49]	Antimuscarinic agent	Direct antimuscarinic activity of the M1, M3, and M2 receptors; and partially through antagonism of bradykinin and histamine; noncompetitively inhibits the action of bradykinin and histamine	Direct action on the smooth muscle, and decreased strength of contractions seen in spasms of the ileum	Used to treat IBS
Valethamate[50]	Anticholinergic		Symptomatically manages conditions involving smooth muscle spasms	Usually used to manage the conditions involving spastic constipation, dysmenorrhea, and gastrointestinal tract cramping
Pirenzepine[51]	Antimuscarinic agent	Muscarinic receptor antagonist and binds to the muscarinic acetylcholine receptor. The muscarinic acetylcholine receptor mediates various cellular responses, including inhibition of adenylate cyclase, breakdown of phosphoinositides and modulation of potassium channels through the action of G proteins	Relieves cramps or spasms of the stomach, intestines, and bladder.	Used to treat peptic ulcers, gastric ulcers, and duodenal ulcers

Oxybutynin[52]	Antimuscarinic agent	Inhibiting the muscarinic action of acetylcholine on smooth muscle, and not skeletal muscle. Competitively inhibits the postganglionic type 1, 2, and 3 muscarinic receptors.	Reduces detrusor muscle activity, relaxing the bladder and preventing the urge to void	Used to treat the symptoms of overactive bladder
Flavoxate[53]	Muscarinic antagonist	Direct antagonist at muscarinic acetylcholine receptors in cholinergically innervated organs	Symptomatic relief of conditions associated with lack of muscle control in the bladder	Used in various urinary syndromes and as an antispasmodic
Tolterodine[54]	Muscarinic receptor antagonist	Competitive antagonists at muscarinic receptors	Tolterodine acts on M2 and M3 subtypes of muscarinic receptors	Used to treat overactive bladder with urinary incontinence, urgency, and frequency
Trihexyphenidyl[55]	Muscarinic antagonist	Nonselective muscarinic acetylcholine-receptor antagonist, but binds with higher affinity to the M1 subtype	Drug-induced extrapyramidal symptoms	Used as an adjunct drug in the management of parkinsonism and as a treatment for extrapyramidal symptoms caused by drugs affecting the CNS
Procyclidine[56]	Muscarinic antagonist	Acts by blocking central cholinergic receptors	Used to treat symptomatic Parkinsonism and extrapyramidal dysfunction caused by antipsychotic agents	Used to treat parkinsonism of various types and in the treatment of extrapyramidal symptoms
Biperiden[57]	Muscarinic receptor antagonist	Competitive antagonism of acetylcholine at cholinergic receptors in the corpus striatum, which then restores the balance	Antisecretory, antispasmodic, and mydriatic effects	Used to treat Parkinsonism and control extrapyramidal side effects of neuroleptic drugs

CNS, Central nervous system; *COPD*, chronic obstructive pulmonary disease; *IBS*, inflammatory bowel syndrome.

Conclusion

This chapter presents an overview of some chemical agents or drugs that act on a specific receptor and regulate the normal physiological and biochemical balance, which in turn regulates the autonomic system of the body and maintains the balance with CNS and other biochemical pathways. Some scientific studies have already proved that neurotransmitters play a vital role in cardiovascular, smooth muscles, glands, CNS, blood vessels, and ganglia. Sometimes neurotransmitter-blocking agents also exhibit vital pharmacological effects, and the enzyme that converts the neurotransmitter into an inactive form also has pharmacological effects.

References

1. Katzung BG, Masters SB Trevor, AJ, eds. (2004). *Basic & Clinical Pharmacology*.
2. Becker DE. Basic and clinical pharmacology of autonomic drugs. *Anesthesia Prog*. 2012;59(4):159–169.
3. Sternini C. Organization of the peripheral nervous system: autonomic and sensory ganglia. *J Invest Dermatol Symp Proc*. 1997;2(1):1–7.
4. Koopman FA, Stoof SP, Straub RH, Van Maanen MA, Vervoordeldonk MJ, Tak PP. Restoring the balance of the autonomic nervous system as an innovative approach to the treatment of rheumatoid arthritis. *Mol Med*. 2011;17(9):937–948.
5. Kenney MJ, Ganta CK. Autonomic nervous system and immune system interactions. *Compr Physiol*. 2014;4(3):1177.
6. Scott GD, Fryer AD. *Role of parasympathetic nerves and muscarinic receptors in allergy and asthma. Allergy and the Nervous System*. Vol. 98. Karger Publishers; 2012:48–69.
7. Aaron CK. Sympathomimetics. *Emerg Med Clin North Am*. 1990;8(3):513–526.
8. Deiana S, Platt B, Riedel G. The cholinergic system and spatial learning. *Behav Brain Res*. 2011;221(2):389–411.
9. Zelikowsky M, Hast TA, Bennett RZ, et al. Cholinergic blockade frees fear extinction from its contextual dependency. *Biol Psychiatry*. 2013;73(4):345–352.
10. Drever BD, Riedel G, Platt B. The cholinergic system and hippocampal plasticity. *Behav Brain Res*. 2011;221(2):505–514.
11. Hausswirth C, Schaal K, Le Meur Y, et al. Parasympathetic activity and blood catecholamine responses following a single partial-body cryostimulation and a whole-body cryostimulation. *PLoS One*. 2013;8(8):e72658.
12. Kawashima K, Fujii T, Moriwaki Y, Misawa H. Critical roles of acetylcholine and the muscarinic and nicotinic acetylcholine receptors in the regulation of immune function. *Life Sci*. 2012;91(21–22):1027–1032.
13. Rollema H, Hurst RS. The contribution of agonist and antagonist activities of $\alpha4\beta2^*$ nAChR ligands to smoking cessation efficacy: a quantitative analysis of literature data. *Psychopharmacology*. 2018;235(9):2479–2505.
14. Du X, Tang Y, Han Y, et al. Acetylcholine suppresses phagocytosis via binding to muscarinic-and nicotinic-acetylcholine receptors and subsequently interfering Ca2 + -and NFκB-signaling pathways in blood clam. *Fish Shellfish Immunol*. 2020;102:152–160.
15. Deneris ES, Connolly J, Rogers SW, Duvoisin R. Pharmacological and functional diversity of neuronal nicotinic acetylcholine receptors. *Trends Pharmacol Sci*. 1991;12:34–40.

16. Hartigan SM, Dmochowski RR. Gender specific pharmacokinetic and pharmacodynamic considerations for antimuscarinic drugs for overactive bladder treatment. *Expert Opin drug Metab Toxicol*. 2020;16(2):103–110.
17. Rosenbaum DM, Rasmussen SG, Kobilka BK. The structure and function of G-protein-coupled receptors. *Nature*. 2009;459(7245):356–363.
18. Bill CA, Vines CM. Phospholipase C. *Calcium Signal*. 2020;215–242.
19. Tarnawski L, Reardon C, Caravaca AS, et al. Adenylyl cyclase 6 mediates inhibition of TNF in the inflammatory reflex. *Front Immunol*. 2018;9:2648.
20. Bagdas D, Gurun MS, Flood P, Papke RL, Damaj MI. New insights on neuronal nicotinic acetylcholine receptors as targets for pain and inflammation: a focus on α7 nAChRs. *Curr Neuropharmacol*. 2018;16(4):415–425.
21. Chevrier S, Abdulnour J, Saint-Pierre M. *Predictors of methacholine challenge testing results: a large retrospective review. TP120. TP120 Asthma: Clinical Studies*. American Thoracic Society; 2021:A4534.
22. Lévesque M, Avoli M. Carbachol-induced theta-like oscillations in the rodent brain limbic system: Underlying mechanisms and significance. *Neurosci Biobehav Rev*. 2018;95:406–420.
23. Padda IS, Derian A. *Bethanechol*. StatPearls; 2021.
24. Matera MG, Rinaldi B, Berardo C, Rinaldi M, Cazzola M. A review of the pharmacokinetics of M3 muscarinic receptor antagonists used for the treatment of asthma. *Expert Opin Drug Metab Toxicol*. 2020;16(2):143–148.
25. Panarese V, Moshirfar M. *Pilocarpine*. StatPearls; 2020 [Internet].
26. Volgin AD, Bashirzade A, Amstislavskaya TG, et al. DARK classics in chemical neuroscience: arecoline. *ACS Chem Neurosci*. 2019;10(5):2176–2185.
27. Arens AM, Shah K, Al-Abri S, Olson KR, Kearney T. Safety and effectiveness of physostigmine: a 10-year retrospective review. *Clin Toxicol*. 2018;56(2):101–107.
28. Eldufani J, Blaise G. The role of acetylcholinesterase inhibitors such as neostigmine and rivastigmine on chronic pain and cognitive function in aging: A review of recent clinical applications. *Alzheimer's Dementia Transl Res Clin Interventions*. 2019;5:175–183.
29. Ahuja NK, Mische L, Clarke JO, Wigley FM, McMahan ZH. Pyridostigmine for the treatment of gastrointestinal symptoms in systemic sclerosis. *Semin Arthritis Rheum*. 2018;48(1):111–116.
30. Naji A, Owens ML. *Edrophonium*. StatPearls; 2021.
31. Patel PH, Gupta V. *Rivastigmine*. StatPearls; 2021.
32. Adlimoghaddam A, Neuendorff M, Roy B, Albensi BC. A review of clinical treatment considerations of donepezil in severe Alzheimer's disease. *CNS Neurosci & therapeutics*. 2018;24(10):876–888.
33. Upadhyay SD, Ahmad Y, Kohli S. A review on pharmacological potential of galantamine. *Pharmacogn Commun*. 2020;10(2):63–66.
34. Przybyłowska M, Kowalski S, Dzierzbicka K, Inkielewicz-Stepniak I. Therapeutic potential of multifunctional tacrine analogues. *Curr Neuropharmacol*. 2019;17(5):472–490.
35. Seetharaman R., Advani M. (2020). *A Summary of Drugs Targeting Enzymes*.
36. Pakala RS, Brown KN, Preuss CV. (2019). *Cholinergic Medications*.
37. Kumar SS, Ghosh P, Malyan SK, Sharma J, Kumar V. A comprehensive review on enzymatic degradation of the organophosphate pesticide malathion in the environment. *J Environ Sci Health C*. 2019;37(4):288–329.
38. Tran HD, Tran YH, Tran TD, Jong M, Coroneo M, Sankaridurg P. A review of myopia control with atropine. *J Ocul Pharmacol Ther*. 2018;34(5):374–379.
39. Wong K, Lim CW, Malvankar-Mehta MS, Hutnik C. Effectiveness of topical cycloplegics as anterior segment analgesics: systematic review and *meta*-analysis. *Can J Ophthalmol*. 2021.

40. Speich B, Thomer A, Aghlmandi S, Ewald H, Zeller A, Hemkens LG. Treatments for subacute cough in primary care: systematic review and *meta*-analyses of randomised clinical trials. *Br J Gen Pract.* 2018;68(675):e694–e702.
41. Anzueto A, Miravitlles M. Tiotropium in chronic obstructive pulmonary disease – a review of clinical development. *Respiratory Res.* 2020;21(1):1–16.
42. Yoon S, Gianturco SL, Pavlech LL, Storm KD, Yuen MV, Mattingly AN. (2020). *Cyclopentolate Hydrochloride: Summary Report.*
43. Hong D, Tripathy K. *Tropicamide.* StatPearls; 2021 [Internet].
44. Chen SY, Ravindran G, Zhang Q, Kisely S, Siskind D. Treatment strategies for clozapine-induced sialorrhea: a systematic review and *meta*-analysis. *CNS Drugs.* 2019;33(3):225–238.
45. Panigrahi BB., Pani MK. *A Review on Compatibility of "Sucralfate" in Bilayer Floating Tablet for Treatment of Ulcer in Pregnancy.*
46. Puasripun S, Thinrungroj N, Pinyopornpanish K, et al. Efficacy and safety of clidinium/chlordiazepoxide as an add-on therapy in functional dyspepsia: a randomized, controlled, trial. *J Neurogastroenterol Motil.* 2020;26(2):259.
47. Ahmad NR, Sulyman EZ. *Development of Kinetic Spectrophotometric Determination of Pipenzolate Methyl Bromide in Pharmaceutical Preparations.*
48. Abdellatif SH. Analytical study on some drugs affecting central nervous system and cardiovascular system. *CU Theses.* 2019;.
49. Kaako A. Probable association of acute pancreatitis with dicyclomine. *Turkish J Gastroenterol.* 2019;30(3):307.
50. Palshetkar NP, Purandare A, Mehta HK, Palshetkar R. Effectiveness and safety of camylofin in augmentation of labor: a systematic review and *meta*-analysis. *J Obstet Gynecol India.* 2020;70:425–439.
51. Takahashi H, Kanase Y, Makino K, et al. Conformational properties and M1 antimuscarinic activity of 4-substituted pirenzepine/telenzepine analogues. *Heterocycles.* 2020;101:273–283.
52. Campanati A, Gregoriou S, Consales V, et al. Combined treatment of palmar hyperhidrosis with botulinum toxin type A and oxybutynin chloride: results of a clinical, multicenter, prospective study. *Dermatol Ther.* 2020;33.
53. Bertoli M, Conti F, Conti M, Cova A, Setnikar I. Pharmacokinetics of flavoxate in man. *Pharmacol Res Commun.* 1976;8(4):417–428.
54. Clemett D, Jarvis B. Tolterodine. *Drugs Aging.* 2001;18(4):277–304.
55. Jilani TN, Sabir S, Sharma S. *Trihexyphenidyl.* StatPearls; 2021 [Internet].
56. Jabor HA. Role of procyclidine use in treatment of antipsychotic side effect among schizophrenic patients. *Syst Rev Pharm.* 2021;12(3):176–178.
57. Bakker C, van Esdonk MJ, Stuurman RFE, et al. Biperiden challenge model in healthy elderly as proof-of-pharmacology tool; a randomized placebo-controlled trial. *J Clin Pharmacology.* 2021;.

Further reading

Karemaker JM. An introduction into autonomic nervous function. *Phys Meas.* 2017;38(5):R89.

McComb MN, Chao JY, Ng TM. Direct vasodilators and sympatholytic agents. *J Cardiovasc Pharmacol Ther.* 2016;21(1):3–19.

Permpikul C, Tongyoo S, Viarasilpa T, Trainarongsakul T, Chakorn T, Udompanturak S. Early use of norepinephrine in septic shock resuscitation (CENSER). A randomized trial. *Am J Respir Crit Care Med.* 2019;199(9):1097–1105.

Chapter 3

Mechanism of action of adrenergic drugs and recent updates

Raisur Rahman[1], Shakir Saleem[2] and Ruqaiyah Khan[3]
[1]*Department of Paediatrics, University Hospitals Plymouth, Plymouth, United Kingdom,* [2]*Department of Public Health, College of Health Sciences, Saudi Electronic University, Riyadh, Saudi Arabia,* [3]*Department of Pharmacology, College of Pharmacy, Princess Noura University, Riyadh, Saudi Arabia*

Background

The pharmacologic effects of adrenergic medications are comparable to those that occur in the organism when the adrenergic nerves and the medulla are stimulated. The heart, blood vessels, and smooth muscles, such as the bronchi, are the principal targets of these medications. Understanding these medications and how they act in the body requires a fundamental understanding of the neurological system.[1]

The Nervous System

The nervous system is a complicated element of the human body responsible for the regulation and coordination of bodily functions such as movement, food processing, sleep, and waste evacuation. The central nervous system (CNS) and the peripheral nervous system (PNS) are the two primary divisions of the nervous system. The divisions of the nervous system are depicted in Fig. 3.1. The CNS receives, integrates, and interprets nerve impulses and is made up of the brain and spinal cord.

All nerves outside the brain and spinal cord are referred to as the PNS. The PNS connects the CNS to all regions of the body.

Peripheral Nervous System

The somatic nervous system and the autonomic nervous system are two subsystems of the PNS. Sensation and voluntary movement are dealt with by the

How Synthetic Drugs Work. DOI: https://doi.org/10.1016/B978-0-323-99855-0.00003-8

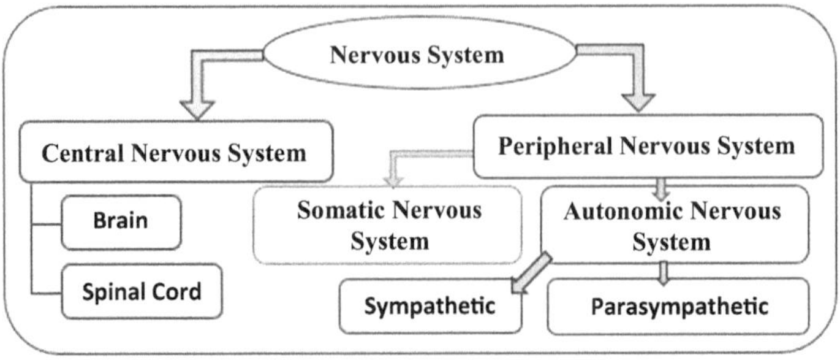

FIGURE 3.1 Divisions of the nervous system.

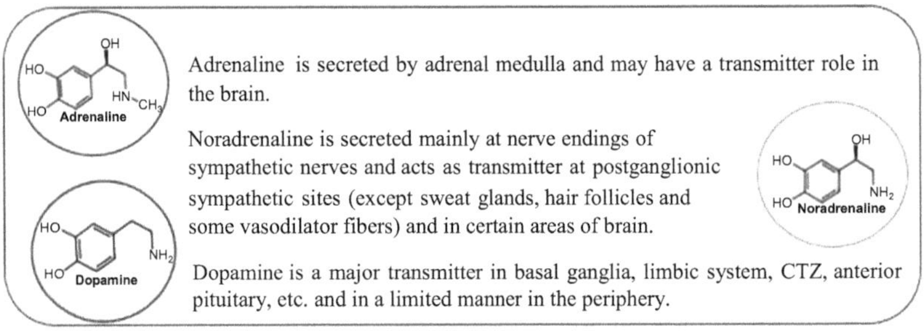

FIGURE 3.2 Chemical structure and function of different endogenous catecholamines.

somatic branch of the PNS. The sensory portion of the somatic nervous system transmits messages to the brain about the internal and external surroundings, such as heat, pain, cold, and pressure feelings. Walking, chewing food, and writing a letter are all voluntary movements of skeletal muscles that the voluntary component of the somatic nervous system is involved with.

Adrenergic Drugs

Adrenergic (or "Noradrenergic") transmission is limited to the sympathetic division of the autonomic nervous system. As shown in Fig. 3.2, there are three endogenous catecholamines (CAs) that are closely linked.

Adrenaline is secreted by adrenal medulla and may have a transmitter role in the brain.

Noradrenaline is secreted mainly at nerve endings of sympathetic nerves and acts as transmitter at postganglionic sympathetic sites (except sweat glands, hair follicles, and some vasodilator fibers) and in certain areas of brain.

Dopamine is a major transmitter in basal ganglia, limbic system, CTZ, anterior pituitary, etc. and in a limited manner in the periphery.

Adrenergic medications imitate sympathetic nervous system activity. These medications are also known as sympathomimetic medicines. Neurohormones—epinephrine and norepinephrine (NE)—are created naturally by the body. In medicine, synthetic formulations of these two neurohormones, which are identical to those produced naturally by the body, are employed. Synthetic adrenergic medications include metaraminol (Aramine), isoproterenol (Isuprel), and ephedrine, among others.

Pharmacological Actions

Adrenergic medications, in general, cause one or more of the following reactions in varied degrees (Fig. 3.3).

Adrenergic Nerve Receptors

α or β receptors can be found on adrenergic nerve fibers. Adrenergic medications can target only α receptors, or only β receptors, or both α receptors and β receptors. For example, phenylephrine (neo-synephrine), isoproterenol, and epinephrine primarily act on receptors. The variance in responses for this group of medicines is due to whether an adrenergic agent works on α or β or both receptors. Table 3.1 shows several types of adrenergic nerve fiber receptors that correlate to each autonomic nervous system effect on the body.

α- and β-adrenergic receptors can further be divided into α_1- and α_2-adrenergic receptors and β_1- and β_2-adrenergic receptors (β_1ARs and β_2ARs). The consequences on the organism when these receptors are stimulated are shown in Table 3.1.

Overall receptors can be distinguished into four types of superfamilies:

- Type 1—Ionotropic or ligand-gated ion channels
- Type 2—Metabotropic receptors or G protein–coupled receptors (GPCRs) or 7-transmembrane (7-TM, serpentine or hepta-helical) receptors
- Type 3—Kinase-linked and related receptors
- Type 4—Nuclear receptors

Adrenoreceptors are part of Type 2 GPCRs. The GCPRs are the most commonly targeted receptors by numerous therapeutic medicines, and they represent the largest receptor family. Besides adrenoreceptors, it includes

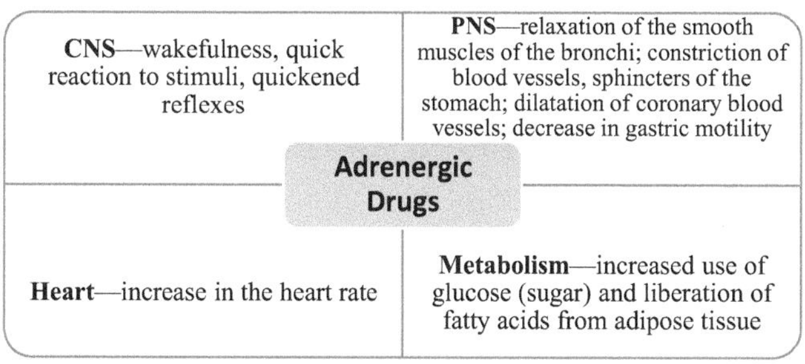

FIGURE 3.3 Major pharmacological activities elucidated by adrenergic drugs.

TABLE 3.1 Shows the list of type of adrenergic receptors and their corresponding pharmacological action on human body.

Types of Adrenergic receptor	Organ and its structures involved	Sympathetic effects	Parasympathetic effects
β	**Heart**	• Increase in heart rate • decrease in muscle contractility • increase in speed of atrioventricular conduction	• Decrease in heart rate • Increase heart muscle contractility
α Cholinergic, β	**Blood Vessels** 1. Skin, mucous membranes 2. Skeletal muscles	• Constriction • Usually, dilatation	
β	**Bronchial muscles**	Relaxation	Contraction
β α	**Gastrointestinal** 1. Muscle motility 2. Sphincters 3. Gallbladder	• Tone decrease • Contraction • Relaxation	• Tone increase • Relaxation • Contraction
β α	**Urinary bladder** 1. Detrusor muscle 2. Trigone, sphincter muscles	• Relaxation • Contraction	• Contraction • Relaxation
α	**Eye** 1. Radial muscle of iris 2. Sphincter muscle of iris 3. Ciliary muscle	• Contraction (pupil dilates)	• Contraction (pupil constricts) • Contraction
Cholinergic α	**Skin** 1. Sweat glands 2. Pilomotor muscles	• Increased activity in localized area • Contraction (gooseflesh)	
β	**Uterus**	• Relaxation	
α	**Salivary glands**	• Thickened secretions	• Copious, watery secretions

(Continued)

TABLE 3.1 (Continued)

Types of Adrenergic receptor	Organ and its structures involved	Sympathetic effects	Parasympathetic effects
β	**Liver**	• Glycogenolysis	
α	**Male reproductive organs**	• Emission	• Erection

dopamine receptors, muscarinic AchRs, 5-HT Serotonin receptors, and many others including receptors for peptides and purines, chemoreceptors related to olfaction, and pheromone sensing.

Molecular structure of G protein–coupled receptor

Several hurdles to understanding the intricacies of structure and function of GCPR have been overcome thanks to improvements in GPCR crystallography, protein engineering, and technological innovations, resulting in improved insights into the molecular biology of GPCR.[2]

Seven transmembrane helices, an extracellular N-terminal region of varied length, and an intracellular C-terminal domain make up the structural characteristic structure. The framework is made up of a single polypeptide chain of 350–400 amino acid residues on average, but up to 1100 in exceptional cases. GPCRs are classified into six classes based on the length of the extracellular N-terminus and the location of the agonist binding domain: Class A—rhodopsin-like receptors, Class B—secretin family, Class C—metabotropic glutamate receptors, Class D—fungal mating pheromone receptors, Class E—cAMP receptors, and Class F—frizzled (FZD) and smoothened (SMO) receptors.[3] Due to their centrality in illnesses, structural availability, and relative ease of accessibility, Class A GPCRs are the most intensively explored GPCR drug targets in the field of pharmacology.

Adrenergic medicines, such as noradrenaline, work by binding to a cleft in the membrane between the helical segments of the class A receptor.

G-proteins

G-protein is a membrane protein that is made up of three subunits (α, β, and γ). The α GTPase activity of the component catalyzes the conversion of GTP to GDP. The β and γ subunits are still complexes of β–γ. Prenylation, a process between the fatty acid chain and the G-protein, holds the γ subunit together. These membrane-bound proteins respond to GPCR activation by relaying the message inside the cell to the effector systems that trigger a physiological response. The transmembrane domain is responsible for signal transmission across cell membranes via three external and three intracellular loops.[4]

Signal transmission appears to be dependent on the rearrangement of transmembrane helices, particularly TM helices 5–7. The conformational change occurs mostly on the intracellular side, but significant alterations also occur in the extracellular and ligand-binding pockets, which are linked to the intracellular helical conformational change.[5]

The G-protein exists as an α–β–γ trimer in the "resting" state, with GDP occupying the spot on the α subunit. The confirmational modifications (described above) open a hole on the intracellular side of the receptor onto which the G-protein can bind when the receptor is triggered by an agonist, resulting in a high-affinity connection between α–β–γ and the receptor.

This agonist-induced interaction of α–β–γ with the receptor occurs in about 50Ms, causing the bound GDP to dissociate and be replaced with GTP (GDP–GTP exchange), which causes dissociation of the G-protein trimer, releasing α-GTP from the β–γ subunits; these are the "active" forms of G-protein, which diffuse in the membrane and can associate with various enzymes and ion channels, causing target activation. Depending on whether G-protein is involved, association of α or β–γ subunits with target enzymes or channels can result in either activation or inhibition.

Because a single agonist–receptor complex can activate numerous G-protein molecules at once, each of them can remain connected with its effector enzyme for long enough to create many molecules of the product, amplification occurs. Before the final cellular response is created, the product is commonly referred to as a "second messenger," and it undergoes further amplification. When the α subunit's natural GTPase activity causes GTP to be hydrolyzed to GDP, signaling is halted. The resultant α-GDP then dissociates from the effector and reunites with β–γ, bringing the cycle to a close.[6–9]

Difference between α and β receptors

	α	β
Agonist's potency	Adr ≥ NA > Iso	Iso > Adr > NA
Antagonist	Phenoxybenzamine	Propranolol
Effector pathway	IP_3/DAG ↑, cAMP↓, K channel ↑	cAMP↓, Ca^{2+} channel ↑
Coupling protein	Gq/Gi/G_0	Gs

The most recent advancements in adrenergic medication mechanism of action.

Drug-related memory reconsolidation in abstinent heroin addicts: effects of β_2-adrenergic receptor inhibition[10]

Reconsolidation is the process of reactivating a consolidated memory and returning it to a labile state. A recent study found that giving humans the β_2AR antagonist propranolol before memory reactivation eliminated the fear memory's behavioral expression 24 h later. In this study, we looked into whether propranolol affects drug-related memory in heroin users by altering the reconsolidation process. On day1, 70 abstinent heroin users learned a word list (which included 10 positive, 10 negative, and 10 neutral terms connected to heroin).

Before retrieval of the word list on day 2, participants were given propranolol, a β_2AR antagonist, or a placebo. On day 3, the free recall of the word list and other psychological and physical responses were tested. In abstinent heroin users, oral administration of propranolol prior to reactivation of the word list hampered reconsolidation of drug-related positive and negative but not neutral terms, and these deficits were dependent on reactivation of the word list. This research backs up previous findings that a β_2AR antagonist alters the drug-induced memory reconsolidation process. Our findings may have substantial implications for the understanding and treatment of abstinent heroin addicts' persisting and aberrant drug-related memories.

The role of the β_2-adrenergic receptor on endothelial progenitor cells dysfunction of proliferation and migration in chronic obstructive pulmonary disease patients[11]

In individuals with moderate-to-severe chronic obstructive pulmonary disease (COPD), cardiovascular disease is the major cause of morbidity and mortality, with more than 44% of these patients having widespread atherosclerosis at autopsy. Endothelial progenitor cells (EPCs) are thought to have a role in the repair of damaged endothelium, hence preventing atherosclerosis.

EPCs are thought to have a role in the repair of damaged endothelium, hence preventing atherosclerosis. T-cell traffic and proliferation are regulated by the β_2AR, which is found on mononuclear cells in peripheral blood and CD_{34}(+) cells in bone. There have been few systematic studies examining β_2AR expression on EPCs in COPD patients' peripheral blood and its involvement in EPC migration and proliferation. As a result, the goal of this study was to investigate the involvement of β_2ARs in EPC function, as well as whether or not this role is altered in COPD patients.

Ficoll density-gradient centrifugation was used to isolate EPCs from 25 COPD and 16 control patients, and fluorescence-activated cell sorting was used to identify them. Western blotting and real-time PCR were used to determine the expression of β_2AR on EPCs.

The migratory potential of EPCs treated with a β_2AR agonist, antagonist, or β_2AR monoclonal antibody was determined using the transwell migration assay. Throughout the cell cycle, the proliferation of EPCs was monitored. Fluorescence microscopy was used to count the number of EPCs treated with siRNA-β_2AR that integrated at the wounded vascular location after arterial injury in NOD/SCID mice. In COPD patients, data revealed a considerable rise in the total number of β_2ARs as well as enhanced expression on early EPCs. When compared to treatment with the β_2AR agonist, NE, COPD EPCs treated with the β_2AR antagonist (ICI 118551) enhanced migration to SDF-1.

These modifications were linked to an increase in $CXCR_4$ on EPCs. Early EPC proliferation was improved after treatment with a β2AR antagonist, which was linked to a reduction in intercellular reactive oxygen species (ROS). Changes in β_2AR in COPD patients affect EPC migration and proliferation, resulting in a reduction in EPC repair capability in this patient group.

α_1-adrenergic drugs affect the development and expression of ethanol-induced behavioral sensitization[12]

According to the incentive sensitization theory, drug-induced sensitization in the brain's meso-cortico-limbic circuits is the primary cause of addiction. Psychomotor sensitization occurs in some animals after repeated ethanol treatment, and it happens at the same time as incentive sensitization. Recent research reveals that NE is involved in substance addiction and that it plays a key part in the ethanol reinforcing characteristics.

The effects of an agonist (phenylephrine) and an antagonist (prazosin) of α_1-adrenergic receptors on the development and manifestation of behavioral sensitization to ethanol were investigated in this study. Male Swiss mice that had previously been given ethanol or saline were given a combination of ethanol (or saline) and α_1-adrenergic medications. The treatment of prazosin (0.1, 0.5, and 1.0 mg/kg) and phenylephrine (1.0 and 2.0 mg/kg) prevented the manifestation of behavioral sensitization to ethanol. In a separate series of tests, mice given 0.5 mg/kg prazosin plus ethanol did not acquire behavioral sensitization. When confronted with ethanol alone, however, they displayed the same levels of sensitized locomotor activity as mice previously treated with ethanol and saline. Treatment with phenylephrine (1.0 mg/kg) had no effect on the development of behavioral sensitization. Based on these findings, we concluded that altering the function of α_1-adrenergic receptors by administering agonists or antagonists affected locomotor sensitization to the stimulant effect of ethanol, implying that the noradrenergic system's normal functioning is critical for its development and expression.

Agonist activation of the β_1-adrenergic receptor in vivo, compound 49b restores insulin receptor signaling[13]

The purpose of this study was to determine whether therapy with compound 49b reduces retinal alterations caused by a lack of 2-adrenergic receptor activation.

The researchers tested the effects of adrenergic agonists acting solely on β_1-adrenergic receptors due to the absence of β_2ARs using retinas from 3-month-old 2-adrenergic receptor–deficient mice treated with our novel β_1-/β_2AR agonist, compound 49b.

In the process, β_1-adrenergic receptor and β_2ARs, as well as critical insulin-resistant proteins such as TNF-α, SOCS3, IRS-1Ser307, and IRTyr960, were analyzed using Western blotting or enzyme-linked immunosorbent assay. Key anti- and proapoptotic proteins such as Akt, Bcl-xL, Bax, and caspase 3 were also studied. Functional alterations were assessed using electroretinograms, whereas changes in retinal thickness were assessed using histological methods.

The β_2AR-deficient mice was treated for two months with eye drops of 1 mM compound 49b, which is a novel β_1-adrenergic receptor and β_2AR agonist, reversed insulin-resistant markers (TNF-α and $SOCS_3$) and increased morphological integrity (retinal thickness) and functional responses (electroretinogram amplitude). These findings imply that activating β_1AR on retinal endothelial cells or Müller cells can compensate for the loss of β_2AR signaling on Müller cells, restore insulin signaling, decrease retinal apoptosis, and improve retinal function.

Since, the authors found in their previous studies with β_1AR knockout mice which showed that the opposite can also happen (i.e., stimulation of the β_2AR can compensate for the loss of Î²1-adrenergic receptor activity), so they assumed that increased activity in either of these pathways is enough to prevent insulin resistance–induced retinal cell apoptosis.

In an animal model of attention deficit hyperactivity disorder, stimulation of the postsynapse adrenergic α2A receptor enhances attention and cognition.[14]

The spontaneously hypertensive rat (SHR) pups were employed as an animal model of attention deficit hyperactivity disorder (ADHD) in a 5-trial inhibitory avoidance test. However, in this model, the involvement of noradrenergic systems, which are important in the pathophysiology of ADHD, have not been examined. The effects of adrenergic α_2 receptor stimulation, which has been shown to be an effective treatment for ADHD, on attention and cognition performance in this model were studied. In addition, neural pathways mediated by adrenergic α_2 receptors were studied. Using a 5-trial inhibitory avoidance test with SHR pups, we assessed the effects of both clonidine, a nonselective adrenergic α_2 receptor agonist, and guanfacine, a selective adrenergic α_{2A} receptor agonist. When compared to juvenile Wistar Kyoto (WKY) rats, SHR rats had a lower transfer delay. Clonidine and guanfacine both dramatically increased the delay of SHR transfer in juveniles. Pretreatment with an adrenergic α_{2A} receptor antagonist dramatically reduced the effects of clonidine and guanfacine. Pretreatment with an adrenergic α_{2B} receptor antagonist or an adrenergic α_{2C} receptor antagonist did not reduce the efficacy of clonidine, but it did reduce the effect of a nonselective adrenergic α_2 receptor antagonist. Pretreatment with a selective noradrenergic neurotoxin did not prevent the effects of either clonidine or guanfacine. These findings imply that stimulating the adrenergic α_{2A} receptor improves the attention/cognition performance of juvenile SHR in the 5-trial inhibitory avoidance test and that this effect is mediated by the postsynaptic, not the presynaptic, adrenergic α_{2A} receptor.

In a mouse model of Down syndrome, formoterol, a long-acting 2-adrenergic agonist, enhances cognitive function and promotes dendritic complexity.[15]

Down syndrome is linked to a considerable decline in cognitive ability. In the Ts65Dn mouse model of Down syndrome, we previously discovered age-dependent degeneration of the locus coeruleus, a key actor in contextual learning. They wanted to see if medications that are already approved for human use may help these mice improve their cognitive performance. Targeting β_2ARs appears to be an efficient technique for restoring synaptic plasticity and cognitive function in these animals, according to their findings. Formoterol or similar β_2AR agonists with the ability to cross the blood–brain barrier may be attractive candidates for clinical trials to improve cognitive function in individuals with Down syndrome, given their widespread use in humans and positive effects on cognition in Ts65Dn mice.

Diadenosine tetraphosphate improves adrenergic anti-glaucomatous drug delivery and efficiency[16]

The ability of the dinucleotide P(1), P(4)-Di (adenosine-5′) tetraphosphate (Ap4A) to improve adrenergic anti-glaucomatous delivery by changing corneal epithelial tight junction proteins was investigated. TJ protein levels and barrier function were determined using Western blotting and transepithelial electrical resistance (TEER), respectively, after stratified human corneal epithelial cells (HCLE) were treated with Ap4A (100 M) for 5 minutes.

When compared to nontreated (control) cells, Western blot studies revealed a considerable drop in ZO-1 and occludin protein levels after 2 h (45% reduction of ZO-1 and 65% reduction of occludin protein levels). TEER values were dramatically lowered [65% as compared to control levels (*P* .001)] 2 h after Ap4A therapy, demonstrating an increase in ocular barrier permeability.

Topical application of Ap4A to New Zealand White rabbits 2 h before instillation of hypotensor compounds (brimonidine, an α_2-adrenergic receptor agonist, and timolol, a β-adrenergic receptor antagonist) improved the delivery of these compounds to the anterior chamber as well as their hypotensive effect on intraocular pressure. When Ap4A was administered topically 2 h before the adrenergic drugs, the concentration of brimonidine in the aqueous humor increased from 64.3 5.3 to 240.6 8.6 nM, and in the case of timolol, it rose from 58.9 9.2 to 183.7 6.8 nM, resulting in a more dramatic impact on IOP. As a result of increased corneal epithelial barrier permeability, Ap4A therapy improves the entry of adrenergic anti-glaucomatous chemicals into the eye, resulting in greater therapeutic efficiency.

α_{1B}-Adrenergic Receptors Differentially Associate with Rab Proteins during Homologous and Heterologous Desensitization[17]

Agonists or other stimuli can cause the internalization of GPCRs. Within seconds of cell stimulation, the process begins and adds to receptor desensitization. Endocytosis, vesicular trafficking, and endosomal fusion are all controlled by the Rab GTPase family. The varied distribution of their members on the surface diverse organelles is one of their noteworthy traits. Rab 5 regulates traffic from the plasma membrane to early endosomes in the endocytic pathway, whereas Rab 4 and Rab 11 control rapid and slow recycling from early endosomes to the plasma membrane, respectively. Rab 7 and Rab 9 also control traffic between late endosomes and lysosomes, as well as recycling to the trans-Golgi. We investigate whether different Rab proteins are involved in α_{1B}-adrenergic receptor internalization triggered by agonists (homologous) and unrelated stimuli (heterologous). Using cells coexpressing α_{1B}-adrenergic receptors labeled with the red fluorescent protein, DsRed, and various Rab proteins tagged with the green fluorescent protein, fluorescence resonance energy transfer (FRET) was used to investigate this potential.

When α_{1B}-adrenergic receptors were triggered with noradrenaline, it was shown that the receptors interacted with proteins found in early endosomes, such as antigen 1, Rab 5, Rab 4, and Rab 11, but not with late endosome markers, such as Rab 9 and Rab 7.

Sphingosine 1-phosphate stimulation, on the other hand, generated a brief and transient α_{1B}-adrenergic receptor connection with Rab 5 and a more significant and continuous interaction with Rab 9; interaction was also detected with Rab 7.

Furthermore, the Rab proteins' GTPase activity appears to be necessary, as no FRET was seen when dominant-negative Rab mutants were used. These findings suggest that depending on the type of desensitization, α_{1B}-adrenergic receptors are directed to distinct endocytic vesicles (homologous vs heterologous).

Molecular Docking and Drug Discovery in β-Adrenergic Receptors[18]

Improved molecular simulations with critical applications in virtual high-throughput screening and drug discovery have resulted from advancements in computer engineering, increased data availability, and the development of novel and rapid docking techniques and software. Furthermore, molecular docking study of protein–ligand recognition has become an important tool in drug development. The application of molecular docking to a specific family of GPCRs, the β-adrenergic receptors, is the topic of this paper. These receptors are important targets in the clinic for the treatment of asthma and cardiovascular illnesses. We describe the binding site in β-adrenergic receptors to better understand important aspects of ligand recognition and protein activation. Furthermore, we concentrate on the identification of novel lead compounds that bind receptors, the evaluation of virtual screening utilizing active/inactive binding site states, and the structural optimization of known binder families to improve β-adrenergic affinity. We also talked about the advantages and disadvantages of using molecular docking in β-adrenergic receptors. Molecular docking is a useful technique in computational chemistry for analyzing ligand recognition in depth, and it has led to significant advances in the field of β-adrenergic receptor drug discovery and design.

The axis of β_2-adrenergic receptor-ROS signaling: An underappreciated aspect of β2AR function?[19]

Clinically, β_2AR agonists are used to elicit rapid bronchodilation for the treatment of bronchospasms in pulmonary diseases like asthma and COPD, which both have high levels of ROS due to overexpression of ROS-generating enzymes and chronically heightened inflammation.

Interestingly, despite the fact that β_2AR has long been connected to ROS, the role of ROS in β_2AR function has not been examined as thoroughly as other aspects of β_2AR signaling. The existing body of evidence tying β_2AR activation to intracellular ROS formation, as well as the role of ROS in regulating β_2AR function, is discussed in this chapter. The reciprocal interaction between the β_2AR and ROS appears to give this receptor with the potential to self-regulate signaling efficacy and ligand binding, revealing a redox-axis that may be negatively altered in disease progression and therapeutic treatment responses.

Recent advancements in the discovery of agonists for the β_2-adrenergic receptor[20]

GPCRs mediate the bulk of cellular responses to external stimuli, and the β_2AR is one of them. Because the agonists can relax smooth muscle, numerous β_2AR agonists have been created specifically for the treatment of pulmonary illnesses such as asthma and chronic obstructive lung disease (COPD). Over the last 5 years, many new natural and synthetic substances have been discovered and produced as novel β_2AR agonists. For the treatment of asthma and COPD, β_2AR agonists have been extensively developed. Novel agonists have been created extensively in the last 5 years, using both natural and synthetic approaches. Compounds that function as both a muscarinic receptor antagonist and a β_2AR agonist are a new trend in this field since they may be able to act in a synergistic manner, relieving patients' symptoms through two different pathways.

The significance of β_2-adrenergic receptors in chronic obstructive pulmonary disease is critical[21]

β_2ARs play a key role in the etiology and therapy of COPD. Progress has been made in the study of β_2ARs in recent years. Here, we cover the fundamentals of β_2ARs, associated pathways, and the use of β_2ARs blockers/agonists, as well as β_2ARs auto-antibodies in COPD. Drugs that target the β_2ARs are fast being developed, and we expect them to ameliorate COPD patients' symptoms and prognosis in the future.

Conclusion

The discovery of newer adrenergic receptors using molecular tools and employment of OMICS study has ushered a new chapter in the management of different classes of diseases. This chapter has brought to light newer advancements in this field.

References

1. McCorry LK. Physiology of the autonomic nervous system. *Am J Pharm Educ*. 2007;71 (4):78. Available from: https://doi.org/10.5688/aj710478.
2. Hilger D. The role of structural dynamics in GPCR-mediated signaling. *FEBS J*. 2021;288 (8):2461–2489. Available from: https://doi.org/10.1111/febs.15841. Available from: 33871923.
3. Basith S, Cui M, Macalino SJY, et al. Exploring G protein-coupled receptors (GPCRs) ligand space via cheminformatics approaches: impact on rational drug design. *Front Pharmacol*. 2018;9:128. Available from: https://doi.org/10.3389/fphar.2018.00128.
4. Sprang SR. Invited review: activation of G proteins by GTP and the mechanism of Gα-catalyzed GTP hydrolysis. *Biopolymers*. 2016;105(8):449–462. Available from: https://doi.org/10.1002/bip.22836.
5. Moro S, Hoffmann C, Jacobson KA. Role of the extracellular loops of G protein-coupled receptors in ligand recognition: a molecular modeling study of the human P2Y1 receptor. *Biochemistry*. 1999;38(12):3498–3507. Available from: https://doi.org/10.1021/bi982369v.
6. Smrcka AV. G protein βγ subunits: central mediators of G protein-coupled receptor signaling. *Cell Mol Life Sci*. 2008;65(14):2191–2214. Available from: https://doi.org/10.1007/s00018-008-8006-5.
7. Dupré DJ, Robitaille M, Rebois RV, Hébert TE. The role of Gbetagamma subunits in the organization, assembly, and function of GPCR signaling complexes. *Annu Rev Pharmacol Toxicol*. 2009;49:31–56. Available from: https://doi.org/10.1146/annurev-pharmtox-061008-103038. PMID: 18834311.
8. Khan SM, Sung JY, Hébert TE. Gβγ subunits – different spaces, different faces. *Pharmacol Res*. 2016;111:434–441. Available from: https://doi.org/10.1016/j.phrs.2016.06.026, Epub 2016 Jul 1. Available from: 27378564.
9. Davis TL, Bonacci TM, Sprang SR, Smrcka AV. Structural and molecular characterization of a preferred protein interaction surface on G protein beta gamma subunits. *Biochemistry*. 2005;44(31):10593–10604. Available from: https://doi.org/10.1021/bi050655i. Available from: 16060668.
10. Zhao LY, Sun LL, Shi J, Li P, Zhang Y, Lu L. Effects of β-adrenergic receptor blockade on drug-related memory reconsolidation in abstinent heroin addicts. *Drug Alcohol Depend*. 2011;118(2–3):224–229. Available from: https://doi.org/10.1016/j.drugalcdep.2011.03.025. Epub 2011 Apr 29. PMID: 21531091.
11. Liu X, Tan W, Liu Y, Lin G, Xie C. The role of the β2 adrenergic receptor on endothelial progenitor cells dysfunction of proliferation and migration in chronic obstructive pulmonary disease patients. *Expert Opin Ther Targets*. 2013;17(5):485–500. Available from: https://doi.org/10.1517/14728222.2013.773975, Epub 2013 Mar 1. Available from: 23448263.
12. Kim AK, Souza-Formigoni ML. Alpha1-adrenergic drugs affect the development and expression of ethanol-induced behavioral sensitization. *Behav Brain Res*. 2013;256:646–654. Available from: https://doi.org/10.1016/j.bbr.2013.09.015, Epub 2013 Sep 12. Available from: 24036170.

13. Jiang Y, Zhang Q, Ye EA, Steinle JJ. β1-adrenergic receptor stimulation by agonist Compound 49b restores insulin receptor signal transduction in vivo. *Mol Vis.* 2014;20:872–880.
14. Kawaura K, Karasawa J, Chaki S, Hikichi H. Stimulation of postsynapse adrenergic α2A receptor improves attention/cognition performance in an animal model of attention deficit hyperactivity disorder. *Behav Brain Res.* 2014;270:349–356. Available from: https://doi.org/10.1016/j.bbr.2014.05.044, Epub 2014 May 29. Available from: 24882610.
15. Dang V, Medina B, Das D, et al. Formoterol, a long-acting β2 adrenergic agonist, improves cognitive function and promotes dendritic complexity in a mouse model of Down syndrome. *Biol Psychiatry.* 2014;75(3):179–188. Available from: https://doi.org/10.1016/j.biopsych.2013.05.024, Epub 2013 Jul 1. Available from: 23827853.
16. Loma P, Guzman-Aranguez A, Perez de Lara MJ, Pintor J. Diadenosine tetraphosphate improves adrenergic anti-glaucomatous drug delivery and efficiency. *Exp Eye Res.* 2015;134:141–147. Available from: https://doi.org/10.1016/j.exer.2015.02.014, Epub 2015 Feb 19. Available from: 25701803.
17. Castillo-Badillo JA, Sánchez-Reyes OB, Alfonzo-Méndez MA, Romero-Ávila MT, Reyes-Cruz G, García-Sáinz JA. α1B-adrenergic receptors differentially associate with Rab proteins during homologous and heterologous desensitization. *PLoS One.* 2015;10(3):e0121165. Available from: https://doi.org/10.1371/journal.pone.0121165. Published 2015 Mar 23.
18. Vilar S, Sobarzo-Sanchez E, Santana L, Uriarte E. Molecular docking and drug discovery in β-adrenergic receptors. *Curr Med Chem.* 2017;24(39):4340–4359. Available from: https://doi.org/10.2174/0929867324666170724101448. Available from: 28738772.
19. Rambacher KM, Moniri NH. The β2-adrenergic receptor-ROS signaling axis: an overlooked component of β2AR function? *Biochem Pharmacol.* 2020;171:113690. Available from: https://doi.org/10.1016/j.bcp.2019.113690. Epub 2019 Nov 5. PMID: 31697929; PMCID: PMC6917825.
20. Xing G, Yi C, Dou P, Zhi Z, Lin B, Cheng M. Recent progress in the development of β2 adrenergic receptor agonists: a patent review (2015–2020). *Expert Opin Ther Pat.* 2021;31(3):239–246. Available from: https://doi.org/10.1080/13543776.2021.1865312, Epub 2020 Dec 23. Available from: 33320034.
21. Yang A, Yu G, Wu Y, Wang H. Role of β2-adrenergic receptors in chronic obstructive pulmonary disease. *Life Sci.* 2021;265:118864. Available from: https://doi.org/10.1016/j.lfs.2020.118864, Epub 2020 Dec 7. Available from: 33301808.

Chapter 4

Insight into the mechanism of steroidal and non-steroidal anti-inflammatory drugs

Kazi Asraf Ali[1], Arindam Maity[2], Sanhati Dutta Roy[3], Siddhartha Das Pramanik[4], Partha Pratim Das[5] and Md. Adil Shaharyar[6]

[1]*Department of Pharmaceutical Technology, Maulana Abul Kalam Azad University of Technology, Haringhata, West Bengal, India,* [2]*Department of Pharmaceutical Technology, JIS University of Technology, Kolkata, West Bengal, India,* [3]*Department o Pharmaceutical Technology, NSHM Knowledge Campus, Kolkata, West Bengal, India,* [4]*Department of Pharmaceutical Technology, School of Medical Science, Adamas University, Barasat, West Bengal, India,* [5]*Department of Pharmaceutics, Bengal School of Technology, Chinsurah, Hooghly, West Bengal, India,* [6]*Bioeuivalence Study Centre, Department of Pharmaceutical Technology, Jadavpur University, Kolkata, West Bengal, India*

Introduction to inflammation and its role

The term "inflammation" has been derived from a Latin term *inflammare* (to burn) (*de oliveira*). It is a highly dynamic process of body, which is specified as the first line defence response of our immunological system. Inflammation is a commutable response that is incited by external stimuli and conditions, such as infection and tissue damage.[1,2] Several advancements have been made in identifying the cellular and molecular occasions that worried inside the extreme inflammation reaction during the course of any kind of tissue injury, infection and cardiac infraction. Inflammation process is one of the predominant intensively investigated regions of experimental medicine. Starting with Adami at McGill University,[1] medical textbooks focused on the main part of inflammation, and today, many textbooks and colloquium proceedings are fully dedicated to this topic.[3] Microcirculation is most important event in inflammation process that has been studied and analyzed. Benjamin W. Zweifach, one of the founders of modern bioengineering from University of California, San Diego (UCSD), is a pioneer in the field of microvascular research[4] and has developed new quantitative methods to study inflammation.

The immediate goal of inflammation is shielding against external parasitological intrusions, alleyway of antigens, any damage or injury of cells and

How Synthetic Drugs Work. DOI: https://doi.org/10.1016/B978-0-323-99855-0.00004-X

tissues. It covers the complex interplay between soluble biological mediators, resident and infiltrating cells, and molecules belonging to the extracellular matrix. Inflammatory response has a different kind of physiological motive as well as pathological consequences depending on the triggering factors or inflammatory mediators as shown in Fig. 4.1.[5]

Effective and controlled provocative reaction is a valuable interaction that prompts elimination of harmful stimuli and the restoration of normal physiology, which is precisely controlled by a complex molecular event.[2] In many cases, it was found that controlled inflammation is preferable (for instance, in protection against germs). However, it can become unsuitable if dysregulated (for instance, septic shock).[5] The physiological causes of inflammation that are governed by the process of infection are very much clear. There exist several other types of inflammatory cascades only found under prominent pathological conditions, but there is a lack of clear understanding of their physiological effects. The most prominent initiators of an inflammatory reaction are infection and tissue damage. A variety of factors can trigger inflammation process and trigger the recruitment of white blood cells as well as plasma proteins in the affected tissues.[6] Tissue stress or tissue dysfunction can also cause an adaptive response, which is referred to as para-inflammation. Inflammation can be broadly divided into two categories. The first is acute inflammation, characterized by short duration and fast onset. It is exhibited with transudation of fluid and plasma proteins and emigration of leukocytes, mainly neutrophils. The second is chronic inflammation, characterized by longer duration of inflammation and histological

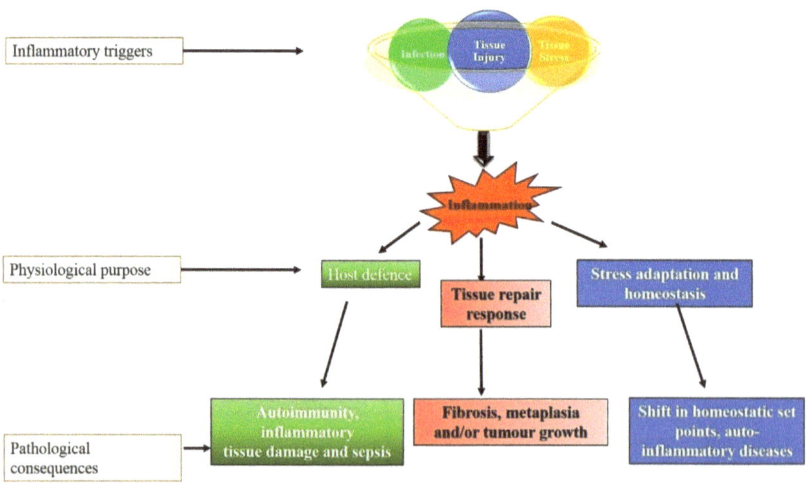

FIGURE 4.1 Different triggers and physiological and pathological consequences of inflammatory reaction in body.[5]

manifestation identified by the presence of lymphocytes and macrophages, blood vessels, fibrosis, and tissue necrosis.[7]

This response, which occurs between the initial homeostatic state and the classic inflammatory response, is primarily based on macrophages residing in the tissue. The cause of the chronic inflammatory situation in modern human diseases is likely to be associated with para-inflammation.[5] Furthermore, the events that cause local chronic inflammation, particularly in chronic infections and autoimmune diseases, are still unclear, whereas the causes and mechanisms of chronic systemic inflammation, which occurs in many diseases, are poorly understood.[8]

Pathophysiology of inflammation and inflammatory pathway

Multiple mediators form a complex regulatory network that coordinates the inflammatory response. Any inflammatory event is distinguished by five cardinal events: (1) redness (rubor), which occurs as a result of increased vascularity, (2) swelling (tumor), which occurs as a result of fluid exudation, (3) heat generation (calor), which occurs at the site of inflammation as a result of increased blood flow and the release of inflammatory mediators, (4) pain (dolor), which is caused by inflammatory exudates stretching pain receptors and nerves and the release of chemical mediators, and (5) loss of function.[7] It is useful to classify these signals into functional categories and distinguish inducers and inflammatory mediators in order to analyze these extremely complex networks. An inducer is a signal that triggers an inflammatory response. They trigger special sensors, which then trigger certain inflammatory mediators and change the functional state of tissues and organs (which is a crucial factor of inflammation), so that they can adapt to the conditions indicated by the specific inflammation triggering conditions. Therefore, the natural "pathway" of inflammation is composed of sensors, mediators, and effectors. Each component determines the type of inflammatory response; inflammation inducer can be divided into exogenous and endogenous; inflammation inducers trigger the generation of many inflammatory mediators, which causes alteration of functions of many tissues and organs.[5] Many of these inflammatory mediators have a common effect on vasculature and white blood cell conscription. Tissues and cells are the effectors of an inflammatory response, and their functional states are specifically affected by inflammatory mediators.[9] Responsiveness to certain inflammatory mediators (such as tumor necrosis factor alpha (TNF-α) and IL-1) is almost ubiquitous, although these mediators have very distinguished effects in different tissue and cell types; the inflammatory response is triggered by two stages: (1) acute and (2) chronic, each stage seems to be mediated by different mechanisms.[10]

Diagrammatic representation of inflammation and inflammatory response to cells is presented in Fig. 4.2.[10]

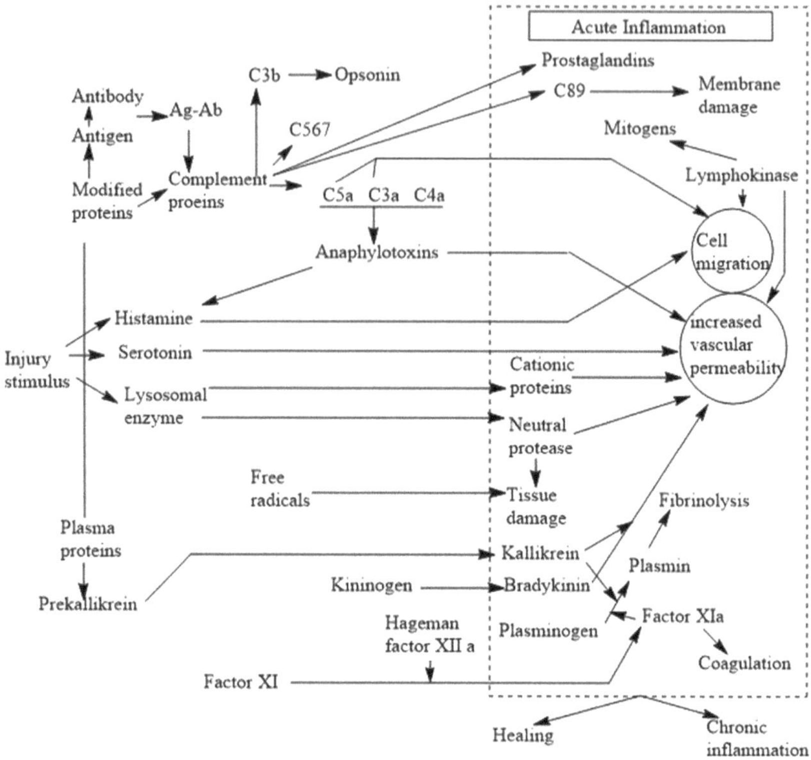

FIGURE 4.2 Inflammatory response pathway.

In acute inflammation, the complex immune response can be divided into two types: vascular and cellular.[11] The responses that occur in the microvasculature normally occur within a few minutes of tissue injury or microbial infection in the presence of other inflammatory stimuli and are referred to as vascular events[11] These processes occur quickly and eventually lead to vasodilation, which subsequently leads to increased vascular permeability. These processes lead to the penetration of inflammatory mediators and interstitial edema.[12] The circulatory system plays a very important role in the inflammatory response.[13,14] A group of chemotactic agents, such as microbial endotoxins containing N-terminal N-formylmethylthio, complement fragment C5a and interleukins, and secretion of basophils (such as platelet-activating factor, histamine, and leukotriene B) stimulate strong leukocyte infiltration.[7] Neutrophils are the first inflammatory cells to become the focal point of acute inflammation among white blood cells.[15] The infiltration of immune cells is triggered by a complex mechanism in which white blood cells collaborating with the endothelium in the post capillary venules.[16] The capture, trundling, and firming of an adhesion to the microvascular endothelium are all cellular events.[17] These events in the mobilization pathway are organized by cell adhesion molecules (CAM). Intracellular adhesion molecules ICAM-1, ICAM-2, integrins, and selectins are examples of CAMs. Three families of selectin are there, namely, P-selectin, E-selectin (produced by endothelial cells) and L-selectin (produced by white blood cells).[18] The high-affinity adhesion of leukocytes to endothelium is mediated by the interaction between integrins (CDII/CDI8) expressed in leukocytes or endothelial cells and adhesion molecules (CAM-1 and CAM-2).[19] White blood cells can escape from the post capillary venules by extending pseudopods spread between endothelial cells and reaching the subendothelial space after a stage of static adhesion. White blood cell extravasations and transendothelial migration are two terms used to describe this complex process.[20] Chronic inflammation is characterized by the infiltration of mononuclear cells (such as monocytes and lymphocytes), the proliferation of fibroblasts, collagen fibers, and the formation of connective tissue, all of which result in 2-mm granuloma formation.[21] Tissue degeneration in chronic inflammation is typically mediated by nitrogenous spices, proteases, and other reactive oxygen species.[22] However, in addition to cancer, p53 genomic changes have been recognized as the cause of many chronic inflammatory diseases [e.g., inflammatory bowel disease (IBD) and rheumatoid arthritis (RA)].[23–25]

Inflammatory mediators

Inflammation is caused by a series of organized dynamic responses involving cellular and vascular events as well as specific humoral secretion. These pathways include changes in the physical location of white blood cells (monocytes, basophils, eosinophils, and neutrophils), plasma, and body fluids in the areas of inflammation.[4] Immune cells release a set of secreted mediators and other signaling molecules (such as histamine, prostaglandins (PGs), leukotrienes, oxygen, nitrogen-free radicals, and serotonin) through various mechanisms and are involved during inflammation.[5,7] Usually, these mediators are two types either cell-derived factors and plasma protein–derived factors. Inflammatory mediators (Table 4.1) are classified in different categories depending on their function and chemical nature as shown in Fig. 4.3.[26]

Inflammatory diseases

Inflammation in body in response to self or non-self inducer molecules results in the development of several critical diseases. We will discuss few of them below and define the role of inflammation in their disease progression.

TABLE 4.1 Summary of inflammatory mediators and their functions.

Sl. No.	Mediators	Functions
1	IL-1	Macrophages activation and T-cell activation, fever, hypotension
2	IL-6	Acute-phase protein production, Naïve B-cell and T-cell proliferation
3	IL-8	Chemotactic signals for T-cells and neutrophils
4	TNF-α	Activation of PMN and endothelial cells, shock-like syndrome
5	PAF	Activation of endothelial cells and platelets, histamine release from platelets
6	NO	Smooth muscle relaxation, generation o cytotoxic peroxynitrile
7	PGE_2 and PGI_2	Vasodilatation
8	TXA_2	Increased pulmonary resistance
9	LTC_4, LTD_4, LTE_4,	Increased pulmonary capillary permeability

IL, Interleukin; *TNF-α*, tumor necrosis factor alpha; *PAF*, platelet activating factor; *NO*, nitric oxide; *PGE_2*, prostaglandin E2; *PGI*, prostacycline; *TXA*, thrombaxone; *LTC*, leukotrine C; *LTD*, leukotrine D; *LTE*, leukotrine E.

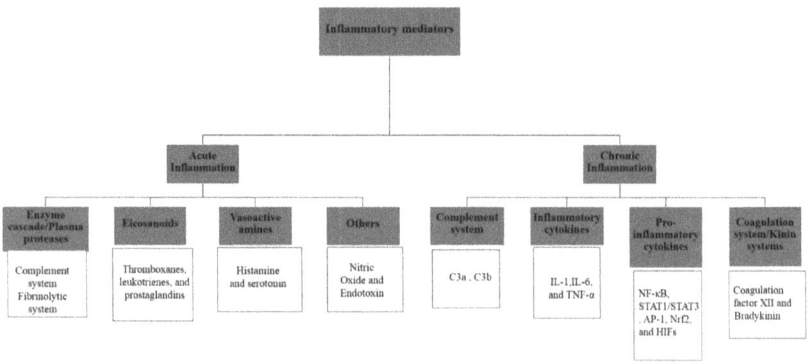

FIGURE 4.3 Classification of inflammatory mediators.[26]

Rheumatoid arthritis (RA)

RA is a chronic autoimmune and systemic inflammatory disease of unknown etiology that mainly affects joints. It is distinguished by symmetrical synovial inflammation, which results in articular cartilage destruction, severe pain,[27] and severe disability.[28] RA affects 1% of the population[29] and is more common in women over 65 years of age. Patients with RA usually have a higher erythrocyte sedimentation rate or C-reactive protein (CRP), which indicates that there is an inflammatory process in the body.[30] Pro-inflammatory cytokine IL-1 is widely involved in the pathogenesis of this disease. It persuades an inflammatory response that activates or increases the expression of other pro-inflammatory mediators that contribute to joint damage.[30] Antibodies to citrullinated protein antigens (ACPAs) are used as a marker of RA and play an important role in the disease's pathogenesis. The calcium-dependent enzyme peptidyl arginine deiminase catalyzes citrullination, which converts positively charged arginine into polar but neutral citrulline via post-translational modification.[31] Compared with ACPA-positive subgroups, RA has a distinct genetic association pattern, as well as distinct immune cell responses to citrullinated antigens.[32]

Asthma

Asthma is a multifactorial disorder of the conducting airways characterized by chronic airway inflammation, declining airway function, and tissue remodeling; activation of eosinophils, mast cells, and T lymphocytes are well-known feature of asthma. Asthma is believed to be caused by a complex interaction between genetic makeup and environmental factors (such as the time and dose of allergens) and the combined effects of infection.[33] As a result, helper T-type (Th-2) lymphocyte-mediated inappropriate inflammatory response to normally harmless allergens in the air was shown.[34] Although no single gene or environmental factor can explain asthma, genetic susceptibility to local immunoglobulin (IgE) mucosal response (referred to as atopy) is the most important risk factor for the disease's development. The initial allergen exposure causes the activation of allergen-specific Th-2 cells and the production of IgE (sensitization).[35] Subsequent exposure to allergens induces the recruitment, activation, and release of inflammatory cell mediators. Mast cells that have been sensitized to IgE and express high-affinity IgE receptors (Fc RI) degranulate and release pre-formed and newly synthesized mediators such as histamine, leukotrienes, and cytokines, as shown in Fig. 4.4.[36] These mediators promote smooth muscle contraction, vascular permeability, and mucus production.

Chronic obstructive pulmonary disease

Chronic obstructive pulmonary disease (COPD) is an inflammatory disease. During most COPD exacerbations, lung and systemic inflammation increase. The characteristics of pneumonia in COPD are different from those in asthma, which affects the choice of treatment. In COPD, chronic inflammation leads to the destruction of lung parenchyma and narrows the small/

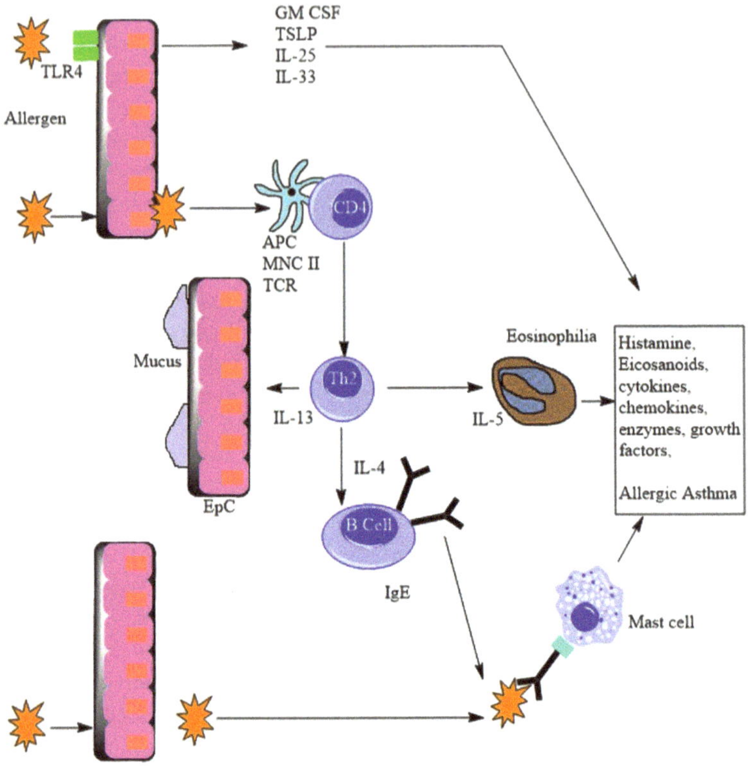

FIGURE 4.4 Involvement of different immune cells and different mediators responsible for asthma.

peripheral airways, leading to progressive airway obstruction that is not completely reversible.[37] The thickening of the membrane and the increase in smooth muscle mass mainly occur in the central/large tract, leading to intermittent and reversible obstruction of airflow.

Inflammatory bowel disease (IBD)

Inflammation of the inner wall of intestinal tract and further worsening and disappearance over time is a critical attribute of IBD. IBD causes severe intestinal inflammation, which is accompanied by an acute phase reaction that can be detected in serum and blood. This acute phase response is of exceptional quality. Proteins that are involved in coagulation and fibrinolysis include plasminogen, fibrinogen, prothrombin, and coagulation factor components of the complement system, such as (C1–C4) inhibitor pro-inflammatory cytokine serum levels, many of which stimulate the acute phase response elevated.[38]

Multiple sclerosis

Multiple sclerosis (MS) is characterized by inflammatory infiltration of specific myelin blood T cells, B cells, which secrete antibodies against myelin components, and a variety of nonspecific monocyte effector cells that attack non-myelinated neuronal cells. MS is a chronic inflammatory, autoimmune, and demyelinating disease of the central nervous system.[39] Inflammatory reactions in MS are caused by the in-situ production of pro-retention and pro-survival factors, which prevent the clearance of blood-borne inflammatory cells involved in invading the central nervous system. Several chemokines have pro-retention activity; inflammatory cytokines were actively found in active MS plaques.[40]

Allergic rhinitis

Allergic rhinitis is a common but underestimated inflammatory disease of the nasal mucosa, characterized by cleanliness, sneezing, runny nose, and nasal congestion. Although allergic rhinitis is often seen as a simple seasonal problem, it can cause persistent, mild inflammation of the mucous membranes associated with infectious microbial infections. Thus, patients with allergic rhinitis have additional difficulties with viral colds. During the pollen season, there are no siblings, and kindergarten or pre-school education is delayed (for example, from 4 years old), mothers who smoke a lot in the first year after delivery, any exposure to animal hair, house dust, mites and other household allergens, and have high serum IgE values (under 6 years old) is >100 IU/mL.[41] In adults, excessive drinking is also a risk factor. Studies have shown that early exposure to various infective agents, such as hepatitis A, mycobacteria, *Toxoplasma gondii*, products of these pathogens (such as endotoxin and lipopolysaccharide), or combinations thereof, can prevent the development of atopy.[42]

Inflammatory disease and their treatments

The treatments of various diseases such as RA, gout, migraine, asthma, and others are described in Table 4.2.

Classification of non steroidal anti-inflammatory drugs and corticosteroids in broad category

In order to treat inflammatory condition, generally the most preferred treatment options include the use of nonsteroidal anti-inflammatory drugs (NSAIDs) and corticosteroids. The former is basically a non-narcotic pain reliever and the latter is a group of synthetic hormones (steroid) capable of reducing inflammation. NSAIDs are also used for reducing fever or pain.

TABLE 4.2 Inflammatory disease and their treatment.

Disease name	Treatment	Comment
Rheumatoid arthritis (RA)	*NSAIDS* Ibuprofen, naproxen, celecoxib, meloxicam, piroxicam aspirin, etodolac, diclofenac, indomethacin, ketoprofen[43]	In the treatment of RA, traditional NSAIDs are widely used For a prolonged action, novel drug delivery systems such as microsphere, transdermal patch, alginate beads, nanoparticles, etc. are preferred over conventional dosage forms[43] For a patient below 65 years, without any major complications traditional NSAIDs are chosen. But for a high risk older patients having age over 65 years (with renal and cardiovascular disease) a safer treatment plan is done with a daily dose of Acetaminophen (<3 g/day), which may be followed up by celecoxib or naproxen if required. But extended release formulations should be avoided in terms of patient safety[44]
	Corticosteroid Glucocorticoid (dexamethasone, methylprednisolone, prednisolone, prednisone)	Glucocorticoid is used along with Methotrexate as the first line treatment in the case of RA[45]
Gout	*NSAIDs* Indomethacin, Etoricoxib, Diclofenac, Naproxen, Aspirin	In the treatment of gout, NSAIDS are given as first line therapy to healthy patients with no hepatic or gastrointestinal problems[46] NSAIDs can be used alone or NSAIDs treatment can be followed by intra- articular corticosteroid injection or prednisolone (oral)[46]
	Corticosteroids (prednisolone, betamethasone, triamcinolone)	Corticosteroids can be given through various routes such as oral, intra-articular, intravenous, intramuscular Corticosteroids can be used either along with NSAIDs or alone if the patients have contraindications to the NSAIDs[47]
Migraine	*NSAIDs* Aspirin, ibuprofen, Acetaminophen, tolfenamic acid, naproxen, diclofenac, flurbiprofen, ketoprofen, rofecoxib.	NSAIDs are the over-the-counter products used for the treatment of migraine. Acetaminophen has been observed to be comparatively less effective than other NSAIDs in the treatment of migraine For emergency condition, more effective NSAIDs are given as rectal, parenteral, or intramuscular injection[48]

(*Continued*)

TABLE 4.2 (Continued)

Disease name	Treatment	Comment
	Corticosteroids Dexamethasone, methylprednisolone, prednisolone	Though corticosteroids can reduce both the recurrent and acute migraine headache, but in the former one, it is slightly more efficient[49]
Asthma	*Corticosteroids* Prednisone, prednisolone, methylprednisolone, triamcinolone, budesonide, fluticasone	Acute incidents of asthma can be treated with inhaled corticosteroids followed by oral therapy[50] In the treatment of asthma, usually NSAIDs are not advisable. Most asthmatic patients have been found to be allergic to NSAIDs. By causing bronchospasm, NSAIDs can even make asthma worse[51]
Allergic rhinitis	*Corticosteroids* Prednisone, prednisolone, methylprednisolone, beclomethasone, triamcinolone, mometasone	Rhinitis is of two types, allergic and non-allergic, and for both the cases, corticosteroids are preferred the most. In this case, corticosteroids are given through nasal route and known as INCS (intra nasal corticosteroids). This is used as symptomatic treatment and after 7 h of starting therapy, effect can be observed. Regular use up to two weeks shows maximum efficacy[52]
Addison's disease	*Corticosteroids* Hydrocortisone, prednisone, fludrocortisone, prednisolone	In order to balance the missing cortisol, the most suitable therapy for Addison's disease is to give a continuous therapy with corticosteroids (glucocorticoids)
COPD (chronic obstructive pulmonary disease)	*Corticosteroids* Prednisone, hydrocortisone, prednisolone, methylprednisolone, dexamethasone	With the treatment of corticosteroids, an improvement has been observed in COPD patients as it can reduce inflammation by reacting on the protein named as C- reactive[53]
Multiple sclerosis	*NSAIDs* Paracetamol, ibuprofen, diclofenac, etc. *Corticosteroids* Prednisone, methylprednisolone, hydrocortisone	A supportive treatment to the pain management in case of severe MS can be given by NSAIDs Corticosteroid has been reported to reduce the occurrence of relapse[54]

Corticosteroids can be mainly classified into two major subclasses:[55] glucocorticoids and mineralocorticoids (MRs). Glucocorticoids are mainly used in the treatment of inflammation and as an immunosuppressive agent. The MRs are also known as salt-retaining agents, as balancing the mineral and salt in the body is also done by them. Nonsteroidal anti-inflammatory drugs show their action by inhibiting the cyclooxygenase enzyme system (both I and II).

Prolonged use of both corticosteroids and NSAIDs result in severe toxicity. Thus, a controlled and monitored therapy pattern is always suggested for these two.

Classification of NSAIDs

NSAIDs are classified into six major groups (depending upon the different chemical structures) which are mentioned in Table 4.3 along with the examples against each class.[56]

As NSAIDs show its function mainly on cyclooxygenase enzyme system (both I and II), depending upon the selectivity of the NSAIDs in respect to

TABLE 4.3 NSAID classification (with example).

Sl. No.	Chemical group	Examples
1	Salicylic acid derivative	Diflunisal salicylsalicylic acid acetylsalicylic acid (aspirin) sulfasalazine olsalazine sodium salicylate
2	Oxicams or enolic acid derivative	Meloxicam Tenoxicam Piroxicam
3	Para-amino phenol derivative	Acetominophen
4	Heteroaryl acetic acid derivatives	Ketoprofen Ibuprofen Neproxen Fenoprofen Oxaprozine Flurbiprofen
5	Fenemates or anthranilic acid derivatives	Meclofenamic acid Mefenamic acid
6	Indole and indene acetic acid derivative	Etodolac Sulindac Indomethacin

these two types of cyclooxygenases (COX) enzymes, they can be classified as follows:

Nonselective COX inhibitor

These NSAIDs are called as nonselective because irrespective of class I or II, this particular group blocks both the types of cyclooxygenase enzymes. Examples include acetylsalicylic acid (aspirin), ketoprofen, ibuprofen, indomethacin, phenyl butazone, etc.

Food Drug and Administration (FDA) has approved some of the popular nonselective COX inhibitors, including ketorolac, diclofenac, ibuprofen, mefenamic acid, and meloxicam.

Preferential cyclooxygenase II inhibitor

Some COX inhibitors in low dose show preferential inhibition on COX-2 enzymes. Examples include meloxicam, nimesulide, etodolac, and others.

Selective COX-2 inhibitor

Though NSAIDs show their actions by blocking both the cyclooxygenase enzymes (I and II), but inhibiting the former one leads to irritation in stomach (which is considered as NSAID's side effect), while inhibition of the latter one gives the therapeutic effectivity of NSAIDs against inflammation. Presently, selective NSAIDs are widely used as they show the same activity as the nonselective one but surely lesser or no gastric irritability. Examples include celecoxib, parecoxib, etoricoxib etc.[57]

Among the selective NSAIDS, rofecoxib and valdecoxib were taken up from market because of their undesired pharmacokinetic profile in the year 2004 and 2005 respectively.

All NSAIDs are not capable of showing enough anti-inflammatory action. The following drugs belong to the class of NSAIDs, but mainly they are good analgesic and antipyretic but are very poor anti-inflammatory agents. Examples include paracetamol, nefopam, metamizol etc.

Newly approved NSAID drugs as per United States Food and Drug Administration (USFDA)

Newly approved NSAID drugs as per USFDA include Rinvoq, Xenleta, Ubrelvy, Zeposia, Vyepti, Ponvory, Lupkynis and Mayzent.

Classification of corticosteroids

Corticosteroids are mainly classified into two major classes: glucocorticoids and MRs.[58]

Glucocorticoids

This kind of corticosteroid has a direct effect on carbohydrate, protein, and fat metabolism. It acts as an anti-inflammatory agent by either blocking the mediators for inflammation or by inducing anti-inflammatory mediators. This group of corticoids also has immunosuppressant activity.

Glucocorticoids are further classified into:

1. Short acting glucocorticoids: This kind of glucocorticoid has a half-life lesser than 12 h. Examples include hydrocortisone and hydrocortisone acetate.
2. Intermediate acting glucocorticoids: These have a biological half-life of 12–36 h. Examples include methylprednisolone, prednisolone, triamcinolone, etc.
3. Long acting glucocorticoids: Their biological half-life is more than 36 h. Examples include betamethasone, dexamethasone.

Mineralocorticoids

This is the class of corticosteroids that is produced from adrenal cortex and is mainly involved in salt and electrolytes balance. The name mineralocorticoids was derived from "minerals," as the main function of these steroidal hormone is to balance electrolytes in our body. Examples include aldosterone, fludrocortisone, desoxycorticosterone acetate etc.

Mechanism of action of corticosteroids and non steroidal anti-inflammatory drugs

Molecular mechanism of action of each class of NSAIDs

Nonselective COX inhibitors

Pyrazolone derivative—oxyphenylbutazone, phenylbutazone

Phenylbutazone is a synthetic pyrazolone moiety showing very good antipyretic and nonhormonal anti-inflammatory activity, specifically for controlling of inflammatory disease. Because of similar type of mechanism, it also shows noticeable analgesic property by reducing the production of prostacyclin and prostaglandin H. Inside the system, these two are bound with the drug and inactivated through peroxide (H_2O_2)-mediated deactivation, that is, by inhibiting COX-1 and COX-2 isoenzymes. Simultaneous production of prostaglandin decreases results in lowering inflammation toward surrounding tissues.[59] Oxyphenbutazone is a parahydroxylated analog of phenylbutazone and is one of its active metabolites. This active metabolite is also responsible for bone marrow suppression and the risk of Stevens–Johnson syndrome, leading to withdrawal of the drug from market worldwide in the mid-1980s.[60]

Acetic acid derivative—indomethacin, nebumetone, ketorolac

Indomethacin is an NSAID drug having family of indoles or indene acetic acids. It acts as a nonspecific inhibitor of the COX enzymes. Out of all other NSAID drugs, indomethacin has a strong ability to cross the blood–brain barrier efficiently compared to naproxen and ibuprofen,[61,62] making a central action in headache treatment plausible.[63] They are also involved in maintaining platelet activity-inhibition, gastrointestinal mucosa, and renal function. In vitro studies have also revealed that indomethacin has a time-dependent tight-binding kinetic profile, whereas naproxen has a time-dependent weak-binding profile, and ibuprofen inhibits COX-1 and COX-2 via competitive inhibition.[64] Indomethacin inhibits the glutathione S-transferase, which demonstrates additional mechanism for COX and phospholipase A2 inhibition in in vitro studies.[65] Symptoms such as dysmenorrhea, fever, arthritis, and other headache syndromes are among the indications for NSAIDs, particularly for indomethacin. In addition, indomethacin is used to close a patent ductus arteriosus.

Nabumetone is a methyl ketone that is 2-butanone with a 6-methoxy-2-naphthyl group in place of one of the methyl hydrogens at position 4. After oral treatment, a prodrug is transformed to the active metabolite, 6-methoxy-2-naphthylacetic acid (6MNA). 6MNA reduces the activity of the enzymes cyclooxygenase I and II, resulting in less synthesis of prostaglandin and thromboxane precursors. The therapeutic effects of nabumetone are due to the decrease in prostaglandin production. The production of thromboxane A2 by thromboxane synthase is also inhibited, resulting in platelet aggregation inhibition. It has been shown to have a lower risk of gastrointestinal side effects than the majority of NSAIDs.

Ketorolac is an FDA-approved pain reliever that is used to treat moderate to severe acute pain.[66] It is versatile because it comes in a variety of dosage forms, including oral, nasal spray, intravenous, and intramuscular. It is commonly used to manage pain after surgery. Ketorolac's exact method of action is unknown. Like other NSAIDs, ketorolac inhibits COX enzymes that convert arachidonic acid into prostaglandins (PGs), prostacyclin, and thromboxane. These chemicals are inhibited, which decreases inflammation, fever, and pain.[67] Both COX-1 and COX-2 are inhibited by ketorolac. It has demonstrated to be more potent than the most NSAIDs.[68]

Salicylates—aspirin

The most extensively used medicine worldwide is aspirin. Taking aspirin twice a day increases one's chances of living a long life. Studies have shown that taking aspirin on a regular basis can lessen the risk of several diseases connected with aging and help people live longer. Aspirin was being used for several thousands of years by the decoctions method of the plants that contain salicylate. Heinrich Dreser, Bayer's chief pharmacologist, gave the new medicine the name “aspirin” because he wanted a name that would not be confused with salicylic acid.[69]

In 1976, COX or prostaglandin endoperoxide synthase (PGHS) was isolated as a homogenous, enzymatically active enzyme.[70] Aspirin acetylates the hydroxyl group of one serine residue (Ser 530), which is positioned 70 amino acids from the COX enzyme’s C terminus.[71] Because acetylation causes irreversible COX inhibition, a new enzyme must be created before further prostanoids may be made. Only the COX, and not the hydroperoxidase, is inhibited when the pure enzyme is acetylated, as shown in Fig. 4.5. This process has a 1:1 stoichiometry, meaning that one acetyl group is transferred per enzyme monomer of this dimeric protein. Aspirin acetylates prostaglandin endoperoxide-H synthase (PGHS) fast (within minutes) and selectively at low concentrations. At high dosages and for prolonged periods of time, aspirin will non-specifically acetylate a number of proteins and nucleic acids.[72] Aspirin acetylation of the enzyme results in a bulky substituent on the Ser 530 oxygen, which prevents arachidonic acid binding.[73] According to a recent study by a research group[74] a third cyclooxygenase (COX-3) is selectively inhibited not only by paracetamol but also by modest doses of NSAIDs like aspirin.[74]

Fenamate—mephenemic acid

Mefenamic acid is an anti-inflammatory, antipyretic, and analgesic anthracitic acid and an NSAID. It reduces the synthesis of precursors to PGs and thromboxanes by inhibiting the activity of the enzymes COX-1 and COX-2. The decrease in prostaglandin synthesis caused by prostaglandin synthase is what causes the therapeutic effects of mefenamic acid. Mefenamic acid also prevents platelet aggregation by decreasing the generation of thromboxane A2 by thromboxane synthase.[75]

Chemically, mefenamic acid is an aminobenzoic acid (anthralinic acid) with a 2,3-dimethylphenyl group replacing one of the hydrogens linked to the nitrogen. Despite the fact that it is classified as an NSAID, its anti-inflammatory activities are thought to be insignificant. It is mostly used to treat mild to moderate pain, including as headaches, dental pain, osteoarthritis, and RA, among others.[76]

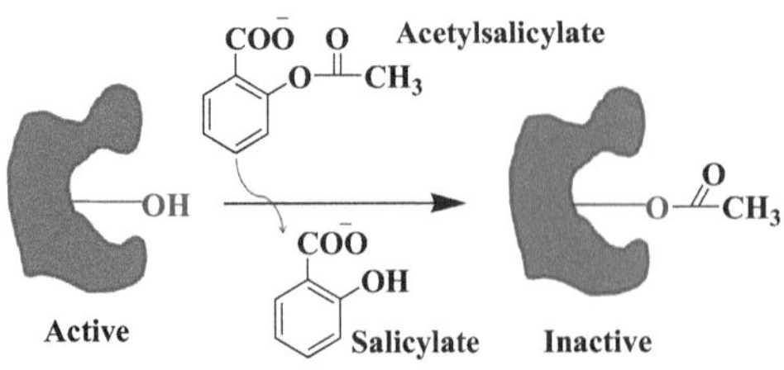

FIGURE 4.5 Inactivation of acetylsalicylic acid (aspirin).

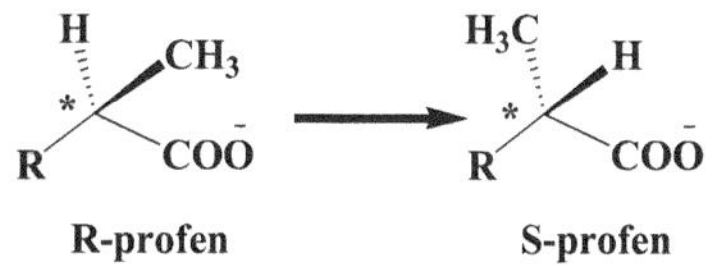

FIGURE 4.6 Basic R- and S-profen structures. The chiral centers are depicted*. Some profens' R-enantiomers are metabolically inverted to S-enantiomers.

Propionic acid derivative—ketoprofen, flurbiprofen, ibuprofen, naproxen

Profens (propionic acid derivative drugs) are a category of nonselective, NSAIDs. They diminish pain (analgesia), fever body temperature (antipyresis), inflammation symptoms (anti-inflammatory action), and cancer formation in rats. Profens are 2-phenylpropanoic acid derivatives. All of them have a chiral core, which causes the creation of two enantiomers (R and S) of each profen (Fig. 4.6). They are mostly found as racemates, which are equal mixtures of the R and S stereoisomers. The most notable exception is naproxen, which is available as its pure S-enantiomer; however, ketoprofen and ibuprofen are also available as their pure S-enantiomers, which are known as dexketoprofen and dexibuprofen, respectively.

S-profens are nonselective NSAIDs that block the production of PGs and thromboxane A2. As a result, S-profens exhibit analgesic, antipyretic, anti-inflammatory, and platelet-aggregation inhibiting properties. S-ibuprofen has a therapeutic (total) plasma concentration of about 25 mmol/L. In a cellular COX-2 system in human blood, the IC50 value of S-ibuprofen is 1.6 mmol/L,[77] which is adequate to produce a very high level of prostaglandin production inhibition in vivo. For many years, R-profens were thought to be pharmacologically inert because they are weak inhibitors of the synthesis of prostaglandins from arachidonic acid in vitro. A recent discovery, however, explains why R-enantiomers exhibit anti-inflammatory and analgesic properties. R-profens have been discovered to reduce endocannabinoid oxidation (Fig. 4.7).[78] Arachidonoylglycerol and anandamide (*N*-arachidonoyl ethanolamine) are the two most important endocannabinoids, and they are both conjugates of arachidonic acid. Endocannabinoids are involved in dampening pain pathways in the central nervous system, and maintaining endocannabinoid levels is now thought to be necessary for the R-profens' analgesic and anti-inflammatory effects.

Enolic acid derivative—piroxicam, tenoxicam

Oxicams are 4-hydroxy-1,2-benzothiazine 3-carboxamide derivatives of the enolic acid class, which have the fewest structural components in common with other NSAIDs. The United States Adopted Names (USAN) Council chose the term "oxicam" to describe NSAIDs in this category. They decrease the action of the two COX isoforms, COX-1 and COX-2 in the treatment of

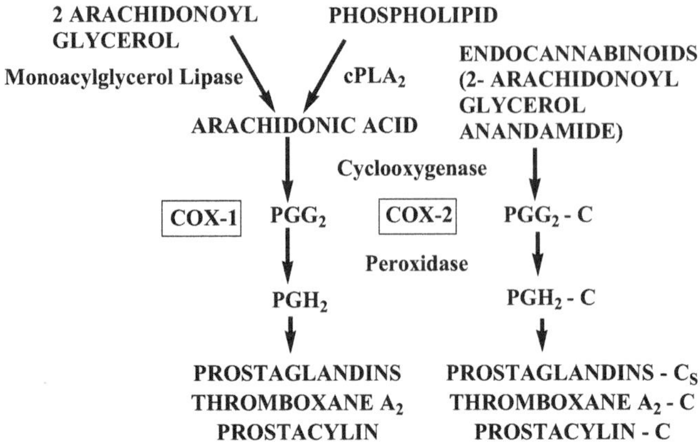

FIGURE 4.7 Synthesis of prostaglandins and related compounds. COX-1 and COX-2 are bifunctional enzymes that perform both cyclooxygenase and peroxide activities. COX-1 catalyzes the formation of PGG2 and PGH2 prostaglandin (PG) intermediates. COX-2 catalyzes the synthesis of PG intermediates as well as PG cannabinoid intermediates from arachidonic acid (PGG2-C and PGH2-C). S-profens, like other nonselective NSAIDs, prevent COX-1 and COX-2 from forming PG intermediates. The R-profens do not stop the production of prostaglandin intermediates, but they do stop COX-2 from producing PGH2-C. Specific enzymes are responsible for the final synthesis of PGs and PG-Cs.

both acute and chronic inflammation (COX-2). Piroxicam, the first member of this class, was released in the United States as Feldene (Pfizer) in 1982 and quickly acquired commercial appeal, becoming one of the top 50 prescribed drugs for several years. Other oxicams, such as tenoxicam, lornoxicam, isoxicam, and meloxicam, were introduced after piroxicam.

Until recently, the structural basis for oxicams' binding to COX was unknown.[79] Meloxicam and tenoxicam may bind to the COX site in a fashion that places the benzothiazine ring near to the catalytic Try-385 and the 3-carboxamide directly above the constriction at the active site's entrance, according to two different computational simulations.[80,81] However, neither prediction explained why the S530A, R120A, and Y355F COX-2 mutants were not inhibited by piroxicam.[82]

Oxicams have a planar conformation in the COX active site, which leads to an intramolecular hydrogen bond between the carboxamide's nitrogen atom and the benzothiazine's 4-hydroxyl group. Many hydrophobic contacts and a single instantaneous hydrogen bond between the oxicam 4-hydroxyl group and Ser-530 of the enzyme allow oxicams to bind to the active site channel. At the catalytic apex and the constriction site, two highly organized water molecules in the active site provide additional polar bridges between oxicams and COX residues.

Inhibition of microsomal prostaglandin E synthase-1 (mPGES-1), which results in a decrease in PGE2 production, has emerged as a therapeutic technique for the treatment of inflammatory illnesses that avoids the common side effects of NSAIDs. The widespread inhibition of prostanoid production has been blamed for these side effects, which include gastrointestinal, renal, and cardiovascular damage.[83]

In a high-throughput screen for human mPGES-1 inhibitors, a series of benzothiopyran S-dioxides were discovered as lead compounds. With an IC50 of 1.68 M against human recombinant mPGES-1, the most powerful molecule in this series showed considerable inhibition, and in the IL-1-stimulated fetal fibroblast cell assay, it showed over 26-fold selectivity for PGE2 decrease (IC50 of 3.4 M) over $PGF_{2\alpha}$ ($IC_{50} > 90\ \mu M$).[84]

Preferential COX II inhibitors—nimesulide, diclofenac, aceclofenac, meloxicam, etodolac

Nimesulide belongs to the sulfonanilide class of NSAIDs. Its anti-inflammatory, antipyretic, and analgesic properties have been demonstrated in a variety of animal models as well as clinical trials. Nimesulide exerts its effects through various mechanisms by the inhibition of COX-2 and selectively and weakly inhibits prostaglandin synthesis. Thus, it generates weaker analgesic properties. It has a potent anti-inflammatory activity, which results in the inhibition of superoxide anion formation in vitro by an activated neutrophil. It also inhibits the release of histamine from tissue mast cells and basophils. It reduces oxidant production from active neutrophils and acts as a scavenger for hypochlorous acid without impairing neutrophil activity. Nimesulide also decreases the synthesis of platelet-activating factor by human basophils and reduces histamine release from tissue mast cells. Furthermore, when nimesulide is introduced to human articular chondrocyte cultures in vitro, it inhibits the production of stromelysin and limits metalloproteinase activity.

Diclofenac is an NSAID with analgesic, antipyretic, and anti-inflammatory effects that is often administered. It works well for a number of acute and chronic pain and inflammatory conditions. Diclofenac inhibits COX-1 and COX-2 in roughly equal amounts, but evidence suggests that COX-2 inhibition is about four times more selective than COX-1 inhibition during in vitro studies. This number is distant from the more specific COX-2 medicines such as rofecoxib's stated 20-fold selectivity of COX-2 inhibition, but diclofenac's action can be compared more appropriately to that of celecoxib.[85,86] Diclofenac and other NSAIDs inhibit the synthesis of thromboxanes, particularly thromboxane-B2 (TX-B2). The principal prostanoids are raised during an inflammatory reaction, and diclofenac is one of the most efficient inhibitors of their production.[87] However, extensive research indicates that diclofenac's pharmacologic efficacy extends beyond COX inhibition to encompass multimodal and, in some cases, new modes of action.

Meloxicam's ability to inhibit COX-2 preferentially is largely dependent on the drug's structure. Meloxicam's selectivity against COX-2 was significantly reduced when it was converted to the 4′-isomer (the methyl substitution on the thiazole group occurs at position 4 rather than position 5). The 4′-isomer showed COX-1 selectivity.[88] Meloxicam's anti-inflammatory properties were compared to those of other well-known NSAIDs in a rat model of progressive and destructive joint disease. The acute symptoms of adjuvant-induced arthritis in rats are linked to COX-2 expression,[89] and inflammation is also immunologically mediated. Meloxicam is more effective at reducing inflammation than the other drugs examined in this study.[90,91] Meloxicam, in low doses, avoided not just edema but also the degradation of bone and cartilage. Piroxicam, on the other hand, showed similar activity at larger doses, but diclofenac and tenidap were only marginally effective in preventing bone and cartilage degradation at levels that controlled swelling.[90,91]

Etodolac demonstrated a remarkable anti-inflammatory impact in a variety of experimental settings, including UV erythema, carrageenin-induced edema, and adjuvant arthritis swelling. In these models, the effective dose of etodolac was several folds higher that of indomethacin. Etodolac attenuated prostaglandin E2 formation in a concentration-dependent manner, and its inhibitory potency was about one-fifth of that of indomethacin. Etodolac also caused a marked reduction of granuloma formation and leukocyte functions such as lysosomal enzyme release, active oxygen generation and chemotaxis. These effects of etodolac were observed at similar doses of indomethacin. Etodolac suppressed inflammatory pain but not non-inflammatory pain, and had an antipyretic effect but did not lower normal rectal temperature.

Selective COX-2 inhibitors—celecoxib, etoricoxib, parecoxib

Medicines with names that end in "coxib," such as celecoxib or etoricoxib, are thought to have the highest selectivity in their effect on COX-2 enzymes and were developed to reduce gastrointestinal toxicity associated with the use of traditional NSAIDs, but they have been criticized by some for having less favorable cardiovascular effects than nonselective agents.[92] The name coxib has no pharmacological significance. The results of several in vitro assay techniques that measure selectivity ratios for COX-1 and COX-2 enzymes might be quite varied.[64,93]

Celecoxib is used in anti-inflammatory, analgesic, and antipyretic nonsteroidal anti-inflammatory medication (NSAID). Ankylosing spondylitis, osteoarthritis, RA, and acute pain are among the conditions for which it has been approved.[94,95] Celecoxib's anti-inflammatory and pain-relieving actions are due to its specific suppression of prostaglandin (PG) synthesis via PG G/H synthase-2 (encoded by gene PTGS2). Although the two PTGS isoforms, PTGS1 and PTGS2, are bifunctional enzymes that have both COX and hydroperoxidase activity, they are often referred to as COX enzymes.[86,96] Celecoxib belongs to the COX-2-selective inhibitors subclass of NSAIDs, sometimes known as coxibs.[97,98]

Merck Frosst introduced rofecoxib into medical practice in 1999.[99] It easily passes through the central nervous system and has strong analgesic, antipyretic, and anti-inflammatory properties. The ratio of IC50 against COX-1 in platelets to IC50 against COX-2 in monocytes in the human whole blood assay is 38, indicating strong selectivity for COX-2 over COX-1.[100]

In several European nations, etoricoxib is prescribed to treat osteoarthritis, RA, and gout episodes. Etoricoxib has been studied in a number of clinical trials for these conditions, as well as ankylosing spondylitis, low back pain, and various types of acute pain. Etoricoxib was no more efficacious than other NSAIDs such ibuprofen, naproxen, or diclofenac in these conditions. In comparison to naproxen, etoricoxib had a greater overall fatality rate in clinical trials.

Parecoxib is the first injectable COX-2-selective inhibitor and is used to treat immediate postoperative pain. It is a prodrug that hydrolyzes to valdecoxib, which has selectivity for COX-2 that is comparable to rofecoxib. Both intravenous and intramuscular administrations of parecoxib at a starting dose of 40 mg has been approved.[101]

Aniline derivatives (analgesics and antipyretics)

Paracetamol, metamizole, propiphenazone, nefopam

Peripherally acting, non-opioid (non-narcotic) or moderate analgesics account for more than 90% of the analgesics used. Aspirin and other acidic NSAIDs, non-acidic pyrazole medications like propyphenazone and dipyrone (metamizole), and aniline derivatives like paracetamol are all derived from three categories of chemicals (acetaminophen).

Although paracetamol is nearly as effective as aspirin as an analgesic and antipyretic, it is not a real anti-inflammatory medication. Thus, aspirin and other NSAIDs are significantly preferable for RA and dental pericoronitis. For people who are allergic to aspirin or other NSAIDs, acetaminophen is often the medicine of choice.[102] Paracetamol and other aniline derivatives are not very effective analgesics, but they are good antipyretics.[103]

Antipyretic analgesics are thought to be unlikely to cause stomach irritation, bleeding, or perforations at therapeutic levels, which are common side effects of aspirin-like medicines. Furthermore, unlike NSAIDs, these medications have no effect on platelet aggregation or bleeding time in patients.[104,105] They also have little or limited anti-inflammatory properties. As a result, it has been proposed that acetaminophen is a modest inhibitor of peripheral COX-1 and COX-2, with the majority of its therapeutic effect focused on the central nervous system[106,107] (Table 4.4).

TABLE 4.4 Newly approved drugs as per USFDA with their mechanism of action and use.

Sl No	Drug	Mechanism	Uses
1	Rinvoq	Janus kinase (JAK) inhibitor preventing the phosphorylation and activation of signal transducers and activators of transcription (STATs)	Treatment of adults with moderately to severely active rheumatoid arthritis who have had an inadequate response or intolerance to methotrexate
2	Xenleta	Inhibits bacterial protein synthesis through interactions with the A- and P-sites of the peptidyl transferase center in domain V of the 23s rRNA of the 50S subunit	Treatment of adults with community-acquired bacterial pneumonia caused by susceptible microorganisms
3	Ubrelvy	Calcitonin gene-related peptide receptor antagonist	Indicated for the acute treatment of migraine with or without aura in adults
4	Zeposia	Sphingosine 1-phosphate receptor modulator	Treatment of relapsing forms of multiple sclerosis (MS)
5	Vyepti	Calcitonin gene-related peptide antagonist	Indicated for the preventive treatment of migraine in adults
6	Ponvory	Sphingosine 1-phosphate receptor modulator	Treatment of relapsing forms of MS
7	Lupkynis	Calcineurin-inhibitor immunosuppressant	Treatment of adult patients with active lupus nephritis
8	Mayzent	Sphingosine 1-phosphate receptor modulator	The relapsing forms of MS

Anti-inflammatory mechanism of corticosteroids

The adrenal glands manufacture and secrete corticosteroids in response to pituitary adrenocorticotropic hormone, which is regulated by hypothalamic corticotropin releasing hormone. Major endocrine system activities, such as stress management and homeostasis control, are governed by these hormones. Cortisol (glucocorticoids) and aldosterone are the major corticosteroids generated by the adrenal cortex (MRs).

Residents cells, notably mast cells and resident macrophages, induce inflammation at the site of damage by releasing pro-inflammatory mediators such as bioactive amines, lipid mediators, and cytokines such as IL-1 and TNF-α. These mediators increase capillary permeability, vasodilation, and leukocyte emigration into wounded tissues, causing redness, swelling, discomfort, and heat, as well as establishing a chemotactic gradient to guide and activate recruited cells to the injury site.

A new evaluation of the anti-inflammatory effects of glucocorticoid-induced genes was published.[108] Dual Specificity Phosphatase 1 (DUSP1) and IκB class of genes includes IL-10, a potent immunomodulatory and anti-inflammatory cytokine,[109] Glucocorticoid-induced leucine zipper (GILZ), a protein whose mechanism of action (Fig. 4.8) is unknown but which interacts with, and inhibits the function of annexin AI (AnxA1), a calcium-dependent phospholipid binding protein[110] and AP-1 and NF-κB.[111] Although GILZ knockout mice have not been reported, AnxA1-deficient mice exhibit defective glucocorticoid suppression of inflammation in zymosan-induced peritonitis, antigen-induced arthritis, and carrageen-induced edema.[112]

The ability of glucocorticoid receptors (GRs) to inhibit the activity of NF-κB and AP-1, as well as other important immunomodulatory

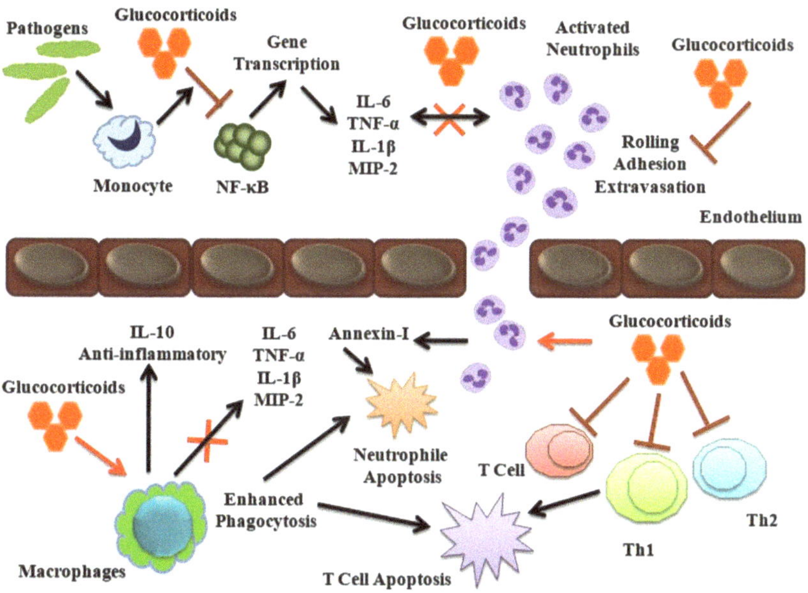

FIGURE 4.8 Glucocorticoids' anti-inflammatory properties- Manifestation to pathogens ends up in a quick activation of the immune reaction. Glucocorticoids suppress the expression of pro-inflammatory cytokines by immune cells, therefore modulating the inflammatory response. Furthermore, glucocorticoids can suppress the production of adhesion molecules, preventing neutrophils from rolling, adherence, and extravasation to the site of inflammation. Annexin-1 expression is also induced by glucocorticoids. Neutrophil detachment and apoptosis are aided by the production of annexin-1. Chronic glucocorticoid exposure changes the gene expression profile of resident macrophages from pro- to anti-inflammatory, and promotes macrophage phagocytic activity. Finally, glucocorticoids affect T cells by inhibiting the generation of Th1- and Th2-derived cytokines and causing necrobiosis.

transcription factors, has been a major focus of research into the mechanisms behind glucocorticoids' anti-inflammatory actions. Although transactivation by GR was implicated in NF-κB repression—promoting production of the NF-κB inhibitor proteins (IκB),[113,114] this was limited to select cell types and did not appear to be a universal mechanism.[113–116]

Glucocorticoids reduce the severity of several of the early stages of an inflammatory reaction. They also promote inflammation resolution, albeit the mechanisms by which they do so have gotten less attention than those linked to inhibition of the initial reaction.[117] Many of glucocorticoids' anti-inflammatory and immunosuppressive effects are due to the transcriptional effects of glucocorticoid receptor agonism, which changes the transcription of several genes in leukocytes, either directly or indirectly.[118]

Corticosteroids have anti-inflammatory and immunosuppressive effects by disrupting numerous processes in the immune system's upregulation. The majority of their suppressive activity is limited to cell-mediated immunity. Corticosteroids are thought to suppress cytokine synthesis, antigen presentation, and lymphocyte proliferation via binding to GRs found all over the body.[119] When corticosteroids are given, they cause lymphocytopenia, which causes circulating lymphocytes to be redistributed to other lymphoid compartments. Within 4 h of delivery, a single dose of corticosteroids causes lymphocytopenia, which normalizes within 24–48 h through redistribution into the circulation away from the periphery, rather than destruction. Monocytes and eosinophils, which ordinarily collect at the inflammatory site, also decrease when corticosteroids are administered. Corticosteroids cause neutrophilia by releasing neutrophils from the bone marrow into the bloodstream, reducing neutrophil migration out of the bloodstream, and demarginating neutrophils from the vascular lining.[120]

MRs are a group of hormones that originate in the adrenal cortex (Fig. 4.9A). These hormones maintain electrolyte and water balance. They also control sodium and potassium retention in the kidneys within the body. Generally, aldosterone is the only functioning natural MR found in humans.

Aldosterone is a steroid hormone that binds to the MR receptor in the body. Changes in blood perfusion, which are sensed by main cells in the juxtaglomerular apparatus, potently boost hormone production and secretion.[121] Cholesterol is the precursor of aldosterone production, which is primarily driven by angiotensin II. This leads to increase in sodium retention by the kidneys. The actions of aldosterone are mediated by binding to the MR in target tissues, mainly in the kidney. When aldosterone is produced and secreted, epithelial cells in the renal tubule[122] or vascular smooth muscle cells[123] respond by inducing the expression of water-absorption genes like epithelial sodium channel (ENaC), sodium-potassium ATPase, and serum/glucocorticoid regulated kinase 1 (SGK1).[124,125]

In terms of immunological response, aldosterone stimulation has been shown to increase pro-inflammatory responses (Fig. 4.9B) in a variety of

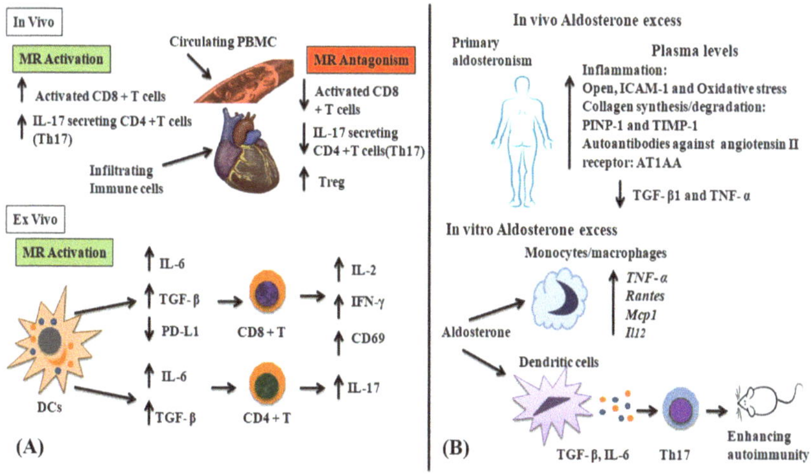

FIGURE 4.9 (A) Excess MR activation has negative effects on circulating and intra-tissue immune cells. In circulating peripheral blood mononuclear cells (PBMCs) and immune cells invading the heart, over activation of MR increases CD8 + T cells and T helper 17 (Th17) cells. MR antagonism, on the other hand, can reduce Th17 polarization and increase the T regulatory cell (Treg) phenotype. Dendritic cells stimulate these subgroups of cells (DCs). Dendritic cells express MR and are encouraged to create polarizing cytokines by aldosterone, which can activate CD8 + T cells and stimulate CD4 + T cells to adopt the Th17 phenotype. PD-L1 stands for programmed death ligand 1; IFN-gamma stands for interferon gamma; IL stands for interleukin; TGF-beta stands for transforming growth factor beta. (B) Pro-inflammatory effect of aldosterone. Excess aldosterone has been linked to an inflammatory phenotype in the past. Aldosterone promotes inflammatory and oxidative alterations in patients with primary aldosteronism, whereas MR antagonism or regulating aldosterone levels promotes to a return to homeostatic conditions. In vitro tests show that aldosterone stimulates the production and production of proinflammatory cytokines in myeloid immune cells. The polarization of adaptive immune response toward the Th17 phenotype is directly affected by this regulation of innate immune cells.

tissues.[126,127] T and B lymphocytes, monocytes, neutrophils, and CD34 + hematopoietic progenitors have all been found to exhibit MR in human leukocytes.[128] Furthermore, clinical investigations have shown that MR antagonistic therapy can improve patient outcomes in cardiovascular illnesses, owing to the avoidance of inflammatory damage.[129]

The existing literature links aldosterone-induced MR activation to the promotion of inflammation and fibrosis, but the majority of these studies focused on the development of hypertension or the generation of inflammatory mediators. Animal models, on the other hand, frequently show elevated levels of circulating aldosterone.[130] Because detrimental effects were avoided only when MR antagonists, rather than GR antagonists, were utilized, it is critical to emphasize that GCs can produce tissue damage and hypertension as a result of MR activation.[131,132] In conclusion, the inflammatory profile is directly linked to MR activation, and evidence suggests that MR activation is associated to other diseases such as chronic kidney disease, obesity, and autoimmune.

Patients with aldosterone-producing adenomas and resistant arterial hypertension released considerably higher quantities of IFN-γ, IL-2, and TNF-α from lymphocytes and IL-6, TNF-α, and IL-1 from monocytes produced at the start of the trial, according to a recent study.[133] During the 24 months of the clinical investigation, there was a considerable decrease in the levels of all cytokines, all the way down to levels corresponding to essential hypertensive (EH) and healthy controls, after two months of spironolactone, eplerenone, or adrenal ectomization therapy.[134] Irita et al. found that primary aldosteronism (PA) patients had greater levels of osteopontin (OPN) than EH patients, with no differences in other markers of systemic inflammation such TNF-α, IL-6, or CRP.[135] Furthermore, when compared to EH patients, PA patients had higher serum levels of IL-10 and TNF-α, as well as lower blood levels of Transforming growth factor beta-1 (TGF-β1). Spironolactone treatment restored serum levels of all three cytokines in PA patients.[136] Furthermore, when compared to EH patients, normotensive and normal pregnant women, PA patients, and pre-eclamptic women had greater titers of autoantibodies against angiotensin II receptor 1 (AT1AA) in their serum.[137,138]

Contraindications of corticosteroids

Corticosteroids are immensely used nowadays to sake the damaged critical body organs. Though it is used to save the organs, it has some contraindications too. Some diseases are exacerbated by the corticosteroids.[139] These diseases are (1) congestive heart failure (CHF), (2) psychosis, (3) renal failure, (4) epilepsy, (5) herpes simplex keratitis, (6) osteoporosis, (7) diabetes mellitus, (8) tuberculosis and other infections, (9) hypertension, (10) viral and fungal infections, and (11) Peptic ulcer.

Contraindications of nonsteroidal anti-inflammatory drugs

After prolonged used of NSAIDs, humans may suffer from various diseases. People should cautious with the following conditions to use of NSAIDs: (1) upsetting of bowel syndrome, (2) persons who have had past gastrointestinal problems (or have a family history) and also the over age of 50, (3) peptic ulcer/stomach bleeding, (4) acute hypertension, (5) Crohn's disease, (6) cardiovascular disease history such as ischemic attack, stroke, coronary artery disorder, coronary artery bypass surgery, CHF, (7) in third trimester of pregnancy, (8) allergic or anti-allergic-type NSAID hypersensitivity, and (9) kidney disease.

Conclusion

In the treatment of inflammation the discovery of COX iso-enzyme are highly useful. COX-1 and COX-2 both have an important role in the recent advancement of treatment of inflammation. COX-1 is important for the synthesis of prostaglandin in the gastrointestinal tract, and COX-2[140] maintains the mucosal integrity of gastrointestinal tract, derived from prostaglandin. COX-2 is used to inhibit selectively renal and cardiovascular toxicity whereas, COX-1 is for tissue homeostasis and cytoprotection.

One of the promising mechanisms of action of glucocorticoids are to inhibit the transcriptional effects of NF-κB and another one is to inhibit IKK2 (inhibitor kappa B kinase 2) by small molecules. From these mechanisms, IKK2 inhibitors have more promising effects in the treatment which are act indirectly by inhibiting NF-κB also. It is identified that IKK2 has more significant clinical benefits than the inhibitors of NF-κB. Inhibitors of NF-κB shows some side effects, while the inhibitors of IKK2 shows less times of side effects in the treatment of inflammation in high doses, topical uses and systemic uses of corticosteroids. To reduce the side effects of corticosteroids, transactivation events of anti-NF-κB has been reported in research scientific studies. Clinical studies are being conducted to reduce the side effects potential of drugs and new compounds in the treatment of inflammations, and results are eagerly expected.

References

1. Adami JG. *Inflammation: An Introduction to the Study of Pathology*. Macmillan; 1909.
2. Daniyal M, Wang W. *Molecular pharmacology of inflammation: medicinal plants as anti-inflammatory agents. InInflammation and Natural Products*. Academic Press; 2021:21–63.
3. Goldstein IM, Snyderman R, Gallin JI, eds. *Inflammation: Basic Principles and Clinical Correlates*. Raven press; 1992.
4. Zweifach BW, Grant L, McCluskey RT, eds. *The Inflammatory Process*. Academic Press; 2014.
5. Medzhitov R. Origin and physiological roles of inflammation. *Nature*. 2008;454 (7203):428–435.
6. Henry G, Garner WL. Inflammatory mediators in wound healing. *Surg Clin*. 2003;83 (3):483–507.
7. Kumar V, Abbas AK, Aster JC. *Robbins Basic Pathology e-Book*. Elsevier Health Sciences; 2017.
8. Pober JS, Sessa WC. Evolving functions of endothelial cells in inflammation. *Nat Rev Immunol*. 2007;7(10):803–815.
9. Kumar V, Abbas AK, Aster JC, Robbins SL. *Inflammation and repair. Robbins Basic Pathology*. Philadelphia, London: Saunders; 2012:p29–p74.
10. Serhan CN, Dalli J, Colas RA, Winkler JW, Chiang N. Protectins and maresins: new pro-resolving families of mediators in acute inflammation and resolution bioactive metabolome. *Biochim Biophys Acta (BBA)—Mol Cell Biol Lipids*. 2015;1851(4):397–413.
11. Nguyen TT. *Systems Biology Approaches to Corticosteroid Pharmacogenomics and Systemic Inflammation* [Doctoral dissertation]. New Brunswick: Rutgers University-Graduate School; 2012.
12. Porter S. *Tidy's Physiotherapy E-Book*. Elsevier Health Sciences; 2013.
13. Bitencourt CS, Bessi VL, Huynh DN, et al. Cooperative role of endogenous leucotrienes and platelet-activating factor in ischaemia–reperfusion-mediated tissue injury. *J Cell Mol Med*. 2013;17(12):1554–1565.

14. Goljan EF. *Rapid Review Pathology: With Student Consult Online Access*; 2013.
15. Curcic S, Holzer M, Frei R, et al. Neutrophil effector responses are suppressed by secretory phospholipase A2 modified HDL. *Biochim Biophys Acta (BBA)—Mol Cell Biol Lipids*. 2015;1851(2):184–193.
16. McDonald B, Kubes P. *Leukocyte trafficking. Inflammatory Diseases of Blood Vessels*. Canada: Department of Physiology and Pharmacology, Faculty of Medicine, University of Calgary; 2012. Chapter 3: 28.
17. Nourshargh S, Hordijk PL, Sixt M. Breaching multiple barriers: leukocyte motility through venular walls and the interstitium. *Nat Rev Mol Cell Biol*. 2010;11(5):366–378.
18. Springer TA, Anderson DC, Rosenthal AS, Rothlein R. September 28–October 2 *Leukocyte Adhesion Molecules: Proceedings of the First International Conference on: "Structure, Function and Regulation of Molecules Involved in Leukocyte Adhesion"*. West Germany: Held in Titisee; 1988.
19. Ogra PL, Mestecky J, Lamm ME, Strober W, McGhee JR, Bienenstock J. *Handbook of Mucosal Immunology*. Academic Press; 2012.
20. Sies H. *Oxidative stress: impact in neuroscience research. Studies on Alzheimer's Disease*. Totowa, NJ: Humana Press; 2013:3–7.
21. Gleeson M, Bishop NC, Stensel DJ, Lindley MR, Mastana SS, Nimmo MA. The anti-inflammatory effects of exercise: mechanisms and implications for the prevention and treatment of disease. *Nat Rev Immunol*. 2011;11(9):607–615.
22. Murakami M, Hirano T. The molecular mechanisms of chronic inflammation development. *Front Immunol*. 2012;3:323.
23. Kong AN, ed. *Inflammation, Oxidative Stress, and Cancer: Dietary Approaches for Cancer Prevention*. CRC Press; 2013.
24. Niederhuber JE, Armitage JO, Doroshow JH, Kastan MB, Tepper JE. *Abeloff's Clinical Oncology e-Book*. Elsevier Health Sciences; 2013.
25. Ogrunc M, Di Micco R, Liontos M, et al. Oncogene-induced reactive oxygen species fuel hyperproliferation and DNA damage response activation. *Cell Death Differ*. 2014;21(6):998–1012.
26. Ansar W, Ghosh S. *Inflammation and inflammatory diseases, markers, and mediators: role of CRP in some inflammatory diseases. Biology of C Reactive Protein in Health and Disease*. New Delhi: Springer; 2016:67–107.
27. Klarenbeek NB, Kerstens PJ, Huizinga TW, Dijkmans BA, Allaart CF. Recent advances in the management of rheumatoid arthritis. *BMJ*. 2010;341.
28. Plum SM, Park EJ, Strawn SJ, Moore EG, Sidor CF, Fogler WE. Disease modifying and antiangiogenic activity of 2-methoxyestradiol in a murine model of rheumatoid arthritis. *BMC Musculoskelet Disord*. 2009;10(1):1–3.
29. Wolfe F. The epidemiology of drug treatment failure in rheumatoid arthritis. *Bailliere's Clin Rheumatol*. 1995;9(4):619–632.
30. Guo Q, Wang Y, Xu D, Nossent J, Pavlos NJ, Xu J. Rheumatoid arthritis: pathological mechanisms and modern pharmacologic therapies. *Bone Res*. 2018;6(1):1–4.
31. Bizzaro N, Bartoloni E, Morozzi G, et al. Anti-cyclic citrullinated peptide antibody titer predicts time to rheumatoid arthritis onset in patients with undifferentiated arthritis: results from a 2-year prospective study. *Arthritis Res Ther*. 2013;15(1):1–9.
32. Malmström V, Catrina AI, Klareskog L. The immunopathogenesis of seropositive rheumatoid arthritis: from triggering to targeting. *Nat Rev Immunol*. 2017;17(1):60.

33. Louis R, Lau LC, Bron AO, Roldaan AC, Radermecker M, Djukanovic R. The relationship between airways inflammation and asthma severity. *Am J Respir Crit Care Med.* 2000;161 (1):9–16.
34. Nelson HS. The importance of allergens in the development of asthma and the persistence of symptoms. *Disease-a-Month.* 2001;47(1):5–15.
35. Holgate ST, Davies DE, Powell RM, Howarth PH, Haitchi HM, Holloway JW. Local genetic and environmental factors in asthma disease pathogenesis: chronicity and persistence mechanisms. *Eur Respir J.* 2007;29(4):793–803.
36. Murdoch JR, Lloyd CM. Chronic inflammation and asthma. *Mutat Res/Fund Mol Mech Mutagen.* 2010;690(1–2):24–39.
37. Sköld CM. Remodeling in asthma and COPD—differences and similarities. *Clin Respir J.* 2010;4:20–27.
38. Sands BE. Biomarkers of inflammation in inflammatory bowel disease. *Gastroenterology.* 2015;149(5):1275–1285.
39. Lucchinetti CF, Brück W, Rodriguez M, Lassmann H. Distinct patterns of multiple sclerosis pathology indicates heterogeneity in pathogenesis. *Brain Pathol.* 1996;6(3):259–274.
40. Kieseier BC, Storch MK, Archelos JJ, Martino G, Hartung HP. Effector pathways in immune mediated central nervous system demyelination. *Curr OpNeurol.* 1999;12 (3):323–336.
41. Scadding GK, Durham SR, Mirakian R, et al. BSACI guidelines for the management of allergic and non-allergic rhinitis. *Clin Exp Allergy.* 2008;38(1):19–42.
42. Bendtsen P, Grønbaek M, Kjaer SK, Munk C, Linneberg A, Tolstrup JS. Alcohol consumption and the risk of self-reported perennial and seasonal allergic rhinitis in young adult women in a population-based cohort study. *Clin Exp Allergy.* 2008;38(7):1179–1185.
43. Thakur S, Riyaz B, Patil A, Kaur A, Kapoor B, Mishra V. Novel drug delivery systems for NSAIDs in management of rheumatoid arthritis: an overview. *Biomed Pharmacother.* 2018;106:1011–1023.
44. Crofford LJ. Use of NSAIDs in treating patients with arthritis. *Arthritis Res Ther.* 2013;15 (3):1–10.
45. Aletaha D, Smolen JS. Diagnosis and management of rheumatoid arthritis: a review. *JAMA.* 2018;320(13):1360–1372.
46. Schlesinger N, Dalbeth N, Perez-Ruiz F. Gout—what are the treatment options? *Expert Opin Pharmacother.* 2009;10(8):1319–1328.
47. Billy CA, Lim RT, Ruospo M, Palmer SC, Strippoli GF. Corticosteroid or nonsteroidal antiinflammatory drugs for the treatment of acute gout: a systematic review of randomized controlled trials. *J Rheumatol.* 2018;45(1):128–136.
48. Pardutz A, Schoenen J. NSAIDs in the acute treatment of migraine: a review of clinical and experimental data. *Pharmaceuticals.* 2010;3(6):1966–1987.
49. Woldeamanuel YW, Rapoport AM, Cowan RP. What is the evidence for the use of corticosteroids in migraine? *Curr Pain Headache Rep.* 2014;18(12):464.
50. Alangari AA. Corticosteroids in the treatment of acute asthma. *Ann Thorac Med.* 2014;9(4):187.
51. Lo PC, Tsai YT, Lin SK, Lai JN. Risk of asthma exacerbation associated with nonsteroidal anti-inflammatory drugs in childhood asthma: a nationwide population-based cohort study in Taiwan. *Medicine.* 2016;95(41).
52. May JR, Dolen WK. Management of allergic rhinitis: a review for the community pharmacist. *Clin Ther.* 2017;39(12):2410–2419.

53. Falk JA, Minai OA, Mosenifar Z. Inhaled and systemic corticosteroids in chronic obstructive pulmonary disease. *Proc Am Thorac Soc.* 2008;5(4):506–512.
54. Myhr KM, Mellgren SI. Corticosteroids in the treatment of multiple sclerosis. *Acta Neurol Scandinavica.* 2009;120:73–80.
55. Demoly P, Chung KF. Pharmacology of corticosteroids. *Respir Med.* 1998;92(3):385–394.
56. Kowalski ML, Makowska JS. Seven steps to the diagnosis of NSAIDs hypersensitivity: how to apply a new classification in real practice? *Allergy Asthma Immunol Res.* 2015;7 (4):312.
57. Zarghi A, Arfaei S. Selective COX-2 inhibitors: a review of their structure-activity relationships. *Iran J Pharm Res: IJPR.* 2011;10(4):655.
58. Samuel S, Nguyen T, Choi HA. Pharmacologic characteristics of corticosteroids. *J Neurocrit Care.* 2017;10(2):53–59.
59. Sturge RA, Scott JT, Hamilton EB, et al. Multicentre trial of naproxen and phenylbutazone in acute gout. *Ann Rheum Dis.* 1977;36(1):80–82.
60. Dwivedi AK, Gurjar V, Kumar S, Singh N. Molecular basis for nonspecificity of nonsteroidal anti-inflammatory drugs (NSAIDs). *Drug Discov Today.* 2015;20(7):863–873.
61. Eriksen JL, Sagi SA, Smith TE, et al. NSAIDs and enantiomers of flurbiprofen target γ-secretase and lower Aβ42 in vivo. *J Clin Investig.* 2003;112(3):440–449.
62. Parepally JM, Mandula H, Smith QR. Brain uptake of nonsteroidal anti-inflammatory drugs: ibuprofen, flurbiprofen, and indomethacin. *Pharm Res.* 2006;23(5):873–881.
63. Summ O, Andreou AP, Akerman S, Goadsby PJ. A potential nitrergic mechanism of action for indomethacin, but not of other COX inhibitors: relevance to indomethacin-sensitive headaches. *J Headache Pain.* 2010;11(6):477–483.
64. Gierse JK, Koboldt CM, Walker MC, Seibert K, Isakson PC. Kinetic basis for selective inhibition of cyclo-oxygenases. *Biochem J.* 1999;339(3):607–614.
65. Hayeshi R, Chinyanga F, Chengedza S, Mukanganyama S. Inhibition of human glutathione transferases by multidrug resistance chemomodulators in vitro. *J Enzyme Inhibition Med Chem.* 2006;21(5):581–587.
66. Gillis JC, Brogden RN. Ketorolac. A reappraisal of its pharmacodynamic and pharmacokinetic properties and therapeutic use in pain management. *Drugs.* 1997;53(1):139–188.
67. Hiľovská L, Jendželovský R, Fedoročko P. Potency of non-steroidal anti-inflammatory drugs in chemotherapy. *Mol Clin Oncol.* 2015;3(1):3–12.
68. Vacha ME, Huang W, Mando-Vandrick J. The role of subcutaneous ketorolac for pain management. *Hospital Pharm.* 2015;50(2):108–112.
69. Dreser H. Pharmacologischesüber aspirin (acetylsalicyl-saüre). *Pflug Arch.* 1899;76:306–318.
70. Hemler M, Lands WEM, Smith WL. Purification of the cyclooxygenase that forms prostaglandins: demonstration of two forms of iron in the holoenzyme. *J Biol Chem.* 1976;251:5575–5579.
71. Roth GJ, Majerus PW. The mechanism of the effect of Aspirin on human platelets: 1 Acetylation of a particulate fraction protein. *J Clin Invest.* 1975;56:624–632.
72. Smith WL. The eicosanoids and their biochemical mechanisms of action. *Biochem J.* 1989;259:315–324.
73. De Witt DL, El-Harith EA, Kraemer SA, et al. The aspirin and heme-binding sites of ovine and murine prostaglandin endoperoxide synthases. *J Biol Chem.* 1990;265:5192–5198.
74. Chandrasekharan NV, Dai H, Roos KL, et al. COX-3, a cyclooxygenase-1 variant inhibited by acetaminophen and other analgesic/antipyretic drugs: cloning, structure and expression. *Proc Natl Acad Sci U S A.* 2002;99:13926–13931.

75. Cimolai N. The potential and promise of mefenamic acid. *Expert Rev Clin Pharmacol.* 2013;6(3):289–305.
76. Myles AB, Bacon PA, Williams KA. Mefenamic acid in rheumatoid arthritis. *Ann Rheum Dis.* 1967;26(6):494.
77 Rainsford KD. Profile and mechanisms of gastrointestinal and other side effects of nonsteroidal anti-inflammatory drugs (NSAIDs). *Am J Med.* 1999;107(6):27–35.
78. Duggan KC, Hermanson DJ, Musee J, et al. (R)-Profens are substrate-selective inhibitors of endocannabinoid oxygenation by COX-2. *Nat Chem Biol.* 2011;7(11):803–809.
79. Xu S, Hermanson DJ, Banerjee S, et al. Oxicams bind in a novel mode to the cyclooxygenase active site via a two-water-mediated H-bonding network. *J Biol Chem.* 2014;289 (10):6799–6808.
80. Park H, Lee S. Free energy perturbation approach to the critical assessment of selective cyclooxygenase-2 inhibitors. *J Comput Mol Des.* 2005;19(1):17–31.
81. Kothekar V, Sahi S, Srinivasan M, Mohan A, Mishra J. Recognition of cyclooxygenase-2 (COX-2) active site by NSAIDs: a computer modelling study. *Indian J Biochem Biophys.* 2001;38:56–63.
82. Rowlinson SW, Kiefer JR, Prusakiewicz JJ, et al. A novel mechanism of cyclooxygenase-2 inhibition involving interactions with Ser-530 and Tyr-385. *J Biol Chem.* 2003;278 (46):45763–45769.
83. Samuelsson B, Morgenstern R, Jakobsson PJ. Membrane prostaglandin E synthase-1: a novel therapeutic target. *Pharmacol Rev.* 2007;59(3):207–224.
84. Wang J, Limburg D, Carter J, Mbalaviele G, Gierse J, Vazquez M. Selective inducible microsomal prostaglandin E2 synthase-1 (mPGES-1) inhibitors derived from an oxicam template. *Bioorg Med Chem Lett.* 2010;20(5):1604–1609.
85. Altman R, Bosch B, Brune K, Patrignani P, Young C. Advances in NSAID development: evolution of diclofenac products using pharmaceutical technology. *Drugs.* 2015;75 (8):859–877.
86. Grosser T, Fries S, FitzGerald GA. Biological basis for the cardiovascular consequences of COX-2 inhibition: therapeutic challenges and opportunities. *J Clin Investig.* 2006;116 (1):4–15.
87. Gan TJ. Diclofenac: an update on its mechanism of action and safety profile. *Curr Med Res Opin.* 2010;26(7):1715–1731.
88. Pairet M, Engelhardt G. The preferential inhibition of COX-2 by meloxicam is highly dependent on the structure of the drug. *Rheumatol Eur.* 1995;24(Suppl. 3):D204.
89. Sano H, Hla T, Maier JA, et al. In vivo cyclooxygenase expression in synovial tissues of patients with rheumatoid arthritis and osteoarthritis and rats with adjuvant and streptococcal cell wall arthritis. *J Clin Investig.* 1992;89(1):97–108.
90. Engelhardt G, Homma D, Schlegel K, Utzmann R, Schnitzler C. Anti-inflammatory, analgesic, antipyretic and related properties of meloxicam, a new non-steroidal anti-inflammatory agent with favourable gastrointestinal tolerance. *Inflamm Res.* 1995;44(10):423–433.
91. Engelhardt G, Homma D, Schnitzler CH. Meloxicam: a potent inhibitor of adjuvant arthritis in the Lewis rat. *Inflamm Res.* 1995;44(12):548–555.
92. Schmidt M, Lamberts M, Olsen AM, et al. Cardiovascular safety of non-aspirin non-steroidal anti-inflammatory drugs: review and position paper by the working group for Cardiovascular Pharmacotherapy of the European Society of Cardiology. *Eur Heart J.* 2016;37(13):1015–1023.
93. Warner TD, Giuliano F, Vojnovic I, Bukasa A, Mitchell JA, Vane JR. Nonsteroid drug selectivities for cyclo-oxygenase-1 rather than cyclo-oxygenase-2 are associated with

human gastrointestinal toxicity: a full in vitro analysis. *Proc Natl Acad Sci*. 1999;96 (13):7563–7568.
94. Clemett D, Goa KL. Celecoxib: a review of its use in osteoarthritis, rheumatoid arthritis and acute pain. *Drugs*. 2000;59(4):957–980.
95. Fort J. Celecoxib, a COX-2--specific inhibitor: the clinical data. *Am J Orthoped (Belle Mead, NJ)*. 1999;28(3 Suppl.):13–18.
96. Davies NM, McLachlan AJ, Day RO, Williams KM. Clinical pharmacokinetics and pharmacodynamics of celecoxib. *Clin Pharmacokinet*. 2000;38(3):225–242.
97. Lanas A, Sopeña F. Nonsteroidal anti-inflammatory drugs and lower gastrointestinal complications. *Gastroenterol Clin*. 2009;38(2):333–352.
98. Lanas A. Clinical experience with cyclooxygenase-2 inhibitors. *Rheumatology (Oxf)*. 2002;41(Suppl. 1):16–22.
99. Bombardier C, Laine L, Reicin A, et al. Comparison of upper gastrointestinal toxicity of rofecoxib and naproxen in patients with rheumatoid arthritis. *N Engl J Med*. 2000;343:1520–1528.
100. Prasit P, Riendeau D, Chan CC. Discovery of Vioxx (rofecoxib). In: Vane JR and Botting RM, eds. *Therapeutic Roles of Selective COX-2 Inhibitors*; 2001:60–75.
101. Colanardi MC, Nettis E, Traetta P, Delle Donne P, Ferrannini A, Vacca A. Parecoxib as an alternative in COX-2 hypersensitivity. *Int J Immunopathol Pharmacol*. 2008;21 (1):233–235.
102. Botting R, Ayoub S, Colville-Nash P, Willoughby D. Analgesia with paracetamol: a peripheral or central action. *Pharmacologist*. 2002;44(2). Suppl. 1, A54 (Abstract).
103. Brune K. Prostaglandins and the mode of action of antipyretic analgesic drugs. *Am J Med*. 1983;75(5):19–23.
104. Woodbury DM, Fingl E. Analgesic-antipyretics, anti-inflammatory agents, and drugs employed in the therapy of gout. In: 5th ed. Goodman LS, Gilman A, eds. *The Pharmacological Basis of Therapeutics*. 5. New York: Macmillan Publishing Co. Inc.; 1975:325–358.
105. Roberts II LJ, Morrow JD. Analgesic-antipyretic and anti-inflammatory agents and drugs employed in the treatment of gout. In: Hardman JG, Limbird LE, eds. *The Pharmacological Basis of Therapeutics*. New York: McGraw Hill; 2001:687–732.
106. Botting RM. Mechanism of action of acetaminophen: is there a cyclooxygenase 3? *Clin Infect Dis*. 2000;31(Suppl. 5):S202–S210.
107. Flower RJ, Vane JR. Inhibition of prostaglandin synthetase in brain explains the antipyretic activity of paracetamol (4-acetamidophenol). *Nature*. 1972;240(5381):410–411.
108. Clark AR. Anti-inflammatory functions of glucocorticoid-induced genes. *Mol Cell Endocrinol*. 2007;275(1–2):79–97.
109. Couper KN, Blount DG, Riley EM. IL-10: the master regulator of immunity to infection. *J Immunol*. 2008;180(9):5771–5777.
110. Perretti M, D'acquisto F. Annexin A1 and glucocorticoids as effectors of the resolution of inflammation. *Nat Rev Immunol*. 2009;9(1):62–70.
111. Ayroldi E, Riccardi C. Glucocorticoid-induced leucine zipper (GILZ): a new important mediator of glucocorticoid action. *FASEB J*. 2009;23(11):3649–3658.
112. Hannon R, Croxtall JD, Getting SJ, et al. Aberrant inflammation and resistance to glucocorticoids in annexin $1^{-/-}$ mouse. *FASEB J*. 2003;17(2):253–255.
113. Scheinman RI, Cogswell PC, Lofquist AK, Baldwin AS. Role of transcriptional activation of IκBα in mediation of immunosuppression by glucocorticoids. *Science*. 1995;270 (5234):283–286.

114. Auphan N, DiDonato JA, Rosette C, Helmberg A, Karin M. Immunosuppression by glucocorticoids: inhibition of NF-κB activity through induction of IκB synthesis. *Science.* 1995;270(5234):286–290.
115. Wissink S, Van Heerde EC, Van der Burg B, Van der Saag PT. A dual mechanism mediates repression of NF-κB activity by glucocorticoids. *Mol Endocrinol.* 1998;12 (3):355–363.
116. Heck S, Bender K, Kullmann M, Göttlicher M, Herrlich P, Cato AC. IκBα-independent downregulation of NF-κB activity by glucocorticoid receptor. *EMBO J.* 1997;16 (15):4698–4707.
117. Ashwell JD, Lu FW, Vacchio MS. Glucocorticoids in T cell development and function. *Annu Rev Immunol.* 2000;18(1):309–345.
118. McEwen BS, Biron CA, Brunson KW, et al. The role of adrenocorticoids as modulators of immune function in health and disease: neural, endocrine and immune interactions. *Brain Res Rev.* 1997;23(1–2):79–133.
119. Fauci AS. Mechanisms of the immunosuppressive and anti-inflammatory effects of glucorcorticosteroids. *J Immunopharmacol.* 1978;1(1):1–25.
120. Coutinho AE, Chapman KE. The anti-inflammatory and immunosuppressive effects of glucocorticoids, recent developments and mechanistic insights. *Mol Cell Endocrinol.* 2011;335(1):2–13.
121. Simpson SA, Tait Jf, Von Euw J. Isolation from the adrenals of a new crystalline hormone with especially high effectiveness on mineral metabolism. *Experientia.* 1953;9 (9):333–335.
122. Marver D, Kokko JP. Renal target sites and the mechanism of action of aldosterone. *Miner Electrolyte Metab.* 1983;9(1):1–18.
123. Jaffe IZ, Mendelsohn ME. Angiotensin II and aldosterone regulate gene transcription via functional mineralocortocoid receptors in human coronary artery smooth muscle cells. *Circ Res.* 2005;96(6):643–650.
124. Derfoul A, Robertson NM, Lingrel JB, Hall DJ, Litwack G. Regulation of the human Na/K-ATPase β1 gene promoter by mineralocorticoid and glucocorticoid receptors. *J Biol Chem.* 1998;273(33):20702–20711.
125. Náray-Fejes-Tóth A, Fejes-Tóth G. The sgk, an aldosterone-induced gene in mineralocorticoid target cells, regulates the epithelial sodium channel. *Kidney Int.* 2000;57 (4):1290–1294.
126. Herrada AA, Campino C, Amador CA, Michea LF, Fardella CE, Kalergis AM. Aldosterone as a modulator of immunity: implications in the organ damage. *J Hypertension.* 2011;29(9):1684–1692.
127. Munoz-Durango N, Barake MF, Letelier NA, Campino C, Fardella CE, Kalergis AM. Immune system alterations by aldosterone during hypertension: from clinical observations to genomic and non-genomic mechanisms leading to vascular damage. *Curr Mol Med.* 2013;13(6):1035–1046.
128. Grafte-Faure S, Leveque C, Vasse M, Soria C, Norris V, Vannier JP. Effects of glucocorticoids and mineralocorticoids on proliferation and maturation of human peripheral blood stem cells. *Am J Hematol.* 1999;62(2):65–73.
129. Rossignol P, Ménard J, Fay R, Gustafsson F, Pitt B, Zannad F. Eplerenone survival benefits in heart failure patients post-myocardial infarction are independent from its diuretic and potassium-sparing effects: insights from an EPHESUS (Eplerenone Post-Acute Myocardial Infarction Heart Failure Efficacy and Survival Study) substudy. *J Am Coll Cardiol.* 2011;58(19):1958–1966.

130. Brilla CG, Weber KT. Mineralocorticoid excess, dietary sodium, and myocardial fibrosis. *J Lab Clin Med.* 1992;120(6):893–901.
131. Young MJ, Morgan J, Brolin K, Fuller PJ, Funder JW. Activation of mineralocorticoid receptors by exogenous glucocorticoids and the development of cardiovascular inflammatory responses in adrenalectomized rats. *Endocrinology.* 2010;151(6):2622–2628.
132. Hattori T, Murase T, Iwase E, et al. Glucocorticoid-induced hypertension and cardiac injury: effects of mineralocorticoid and glucocorticoid receptor antagonism. *Nagoya J Med Sci.* 2013;75(1–2):81.
133 Kim YK, Jung HG, Myint AM, Kim H, Park SH. Imbalance between pro-inflammatory and anti-inflammatory cytokines in bipolar disorder. *Journal of affective disorders.* 2007;104(1–3):91–95.
134. Krysiak R, Okopien B. The effect of treatment on monocyte and lymphocyte cytokine release in patients with aldosteronoma. *Hypertension Res.* 2012;35(1):123–125.
135. Irita J, Okura T, Manabe S, et al. Plasma osteopontin levels are higher in patients with primary aldosteronism than in patients with essential hypertension. *Am J Hypertension.* 2006;19(3):293–297.
136. Carvajal CA, Herrada AA, Castillo CR, et al. Primary aldosteronism can alter peripheral levels of transforming growth factor β and tumor necrosis factor α. *J Endocrinol Investig.* 2009;32(9):759–765.
137. Rossitto G, Regolisti G, Rossi E, et al. Elevation of angiotensin-II type-1-receptor autoantibodies titer in primary aldosteronism as a result of aldosterone-producing adenoma. *Hypertension.* 2013;61(2):526–533.
138. Kem DC, Li H, Yu X, Benbrook A, Cicala MV, Mantero F. AT1R activating autoantibodies occur in both aldosterone producing adenoma and idiopathic adrenal hyperplasia subgroups in primary aldosteronism. *Endocr Rev.* 2014;35(3).
139. Tripathi KD. *Corticosteroids, Essentials of Medical Pharmacology.* 7th ed. New Delhi; 2013:282–295.
140 Barik R, Sarkar R, Biswas P, et al. 5,7-dihydroxy-2-(3-hydroxy-4, 5-dimethoxy-phenyl)-chromen-4-one-a flavone from Bruguiera gymnorrhiza displaying anti-inflammatory properties. *Indian J Pharmacol.* 2016;48(3):304–311. Available from: https://doi.org/10.4103/0253-7613.182890.27298502.

Chapter 5

Insight into the mechanism of action of anti-diabetic drugs

Gayatri Thapa[1], Amrita Kumari[2], Debankini Dasgupta[3], Shwetlana Bandyopadhy[3], Nilanjan Sarkar[3], Kalyan Roy[4], Gauthaman Karunakaran[4], Imran Kazmi[5], Samit Karmakar[6] and Mainak Chakraborty[3]

[1]*Himalayan Pharmacy Institute, Rangpo, Sikkim, India,* [2]*Ranchi College of Pharmacy and Research Centre, Ranchi, Jharkhand, India,* [3]*Department of Pharmaceutical Technology, NSHM Knowledge campus Kolkata, Group of Institutions, Kolkata, West Bengal, India,* [4]*Government Pharmacy College, Gangtok, Sikkim, India,* [5]*Department of Biochemistry, Faculty of Science, King Abdulaziz University, Jeddah, Saudi Arabia,* [6]*Medical College Kolkata, Kolkata, West Bengal, India*

Introduction

Diabetes mellitus, a metabolic disorder in which a person has high blood glucose level, has become a matter of serious concern because of its worldwide prevalence. Depending upon the etiology, diabetes mellitus is of different types:

- Type 1 diabetes is insulin-dependent diabetes mellitus;
- Type 2 diabetes is non-insulin-dependent diabetes mellitus.
- Gestational diabetes is another type of diabetes that occurs during pregnancy. [1]

Biochemical background of diabetes mellitus

In the human body, glucose is the primary source of energy, which is required by the cell to function, which circulates in the blood as a source of mobilizable fuel for the cells. The release of insulin, a pancreatic hormone, maintains the blood glucose level in the body. The hormone binds to its receptor sites on the peripheral site of the cell membranes. It helps the entry of glucose into respiring cells and tissues via the requisite channels. Then the catabolic process takes place where the insulin converts the glucose into pyruvate through glycolysis. It also upregulates glycogenesis from excessive cytosolic glucose and lipogenesis from excessive cytosolic acetyl coenzyme A (acetyl-COA).

How Synthetic Drugs Work. DOI: https://doi.org/10.1016/B978-0-323-99855-0.00005-1

The hormone glucagon antagonizes these actions of insulin. Below threshold level, glucose remains in the systemic circulation instead of entering the cells. The body attempts to arrest hyperglycemia by drawing water out of the cells and into the bloodstream. The excess sugar is excreted through urine. Thus, diabetes is accompanied with constant thirst and polyuria as the cells try to get rid of the extra glucose, which ultimately leads to glucosuria. With the prolonged persistence of hyperglycemia, the body cells remain devoid of glucose because of the lack of insulin. This ultimately forces the cells to seek alternative mobilizable energy sources. At this point, the cells uptake the fatty acids stored in adipose tissue. The fats are not fuel source for the red blood cells, kidney cortex, and the brain because red blood cells lack mitochondria in which beta-oxidation pathway rests. Also, the fatty acids cannot pass through blood–brain barrier. To provide energy to such cells and tissues, the acetyl-CoA arising from catabolism of fatty acids is diverted to ketogenesis to generate ketone bodies, which can serve as alternative fuel sources for such cells and tissues. These ketone bodies are also passed through the urine, thereby leading to ketonuria, which characterizes diabetes mellitus. Build-up of ketone bodies in the blood produces ketosis.[2–9]

Classification of diabetes

Type 1 diabetes mellitus

β cells' destruction in the pancreas leads to the development of type 1 diabetes mellitus (T1DM), which accounts for approximately 10% of all patients with DM. There are two forms of T1DM. One is an immune-mediated disease with autoimmune markers such as islet cell antibodies, insulin autoantibodies, and autoantibodies to glutamic acid decarboxylase. As many as 85 – 90% of patients with fasting hyperglycemia are positive for one or more of these markers. Strong human leukocyte antigen (HLA) associations also exist.

A second form of T1DM, now called idiopathic diabetes, has no known cause. Only a minority of patients fall into this group.

Idiopathic diabetes is genetic disorder, but it lacks autoimmune markers and is not associated with HLA. Although it can occur at any age, T1DM. The rate of pancreatic destruction is variable and is generally more rapid in infants and children and slower in adults.[10] (Fig. 5.1)

Pathophysiology of type-1 diabetes

Type 2 diabetes mellitus

Type 2 diabetes mellitus (T2DM) is a metabolic disorder that occurs as a result of either insulin resistance and/or insulin deficiency.[11]

Excess calorie intake is also a major cause of metabolic disorder, which ultimately leads to abnormal insulin secretion or insulin resistance. To retain

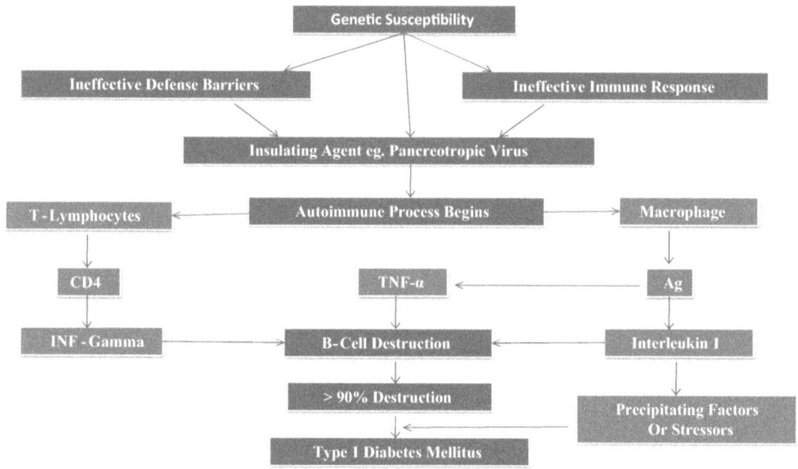

FIGURE 5.1 Pathophysiology of type-1 diabetes.

glucose homeostasis, the body demands insulin, and if pancreatic β-cells are unable or fail to secrete enough insulin to compensate the demand, the blood glucose level will be elevated gradually. Chronic hyperglycemia, which is strongly associated with long-term damage, dysfunction, and failure of different organs, especially the eyes, kidneys, nerves, heart, and blood vessels results in increasing levels of morbidity and mortality. Poor lifestyle, progressive reduction of physical activity, and changes of dietary habits are the primary factors leading to the development. The vast majority of patients with diabetes suffer from T2DM.[12]

Pathophysiology of Type 2 diabetes

Baynes.[13] (Fig. 5.2)

Other specific types of diabetes[14]

Genetic defects in insulin action

1. Type A insulin resistance
2. Leprechaunism
3. Rabson–Mendenhall syndrome
4. Lipoatrophic diabetes

Diseases of the exocrine pancreas

1. Pancreatitis
2. Trauma/pancreatectomy

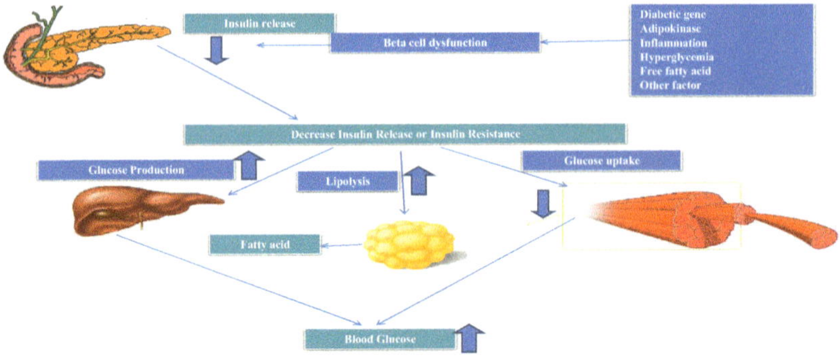

FIGURE 5.2 Pathophysiology of type-2 diabetes.

3. Neoplasia
4. Cystic fibrosis
5. Hemochromatosis
6. Fibrocalculous pancreatopathy
7. Others

Endocrinopathies

1. Acromegaly
2. Cushing's syndrome
3. Glucagonoma
4. Pheochromocytoma
5. Hyperthyroidism
6. Somatostatinoma
7. Aldosteronoma
8. Others

Drug or chemical-induced

1. Vacor
2. Pentamidine
3. Nicotinic acid
4. Glucocorticoids
5. Thyroid hormone
6. Diazoxide
7. Adrenergic agonists
8. Thiazides
9. Dilantin
10. Interferon
11. Others

Infections

1. Congenital rubella
2. Cytomegalovirus
3. Others

Uncommon forms of immune-mediated diabetes

1. "Stiff-man" syndrome
2. Anti-insulin receptor antibodies
3. Others

Other genetic syndromes sometimes associated with diabetes

1. Down's syndrome
2. Klinefelter's syndrome
3. Turner's syndrome
4. Wolfram's syndrome
5. Friedreich's ataxia
6. Huntington's chorea
7. Laurence–Moon–Biedl syndrome
8. Myotonic dystrophy
9. Porphyria
10. Prader–Willi syndrome
11. Others

Gestational diabetes mellitus

This condition occurs during pregnancy, and normalizes after parturition. Females who develop T1DM during pregnancy and females with undiagnosed asymptomatic T2DM that is discovered during gestational period are classified with gestational diabetes mellitus (GDM). This disorder has its onset in the third trimester of the pregnancy.[13] (Fig. 5.3)

Etiology

Genetic component

Genetic connection plays an important role in T2DM. Concordance among monozygotic twins is close to 100%, and about 25% of those with the disease have a family history of diabetes mellitus. Recently, genes discovered to be significantly associated with developing T2DM include *TCF7L2*, *PPARG*, *FTO*, *KCNJ11*, *NOTCH2*, *WFS1*, *CDKAL1*, *IGF2BP2*, *SLC30A8*, *JAZF1*, and *HHEX*. *KCNJ11* (potassium inwardly rectifying channel, subfamily J, member 11), encodes the islet adenosine triphosphate (ATP)-sensitive potassium channel Kir6.2, and *TCF7L2* (transcription factor 7-like 2)

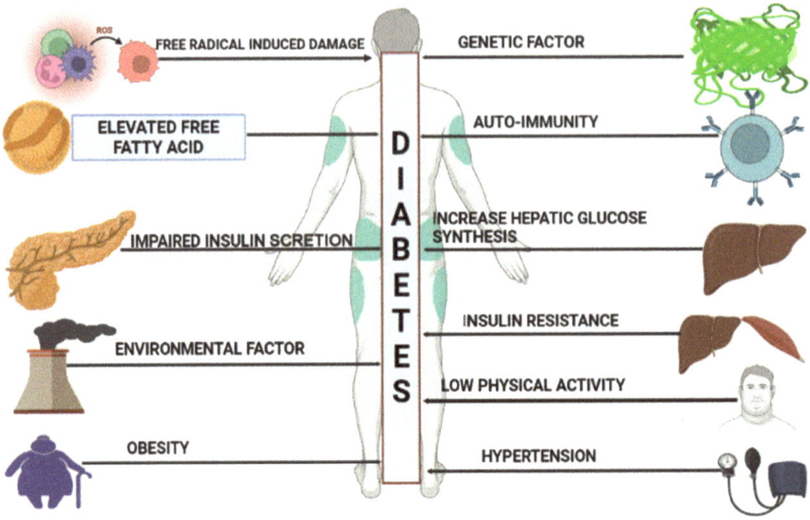

FIGURE 5.3 Etiology of diabetes.

regulates proglucagon gene expression and thus the production of glucagon-like peptide-1.[15]

Susceptibility loci

In addition to a considerable number of genetic components associated with T2DM, segregation analysis also suggests the polygenic nature of T2DM. Numerous genome-wide association studies conducted in different countries and ethnic groups have reported linkage signals at the same or different chromosomes with T2DM and have successfully identified approximately 75 susceptibility loci related to T2DM.[16]

Obesity and Physical Inactivity

A strong correlation exists between lifestyle and diabetes mellitus. Lifestyle-related factors plays an important role in the development of T2DM, such as sedentary lifestyle, physical inactivity, smoking, and alcohol consumption.

Development of T2DM diet is also considered to be a risk factor. Studies have shown that a low-fiber diet with a high glycemic index is positively associated with a higher risk of T2DM, and specific dietary fatty acids may affect insulin resistance and the risk of diabetes in varying degrees.[16]

Insulin resistance

An increase in free fatty acid (FFA) concentration has important physiological consequences of T2DM. During pregnancy, FFA level is increased, which induces insulin resistance, and glucose is conserved for the developing fetus. Thus, FFA plays both physiological and pathological role in the body. Excess amount of FFA in blood may cause serious metabolic syndrome. More than 80% of people with T2DM are obese and insulin resistant. Obesity and insulin resistance may be linked with some mediators including FFA, tumor necrosis factor-α (TNF-α), leptin, and adiponectin. Adipocytes are considered to be a site of insulin resistance. Insulin resistance leads to lipolysis and increased concentration of circulating FFA and development of insulin resistance in skeletal muscles and liver. Thus, there is a strong association between increased plasma FFA, intra-myocellular lipid accumulation, and insulin resistance.[17]

Oxidative stress in diabetes mellitus

Oxidative stress plays an important role in the development of vascular complications mainly in T2DM. Reactive oxygen species (ROS) level elevates in diabetes because of decrease in destruction and increase in the production of enzymatic and non-enzymatic antioxidant defense system, for example, catalase (enzymatic/non-enzymatic, superoxide dismutase, and glutathione peroxidase GSH−Px). The alteration in the level of these enzymes makes the tissues susceptible to oxidative stress, leading to the development of diabetic complications. According to epidemiological studies, diabetic mortalities can be explained notably by an increase in vascular diseases other than hyperglycemia.

Pathophysiology of oxidative stress in diabetes

Scientific evidence supports the role of oxidative stress in the pathogenesis of both types of diabetes. Generation of free radicals in diabetes by non-enzymatic glycation of proteins, glucose oxidation, and increase in lipid peroxidation lead to damage of enzymes and cellular machinery, as well as increase insulin resistance because of oxidative stress. According to the latest research, lipid is the apolipoprotein component of low-density lipoprotein (LDL) that forms insoluble aggregates oxidatively because of hydroxyl radical-induced cross-linkage between apo-B monomers responsible for oxidative damage in diabetic complications. For a diabetes mellitus patient, the main source of free radicals is oxidative stress in mitochondria. During this process, a component of the used oxygen is reduced to water, and the remaining oxygen is transformed to oxygen free radical (O.), which is an important ROS that is converted to other RSs such as $ONOO^-$, OH, and H_2O_2. Insulin signaling is modulated by ROS/reactive nitrogen species (RNS) in two ways. In response to insulin, the ROS/RNS are produced to exert its full physiological function and the ROS and RNS have got negative regulation on insulin signaling, interpreting them to the development of insulin resistance.[18]

The metabolic syndrome (MetS) is a major and escalating public health and clinical challenge worldwide and is caused by surplus energy intake, increasing obesity, and sedentary life habits. MetS confers a fivefold increase in the risk of T2DM and twofold the risk of development of cardiovascular diseases. Patients with the MetS are at two- to fourfold increased risk of cerebrovascular accident, a three- to fourfold increased risk of myocardial infarction, and twofold the risk of death as compared to those without the syndrome regardless of a previous history of cardiovascular events. MetS is considered to be the first-order risk factor for atherothrombotic complications.[19] (Table 5.1)

β-cell demise and dysfunction

β-cell destruction or dysfunction occurs because of cytokine-induced inflammation, obesity, insulin resistance, and overconsumption of saturated fat and FFAs. A progressive decline or destruction of β-cell, leads to β-cell exhaustion and precedes β-cell demise. Loss of β-cell mass and function are central to the development of both types of diabetes.[20]

Classification of antidiabetic drugs

TABLE 5.1 Classification of anti-diabetic drugs and their probable mechanism of action.

Nature of treatment	Drugs	Mechanism of actions
Oral class		
Sulfonylureas	Glimepiride Glipizide Glyburide	K_{ATP} – Channel blockers. Enhance insulin secretion.
Biguanides	Metformin	AMPK activator. Decreased hepatic glucose metabolism
Meglitinide/ Phenylalanine	Repaglinide Nateglinide	K_{ATP} – Channel blockers. Short lasting insulinemic action.
α- Glucosidase inhibitors	Acarbose Miglitol Voglibose	Decrease GI glucose absorption.
Dipeptidyl peptidase-4 inhibitors	Sitagliptin Alogliptin Linagliptin, Vildagliptin.	Prolong and potentiate the action of GLP-1.
Thiazolidindiones	Pioglitazone Rosiglitazone troglitazone	PPARγ (Peroxisome proliferator-activated receptor gamma) activators Decrease insulin resistance Increase glucose utilization.

(Continued)

TABLE 5.1 (Continued)

Nature of treatment	Drugs	Mechanism of actions
Dopamine (D_2) receptor agonist	Bromocriptine	Increases renal glucose excretion.
SGLT-2 inhibitors	Dapagliflozine Canagliflozin Empagliflozin	Reduce insulin resistance by acting on hypothalamic dopaminergic control of the circadian rhythm of hormone. Lower HbA_{1c} level.
Parenteral drugs		
Insulin	Regular insulin Lispro Aspart Glargine Degludec	Increases glucose utilization, decreases hepatic glucose production, and other anabolic actions
GLP-1R (glucagon-like peptide-1 receptor) agonists	Liraglutide Albiglutide Semaglutide Exenatide	Increase insulin, decrease glucagon, slow gastric emptying, satiety.
Amylin agonist	Pramlintide	Slow gastric emptying, decreases glucagon
Other treatment		
Medical nutrition therapy and physical activity	Diabetic diet	Decrease insulin resistance, increase insulin secretion.
Inhaled insulin	Afrezza (insulin regular human)	Increases glucose utilization, decreases hepatic glucose production, and other anabolic actions

Sulfonylureas

Sulfonylureas (SUs) stimulate the quick release of insulin from pancreas at any concentration of glucose by binding to a specific site on the β-cell K_{ATP} channel complex. The binding of SU causes the inhibition of the K_{ATP} channel, which leads to depolarization of the cell membrane and a series of events that follow insulin secretion. In this event, SU inhibits the sulfonylurea receptor (SUR), which is a subunit of ATP-sensitive K^+ channel in the pancreatic β-cell membrane. Normally, at a hyperpolarized state, insulin is not secreted, but when there is plasma glucose elevation, glucose enters the cell and because of enhanced glucose metabolism, cellular ATP increases. This causes the decrease in the K^+ conductance followed by depolarization brought about by the activation of Na^+ and Ca^+ channels. Ca^+ augmentation causes the vesicular insulin present inside the membrane to be released by exocytosis.[21] The exocytosis can be enhanced by the activation of cAMP pathway where elevated cAMP leads to inhibition of the K_{ATP} channel. SU, therefore, acts on this particular SUR-1 and blocks them, further inhibiting the hyperpolarization and facilitating the depolarization of the pancreatic β-cell membrane to augment the release of insulin. It is also mediated by Ca^{2+}/calmodulin-dependent protein kinase II (CaMK II).[22] These enzyme phosphorylates proteins such as synapsin-I, microtubule-associated protein (MAP-2), soluble NSF (N-ethylmaleimide-sensitive furoin protein), attachment protein, i.e., SNAP, vesicle-associated membrane protein, and other unknown components that regulate the SNAP receptor/fusion protein complex. Critically, the regulation of the interaction between the granules and the cytoskeleton is presumed to be via CaMKII-dependent phosphorylation of synapsin-I.[23] SU causes the brisk release of insulin at any concentration of glucose, which develops the risk of precipitating untoward hypoglycemia if the glucose level is low. In T2DM, the kinetics of insulin release in response to glucose or meals is delayed and subdued. The SUs primarily augment the second-phase insulin secretion with little effect on the first phase.[24] The SUR subunit (SUR-1), expressed in glucose-responsive neurons of the hypothalamus and pancreatic cells, is an ATP-binding cassette protein or transport ATPase. It houses about 17 different transmembrane domains (TMD) and two nucleotide-binding folds (NBF). Each of them is constituted by a Walker motif A and B. They are the specific binding sites of (Mg^{2+}) ADP/ATP[25–27] Another SUR subunit, i.e., the KIR6.2 subunits have two TMDs, and they also contribute to the conduction of K^+. SUR2A/B are the variants of the SUR2A gene, and this gene is expressed mainly in cardiac/skeletal muscle cells, whereas SUR2B is expressed in vascular/nonvascular smooth muscle cells. K-channel openers (KCO) bind to SURs at the TMDs 12–17, which surround the central core region of the drug-like tolbutamide-binding site.[28] SURs are responsible for defining the sensitivity of the K_{ATP} complexes with TMDs for its sensitivity toward both SUs and KCOs with SUR1 mediating high sensitivity for SUs and low sensitivity toward KCOs and vice versa, SUR2A/2B mediating low sensitivity for SUs and high sensitivity for KCOs. The cooperative interactions between NBFs 1 and 2 of SUR1 in the open state of the K_{ATP} are disrupted by the conformational change induced by the binding of SUs, for example, glibenclamide embodies TMDs 1–5. This conformational change repositions TMD 2 of KIR6.2, because it is closely associated with TMD 1–5 of SUR1. Thus, SU binding to SUR1 apparently induces an association between SUR1 and KIR6.2, which is required for keeping KIR6.2 in a (partly) open state. Binding of ATP to KIR6.2 facilitates and/or stabilizes the glibenclamide-induced relative dissociation of SUR1 and KIR6.2. Thus, ATP-binding favors the closed state of the K_{ATP}.[29]

Effect of amaryl in adipose cells: regulation of key metabolic proteins/enzymes

Phosphorylation of GLUT4 is a potential mechanism for regulation of the distribution of GLUT4 between the plasma membrane and the intracellular GLUT4 vesicles. Amaryl activates either serine or more specifically threonine-related protein phosphatase, which dephosphorylates GLUT4. The dephosphorylation may reduce the internalization rate of GLUT4. The impaired internalization, in conjunction with the constitutive externalization of GLUT4 even in the absence of insulin, ultimately will lead to a net flux of GLUT4 molecules from the intracellular GLUT4 vesicles to the plasma membrane. The Amaryl-induced GLUT4 dephosphorylation and, in consequence, translocation may be particularly prominent in insulin-resistant adipocytes because of their high content of phosphorylated GLUT4.[30–32] (Figs 5.4–5.6)

Biguanides

As compared to SUs, the occurrence of hypoglycemia with metformin, which is the only member of the biguanide for use today, is rare in diabetic patients. Phenformin and buformin were also there in market, but because of high risk of lactic acidosis, it was withdrawn from the market during the 1970s. Metformin effectively reduces the production of hepatic glucose, which significantly suppresses the gluconeogenesis. Metformin possesses the property to reduce the mitochondrial respiration, which causes the number of

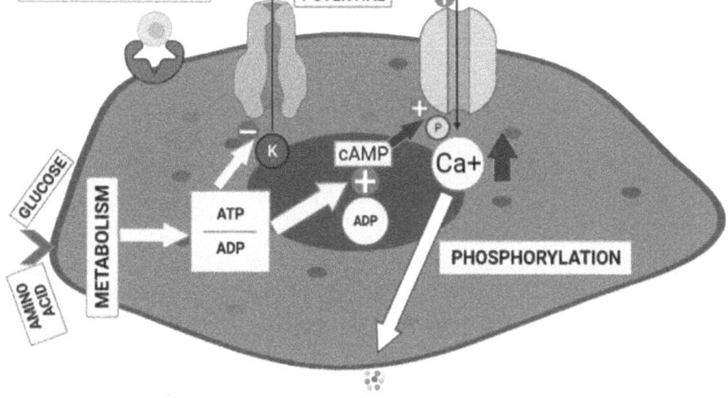

FIGURE 5.4 Depiction of SUR, K_{ATP}-channel, and voltage-gated Ca^{2+} channel in the β-cell. Binding of SU to its receptor closes the K^+ channel because glucose metabolism increases ATP: ADP ratio, which causes the ATP to bind to its specific site and inhibit the entry of K^+. This leads the cell to be in a depolarized state that opens voltage-gated calcium channel. Increase in intracellular calcium triggers exocytosis and release of insulin occurs.

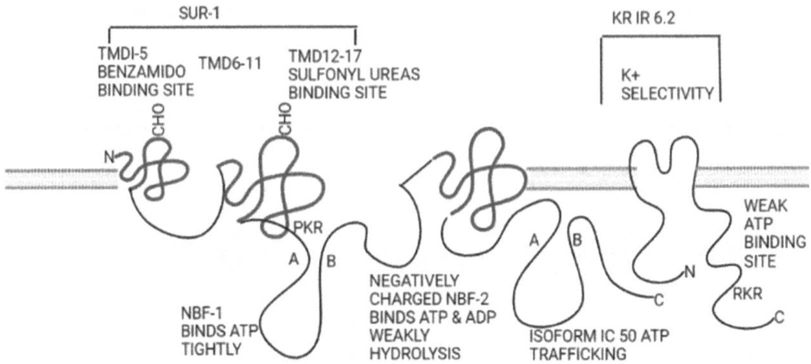

FIGURE 5.5 Properties of K_{ATP} and features of SUR and KIR6.2.

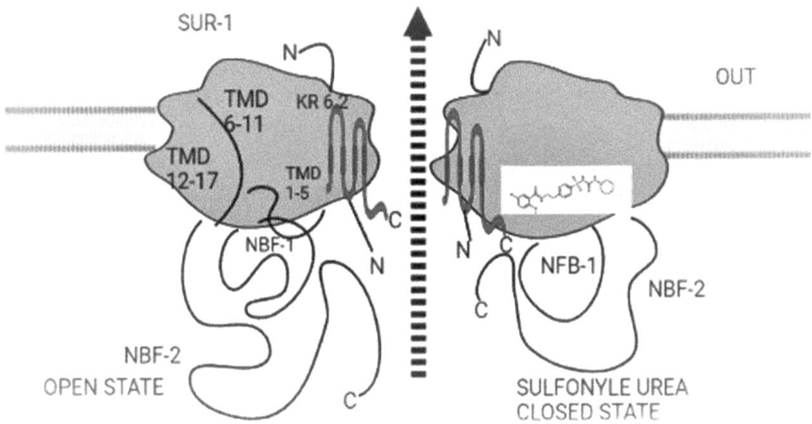

FIGURE 5.6 Theoretical model depicting open and closed state of K_{ATP} channel.

ATP molecules to decrease but AMP molecules to increase. It has been observed recently that metformin causes activation of AMP-dependent protein kinase (AMPK) because of which various actions of metformin are mediated, for example, the elevation of fatty acid oxidation in the liver and decreased lipogenesis in adipose tissues, glucose uptake by skeletal muscles, promotion of peripheral glucose utilization. Metformin interferes with the mitochondrial enzyme, glycerol phosphate dehydrogenase, which changes the redox state of the cell. Recent mechanism observed for metformin includes diminishing the effect of glucagon. This mechanism is thought to be because of the inhibition of conversion of lactate and glycerol to glucose and improving the lipid balance in the liver by reducing the lipid level. In the normal individual whose plasma glucose level is normal, metformin has relatively low effect on blood glucose. Therefore, it does not have a direct effect on pancreatic cells or other hormones for releasing the insulin. This is the reason why hypoglycemia is uncommon with metformin administration. However, if an individual is mildly hyperglycemic, then metformin will definitely lower the blood glucose level. It is due to the reduction of hepatic glucose production and uptake of glucose.[33]

Metformin

The inhibition of gluconeogenesis may also be due to the effects on pyruvate carboxylase and other enzymes, which also accompany the mild mitochondrial inhibition and this effect is ATP-/ADP-/AMP-independent.[34,35] Lactic acidosis is rare with metformin because mitochondrial inhibition due to metformin is a self-limiting process as it depends on the condition of mitochondria being active.[36]

LKB1–AMPK-dependent pathway is a key molecular effector of metformin. Metformin has a signal transduction effect on 5'-AMPK. AMPK has the ability to sense the change in cellular energy and regulate homeostasis of energy. AMPK becomes active whenever there is increase in cellular ADP:ATP and/or AMP:ATP ratios either by decreasing the catabolic production of ATP (e.g., via nutrient deprivation and exposure to mitochondrial toxins) or by promoting ATP consumption (e.g., by muscle contraction). The activation of downstream processes led by AMPK activation (e.g., promotion of glucose uptake and fatty acid oxidation in muscle and inhibition of lipid synthesis in the liver) elevates the therapeutic effects of metformin.[37] The stimulation of AMPK by metformin is in close relation with the inhibition of glucose production. Metformin also decreases the levels of sterol regulatory element-binding protein-1 (SREBP-1), which is an important transcriptor factor in lipogenesis.[38] It is to be noted that AMPK is indirectly activated by metformin. The activation of AMPK takes place when there is an increase in AMP:ATP and ADP:ATP ratios. This has been concluded in one of the studies where the cell line considered expressed AMPK complexes having Arg531.[39] This complex was insensitive to the effects of ADP and AMP on phosphorylation. This proves that the metformin acts indirectly and not by direct phosphorylation.[33]

Metformin and organic cation transporters

Instead of metabolizing, metformin is excreted in the urine and bile in an unchanged form. The active transport of metformin takes place by important organic cation transporters. Although metformin exerts its major effect through inhibition of hepatic glucose production, enhanced glucose disposal has also been described. This is because metformin promotes glucose transport independent of the insulin receptor-mediated proximal signaling pathway in skeletal muscle. In spite the fact that metformin may accumulate in skeletal muscle and tissues over longer periods of time to bring about some effects, the potent and preferential effects of metformin in the liver can be explained by the fact that the drug is supplied directly from the gut by the portal vein, which means that an immense concentration of rally taken metformin reaches the liver than other peripheral organs/tissues. Also, because of the high level of OCT1 (Organic Cation transporter-1) expression, it actively transports metformin to its site of action, in hepatocytes.[40–42]

The fact that metformin suppresses the hepatic gluconeogenesis is because mitochondrial inhibition is widely accepted,[21] but the most recent mouse genetic studies indicate that suppression of gluconeogenesis depends more directly on the mitochondrial respiration and/or on AMPK-independent cellular responses to reductions in ATP availability, such as the recently described effects on cAMP-PKA signaling. In addition, it should be noted that AMPK might play a key role in long-term effects of metformin by improving lipid metabolism and mitochondrial function in the liver. The glycemic response to metformin is highly variable, even after controlling for differences in adherence to medication.[33] (Fig. 5.7)

K_{ATP} channel modulators (nonsulfonyl ureas): meglitinides

Repaglinide

Insulin release is promoted by repaglinide when taken orally. It exhibits its action in a way similar to SUs by inhibiting ATP-sensitive K^+ channel.[43] Its advantage is that it is well absorbed orally and attains high plasma level within 1 h, which then normalizes the meal time glucose fluctuation. Metabolism of repaglinide takes place in the liver with the help of CYP3A4 enzyme. Small amount of drug is also metabolized by the kidney, so it is to be noted that this drug should be dosed carefully in renal insufficient patients. Hypoglycemia is a major drawback of repaglinide. Certain drugs may potentiate the action of repaglinide by displacing it from plasma protein-binding sites (β blockers, chloramphenicol, coumarin, Monoamine oxidase inhibitors, non-steroidal anti-inflammatory drugs, probenecid, salicylates, and sulfonamide) or altering its metabolism (gemfibrozil, itraconazole, trimethoprim, cyclosporine, simvastatin, clarithromycin).[21]

α-Glucosidase inhibitors

α-Glucosidase inhibitors like acarbose reversibly inhibit α-Glucosidase, an enzyme that causes the digestion of carbohydrates in the small intestine.

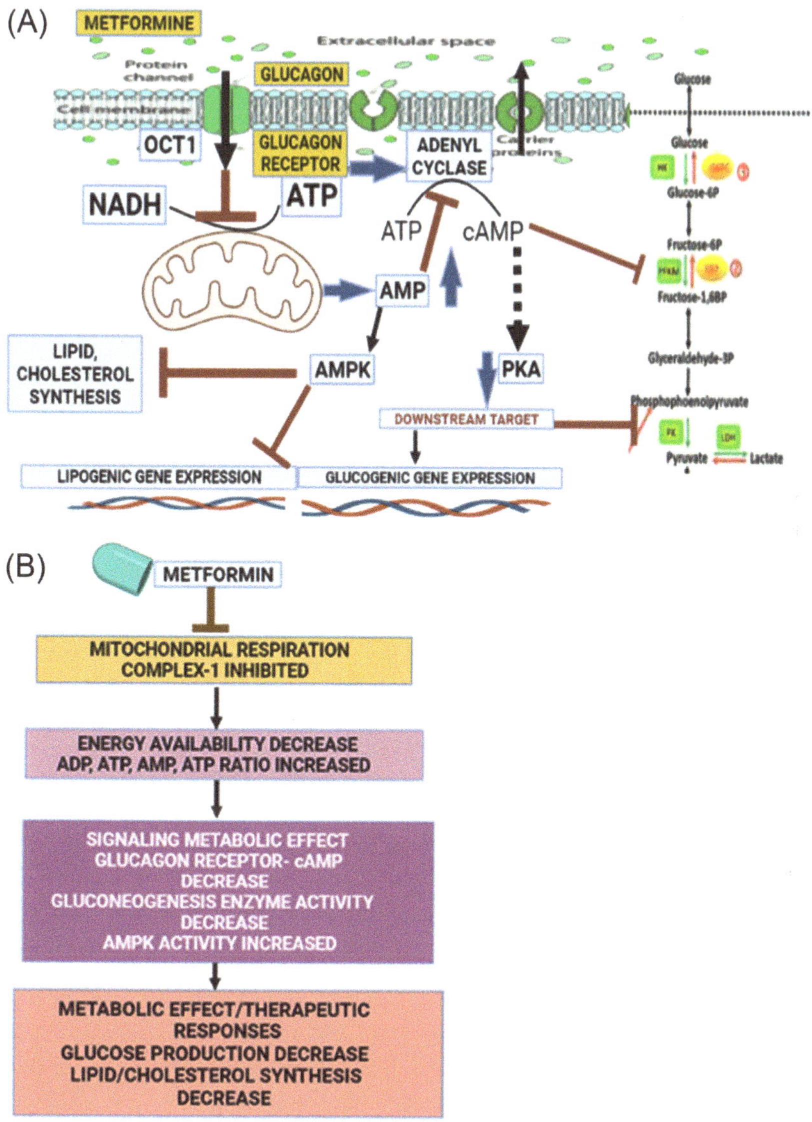

FIGURE 5.7 (A, B) Schematic diagram of the anti-hyperglycemic action of metformin on the liver cell. Part (B) shows a simplified version of (A). Metformin is transported into hepatocytes mainly via OCT1, resulting in an inhibition of the mitochondrial respiratory chain (complex I) through a currently unknown mechanism(s). The resulting deficit in energy production is balanced by reducing the consumption of energy in the cell, particularly reduced gluconeogenesis in the liver. This is mediated mainly in two ways. First, a decrease in ATP and a concomitant increase in AMP concentration occur, which is thought to contribute to the inhibition of gluconeogenesis directly (because of the energy/ATP deficit). Second, increased AMP levels function as a key signaling mediator that has been proposed to (1) allosterically inhibit cAMP−PKA signaling through suppression of adenylate cyclase, (2) allosterically inhibit FBPase, a key of gluconeogenic, and (3) activate AMPK. This leads to inhibition of gluconeogenesis (1 and 2) and lipid/cholesterol synthesis (3), which may contribute to the longer term metabolic and therapeutic responses to the drug. FBPase; fructose-1,6-bisphophatase.

Therefore, α-Glucosidase inhibitors slower down the rate of digestion and absorption of carbohydrates from the brush border of small intestine mucosa.[44] The additional effect of the drug is to facilitate the release of the glucoregulatory hormone glucagon-like peptide (GLP-1) into the circulation, which may be responsible for lowering the glucose level. The drugs in this class are acarbose, miglitol, and voglibose (not available in the U.S.).[21]

Dipeptidyl peptidase-4 inhibitors

Dipeptidyl peptidase-4 (DPP-4) is widely distributed throughout the body. It is a serine protease found on vascular endothelial cells as an ectoenzyme, on the surface of T lymphocytes, and in a circulating form. The structural change in the DPP-4 inactivates GLP-1 and glucose-dependent insulinotropic polypeptide (GIP) and reduces the insulin secretion in T2DM patients. The drugs available in the U.S. such as sitagliptin, saxagliptin, linagliptin, and alogliptin, and vildagliptin in the E. U. inhibits this DPP-4 enzyme. Alogliptin, linagliptin, and sitagliptin are competitive inhibitors of DPP-4; vildagliptin and saxagliptin bind the enzyme covalently. All five drugs can be given in doses that lower measurable activity of DPP-4 by more than 95% for 12 h. This causes a greater than twofold elevation of plasma concentrations of active GIP and GLP-1 and is associated with increased insulin secretion, reduced glucagon levels, and improvements in both fasting and postprandial hyperglycemia. Inhibition of DPP-4 does not appear to have direct effects on insulin sensitivity, gastric motility, or satiety; chronic treatment with a DPP-4 inhibitor also does not affect body weight. DPP-4 inhibitors, used as monotherapy in T2DM patients, reduce A1c levels by an average of about 0.8%.[21]

Mechanism of action

DPP-4 inhibition is a glucose-lowering treatment for T2DM. The classical mechanism for DPP-4 inhibitors is that they inhibit DPP-4 activity in peripheral plasma, which prevents the inactivation of the incretin hormone GLP-1 in the peripheral circulation. This in turn increases circulating intact GLP-1, which results in stimulated insulin secretion and inhibited glucagon secretion. This leads to increased glucose utilization and diminished hepatic glucose production. This brings about the reduction in the postprandial glucose level and reduces HbA1c. However, additional non-classical pleotropic mechanisms of DPP-4 inhibitors have recently been discovered, and it is confirmed that DPP-4 inhibition can reduce hyperglycemia and increase insulin secretion by a mechanism independent of inhibition of DPP-4 activity in peripheral plasma.[45]

Dipeptidyl peptidase-4 inhibition in the gut

The first mechanism is that DPP-4 inhibitors (e.g., sitagliptin) inhibit the action of DPP-4 in the gut (duodenum, jejunum, ileum) where DPP-4 is localized to capillaries, which are in close association with the entero-endocrine cells and the nerve endings in the enteric autonomic nervous system. Inhibition of gut DPP-4 activity thus prevents the inactivation of intact GLP-1 immediately after its release from the L-cells, which raises the active form of the hormone in the tissue level. This in turn may activate the autonomic nerves as well as result in increased portal GLP-1 levels to augment the activation of portal GLP-1 receptors. Therefore, sitagliptin at low doses inhibits DPP-4 in the intestine compartment, which prevents the inactivation of GLP-1 immediately after its release from the L-cells, rather than having an effect on inactivation of GLP-1 in the peripheral circulation by inhibiting DPP-4 activity in peripheral plasma. This will eventually reduce the blood glucose level without inhibiting the circulating peripheral plasma DPP-4 activity.[46]

The second mechanism that contributes the lowering of the glucose level involves inhibition of DPP-4 activity in the islet, which prevents inactivation of locally produced intact GLP-1 in the islets, thereby augmenting insulin secretion and inhibiting glucagon secretion and possibly preventing islet inflammation. There is accumulating evidence that GLP-1 is expressed in islets, which is not surprising considering its coding in the proglucagon sequence in a-cells. It has, however, been thought that proglucagon is processed to glucagon in a-cells because of cell-specific expression of the processing enzymes prohormone convertase. Marchetti et al.[47] recently demonstrated in human islets that GLP-1 may also be expressed in a-cells. It has also been shown that under certain conditions, such as high glucose, GLP-1 production is increased in a-cells because of a specific overexpression of prohormone convertase 1/3. Therefore, in subjects with diabetes, there is a possibility that GLP-1 is produced in islets to such a degree that it will be of relevance after DPP-4 inhibition. This assumption has become even more likely because of accumulating evidence that DPP-4 is also expressed in islets. In line with these observations, Shah et al.[48] recently showed that long term incubation of isolated human islets with high glucose, palmitate, and cytokines increases apoptosis and impairs insulin secretion and that the DPP-4 inhibitor linagliptin prevents this by stabilizing and increasing GLP-1 secretion along with inhibited islet DPP-4 activity. These findings therefore suggest that a local islet mechanism may contribute to the increased insulin secretion during DPP-4 inhibition. A local islet effect may also have anti-inflammatory effects, which may be of importance since local islet inflammation may contribute to the development of b-cell deterioration in T2DM. This may be caused by cytokines released from infiltrating immune cells. An additional mechanism may be that hyperglycemia may cause a secretion of interleukin-1b from b-cells. A recent study by Dobrian et al. reported that sitagliptin reduces expression of inflammatory cytokines in islets from dietary-induced obesity in mice.[49] We also found recently that chronic treatment of high-fat–fed mice with vildagliptin prevented fat-induced pancreatic inflammation and peri-insulitis. This may be mediated by the two incretin hormones since it has been shown that treatment of splenic T-cells with both GLP-1 and GIP diminishes pancreatic infiltration of T-cells after splenic T-cells are injected into nonobese diabetic mice. Hence, in addition to stimulating insulin secretion and inhibiting glucagon secretion through preventing GLP-1 inactivation in islets, DPP-4 inhibition may also prevent islet inflammation as a mechanism for improving islet function.[50]

The third mechanism involves the prevention of the inactivation of other bioactive peptides apart from GLP-1, such as GIP, stromal-derived factor-1a, and pituitary adenylate cyclase-activating polypeptide, which may improve islet function.[51]

Recent studies have suggested that there are islet-independent glycemic effects of GLP-1 mediated by the hepatic portal system. Infusion of GLP-1 was found to reduce hepatic glucose production independent of changes in insulin or glucagon levels. The local prevention of GLP-1 inactivation by DPP-4 inhibition in the gut and hepatic portal system may increase portal GLP-1 levels, allowing for such a direct effect of GLP-1 to suppress hepatic glucose output through activating portal GLP-1 receptors, which is also evident from several experimental studies. Indeed, there is a higher increase in circulating levels of intact GLP-1 in the portal vein than in the peripheral circulation. Altogether, these findings suggest that DPP-4 inhibition may increase portal GLP-1 levels, which reduces hepatic glucose output and increases peripheral glucose utilization by islet hormone–independent mechanisms. Therefore, these pleiotropic effects may contribute to the effects of DPP-4 inhibition.[45]

Thiazolidinediones

Thiazolidinediones are ligands for the PPARγ receptor, a nuclear hormone receptor that has two isoforms and is involved in the regulation of genes related to glucose and lipid metabolism. Two thiazolidinediones are currently available to treat patients with T2DM, rosiglitazone, and pioglitazone; a third, troglitazone, was removed from the market in 2000 due to hepatotoxicity.[21]

Mechanism of action

Thiazolidinediones activate peroxisomal proliferator-activated receptor gamma (PPAR)γ receptors, which are expressed primarily in adipose tissue with lesser expression in cardiac, skeletal, and smooth muscle cells, islet β-cells, macrophages, and vascular endothelial cells. The endogenous ligands for PPARγ include small lipophilic molecules such as oxidized linoleic acid, arachidonic acid, and the prostaglandin metabolite. Ligand binding to PPARγ causes heterodimer formation with the retinoid X receptor and interaction with PPAR response elements on specific genes. The principal response to PPARγ activation is adipocyte differentiation.[52–54] PPARγ activity also promotes uptake of circulating fatty acids into fat cells and shifts of lipid stores from extra-adipose sites to adipose tissue. One consequence of the cellular responses to PPARγ activation is increased tissue sensitivity to insulin. Pioglitazone and rosiglitazone are insulin sensitizers and increase insulin-mediated glucose uptake by 30%–50% in patients with T2DM. Although adipose tissue seems to be the primary target for PPARγ agonists, both clinical and preclinical models support a role for skeletal muscle, the major site for insulin-mediated glucose disposal, in the response to thiazolidinediones. In addition to promoting glucose uptake into muscle and adipose tissue, the thiazolidinediones reduce HGP (hepatic glucose production) and increase hepatic glucose uptake. It is not clear whether thiazolidinedione-induced improvement of insulin resistance is due to direct effects on key target tissues (skeletal muscle and liver), indirect effects mediated by secreted products of adipocytes (e.g., adiponectin), or some combination of these. Thiazolidinediones also affect lipid metabolism. Treatment with rosiglitazone or pioglitazone reduces plasma levels of fatty acids by increasing clearance and reducing lipolysis. These drugs also cause a shift of triglyceride stores from non-adipose to adipose tissues and from visceral to subcutaneous fat depots. Pioglitazone reduces plasma triglycerides by 10%–15%, raises high-density lipoprotein cholesterol levels, and increases LDL cholesterol. In contrast, rosiglitazone has minimal effects on plasma triglycerides, and the only consistent effect on circulating lipids is an increase of LDL cholesterol.[55]

Thiazolidindiones can reduce the hyperglycemic state by 40 mg/dL. Thiazolidinediones reduce insulin resistance associated with nondiabetic conditions such as obesity. PPARγ is a transcription factor that regulates the expression of specific genes of fat cells. This drug primarily acts on the adipose tissue as PPARγ is enormously expressed there. It binds and activates the PPARγ. It is a nuclear receptor that acts as transcription factor upon activation by regulating the transcription and expression of specific genes. There are endogenous ligands of PPARγ such as unsaturated fatty acids and specific prostanoid, which activates the PPARγ and causes heterodimerization with the retinoid X receptor. This leads to the binding of the activated complex resulted from heterodimerization to the specific DNA segments to induce transcription of PPAR- responsive elements (PPRE). Thus, thiazolidinedione also expresses the number of adipocyte-specific genes (lipoprotein lipase, fatty-acid binding protein, glucose FFA, GLUT4, etc.), which concludes that the activation or expression of PPARγ is associated with adipogenic differentiation. Thiazolidinediones selectively stimulate the lipogenic activities in fat cells that results in greater insulin suppression of lipolysis. This would leave less FFAs available for other tissues. Thus, insulin desensitizing effects of FFAs in muscle and liver would be reduced as a result of thiazolidinedione treatment. This is known as "fatty acid steal phenomenon." Thiazolidinediones also alter the expression and release of adipocytokines. It also reduces resistin, leptin, and TNFα which have potential in decreasing insulin sensitivity.[55,56] (Figs. 5.8 and 5.9)

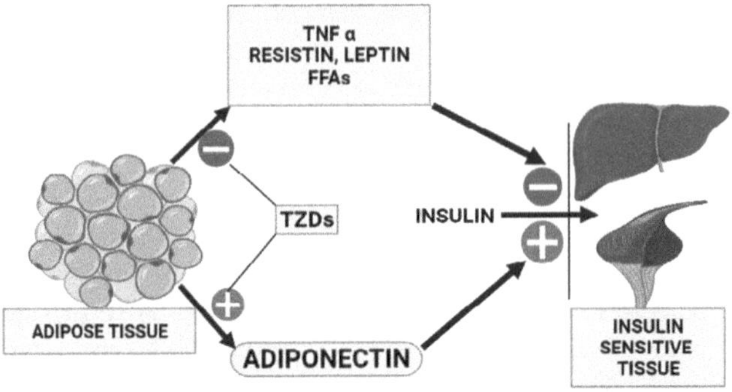

FIGURE 5.8 Interference of thiazolidinediones with factors released from adipose tissue (see text for details).

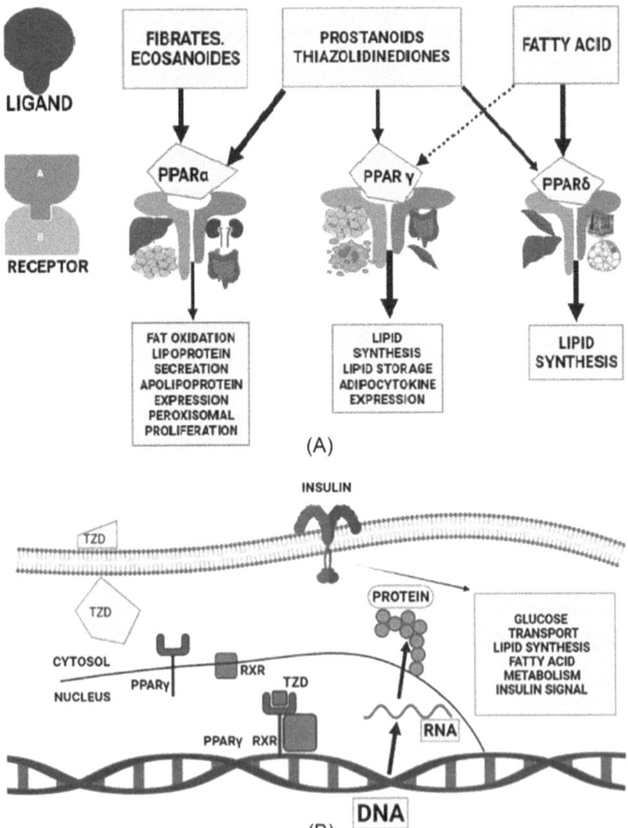

FIGURE 5.9 *Family of PPARs and ligand specificity.* Font size reflects expression levels in specific tissues. *Cellular mechanism of action of thiazolidinediones. Ins,* Insulin; *IR,* insulin receptor; *RXR,* retinoid X receptor; *TZD,* thiazolidinedione; see text for details.

Bromocriptine

It is a dopamine (D2) receptor agonist. This formulation has been approved for the treatment of T2DM. Bromocriptine actually gained importance after its therapeutic effect was established for treating Parkinson's disease and hyperprolactinemia. Bromocriptine has a moderated influence on blood glucose level, and it may also exhibit CNS (central nervous system) action. The dose range for bromocriptine is 1.6 to 4.8 mg, taken with food in the morning within 3 h of awakening. Side effects include nausea, fatigue, dizziness, orthostatic hypotension, vomiting, and headache.[21] Bromocriptine has the ability to activate the inflammatory signal IL-6/JAK2/p-STAT3/SOCS3 and exhibit its action on the molecular level of the muscles. It also enhances the PPAR-γ/adiponectin signaling that results in activation of the insulin signaling pathway (p- IR/p-AKT/GLUT4).[57]

Na + −Glucose transporter-2 inhibitors

Na + −Glucose Transporter-2 (SGLT2) is an Na^+−glucose cotransporter located almost exclusively in the proximal portion of the renal tubule. It is a high-affinity, low-capacity transporter that moves glucose against a concentration gradient from the tubular lumen using energy generated from Na + flux through the epithelial cells. Renal retention of glucose is nearly complete in nondiabetic persons, and SGLT2 accounts for 80%−90% of this reclamation; the remainder is recovered by SGLT1 more distally in the tubule. Early studies in diabetic animals demonstrated that hyperglycemia could be nearly ameliorated by the naturally occurring compound phlorizin, an SGLT inhibitor. In accordance with this proof of principle, drugs that are specific inhibitors of SGLT2 have been developed to treat diabetes.[58] These agents block glucose transport in the proximal tubule and lower blood glucose by promoting urinary loss. SGLT2 inhibitors reduce the rate of glucose reclamation in the proximal tubule and shift the renal threshold for glucose excretion from about 180 to 50 mg/dL (10 to 2.8 mM). In monotherapy, they reduce A1c by 0.7%−1.0%, cause weight loss of 2−4 kg, and decrease blood pressure by 2−4 mm Hg. There are currently three SGLP2 inhibitors available for clinical use—canagliflozin, dapagliflozin, and empagliflozin—with several other members of this class still in development. These agents are indicated for use in combination with other oral agents and insulin; such use leads to an additional decrease of A1c of 0.5%−0.7%. SGLT2 inhibitors are available in combination with metformin and DPP-4 inhibitors; a combined SGLT1/SGLT2 inhibitor is under investigation.[21]

GLP-1 agonist

Insulin secretion is stimulated after meals by gastrointestinal hormones incretins (GLP-1 and GIP). However, GIP stimulates insulin release inefficiently as compared to GLP and lower blood glucose T2DM. Signaling system of

GLP-1 is a major target of GLP-agonists. GLP-1 and glucagon are derived from preproglucagon (a 180–amino acid precursor having five domains, which are processed separately). An amino-terminal signal peptide is followed by glicentin-related pancreatic peptide, glucagon, GLP-1, and GLP-2. Processing of the protein is sequential and occurs in a tissue-specific fashion. Pancreatic α-cells cleave proglucagon into glucagon and a large C-terminal peptide that includes both of the GLPs. Intestinal L-cells and specific hindbrain neurons process proglucagon into a large N-terminal peptide that includes glucagon or GLP-1 and GLP-2. GLP-2 affects the proliferation of epithelial cell lining the gastrointestinal tract. Teduglutide, a GLP-2 analog, is approved for treatment of short-bowel. When GLP-1 agonist is given intravenously to diabetics, GLP-1 stimulates insulin secretion and inhibits glucagon release. It also delays gastric emptying, reduces food intake, and normalizes fasting and postprandial insulin secretion. Natural GLP-1 peptide can also exhibit this function, but DPP-4 enzyme rapidly inactivates GLP-1. Therefore, GLP-1 therapeutic agents are taken for obtaining the benefits of GLP-1. GLP-1 receptor agonists Albiglutide, Dulaglutide, Exenatide, and Liraglutidehave been approved for treatment of diabetic patients in the U.S. Recently, Semaglutide has also been approved.[21,59]

Exenatide

Exendin-4 is a naturally occurring 39–amino acid reptilian peptide with 53% sequence homology to GLP-1. This peptide is a potent GLP-1 receptor agonist (GLP-1RA) that shares many of the physiological and pharmacological effects of GLP-1. It is not metabolized by DPP-4 and thus has extended activity following injection. Synthetic exendin-4, exenatide, is approved for use as monotherapy and as adjunctive therapy for patients with T2DM not achieving glycemic targets with other drugs. Evidence from clinical trials has indicated that exenatide can also be used in conjunction with basal insulin. An extended-release form of exenatide is administered by subcutaneous injection once a week with greater effectiveness than twice-daily treatment.[21]

Liraglutide

The liraglutide peptide is a long-acting GLP-1 agonist. When Lys34Arg substitutes Lys26 with an addition of α-glutamic acid spacer coupled to a C16 fatty acyl group to its structure, it becomes resistant to DPP-4 degradation. The binding of albumin takes place with the fatty acid side chain that extends the half-life, which makes the drug to be administered only once a day. The mechanism may be that the fatty acid offers some protection from cleavage of the N-terminus by DPP-4. The pharmacodynamic profile of liraglutide mimics GLP-1 and exenatide. In clinical trials, liraglutide caused both improvement in glycemic control and weight loss. In a single comparative trial, liraglutide reduced

A1c about 30% more than exenatide. Liraglutide is indicated for adjunctive therapy in patients not achieving glycemic control with oral agents. Liraglutide can be added to oral agents or basal insulin. In a recent report, liraglutide reduced the risk of cardiovascular death, nonfatal myocardial infarction, or nonfatal stroke in patients with T2DM and established cardiovascular disease. Similar positive effects on cardiovascular risk have also been demonstrated in a trial of semaglutide, a compound in development with similarities to liraglutide. Other GLP-1 receptor agonists (exenatide and lixisenatide; approved in E.U.) are neutral with regard to cardiovascular risk in the trials completed to date.

Albiglutide

Albiglutide is a fusion protein that includes two sequential GLP-1 moieties linked to human albumin; the GLP-1 sequences are modified to prevent DPP-4 cleavage. Albiglutide is also indicated for patients with T2DM with suboptimal glucose control and can be used in conjunction with oral agents and basal insulin.

Overall, all GLP-1RAs share a common mechanism, activation of the GLP-1 receptor, a member of glucagon receptor family of GPCRs (class B GPCRs). GLP-1 receptors are expressed by β-cells, cells in the peripheral and central nervous systems, the heart and vasculature, kidney, lung, and gastrointestinal mucosa. Binding of agonists to the GLP-1 receptor activates the cAMP-PKA pathway and several GEFs. GLP-1 receptor activation also initiates signaling via PKC and PI3K and alters the activity of several ion channels. In β-cells, the end result of these actions is increased insulin biosynthesis and exocytosis in a glucose-dependent manner. Activation of GLP-1 receptors in the CNS accounts for the effects of receptor agonists on food intake and gastric emptying and for side effects such as nausea.[60]

Other glucose-lowering agents

Pramlintide: amylin analog

It is the first new class of injectable drug that acts as an amylin analog. It is soluble as compared to natural amylin. Native amylin is an islet amyloid polypeptide that possess a 37−amino acid peptide produced in the pancreatic β-cells and secreted with insulin. A synthetic form of amylin with several amino acid modifications is pramlintide, which improves bioavailability. It has been developed as a drug for the treatment of diabetes. It acts centrally through the amylin receptor in specific regions of the hindbrain. The activation of the amylin receptor results in the reduced secretion of glucagon. It further slows the gastric emptying rate and provides satiety. It is injected subcutaneously with an insulin regimen to control and improve the glycemic control without weight gain. [21,61] (Fig. 5.10)

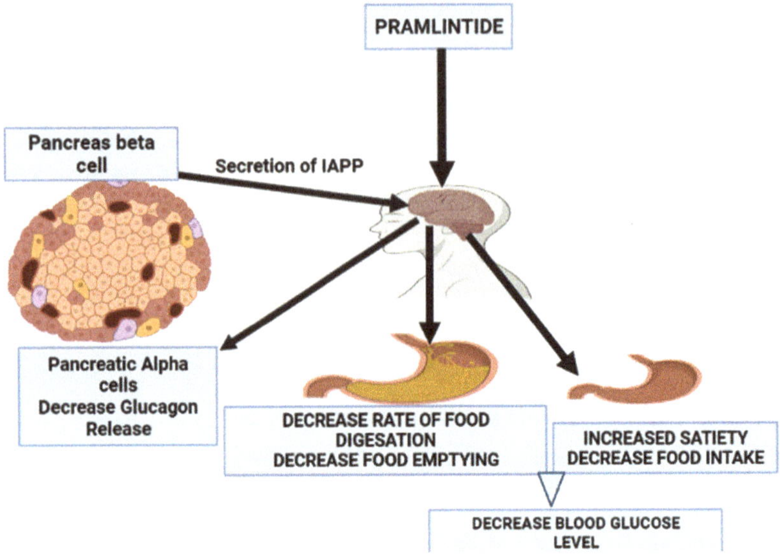

FIGURE 5.10 Action of pramlintide.

References

1. The Expert Committee on the Diagnosis and Classification of Diabetes Mellitus: Report of the Expert Committee on the Diagnosis and Classification of Diabetes Mellitus. Diabetes Care. 1997; 20: 1183–1197.
2. Piero MN, Nzaro GM, Njagi JM. Diabetes mellitus—a devastating metabolic disorder. *AJBPS*. 2014;4(40):1–7.
3. Wang Y, Karmakar T, Ghosh N, Basak S, Gopal Sahoo N. Targeting mangiferin loaded N-succinyl chitosan-alginate grafted nanoparticles against atherosclerosis - a case study against diabetes mediated hyperlipidemia in rat. *Food Chem*. 2022;370:131376. Available from: https://doi.org/10.1016/j.foodchem.2021.131376.
4. Kundu A, Dey P, Sarkar P, et al. Protective effects of Croton hookeri on streptozotocin-induced diabetic nephropathy. *Food Chem Toxicol*. 2020;135:110873. Available from: https://doi.org/10.1016/j.fct.2019.110873.
5. Karmakar T, Chaki R, Ghosh N. Pharmacology and mechanisms of natural medicine in treatment of type 2 diabetes Mellitus. In: Mandal SC, Chakraborty R, Sen S, eds. *Evidence Based Validation of Traditional Medicines*. Singapore: Springer; 2021. Available from: https://doi.org/10.1007/978-981-15-8127-4_49.
6. Chaki R, Ghosh N, Mandal SC. Chapter 6 - Phytopharmacology of herbal biomolecules. In: Mandal SC, Nayak AK, Dhara AK, eds. *Herbal Biomolecules in Healthcare Applications*. Academic Press; 2022:101–119. Available from: https://doi.org/10.1016/B978-0-323-85852-6.00026-3. ISBN 9780323858526.
7. Ghosh N., Ghosh R.C., Kundu, A., Subhash C. Mandal, S.C., Chapter 17 - Herb and drug interaction, In: Mandal S.C., Mandal V., Konishi T., eds. Natural Products and Drug Discovery, Elsevier; 2018:467-490. ISBN 9780081020814, https://doi.org/10.1016/B978-0-08-102081-4.00017-4.

8. Nepal A, Chakraborty M. An overview on medicinal plants of Sikkim Himalayas region with emphasis on antidiabetic: a review. *J Pharm Phytochem.* 2021;10:215–217. Available from: https://doi.org/10.22271/phyto.2021.v10.i4c.14148.
9. Dalui SK, Chakraverty R, Yasmin N, Pattanaik S, Pandit K, Chatterjee S. Effects of DPP4 inhibitors on renal outcomes in diabetes mellitus: a systematic review and meta-analysis. *Indian J Endocrinol Metab.* 2021;25(4):283–292. Available from: https://doi.org/10.4103/ijem.ijem_237_21.
10. Harikumar K, Kumar BK, Hemalatha GJ, Kumar MB, Lado SFS. A Review on Diabetes Mellitus. *IJNTPS.* 2015;5(3):201–217.
11. Hassan BAR. Overview on diabetes mellitus (type 2). *J Chromat Sep Techniq.* 2013;4 (2):1000e114.
12. Zhao Y, Xu G, Wu W, Yi X. Type 2 diabetes mellitus—disease, diagnosis and treatment. *J Diabetes Metab.* 2015;6:533. Available from: https://doi.org/10.4172/2155-6156.1000533.
13. Baynes HW. Classification, pathophysiology, diagnosis and management of diabetes mellitus. *J Diabetes Metab.* 2015;6:541. Available from: https://doi.org/10.4172/2155-6156.1000541.
14. American diabetes association. Diagnosis and classification of diabetes mellitus. *Diabetes Care.* 2008;31(1):55–60.
15. Olokoba AB, Obateru OA, Olokoba LB. Type 2 diabetes mellitus: a review of current trends. *Oman Med J.* 2012;27(4):269–273.
16. Ding Y, Tanaka Y, Zhang W, Wu Y. Risk factors contributing to type 2 diabetes and recent advances in the treatment and prevention. *Int J Med Sci.* 2014;11(11):1185–1200. Available from: https://doi.org/10.7150/ijms.10001.
17. Mukherjee B, Hossain CM, Mondal L, Paul P, Ghosh MK. Obesity and Insulin Resistance: An Abridged Molecular Correlation. *Lipid Insights.* 2013;6:1–11.
18. Ullah A, Khan A, Khan I. Diabetes mellitus and oxidative stress−−a concise review. *Saudi Pharm J.* 2016;24:547–553. INTRODUCTION CHAPTER 1 Page 35.
19. Kaur J. A comprehensive review on metabolic syndrome. *Cardiol Res Pract.* 2014;. Available from: https://doi.org/10.1155/2014/943162.
20. Cerf ME. B cell dysfunction and insulin resistance. *Front Endocrinol.* 2013;4(37):1–12.
21. Brunton L, Knollmann B. In: Goodman, ed. *The Pharmacological Basis of Therapeutics.* 13th ed. McGraw-Hill Education; 2017.
22. Tabuchi H, Yamamoto H, Matsumoto K, et al. Regulation of insulin secretion by overexpression of Ca2 + /calmodulin-dependent protein kinase II in insulinoma MIN6 cells. *Endocrinology.* 2000;141(7):2350–2360. Available from: https://doi.org/10.1210/endo.141.7.7553.
23. Popoli M. Synaptotagmin is endogenously phosphorylated by Ca2 + /calmodulin protein kinase II in synaptic vesicles. *FEBS Lett.* 1993;317(1–2):85–88. Available from: https://doi.org/10.1016/0014-5793(93)81496-M.
24. Tripathi KD. In: Tripathi KD, ed. *Essentials of Medical Pharmacology.* 7th ed. Jaypee; 2013.
25. Aguilar Bryan L, Nichols CG, Wechsler SW, et al. Cloning of the beta cell high-affinity sulfonylurea receptor: a regulator of insulin secretion [see comments] Comments: Comment inScience 1995 Apr 21;268(5209):372-3 *Science.* 1995;268(5209):423–426.
26. Inagaki N, Gonoi T, Clement IV JP, et al. Reconstitution of IKATP: an inward rectifier subunit plus the sulfonylurea receptor. *Science.* 1995;270(5239):1166–1170. Available from: https://doi.org/10.1126/science.270.5239.1166.

27. Ueda K, Komine J, Matsuo M, Seino S, Amachi T. Cooperative binding of ATP and MgADP in the sulfonylurea receptor is modulated by glibenclamide. *Proc Natl Acad Sci U S Am*. 1999;96(4):1268–1272. Available from: https://doi.org/10.1073/pnas.96.4.1268.
28. Uhde I, Toman A, Gross I, Schwanstecher C, Schwanstecher M. Identification of the potassium channel opener site on sulfonylurea receptors. *J Biol Chem*. 1999;274 (40):28079–28082. Available from: https://doi.org/10.1074/jbc.274.40.28079.
29. Müller G. The molecular mechanism of the insulin-mimetic/sensitizing activity of the anti-diabetic sulfonylurea drug amaryl. *Mol Med (Cambridge, Mass*. 2000;(6(11):907–933. Available from: https://doi.org/10.1007/bf03401827.
30. Holman GD, Kasuga M. From receptor to transporter: insulin signalling to glucose transport. *Diabetologia*. 1997;40(9):991–1003. Available from: https://doi.org/10.1007/s001250050780.
31. Muller G, Wied S. The sulfonylurea drug, glimepiride, stimulates glucose transport, glucose transporter translocation, and dephosphorylation in insulin-resistant rat adipocytes in vitro. *Diabetes*. 1993;42(12):1852–1867. Available from: https://doi.org/10.2337/diab.42.12.1852.
32. Pessin JE, Thurmond DC, Elmendorf JS, Coker KJ, Okada S. Molecular basis of insulin-stimulated GLUT4 vesicle trafficking. Location! location! location!. *J Biol Chem*. 1999;274(5):2593–2596. Available from: https://doi.org/10.1074/jbc.274.5.2593. Â© 1999 ASBMB. Currently published by Elsevier Inc; originally published by American Society for Biochemistry and Molecular Biology.
33. Rena G, Pearson ER, Sakamoto K. Molecular mechanism of action of metformin: old or new insights? *Diabetologia*. 2013;56(9):1898–1906. Available from: https://doi.org/10.1007/s00125-013-2991-0.
34. OWEN MR, DORAN E, HALESTRAP AP. Evidence that metformin exerts its anti-diabetic effects through inhibition of complex 1 of the mitochondrial respiratory chain. *Biochemical J*. 2000;348(3):607–614. Available from: https://doi.org/10.1042/bj3480607.
35. Pryor HJ, Smyth JE, Quinlan PT, Halestrap AP. Evidence that the flux control coefficient of the respiratory chain is high during gluconeogenesis from lactate in hepatocytes from starved rats. Implications for the hormonal control of gluconeogenesis and action of hypoglycaemic agents. *Biochemical J*. 1987;247(2):449–457. Available from: https://doi.org/10.1042/bj2470449.
36. Salpeter SR, Greyber E, Pasternak GA, Salpeter EE. Risk of fatal and nonfatal lactic acidosis with metformin use in type 2 diabetes mellitus. *Cochrane Database Syst Rev*. 2010;2017(12). Available from: https://doi.org/10.1002/14651858.CD002967.pub4.
37. Kahn BB, Alquier T, Carling D, Hardie DG. AMP-activated protein kinase: ancient energy gauge provides clues to modern understanding of metabolism. *Cell Metab*. 2005;1 (1):15–25. Available from: https://doi.org/10.1016/j.cmet.2004.12.003.
38. Zhou G, Myers R, Li Y, et al. Role of AMP-activated protein kinase in mechanism of metformin action. *J Clin Investigation*. 2001;108(8):1167–1174. Available from: https://doi.org/10.1172/JCI13505.
39. Hawley SA, Ross FA, Chevtzoff C, et al. Use of cells expressing γ subunit variants to identify diverse mechanisms of AMPK activation. *Cell Metab*. 2010;11(6):554–565. Available from: https://doi.org/10.1016/j.cmet.2010.04.001.
40. Chen Y, Li S, Brown C, et al. Effect of genetic variation in the organic cation transporter 2 on the renal elimination of metformin. *Pharmacogenetics Genomics*. 2009;19(7):497–504. Available from: https://doi.org/10.1097/FPC.0b013e32832cc7e9.

41. Koepsell H, Lips K, Volk C. Polyspecific organic cation transporters: Structure, function, physiological roles, and biopharmaceutical implications. *Pharm Res.* 2007;24 (7):1227–1251. Available from: https://doi.org/10.1007/s11095-007-9254-z.
42. Rena G, Pearson ER, Sakamoto K. Molecular action and pharmacogenetics of metformin: current understanding of an old drug. *Diabetes Manag.* 2012;2(5):439–452. Available from: https://doi.org/10.2217/dmt.12.42.
43. Chen M, Hu C, Jia W. Pharmacogenomics of glinides. *Pharmacogenomics.* 2015;16 (1):45–60. Available from: https://doi.org/10.2217/pgs.14.152.
44. Standl E, S. O. Alpha-glucosidase inhibitors 2012—cardiovascular considerations and trial evaluation. *Diabetes Vasc Dis Res.* 2012;9:163–169.
45. Omar B, Ahrén B. Pleiotropic mechanisms for the glucose-lowering action of DPP-4 inhibitors. *Diabetes.* 2014;63(7):2196–2202. Available from: https://doi.org/10.2337/db14-0052.
46. Waget A, Cabou C, Masseboeuf M, et al. Physiological and pharmacological mechanisms through which the DPP-4 inhibitor sitagliptin regulates glycemia in mice. *Endocrinology.* 2011;152(8):3018–3029. Available from: https://doi.org/10.1210/en.2011-0286.
47. Marchetti P, Lupi R, Bugliani M, et al. A local glucagon-like peptide 1 (GLP-1) system in human pancreatic islets. *Diabetologia.* 2012;55(12):3262–3272. Available from: https://doi.org/10.1007/s00125-012-2716-9. Epub 2012 Sep 11. PMID: 22965295.
48. Shah P, Ardestani A, Dharmadhikari G, et al. The DPP-4 inhibitor linagliptin restores β-cell function and survival in human isolated islets through GLP-1 stabilization. *J Clin Endocrinol Metab.* 2013;98(7):E1163–E1172. Available from: https://doi.org/10.1210/jc.2013-102940.
49. Dobrian AD, Ma Q, Lindsay JW, et al. Dipeptidyl peptidase IV inhibitor sitagliptin reduces local inflammation in adipose tissue and in pancreatic islets of obese mice. *Am J Physiol - Endocrinol Metab.* 2011;300(2):410–421. Available from: https://doi.org/10.1152/ajpendo.00463.2010.
50. Kim SJ, Nian C, Doudet DJ, Mcintosh CHS. Dipeptidyl peptidase IV inhibition with MK0431 improves islet graft survival in diabetic NOD mice partially via T-cell modulation. *Diabetes.* 2009;58(3):641–651. Available from: https://doi.org/10.2337/db08-1101.
51. Liu Z, Stanojevic V, Avadhani S, Yano T, Habener JF. Stromal cell-derived factor-1 (SDF-1)/chemokine (C-X-C motif) receptor 4 (CXCR4) axis activation induces intra-islet glucagon-like peptide-1 (GLP-1) production and enhances beta cell survival. *Diabetologia.* 2011;54(8):2067–2076. Available from: https://doi.org/10.1007/s00125-011-2181-x.
52. Tafuri SR. Troglitazone enhances differentiation, basal glucose uptake, and Glut1 protein levels in 3T3-L1 adipocytes. *Endocrinology.* 1996;137(11):4706–4712. Available from: https://doi.org/10.1210/endo.137.11.8895337.
53. Teboul L, Gaillard D, Staccini L, Inadera H, Amri EZ, Grimaldi PA. Thiazolidinediones and fatty acids convert myogenic cells into adipose- like cells. *J Biol Chem.* 1995;270 (47):28183–28187. Available from: https://doi.org/10.1074/jbc.270.47.28183.
54. Tontonoz P, Hu E, Spiegelman BM. Stimulation of adipogenesis in fibroblasts by PPARγ2, a lipid-activated transcription factor. *Cell.* 1994;79(7):1147–1156. Available from: https://doi.org/10.1016/0092-8674(94)90006-X.
55. Stumvoll M, Häring HU. Glitazones: clinical effects and molecular mechanisms. *Ann Med.* 2002;34(3):217–224. Available from: https://doi.org/10.1080/ann.34.3.217.224.
56. El-Mesallamy HO, Hamdy NM, Sallam AAM. Effect of obesity and glycemic control on serum lipocalins and insulin-like growth factor axis in type 2 diabetic patients. *Acta Diabetologica.* 2013;50(5):679–685. Available from: https://doi.org/10.1007/s00592-012-0373-6.

57. Reda E, Hassaneen S, El-Abhar HS. Novel trajectories of bromocriptine antidiabetic action: Leptin-IL-6/JAK2/p-STAT3/SOCS3, p-IR/p-AKT/GLUT4, PPAR-γ/adiponectin, Nrf2/PARP-1, and GLP-1. *Front Pharmacology*. 2018;9(JUL):1–12. Available from: https://doi.org/10.3389/fphar.2018.00771.
58. Mudaliar S, Polidori D, Zambrowicz B, Henry RR. Sodium-glucose cotransporter inhibitors: effects on renal and intestinal glucose transport from bench to bedside. *Diabetes Care*. 2015;38(12):2344–2353. Available from: https://doi.org/10.2337/dc15-0642.
59. Blundell J, Finlayson G, Axelsen M, et al. Effects of once-weekly semaglutide on appetite, energy intake, control of eating, food preference and body weight in subjects with obesity. *Diabetes, Obes Metab*. 2017;19(9):1242–1251. Available from: https://doi.org/10.1111/dom.12932.
60. Kalra S, Sahay R. *A review on semaglutide: an oral glucagon-like peptide 1 receptor agonist in management of type 2 diabetes mellitus. Diabetes Therapy*. Vol. 11. Springer Healthcare; 2020:1965–1982, Issue 9. Available from: https://doi.org/10.1007/s13300-020-00894-y.
61. Day C. Amylin analogue as an antidiabetic agent. *Br J Diabetes Vasc Dis*. 2005;5(3):151–154. Available from: https://doi.org/10.1177/14746514050050030701.

Chapter 6

Molecular mechanism of action of estrogens, progestins, and androgens

Muhammad Arshad Malik[1] **and Muhammad Shahid Nadeem**[2]
[1]*Department of Biological Sciences, Faculty of Basic & Applied Sciences, International Islamic University Islamabad, Islamabad, Pakistan,* [2]*Department of Biochemistry, Faculty of Science, King Abdulaziz University, Jeddah, Saudi Arabia*

Introduction

Steroid hormones are lipophilic (fat-soluble) molecules that have a significant role in the signal transduction pathway, thus regulate a wide range of cellular processes and biological functions. All classes of steroid hormones are derived from cholesterol precursors, as shown in Fig. 6.1. The major classes of steroid hormones can be classified into corticosteroids (glucocorticoids and mineralocorticoids) and sex hormones (estrogens, progesterone, and androgens). The corticosteroids are secreted from adrenal glands, whereas sex hormones are secreted by gonads (i.e., testes and ovaries, e.g., estrogens, progesterone, and testosterone) as well as the adrenal gland (e.g., androgens). Generally, males and females have similar sex hormones, but their secretion sites, concentration, and site-of-action differ. Testosterone, an androgen, is predominantly a male sex hormone and anabolic steroid secreted from testes. However, the testes and adrenal cortex also secrete a small amount of estrogen (or oestrogen) and progesterone. In females, ovaries and also placenta (during pregnancy) produce estrogen and progesterone, with an additional small amount of testosterone from the ovaries and adrenal gland. Estrogens, progesterone, and androgens are implicated in many vital cellular processes, as described in Table 6.1. The changes in concentration (either too high or too low) of these sex hormones or a deficit in the step of their biosynthesis could lead to serious health issues, including disorders of sexual development, infertility, and cancers.

How Synthetic Drugs Work. DOI: https://doi.org/10.1016/B978-0-323-99855-0.00006-3

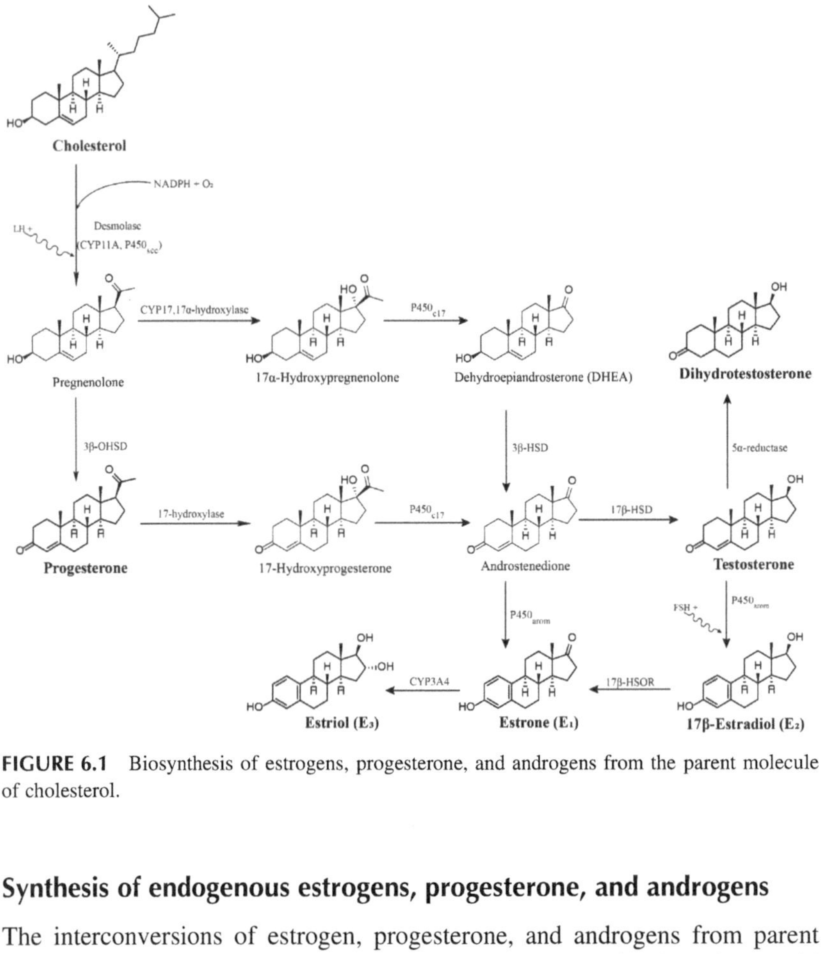

FIGURE 6.1 Biosynthesis of estrogens, progesterone, and androgens from the parent molecule of cholesterol.

Synthesis of endogenous estrogens, progesterone, and androgens

The interconversions of estrogen, progesterone, and androgens from parent cholesterol molecule with intermediates are described in Fig. 6.1. The steroid nucleus undergoes hydroxylation and hydrocarbon side-chain cleavage by cytochrome P450 17A1 (also known as P450c17, CYP17A1, 17α-hydroxylase, 17,20-lyase, or 17,20-desmolase) in presence of NADPH and O_2. The resulting pregnenolone is changed to Progesterone via 3β-hydroxysteroid dehydrogenase (3β-HSD). Pregnenolone also undergoes hydroxylation, in which 17α-hydroxylase introduces hydroxyl group at C-17 position of pregnenolone, leading toward the formation of 17α-hydroxypregnenolone. Similarly, 17α-hydroxylase also catalyzed the hydroxylation of progesterone and forms 17α-hydroxyprogesterone. 17α-Hydroxypregnenolone is converted into dehydroepiandrosterone (DHEA) by the removal of hydrogen from C3-OH, via the catalyzation of 3β-HSD, also known as $\Delta^{5\text{-}4}$ isomerase. The dehydrogenation of DHEA, and androstenedione results in the conversion of Testosterone (by 3β-HSD) or Estrone (by cytochrome P450

TABLE 6.1 Characteristics of estrogen, progesterone, and androgen.

Hormone group	Hormone(s)	Major secretion site	Receptor(s)	Function(s)	Associated disease
Estrogen	Estrone (E1)	Ovaries	ERs: ERα, ERβ, mER (i.e., GPER)	Development of female secondary sexual characters and female fertility: breast, thickening of endometrium and vaginal wall, vaginal lubrication, maturation of follicles, regulates gonadotrophin secretion.	Various types of cancer (breast, ovarian, colorectal, prostate, endometrial), osteoporosis, neurodegenerative diseases, cardiovascular disease, insulin resistance, lupus erythematosus, endometriosis, and obesity
	Estradiol (or 17β-Estradiol) (E2)				
	Estriol (E3)				
	Estetrol (E4)				
Progesterone	Progesterone	Ovaries	PRs (PgR), PR-A, PR-B, and PR-C	Important for menstruation, pregnancy, and sperm production. Prepares the endometrium for the potential of pregnancy after ovulation, development of fetus, breast development, milk production. Implantation and maturation of fertilized ovum.	Irregular menstrual cycle, infertility, obesity, breast cancer, endometrial cancer, liver diseases, cardiovascular diseases, breast tenderness, fibrocystic breasts, gallbladder problems, etc.
		Placenta	mPR (mPRα, mPRβ, mPRγ, mPRδ, and mPRε)		

(*Continued*)

TABLE 6.1 (Continued)

Hormone group	Hormone(s)	Major secretion site	Receptor(s)	Function(s)	Associated disease
Androgen	Testosterone	Gonads (testes and ovaries)	AR; NR3C4, IGF-1R, mARs (GPRC6A and ZIP9)	Development of male secondary sexual characters, including facial hair, body hair growth, and voice change. Stimulates puberty, hair growth in the pubic underarm areas, and spermatogenesis. Stimulates the production of skeletal muscles and bone as well as red blood cells. Masculinization of the fetus.	Androgenic alopecia, Androgen insensitivity syndrome, precocious puberty in boys, hypersexuality, paraphilias, BPH, prostate cancer, and hyperandrogenism in women such as in PCOS.
	Dihydrotestosterone				
	Androstenedione	Adrenal cortex			
	Androsterone				

AR, Androgen receptor; *BPH*, benign prostatic hyperplasia; *ERs*, estrogen receptors; *GPER*, G protein–coupled ER; *IGF-1R*, insulin-like growth factor 1 receptor; *mARs*, membrane ARs; *mER*, membrane ER; *mPR*, membrane progesterone receptor; *NR3C4*, nuclear receptor subfamily 3, group C, member 4; *PCOS*, polycystic ovary syndrome; *PRs*, progesterone receptors.

aromatase). 17α-Hydroxyprogesterone is also converted into androstenedione via cytochrome P450. Testosterone can also be converted into 5α-dihydrotestosterone (DHT) or 17β-Estradiol (E_2), by 5α-reductase and P450c17, respectively. Another estrogen, estrone (E_1) is formed either from estradiol via P450 aromatase or testosterone via 17β-hydroxysteroid oxidoreductase. Estrone is converted into estriol (E_3) and the reaction is catalyzed via cytochrome 450 3A4 (CYP3A4).[1,2]

Mechanism of action of endogenous steroid sex hormones (estrogens, progesterone, and androgens)

Sex hormones, that is, estrogens and progesterone, are transported by the blood from their site of secretion to their targeted cells. Some hormones, for example, testosterone, have specific localized effects through paracrine secretion. Corticosteroid-binding globulin (CBG) (e.g., progesterone) and sex hormone–binding globulin (SHBG) (estrogen and androgen) can act as a nonspecific carrier and reversibly bound to carry the specific steroid hormones. As sex hormones are lipophilic molecules, they can freely diffuse across the phospholipid layer of the plasma membrane of its target cells. On entry of the hormone into the cell, it is bound to its specific receptor localized on the cell membrane or distributed in the cytosol or nucleus (the receptors of the hormones described in Table 6.1) and forms a hormone-receptor complex. (Note: The cells without hormone receptors cannot be influenced by the action of hormones.) This hormone-receptor complex forms a dimer and causes a conformational change in the receptor, revealing its DNA-binding domain. The hormone-receptor complex is translocated to the nucleus, where it binds to the targeted regulatory DNA sequence, referred to as the hormone-response element (HRE).[3] The hormone-receptor complex interacts with HRE through a zinc finger motif and regulates the transcription, synthesis of messenger RNA (mRNA), and protein.[4–6] In addition, coactivators and corepressors also regulate the pathway either by activating or inhibiting the transcription of the specific gene, respectively.

Role of estrogen, progesterone, and androgen in diseases

Hormonal imbalance in females

Menstruation and fertility are significantly controlled by the activity of estrogen and progesterone. Estrogen regulates the menstrual cycle by controlling the growth and maturation of the uterine lining and also the maturation of the egg prior to ovulation. Progesterone balances the effects of estrogen. It is secreted by the corpus luteum in the ovary after ovulation during the second half of the menstruation cycle. It prepares the endometrium, matures the uterine lining, and maintains the possible pregnancy. If the egg is not fertilized, the estrogen decreases and tends to start the menstrual cycle.

Due to the integral role of each hormone, the slight imbalance in the concentration (i.e., too much or too little) of these hormones could disastrously affect normal cellular functioning and physiology of the human body. Such as, in women, the low levels of estrogen typically cause irregular periods or menopause symptoms. Menopause is marked as the end of the menstrual cycle when no menstruation occurs for 12 consecutive months, and women could no longer be pregnant. A woman's hormones level naturally changes throughout life, menstrual cycle, pregnancy, and even at different times of the day.

- Decreased estrogen: The levels of estrogen decrease naturally as woman ages, especially when a woman reaches menopause. The low levels of estrogen at menopause can cause hot flashes, night sweats, vaginal dryness, loss of sex drive, mood swings, etc. The drop in estrogen levels might be a risk factor for cardiovascular disorders, stroke, osteoporosis, and fractures.[7]
- Decreased progesterone: The low levels of progesterone result in irregular or missed periods, difficulty conceiving, ectopic pregnancy, spotting, miscarriage, and infertility.
- Increased estrogen: When the balance of progesterone is inadequate, it tends to increase estrogen levels, causing estrogen dominance. Estrogen dominance could be a risk factor for breast cancer, ovarian cancer, tumors of testes and adrenal glands, liver diseases, acne, loss of sex drive, obesity, and depression.
- Increased progesterone: However, the high levels of progesterone are not associated with any serious medical issues, as during pregnancy, progesterone level increases, although ovarian cancer, ovarian cyst, congenital adrenal hyperplasia, and hydatidiform mole are associated with high progesterone levels.[8]
- Decreased testosterone: The abnormally low levels of testosterone in women can cause muscle weakness, fatigue, stress, sexual dysfunction, irregular menstruation, vaginal dryness, bone loss, weight gain, and fertility issues. The low levels of testosterone in women can cause HSD disorder (HSDD), in which women have a lack of interest in sexual activity, frustration, and lack of self-confidence.[9,10]
- Increased testosterone: On the other hand, increased testosterone level is linked with infertility, obesity, ovarian cancer, or diabetes.

Polycystic ovary syndrome

Polycystic ovary syndrome (PCOS) is a hormonal disorder in teen girls and young women that causes abnormalities in the estrogen and androgens metabolism in the ovaries and produces abnormally uncontrolled increased levels of male sex hormones (androgen), primarily testosterone.[11] PCOS is the common cause of infertility as it disrupts egg development and release, causing anovulation. PCOS could be caused by insulin resistance, in which cells do not properly utilize insulin. The cells of muscles, liver, and liver cannot utilize glucose for energy production. When the blood glucose level increases, it triggers the pancreas to secrete more insulin, causing hyperinsulinemia.[12] Extra insulin contributes to hyperandrogenism, that is, increases production and activity of androgen like testosterone, causing difficulty with ovulation. Several genes are also linked to PCOS, and it runs in families.[13] The abnormality in the functions of hypothalamic–pituitary–gonadal axis and the hypothalamic–pituitary–ovary (HPO) axis is also a pathological factor of PCOS that causes the excessive secretion of adrenal and ovarian androgen. The levels of luteinizing hormone (LH), a hormone responsible for stimulating ovulation, also increase and exert chronic low-grade inflammation also leads to the pathogenesis of PCOS. In PCOS inflammation, C-reactive protein increases, which is also associated with diabetes, insulin resistance, and heart diseases. In PCOS, ovaries may enlarge, or numerous small cysts form in the ovaries. PCOS also causes menstrual dysfunction (irregular menstrual cycle or missed periods). Due to increased androgen levels, women experience male pattern baldness, severe acne, and hirsutism that results in excessive body hairs in male-like patterns on the face, chest, and stomach. PCOS also results in alopecia, acanthosis nigricans (skin darkening around neck, armpits, or breast), diabetes, heart disease, high blood pressure, obesity, and obstructive sleep apnea.

Hormonal imbalance in males

Males also experience natural hormonal imbalance that affects bodily functions. As men age, they are more likely to experience an imbalance in testosterone levels. The changes in androgens, particularly testosterone, considerably affect the sexual activity and erection.[14] The decline in the androgen, specifically testosterone, in aging men causes hypoandrogenism and leads to men's menopause. This condition is also referred to as andropause, late-onset hypogonadism, low testosterone, or androgen decline in the aging male.[15] Testosterone deficiency syndrome or low testosterone level (as less than 300 ng/dL) can cause erectile dysfunction, reduced bone and muscle mass, low sex drive (libido), low semen volume and blood count, decreased energy, strength, loss of body and facial hair, smaller testicle size, increased body fats and breast size (gynecomastia), cognitive decline, depression, and mood changes.

Too much testosterone also causes health complications.[10] The abnormally high testosterone levels in men are associated with low sperm counts, shrinking of the testicles, high blood pressure and cholesterol, heart muscle damage, liver problems, enlargement of the prostate, weight gain, increased appetite, increased muscle mass, blood clotting, acne, aggressive behavior, mood swings, irritability, etc.

As men age, the testosterone level decreases naturally, and estrogen level increases. But abnormally high levels of estrogens are much concern. The high estrogen production causes slow production of sperms and leads to infertility.[16] Too much estrogen also causes gynecomastia, in which male breast enlarges, and breast fat tissue becomes abnormally high. Other complications due to high estrogens level are prostate cancer, low sex drive, erectile dysfunction, slowed growth of body, penis, testicles, reduced body hairs, reduced muscle and body mass, feeling exhausted, hot flashes, etc. The low levels of estrogen in men are not much concerned. Hypogonadism, in which testosterone decreases, also lowers estrogen production and may lead to loss of libido, delayed ejaculation, fat accumulation, bone loss, osteoporosis, insulin resistance, depression, etc.

Progesterone acts as a precursor to synthesize testosterone and balance estrogen levels. If progesterone decreases, the testosterone also decreases. Progesterone also matures sperm cells.[17] The symptoms of decrease in progesterone levels are similar to that of decrease in testosterone levels, that is, erectile dysfunction, low libido, low semen volume, decreased energy, strength, reduced bone and muscles mass, loss of body and facial hair, weight gain, increased body fats, cognitive decline, depression, and mood swings. The increase in progesterone level causes an increase in the estrogen level, thus having similar symptoms as results in high estrogen levels.

Cancer

Estrogen, progesterone, and androgen and their precursors have also been associated with pathophysiology and modulate disease activity. Besides essential roles in the normal physiology of cellular processes, these hormones play a critical role in the etiology of several hormone-sensitive or -dependent cancers. Not all cancers are caused by estrogen, progesterone, and androgen, but only a few cancers are dependent on hormones for growth or survival, including breast cancer,[18] ovarian cancer,[19] uterus/endometrial cancer,[20] and prostate cancer.[21] Steroid hormones, specifically estrogen and progesterone, are essential for breast development and growth at puberty. However, increased lifetime exposure to endogenous estrogen and early menarche (first menstruation cycle), late menopause, estrogen replacement therapy, obesity, or late first full-term pregnancy, are associated with an increased risk of breast cancer in pre- and postmenopausal women.[18]

Estrogen carcinogenesis: Estrogen acting via estrogen receptors (ERs) causes mutation, which errors in DNA replication and induces cancer cell proliferation in breast cancer. Estrogen, their catechol metabolites, and ER-mediated signaling pathways significantly contribute to cancer initiation and development of cancer. In extrahepatic tissues, endogenous estrogens, estrone (E_1) and estradiol [or 17β-estradiol (E_2)], are metabolized into 2-$OHE_1(E_2)$ and 4-$OHE_1(E_2)$. The 2-$OHE_1(E_2)$ and 4-$OHE_1(E_2)$ methylation are catalyzed by the catechol-O-methyltransferase (COMT) at 2-OH, 3-OH [sites of 2-$OHE_1(E_2)$], and 4-OH [site of 4-$OHE_1(E_2)$]. 2-$OHE_1(E_2)$ and 4-$OHE_1(E_2)$ further oxidized to their catechol quinone metabolites, that is, $E_1(E_2)$-2,3-quinones [$E_1(E_2)$-2,3-Q] and $E_1(E_2)$-3,4-quinones [$E_1(E_2)$-3,4-Q], respectively, which covalently bind and react with DNA to form depurinating adducts. $E_1(E_2)$-2,3-Q is less reactive with DNA and produces stable DNA adducts, whereas $E_1(E_2)$-3,4-Q forms higher levels of depurinating DNA adducts. 2-$OHE_1(E_2)$ methylation by COMT has inhibitory effects on cell proliferation, thus reducing genotoxicity. $E_1(E_2)$-3,4-Q reacts with DNA and forms the depurinating estrogen-DNA adducts, 4-$OHE_1(E_2)$-1-N3A, and 4-$OHE_1(E_2)$-1-N7G. These depurinating adducts induce mutation in DNA and oxidative stress, leading toward cancer initiation and development. The glycosyl bond cleavage removes depurinating DNA adducts forming an apurinic site and leading toward the cancer cascade.[22,23]

Progesterone carcinogenesis:

Progesterone acts via binding to its receptor, progesterone receptors (PRs), which dimerize and interact with progesterone response element, and transcription pathway to regulate gene expression. PR has two predominant isoforms: PR-A (94 kDa) and PR-B (116 kDa), which are transcribed by the two promoter regions of a single-same gene, PR gene (*PGR*). Both promoter regions have different transcriptional and functional roles. PR-A is considered a transcriptional inhibitor of PR-B, which functions as a transcriptional activator. In normal tissues, both isoforms of PR are expressed in an equivalent ratio. However, the ratio of PR-A and PR-B is uneven in brain cells, which alters the transcription and thus dysregulates gene expression. The dysregulated transcriptional activities and differential cellular signaling plausibly contribute to the cancer pathology. The precancerous cells have increased kinase activity that phosphorylates PR-B leading to the hyperactivity of PR-B. The PR-B isoform exerts dysplastic phenotypes, induces cell proliferation in breast cancer, and regulates the extracellular signal transduction pathway in response to progesterone.[24,25]

Androgen carcinogenesis: Androgens perform function by binding to the androgen receptors (ARs) and regulating transcription that primarily influences the development of sexual characteristics at puberty and maintenance of the function of the male reproductive system. Androgens are also involved in the development of male-specific phenotype during embryogenesis, regulate spermatogenesis, early prostatic development, and are also responsible for the growth and proper functioning of the prostate gland. Since the activation of ARs by androgens is vital for the development and survival of the prostate, such a pathway is also crucial for the initiation and progression of the oncogenic potential of prostate cancer and metastatic pathway. Low levels of testosterone are associated with a higher risk of prostate cancer and deterioration of metastatic prostate cancer. AR is a ligand-dependent transcription activator, and the AR signaling axis has a significant role in prostate carcinogenesis. In nonmalignant normal prostate, AR activates transcriptional program for genes, such as prostate-specific antigen, required for normal prostate functioning. However, AR is the primary mediator of the cell cycle, growth, and survival of cancerous cells. Increased production of ARs and low circulating testosterone level facilitate the survival and cell proliferation of prostate cancer and depletion of androgens. Increased AR expression could be caused by mutations in the ligand-binding domain (LBD), amino terminus, and DNA-binding domain, resulting in gene amplification and increasing transcriptional pathways. ARs are only activated by testosterone and DHT. However, mutations increase the sensitivity of ARs to low concentrations of androgens, weak adrenal androgens (DHEA), weak androgen precursors, other steroid hormones (estradiol, estrogen, progesterone, and cortisol), and even antiandrogens that results in promiscuous binding and activation of ARs. The binding and activation of ARs by nonsteroid molecules are ligand-dependent activation, and ligand-independent binding activates downstream signaling of the ARs. This type of activation is outlaw activation. Deregulated growth factors, such as epidermal growth factor, insulin-like growth factor, and cytokines (i.e., IL-6), activate the outlaw activation and result in an outlaw pathway, in which growth and survival of cancer are no longer dependent on ARs. The AR-mediated signal transduction pathway is also regulated by coactivators and corepressors that act as signal intermediates between ARs and transcriptional pathways. Alterations in the expression levels of the coactivators and corepressors facilitate aberrant AR activity and lead to the oncogenic potential of cancer. This imbalance in coactivators and corepressors also sensitizes ARs to lower androgen levels. Thus AR signaling transduction initiates and develops prostate cancer. [26,27]

Synthetic estrogens, progestins, and androgens for treatment of hormone-related diseases

Hormonal therapy

Currently, synthetic hormones have been widely used as pharmaceuticals to treat hormonal disorders and diseases caused by hormonal disorders. Exogenous or synthetic steroid hormones are used as pharmaceutical agents in hormone replacement therapy to treat menopausal symptoms and hormonal birth control methods (hormonal contraception). Hormones, either endogenous or synthetic, have potential to treat to treat menopausal symptoms, cancer, hypogonadism, etc. Hormone replacement therapy, or menopausal hormone therapy, treat symptoms associated with female menopause that include vasomotor hot flashes, vaginal dryness, mood swing, depression, anxiety, sleep disturbance, night sweats, osteoporosis, sexual dysfunction, reduced libido, irritability, and others. The main hormonal medications involved in menopausal hormone therapy are estrogen, progesterone, and progestins (synthetic progesterone). Testosterone, sometimes, also are used for postmenopausal therapy. Androgen replacement therapy, also known as testosterone therapy, is used to counter the effects of low testosterone levels or hypogonadism in males. Hormonal therapy is also used to treat various hormone-sensitive cancers, including breast, endometrium, and prostate.[28] Hormone antagonists are utilized in hormone therapy for cancer to inhibit secretion and block the activity of hormones, thereby reducing the development and progression of a cancerous mass. Hormones are also exploiting as contraceptives, that is, for preventing pregnancy, known as hormonal contraception. Hormonal contraceptives contain estrogen and progestins, or a combination of both that inhibits follicle-stimulating hormone (FSH) and LH secretion, suppresses ovulation, and thickens cervical mucus to block sperm penetration.[29] Synthetic hormones are widely used as pharmacological agents and have an almost similar mode of action, just like endogenous hormones.

Mechanism of action of synthetic estrogens

Synthetic estrogens have relatively slightly different chemical structures and properties due to which they are absorbed, metabolized, and secreted by the body differently, as compared to endogenous estrogens. As synthetic estrogens mimic the estrogens (as shown in Table 6.2), they act upon the endogenous ERs to exert their pharmaceutical activity.

Estradiol: One of the classes of estrogen is estradiol, a steroid, and lipophilic compound, which can bind and activate nuclear ERs (ERα, ERβ) and membrane ERs (GPER). Estradiol is considered more potent than estrone and estriol. Estradiol can readily penetrate cell membrane through lipid bilayer via passive diffusion and binds with ERs on a wide variety of tissues in the body. The ERs are mainly expressed in the ovaries, uterus, and breast. The binding of estradiol with ER forms estradiol-bound ER–ER complex and causes homodimerization (ERα–ERα or ERβ–ERβ) or heterodimerization (ERα–ERβ), which binds with a specific DNA sequence called estrogen response elements (ERE). The binding of estradiol-bound ER–ER complex with ERE in promoter regions of estrogen-responsive gene regulates transcriptional program and gene expression (Fig. 6.3). The binding of estradiol with ER causes downregulation of the ERs through ubiquitination and proteasome degradation. Synthetic estrogens also control the pituitary gonadotropin secretion, FSH, and LH via a negative feedback mechanism, inhibiting follicle development and ovulation. Gonadotropin-releasing hormone (GnRH) is the major regulator of FSH and LH, which is released from hypothalamic neurons and binds to receptors expressed on gonadotrophs to stimulate LH secretion. The LH stimulates the secretion of estrogen, progesterone, and testosterone, which in turn inhibiting GnRH secretion.[30,31] This negative feedback mechanism is also utilized by

TABLE 6.2 Properties of synthetic estrogens.

Synthetic estrogen type	IUPAC name	Structure	Form of medication	Medical uses	Side effects
EE	(8R,9S,13S,14S,17R)-17-ethynyl-13-methyl-7,8,9,11,12,14,15,16-octahydro-6H-cyclopenta [a]phenanthrene-3,17-diol	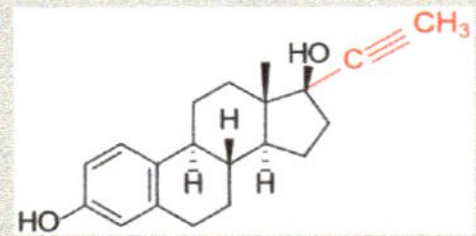	Available in combination with progestins in form of tablets, transdermal contraceptive patch, and contraceptive vaginal ring	Contraception, menopause symptoms, gynecological disorders, hypogonadism, prostate cancer, and breast cancer	Breast enlargement and tenderness, feminization, and hypogonadism
Estrone sulfate	(3aS,3bR,9bS,11aS)-11a-Methyl-1-oxo-2,3,3a,3b,4,5,9b,10,11,11a-decahydro-1H-cyclopenta[a]phenanthren-7-yl hydrogen sulfate	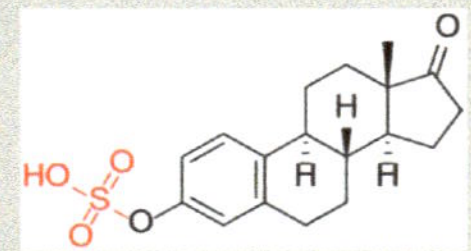	Tablet, cream	Menopausal hormone therapy, hypoestrogenism, underdeveloped female sexual characteristic, vaginal atrophy, cancers	Breast enlargement and tenderness, high blood pressure, ovarian cancer, etc.

Estropipate	[(8R,9S,13S,14S)-13-methyl-17-oxo-7,8,9,11,12,14,15,16-octahydro-6H-cyclopenta [a]phenanthren-3-yl] hydrogen sulfate; piperazine	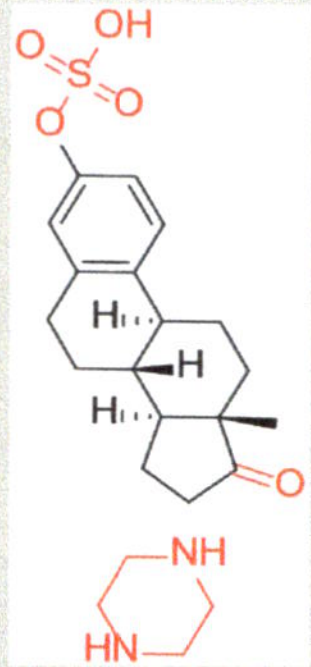	Tablet	Menopausal symptoms, osteoporosis	Breast tenderness or swelling, headache, nausea, etc.
Estradiol valerate	(1S,3aS,3bR,9bS,11aS)-7-hydroxy-11a-methyl-1H,2H,3H,3aH,3bH,4H,5H,9bH,10H,11H,11aH-cyclopenta[a]phenanthren-1-yl pentanoate	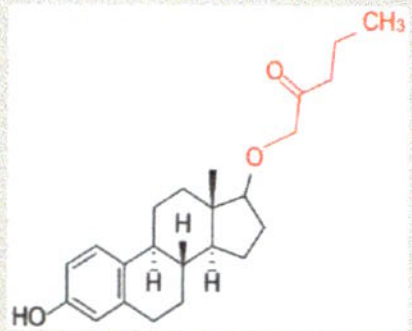	Tablet and intramuscular injection	Menopause, hypoestrogenism, androgen-sensitive prostate cancer, endometriosis	Yeast infection of vagina, decreased appetite, nausea, stomach upset, etc.
Estradiol acetate	(1S,3aS,3bR,9bS,11aS)-1-hydroxy-11a-methyl-1H,2H,3H,3aH,3bH,4H,5H,9bH,10H,11H,11aH-cyclopenta[a]phenanthren-7-yl acetate	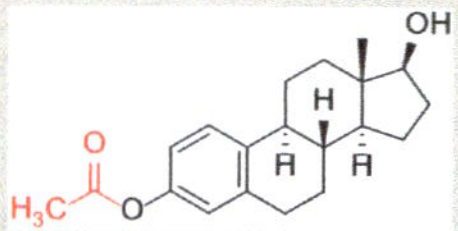	Tablet, vaginal ring	Menopausal symptoms and vaginal atrophy	Nausea, vomiting, weakness, unusual sweating, body pain, etc.

(*Continued*)

TABLE 6.2 (Continued)

Synthetic estrogen type	IUPAC name	Structure	Form of medication	Medical uses	Side effects
Estradiol cypionate	(1S,3aS,3bR,9bS,11aS)-7-hydroxy-11a-methyl-1H,2H,3H,3aH,3bH,4H,5H,9bH,10H,11H,11aH-cyclopenta[a]phenanthren-1-yl 3-cyclopentylpropanoate	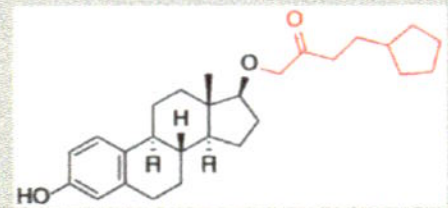	Intramuscular injection	Vasomotor symptoms, hypoestrogenism, hypogonadism	Decreased appetite, nausea, stomach upset, vomiting, weakness, unusual sweating, body pain, etc.
Estradiol benzoate	(1S,3aS,3bR,9bS,11aS)-1-hydroxy-11a-methyl-1H,2H,3H,3aH,3bH,4H,5H,9bH,10H,11H,11aH-cyclopenta[a]phenanthren-7-yl benzoate	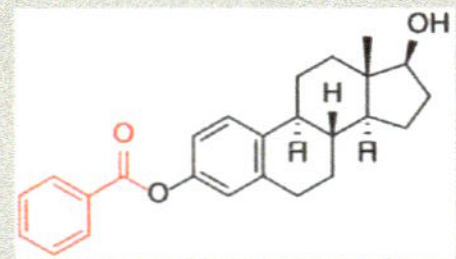	Intramuscular injection and subcutaneous injection	Irregular menstruation, low-estrogen level	Breast swelling, decrease appetite, nausea, stomach upset, vomiting, weakness, unusual sweating, body pain, etc.

Note: Red color in structures shows the difference of synthetic estrogens from endogenous estradiol and estriol. *EE*, Ethinyl estradiol.

synthetic estrogens, due to which FSH and LH decrease and ovulation stopped (Fig. 6.2). This effect of estradiol results in a preovulatory surge in output of FSH and LH and is highly effective in preventing pregnancy, thus utilized for hormonal contraception. However, estradiol is an endogenous hormone and has low oral bioavailability. Thus estradiol is commonly synthesized as prodrug with an ester side chain.

Ethinyl estradiol: One of the classes of synthetic estrogen is ethinyl estradiol (EE), which is used as oral contraceptive progestins to prevent pregnancy. EE is also used as a treatment of symptoms associated with menopause, gynecological disorders, and hormone-dependent cancers. EE is the synthetic derivative of endogenous estradiol, with enhanced bioavailability and decreased metabolism rate. EE is an agonist to both isoforms of nuclear ERs (ERα and ERβ) and GPER. EE binds and activates ERα and

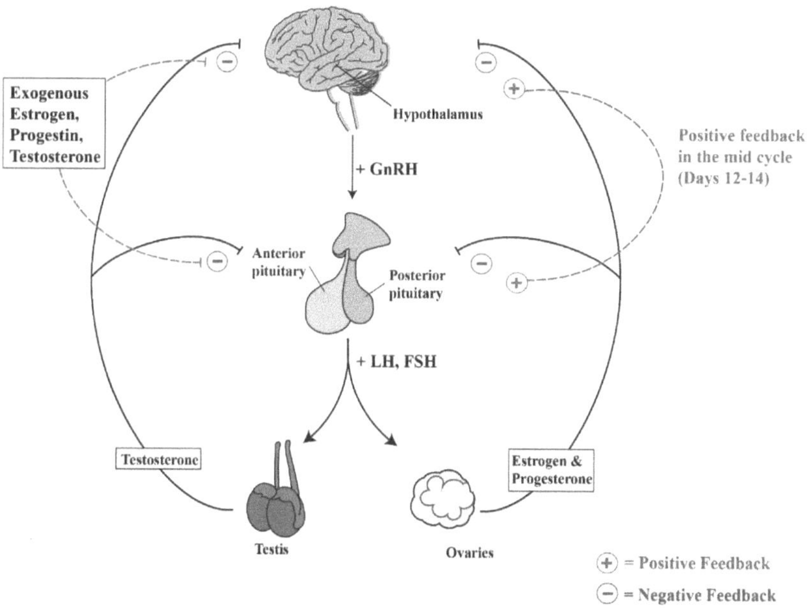

FIGURE 6.2 Hypothalamic–pituitary–ovarian axis and negative feedback mechanism: Hypothalamic neurons secrete GnRH, which triggers the secretion of LH and FSH from anterior pituitary. In males, LH binds to the receptors in Leydig cells in testes and stimulates the secretion of testosterone. In females, FSH triggers estradiol secretion from granulosa cells in primary follicles and LH stimulates theca cells to secrete androgens as estrogen precursors. If fertilization occurs, LH will stimulate the corpus luteum, which produces progesterone to sustain the pregnancy. In negative feedback mechanism, the resulting estradiol, progesterone, and testosterone suppress the secretion of GnRH and also LH and FSH. Moreover, Estrogen and progesterone appear to have positive effects on GnRH and in turn LH and FSH during midmenstrual cycle surge (i.e., day 12th–14th). This negative feedback loop controls menstruation and ovulation. *FSH*, Follicle-stimulating hormone; *GnRH*, Gonadotropin-releasing hormone; *LH*, luteinizing hormone.

exerts its antigonadotrophic and contraceptive effects by inhibiting FSH and LH synthesis, thus negatively interfering follicular development, ovulation, corpus luteum formation, and hence possible pregnancy (Fig. 6.2). EE also exerts antiandrogenic effects by stimulating the synthesis and production of SHBG and inhibiting the pituitary secretion of LH.[32] Through SHBG and LH, the gonadal production of testosterone levels decreases, hence treating acne and hirsutism. The vaginal rings are also used for hormonal contraception that contains ethinyl acetate that releases EE and progestins, which combines with receptors, and receptor-mediated signaling pathway modulates gene expression (Fig. 6.3).

Conjugated equine estrogen and estrone sulfate: Conjugated equine estrogen (CEE), also known as CE, is also an estrogen medication used for hormonal therapy of menopausal symptoms, hypoestrogenism, breast cancer, prostate cancer, and other indications.[18] Conjugated estrogen is the mixture of estrogen hormones and agonists of the ERs, sold under the brand name of PREMARIN (PREgnant MARes' urine). Premarin is made from horse urine and consists of the sodium salts of water-soluble estrogen sulfates. CEEs have 71.5%–92% of estrogens: sodium estrone sulfate and sodium equilin sulfate. The steroid sulfatase acts upon estrone sulfate and converts into estrone, which in turn is converted into estradiol by 17β-dihydroxysteroid dehydrogenase. Sodium estrone is a prodrug of estrone, and estrone is a prodrug of estradiol, whereas sodium equilin sulfate is a prodrug of equilin which, in turn, is a prodrug of 17α-dihydroequilin sulfate. Moreover, synthetic CEEs contain 10 estrogen derivatives, which are derived from plants; sodium estrone sulfate, sodium Δ8,9-dehydroestrone sulfate, sodium equilin sulfate, sodium equilenin sulfate, sodium 17α-dihydroequilin sulfate, sodium 17β-dihydroequilin sulfate, sodium 17α-dihydroequilenin sulfate, sodium 17β-dihydroequilenin sulfate, sodium 17α-estradiol sulfate, sodium 17β-estradiol sulfate. (These plant-derived CEEs are sold as product Cenestin.) All these estrogen derivatives mimic the endogenous estrogen and hence bind ER (Fig. 6.3) and modulate gonadotropin secretions via a negative feedback mechanism, inhibiting FSH and LH synthesis and release (Fig. 6.2). Estropipate, or piperazine estrone sulfate, is a salt of estrone sulfate and piperazine. Estropipate is an estrogen prodrug of estrone and estradiol, which is hydrolyzed into estrone, which, in turn, is converted into estradiol and 17β-hydroxysteroid dehydrogenase (an enzyme that catalyzed steroid metabolism). Hence, it is estrogen and an agonist of ERs. Estropipate treats menopausal symptoms, breast cancer, prostate cancer, infertility, underdevelopment of female sexual characteristics and prevents osteoporosis. CEEs also increase the risk of stroke and decrease the risk of hip fracture.[33]

Estradiol esters: Estradiol valerate, estradiol acetate, estradiol cypionate, and estradiol benzoate are synthetic estradiol esters or estradiol prodrugs, which are used as a medication for hormonal therapy, hormonal contraception, low-estrogen levels, and prostate cancer. When estradiol valerate enters into blood or body tissue, it catalyzes into estradiol by the esterase. Estradiol acetate is also converted into bioidentical estradiol. These estradiol functions similarly as the endogenous estrogen activate ER and modulate gene expression (Fig. 6.3).[34] Estradiol binds with a target cell receptor, and a ligand enters the nucleus of the target cell. The ligand interacts with the estrogen response element, regulating transcriptional cascade and mRNA forms. The mRNA translates into a specific protein that expresses the effects of estradiol upon the target cell. Estradiol also inhibits FSH and LH, which in turn suppresses ovulation, leading toward contraception. Estradiol undecylenate also decreases testosterone levels.

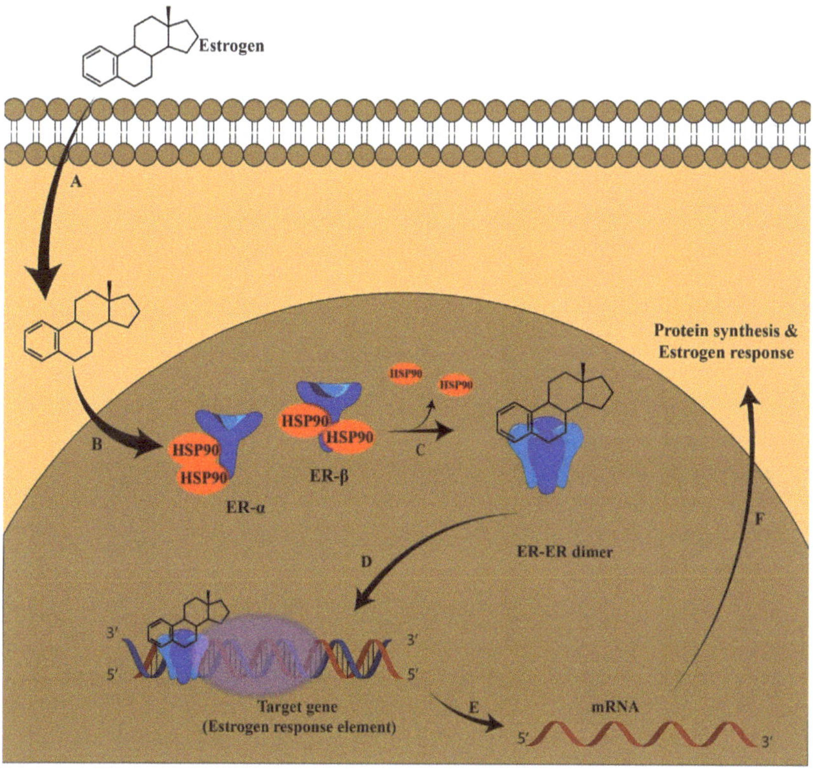

FIGURE 6.3 Mechanism of action of estrogens. (A) Estrogen enters the target cell and penetrates lipid bilayer (the uterus, ovary, breast, bone marrow, and brain) via diffusion due to their small size and lipophilicity. (B) Inactive ERs are located in the nucleus of the cell and bounded with the receptor-associated proteins, such as HSP90. Estrogen then enters the nucleus where it binds ERs (ER-α, ER-β), (C) and receptor-associated proteins dissociate. The binding of estrogen ligands to ERs forms estrogen-receptor complex and causes dimerization, which (D) binds with palindromic ERE and (E) regulates transcription cascade (F) and gene expression, thus exerting its biological function. *ER*, Estrogen receptor; *ERE*, estrogen response elements; *HSP*, heat-shock protein.

Mechanism of action of progestins

The synthetic form of endogenous progesterone is known as progestin. Progestins mimic the body's naturally occurring progesterone and interact with PRs and produce progesterone-like effects. They may also interfere with estrogen and ARs, activating or blocking them, thus causing side effects. Progestins, also known as progestogen, gestogen, progestagen, or gestagen, have been used for menopausal hormone therapy, hormonal contraception, gynecological disorders, infertility, cancers, and supporting pregnancy. Progestins prevent the proliferation of the endometrium, thus supporting pregnancy. Progestins decrease estrogen levels and are used for hormonal therapy in postmenopausal women. Progestins are also used for hormonal birth control by preventing LH surge, suppressing ovulation, thickening cervical mucus, and inhibiting sperm penetration to the uterus. Progestins also exert antigonadotrophic effects by inhibiting the synthesis and release of sex hormones.[28] Synthetic progesterone is used alone or in combination with a synthetic version of estrogen. Estrogen medications are usually taken with progestins to lower the risk of cancer. Progestins could be structural mimics of progesterone (nestorone, cyproterone acetate, etc.) or testosterone (norethindrone, levonorgestrel, etc.) (see Table 6.3).

Progestin generations: Progestins, used in oral contraceptives, are categorized as first to fourth-generation progestins on the basis of first commercial availability (Table 6.3).

- First-generation progestins include norethindrone, norethindrone acetate (NETA), ethynodiol diacetate, and medroxyprogesterone acetate (MPA).
- Second-generation progestins include norgestrel and levonorgestrel.
- Third-generation progestins include desogestrel, gestodene, cyproterone acetate, and norgestimate.
- Fourth-generation progestins include drospirenone, dienogest, and segesterone acetate.

Each of these progestins has a slightly different affinity toward progesterone, estrogen, ARs. The first-generation progestins are less potent and have a less androgenic effect (improve lipid profile by decreasing low-density lipoprotein or LDL and increasing high-density lipoprotein or HDL) than second-generation progestins, which are more potent, and have a high progestational and androgenic effect (increases LDL and decreases HDL). Third- and fourth-generation progestins are more potent than second generation but with less androgenic properties and side effects. Fourth-generation progestins have almost no androgenic activity, such as acne, hirsutism, obesity, and increased libido.

Progestins, being steroids (lipophilic), can pass through plasma and nuclear membrane via passive diffusion. When progestins enter the target cell, they bind freely to the PRs (PR-A, PR-B, and PR-C). Target tissues of

TABLE 6.3 Properties of progestins.

Synthetic estrogen type	IUPAC name	Structure	Form of medication	Medical uses	Side effects
Norethindrone	(8R,9S,10R,13S,14S,17R)-17-ethynyl-17-hydroxy-13-methyl-1,2,6,7,8,9,10,11,12,14,15,16-dodecahydrocyclopenta[a]phenanthren-3-one	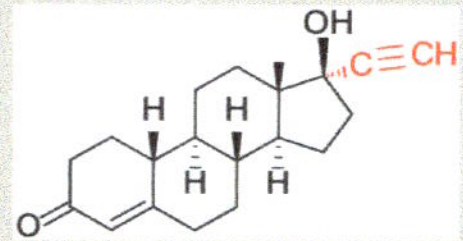	Tablet, film coated	Contraception, Endometrial hyperplasia, endometriosis, hormone therapy,	Hepatic veno-occlusive disease, nausea, vomiting, weakness, unusual sweating, body pain, breast tenderness, irregular periods, etc.
Norethindrone acetate	(8R,9S,10R,13S,14S,17S)-17-ethynyl-13-methyl-3-oxo-2,3,6,7,8,9,10,11,12,13,14,15,16,17-tetradecahydro-1H-cyclopenta[a]phenanthren-17-yl acetate	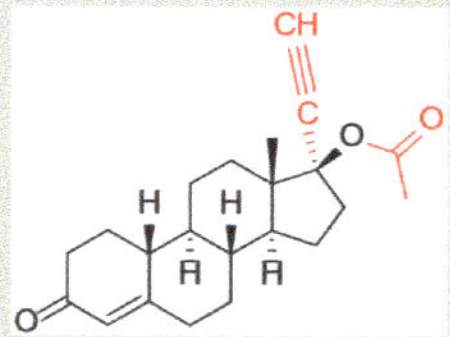	Tablet, transdermal patch, intramuscular injection	Endometriosis, leiomyoma of uterus, contraception, hormone therapy	Acne, nausea, vomiting, weakness, unusual sweating, body pain, breast tenderness, irregular periods, etc.

(*Continued*)

TABLE 6.3 (Continued)

Synthetic estrogen type	IUPAC name	Structure	Form of medication	Medical uses	Side effects
Ethynodiol diacetate	(1S,2R,5S,10R,11S,14R,15S)-5-(acetyloxy)-14-ethynyl-15-methyltetracyclo [8.7.0.0^{2}, ^{7}.0^{11}, ^{15}] heptadec-6-en-14-yl acetate	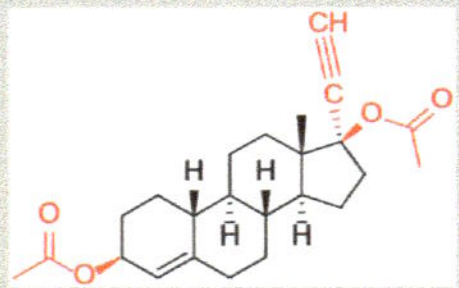	Tablet	Contraception	Acne, increased hair growth, breast pain, nausea, vomiting, water retention, etc.
Medroxyprogesterone acetate	(1S,2R,8S,10R,11S,14R,15S)-14-acetyl-2,8,15-trimethyl-5-oxotetracyclo [8.7.0.0^{2}, ^{7}.0^{11}, ^{15}] heptadec-6-en-14-yl acetate	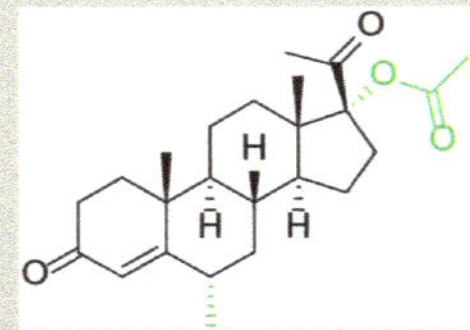	Tablet, intramuscular injection suspension.	Secondary amenorrhea, hormonal birth control, abnormal uterine bleeding, pain from endometriosis, endometrial and renal carcinomas, endometrial hyperplasia, osteoporosis, vasomotor symptoms in menopause paraphilia in males, and GnRH-dependent precocious puberty	Mood changes, swelling in ankles/feet, bone pain, vaginal bleeding, weakness, nausea, vomiting, etc.

Levonorgestrel	(1S,2R,10R,11S,14R,15S)-15-ethyl-14-ethynyl-14-hydroxytetracyclo [8.7.0.0^{2}, ^{7}.0^{11}, ^{15}] heptadec-6-en-5-one	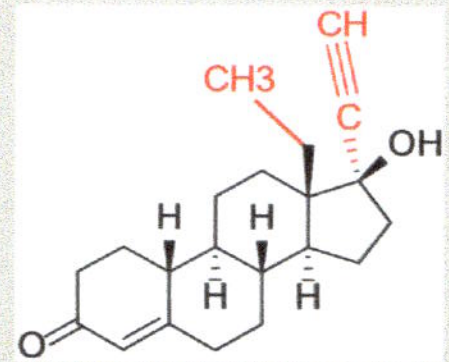	Tablet, IUD, subcutaneous implant, intrauterine insert	Contraception, pregnancy prevention, menopausal hormone therapy	Acne, increased hair growth, breast pain, nausea, vomiting, irregular menstruation, mood changes, etc.
Desogestrel	(1S,2R,10S,11S,14R,15S)-15-ethyl-14-ethynyl-17-methylidenetetracyclo [8.7.0.0^{2}, ^{7}.0^{11}, ^{15}] heptadec-6-en-14-ol	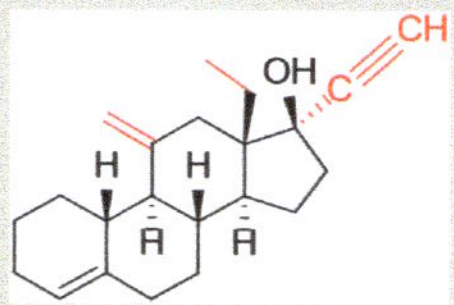	Tablet, kit	Contraception, menopausal hormone therapy.	Irregular menstrual cycle, amenorrhea, headache, nausea, vomiting, mood changes, breast tenderness, etc.
Gestodene	(1S,2R,10R,11S,14R,15S)-15-ethyl-14-ethynyl-14-hydroxytetracyclo [8.7.0.0^{2}, ^{7}.0^{11}, ^{15}] heptadeca-6,12-dien-5-one	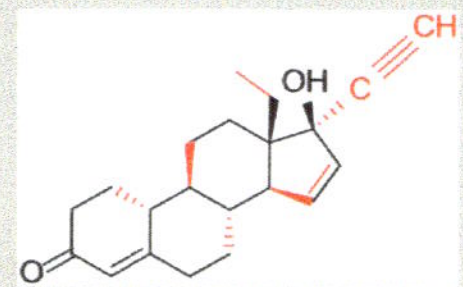	Tablet (delayed release), tablet (film coated), tablet (sugar coated), kit	Contraception, menopausal hormone therapy.	Irregular menstrual cycle, amenorrhea, headache, nausea, vomiting, mood changes, breast tenderness, etc.

(*Continued*)

TABLE 6.3 (Continued)

Synthetic estrogen type	IUPAC name	Structure	Form of medication	Medical uses	Side effects
Cyproterone acetate	(2aR,3aS,3bS,3cS,5aS,6R,8aS,8bR)-6-acetyl-10-chloro-5a-ethyl-3b-methyl-2-oxo-2,2a,3,3a,3b,3c,4,5,5a,6,7,8,8a,8b,9,10-hexadecahydrocyclopenta[a]cyclopropa[g]phenanthren-6-yl acetate	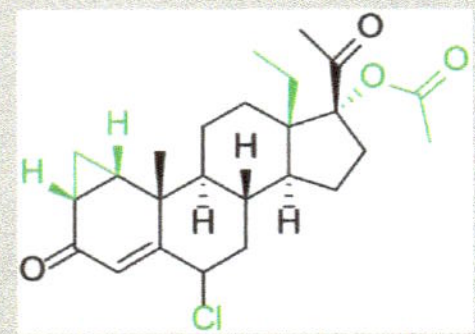	Tablet, intramuscular injection	Prostate cancer, hypersexuality in males, severe acne, hirsutism, and symptoms of androgenization	Gynecomastia and feminization in men, infertility, sexual dysfunction, depression, cardiovascular disorders, etc.
Norgestimate	(1R,3aS,3bR,7E,9aR,9bS,11aS)-11a-ethyl-1-ethynyl-7-(hydroxyimino)-1H,2H,3H,3aH,3bH,4H,5H,7H,8H,9H,9aH,9bH,10H,11H,11aH-cyclopenta[a]phenanthren-1-yl acetate	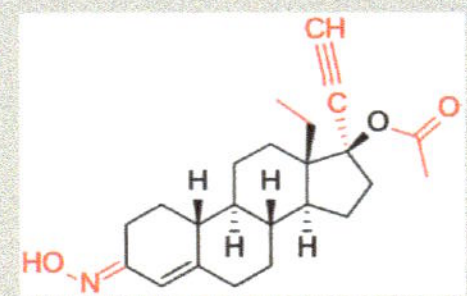	Tablet, kit	Contraception, pregnancy prevention, menopausal hormone therapy	Headache, abdominal pain, vaginal infection, breast tenderness, breast pain, vaginal discharge, mood changes, etc.

Drospirenone	(4aR,4bS,6aS,7S,7aS,8aS,8bS,8cR,8dR, 9aR)-4a,6a-dimethyl- 3′,4,4a,4b,4′,5,6,6a,7a,8,8a,8b, 8c,8d,9,9a-hexadecahydro-5′H-spiro [cyclopropa[4,5] cyclopenta[1,2-a] cyclopropa[l]phenanthrene-7,2′-furan]- 2,5′(3H)-dione	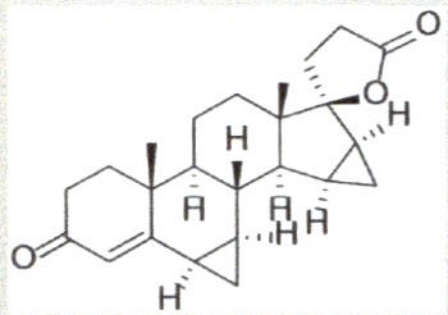	Tablet (film coated)	Contraception, pregnancy prevention, menopausal hormone therapy	Irregular menstrual cycle, amenorrhea, headache, nausea, vomiting, mood changes, breast tenderness, etc.
Dienogest	2-((8S,13S,14S,17R)-17-hydroxy-13-methyl-3-oxo- 2,3,6,7,8,11,12,13,14,15,16,17-dodecahydro-1H-cyclopenta[a] phenanthren-17-yl) acetonitrile	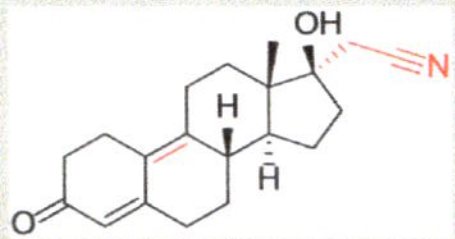	Tablet (film coated)	Contraception, pregnancy prevention, menopausal hormone therapy	Irregular menstrual cycle, amenorrhea, headache, nausea, vomiting, mood changes, breast tenderness, etc.
Segesterone acetate	(8R,9S,10R,13S,14S,17R)-17-acetyl-10,13-dimethyl-16-methylene-17-(prop-1-en-2-yloxy)- 1,2,6,7,8,9,10,11,12,13,14,15,16,17-tetradecahydro-3H-cyclopenta[a] phenanthren-3-one	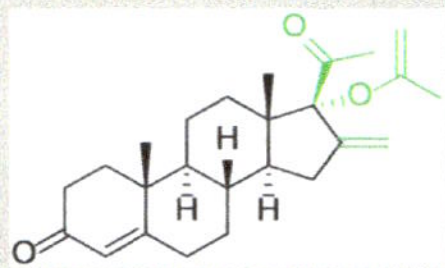	Vaginal ring, subcutaneous implant, transdermal gel	Endometriosis, male and female contraception	Depression, blur eyesight, lump in breast, breast pain, imbalance, trouble speaking or thinking, etc.

Note: Progestins may be created from progesterone or testosterone. The red color in structures shows the difference of progestins from endogenous testosterone, whereas the green color shows a difference of progestins from progesterone.

the progestin may include the brain (pituitary gland, hypothalamus), breast (the mammary glands), and female reproductive tract (uterus, cervix, vagina). Moreover, progestins are also an agonist of the membrane PRs (mPRα, mPRβ, mPRγ, mPRδ, and mPRε). Also, progestins have are weak affinity for the androgen and ERs. The binding of progestin with PR causes a conformational change in receptor converting into a dimer. The dimerization increases the affinity of PR toward DNA and regulates gene transcription leading toward the formation of mRNA. The mRNA interacts with ribosomes to modulate gene expression (Fig. 6.4).[35] The interaction of progestin with PR also suppresses GnRH by the hypothalamus, and gonadotropin (FSH and LH) secretion from the pituitary gland, via a negative feedback mechanism, thus preventing follicular development and maturation, ovulation, and altering or seizing menstrual cycle (Fig. 6.2).[36,37]

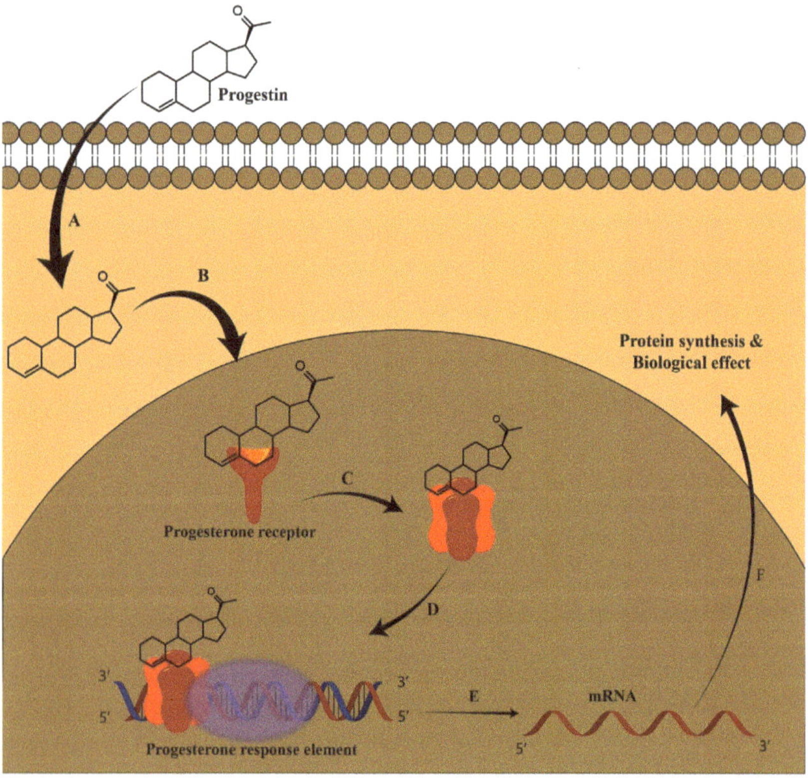

FIGURE 6.4 Mechanism of progestin. (A) Progestins penetrate the cell membrane easily due to steroid nucleus and (B) binds progesterone receptors, (C) causing conformational change and dimerization of progestin receptor complex. (D) The dimer recognizes and binds to DNA in a sequence-specific manner, which regulates (E) transcription. The resulting (E) mRNA translates into the required (F) protein and exerts therapeutic response.

First-generation progestins: Norethindrone, or Norethisterone or NET, was one of the first progestin to be developed. NET is a potent progestin and agonist of PRs with weak androgenic and estrogenic properties. Norethindrone is a progestin and has similar effects and mechanism of action to those of the body's natural progesterone. Some progestins are prodrugs of norethindrone as their structure resembles norethindrone, hence having similar progestogenic effects.[38] NETA is a prodrug of norethindrone, which upon hydrolysis by esterase during intestinal and first-pass hepatic metabolism is converted into norethindrone. Another progestin, ethynodiol diacetate or ethynodiol acetate, is also a prodrug of norethindrone. After oral administration, ethynodiol acetate is catalyzed by esterase into ethynodiol as intermediate and then converted into norethindrone during intestinal and hepatic first-pass metabolism.

MPA, first-generation progestin, works by activating progesterone, androgen, and glucocorticoid receptors.[39] MPA is a derivative of 19-nortestosterone progestin that is structurally related to testosterone. MPA suppresses FSH that inhibits follicular development, and prevention of LH surge prevents ovulation as the primary mechanism of action in preventing pregnancy. MPA also inhibits sperm penetration by cervical mucus thickness, promotes thinning of the endometrium, and reduces the likelihood of implantation.

Second-generation progestins: Norgestrel and its levo isomer, Levonorgestrel, are second-generation progestins. They are agonists of the PRs. Norgestrel and levonorgestrel interact with PRs and regulate GnRH, FSH, and LH secretion in a negative feedback loop manner (Fig. 6.2). Inhibition of LH surge prevents pregnancy by inhibiting ovulation and thickening of cervical mucus interfere with sperm movement and penetration.[40]

Third-generation progestins: Progesterone analogs desogestrel, gestodene, and norgestimate are third-generation oral contraceptives that inhibit ovulation by suppressing the secretion of FSH and LH from the pituitary gland. Desogestrel is an inactive progestin that is rapidly and completely metabolized into a biologically active metabolite, etonogestrel (C3 ketone derivative of desogestrel), in intestinal mucosa and liver. Etonogestrel interacts with PRs and sometimes with ERs and activates gene expression to prevent ovulation. Norgestimate is prodrug of norelgestromin and to a lesser extent of levonorgestrel and levonorgestrel acetate. Levonorgestrel, which is catalyzed by 5α-reductase into 5α-dihydrolevonorgestrel, is an active metabolite of levonorgestrel acetate and norelgestromin. However, gestodene is not a prodrug like desogestrel and norgestimate. Cyproterone acetate, an antiandrogen, binds ARs and suppresses LH production which in turn blocks the synthesis of testosterone and DHT via negative feedback mechanism (Fig. 6.2).[41] By this mechanism, cyproterone acetate treats prostatic cancer.

Fourth-generation progestins: Dienogest is a fourth-generation oral contraceptive progestin and a derivative of 19-nortestosterone with a cyanomethyl rather than ethinyl group at 17 α position. Dienogest prevents the growth of the endometrium by inhibiting angiogenesis, vascularization, and proliferation. Dienogest antagonizes the PR with a weak affinity for PR but high progestogenic activity. Dienogest activates PR and suppresses the hypothalamic–pituitary–ovarian (HPO) axis and gonadotropin secretion with moderate suppression of circulating estradiol and causes anovulation. Dienogest increases the progesterone secretion that enhances the stability of the endometrium. Dienogest treats endometriosis and reduces inflammation. Dienogest also influences prostaglandin E2 (PGE2), which is a common medication for pregnancy termination. PGE2 has a critical role in the pathogenesis of endometriosis, a highly estrogen-dependent and antiapoptotic disease. Increased concentration of PGE2 enhances inflammation and pain hypersensitivity leading toward initiation and development of endometriosis. Dienogest inhibits PGE2 production and aromatase (or estrogen synthase), an enzyme that catalyzes the conversion of androgens into estrogens. Thus dienogest decreases estrogen level and significantly treats endometriosis.[42] The fourth-generation pills, Dienogest, bind PRs and form a dienogest-receptor complex. This dienogest-receptor complex is translocated toward the nucleus, binds to the progesterone response element, and regulates the transcriptional pathway for gene expression. Thus it prevents the LH surge and FSH secretion[43] resulting in anovulation. Dienogest also thickens cervical mucus, inhibiting sperm penetration. Drospirenone is a fourth-generation progestin that resembles natural progesterone more than progestin, and its mode of action is also the same as progesterone. Segesterone acetate, also known as nestorone, is the derivative of 19-norprogesterone that lacks CH3 group radical at position 6. Segesterone acetate differs from progesterone with the presence of 17α-acetoxy and 16-methylene groups. The additional stabilizing contacts form between 17α-acetoxy, 16-methylene groups, and PR LBD, due to which segesterone acetate has a higher potency than progesterone. Segesterone acetate acts as an agonist and transactivator by selectively binding at PR, inhibiting follicular development, preventing LH surge, thereby suppressing ovulation.[44] It can also treat endometriosis and restrain irregular shedding of endometriosis.

Mechanism of action of synthetic Androgens

Synthetic androgens, often testosterone, are used as pharmacological agents to treat male hypogonadism, hypoandrogenism, impotence male, and delayed puberty in boys. It is also used in postmenopausal women to regulate libido and sexual desire, prevent abortion, treat HSDD and breast cancer.[45] Synthetic androgens are also known as Anabolic-androgenic steroids (AAS) or anabolic steroids that are structurally related to testosterone activate ARs on the target cell surface just like endogenous testosterone[46] (Table 6.4). Testosterone replacement therapy is used to treat testosterone deficiency or hypotestosteronemia. AAS or testosterone either exert biological effect by interacting with ARs (directly or metabolites) or by conversion to estradiol

TABLE 6.4 Properties of synthetic androgens (testosterone and dihydrotestosterone).

Synthetic estrogen type	IUPAC name	Structure	Form of medication	Medical uses	Side effects
Testosterone cypionate	(8R,9S,10R,13S,14S,17S)-10,13-dimethyl-3-oxo-2,3,6,7,8,9,10,11,12,13,14,15,16,17-tetradecahydro-1H-cyclopenta[a] phenanthren-17-yl 3-cyclopentylpropanoate	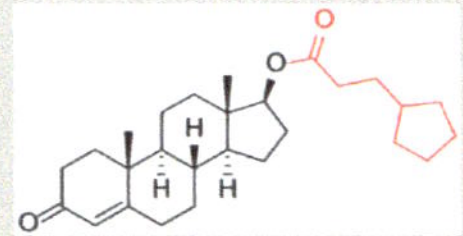	Intramuscular injection	Hypogonadotropic hypogonadism or primary hypogonadism	Virilization or masculinization, prostate gland enlargement, acne, gynecomastia, more frequent painful erections and for longer time (priapism), mood swings, headache, etc.
Testosterone propionate	(8R,9S,10R,13S,14S,17S)-10,13-dimethyl-3-oxo-2,3,6,7,8,9,10,11,12,13,14,15,16,17-tetradecahydro-1H-cyclopenta[a] phenanthren-17-yl propionate	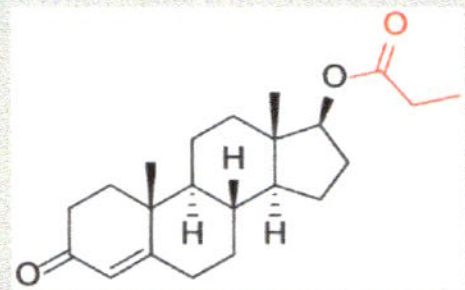	Intramuscular injection	Androgen deficiency in male adults either in hypogonadism or andropause, breast cancer	Virilization, irritable bladder, priapism, irregular menstruation
Testosterone enanthate	(8R,9S,10R,13S,14S,17S)-10,13-dimethyl-3-oxo-2,3,6,7,8,9,10,11,12,13,14,15,16,17-tetradecahydro-1H-cyclopenta[a] phenanthren-17-yl heptanoate	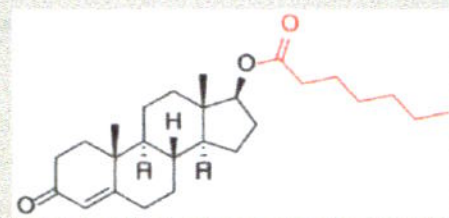	Intramuscular injection, subcutaneous injection	Low or absent testosterone level, hypogonadotropic hypogonadism, or primary hypogonadism	Nausea, vomiting, headache, hair loss, acne, altered sexual interest, skin color change, oily skin, etc.

(*Continued*)

TABLE 6.4 (Continued)

Synthetic estrogen type	IUPAC name	Structure	Form of medication	Medical uses	Side effects
Testosterone undecanoate	(8R,9S,10R,13S,14S,17S)-10,13-dimethyl-3-oxo-2,3,6,7,8,9,10,11,12,13,14,15,16,17-tetradecahydro-1H-cyclopenta[a]phenanthren-17-yl undecanoate	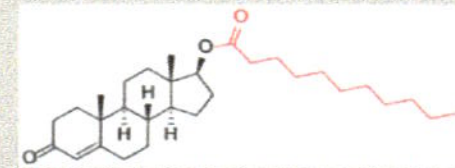	Liquid filled capsule, intramuscular injection	Hypogonadism, low or absent testosterone level	Nausea, vomiting, headache, hair loss, acne, altered sexual interest, skin color change, oily skin, etc.
Methyltestosterone	(8R,9S,10R,13S,14S,17S)-17-hydroxy-10,13,17-trimethyl-1,2,6,7,8,9,10,11,12,13,14,15,16,17-tetradecahydro-3H-cyclopenta[a]phenanthren-3-one	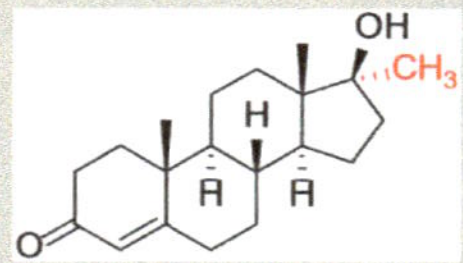	Tablet, capsule	Hypogonadism, breast cancer, menopausal hormonal therapy	Masculinization, acne, increased hair growth, nausea, vomiting, headache, hair loss, altered sexual desire, skin color change, oily skin, etc.
Oxymetholone	(8R,9S,10S,13S,14S,17S, E)-17-hydroxy-2-(hydroxymethylene)-10,13,17-trimethylhexadecahydro-3H-cyclopenta[a]phenanthren-3-one	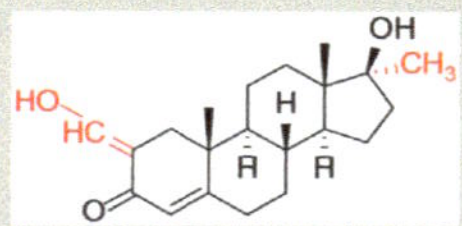	Tablet	Anemia, HIV/AIDS wasting syndrome	Nausea, vomiting, diarrhea, male pattern baldness, breast swelling or tenderness, acne, etc.
Fluoxymesterone	(8S,9R,10S,11S,13S,14S,17S)-9-fluoro-11,17-dihydroxy-10,13,17-trimethyl-1,2,6,7,8,9,10,11,12,13,14,15,16,17-tetradecahydro-3H-cyclopenta[a]phenanthren-3-one	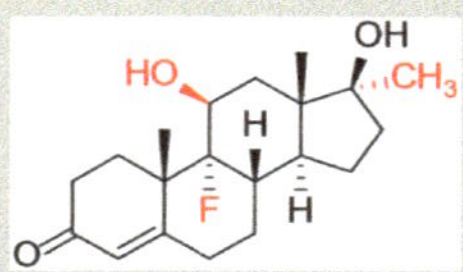	Tablet	Hypogonadism, delayed puberty, breast cancer, anemia	Masculinization, acne, increased hair growth, nausea, vomiting, headache, hair loss, altered sexual desire, skin color change, oily skin, etc.

Danazol	(1R,3aS,3bR,10aR,10bS,12aS)-1-ethynyl-10a,12a-dimethyl-2,3,3a,3b,4,5,10,10a,10b,11,12,12a-dodecahydro-1H-cyclopenta[7,8] phenanthrol[3,2-d] isoxazol-1-ol	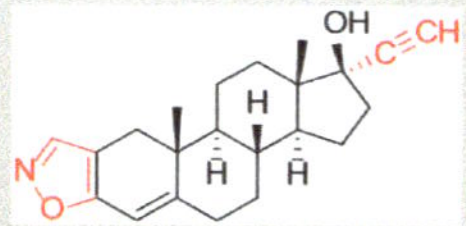	Tablet	Endometriosis, benign fibrocystic breasts disease, hereditary angioedema in males and females	Ace, decreased breast size, vaginal dryness, sweating, oily skin, weight gain, etc.
Oxandrolone	(4aS,4bS,6aS,7S,9aS,9bR)-7-hydroxy-4a,6a,7-trimethyltetradecahydroindeno[4,5-h] isochromen-2(1H)-one	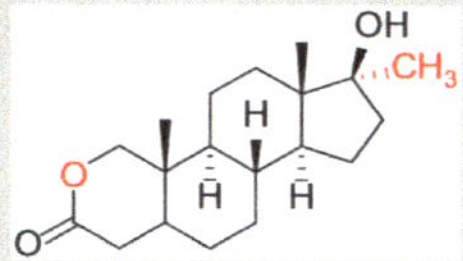	Tablet	Osteoporosis, muscle loss from prolonged corticosteroid treatment, weight gain following surgery or trauma	Masculinization, acne, increased hair growth, nausea, vomiting, headache, hair loss, altered sexual desire, skin color change, oily skin, etc.
Methandrostenolone	(8R,9S,10R,13S,14S,17S)-17-hydroxy-10,13,17-trimethyl-6,7,8,9,10,11,12,13,14,15,16,17-dodecahydro-3H-cyclopenta[a] phenanthren-3-one	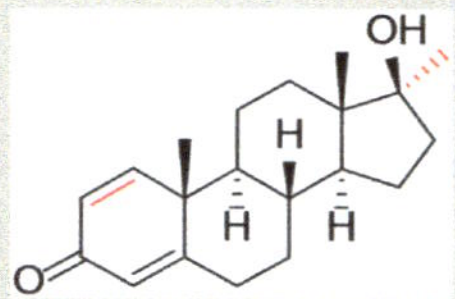	Tablet, intramuscular injection	Anorexia, physique- and performance-enhancing purposes	Masculinization, acne, increased hair growth, nausea, vomiting, headache, hair loss, altered sexual desire, skin color change, oily skin, voice changes, etc.

(*Continued*)

TABLE 6.4 (Continued)

Synthetic estrogen type	IUPAC name	Structure	Form of medication	Medical uses	Side effects
Norethandrolone	(8R,9S,10R,13S,14S,17S)-17-ethyl-17-hydroxy-10,13-dimethyl-1,2,6,7,8,9,10,11,12,13,14,15,16,17-tetradecahydro-3H-cyclopenta[a]phenanthren-3-one	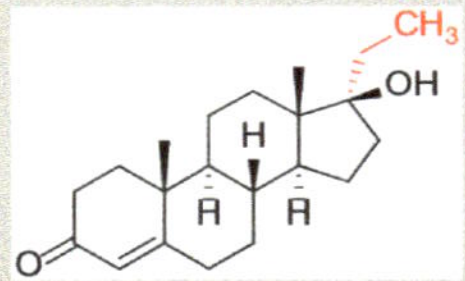	Tablet	Muscle loss, burn, trauma, anemia	Masculinization, acne, increased body hair growth, hair loss, altered sexual desire, voice changes, etc.
Nandrolone decanoate	(8R,9S,10R,13S,14S,17S)-13-methyl-3-oxo-2,3,6,7,8,9,10,11,12,13,14,15,16,17-tetradecahydro-1H-cyclopenta[a]phenanthren-17-yl decanoate	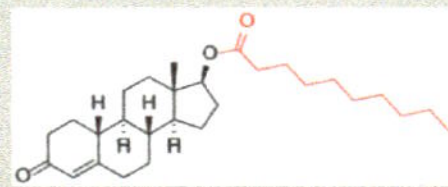	Intramuscular injection	Anemia of renal insufficiency, osteoporosis, wasting syndrome, menopausal therapy	Masculinization, acne, increased body hair growth, hair loss, altered sexual desire, voice changes, etc.
Nandrolone phenylpropionate	(8R,9S,10R,13S,14S,17S)-13-methyl-3-oxo-2,3,6,7,8,9,10,11,12,13,14,15,16,17-tetradecahydro-1H-cyclopenta[a]phenanthren-17-yl 3-phenylpropanoate	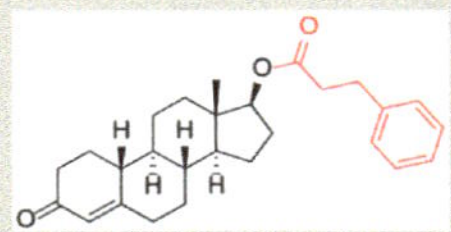	Intramuscular injection	Anemia, breast cancer, hereditary angioedema, antithrombin III deficiency, fibrinogen excess, growth failure, and Turner's syndrome	Gastrointestinal irritation, water retention, diarrhea, jaundice, abdominal pain, irregular menstruation, etc.

and binding with ERs. Testosterone and its active androgenic metabolites, DHT, penetrate the plasma membrane of the target cell and bind with the ARs located in the cytoplasm. In another pathway, testosterone is reduced by 5α-reductase into DHT, which is more potent than testosterone and binds with AR more strongly. The ARs are bounded with heat-shock proteins (HSPs) and chaperones. When testosterone or DHT binds with AR, it forms a testosterone-receptor complex/DHT-receptor complex, an HSP (HSP90) detaches from the receptor, and conformational changes occur.[47] This complex is translocated to the nucleus and binds to the specific HRE initiating transcriptional pathways inducing specific gene expression and androgenic effects of the target tissue(s). Testosterones may also activate ERs, which involve the conversion of testosterone into estradiol catalyzed by aromatase (Fig. 6.5), with nandrolone as intermediate. Androgens can also regulate transcription cascade through activating various cellular pathways, including ERK, Akt, and MAPK.

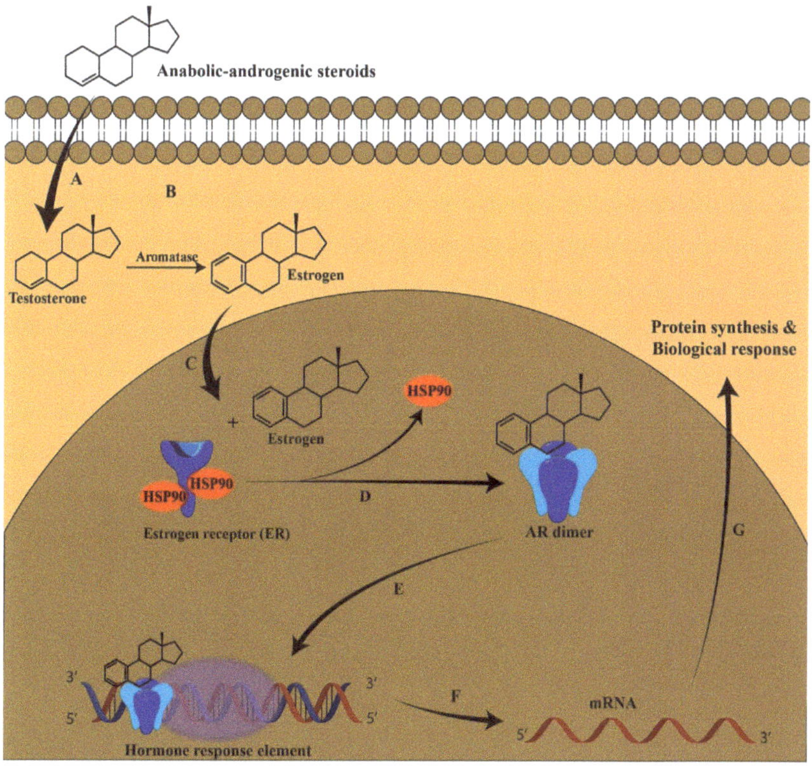

FIGURE 6.5 Mechanism of AAS and diversification pathway. In diversification pathway, synthetic testosterone is converted into an estrogen molecule via activity of aromatase. The estrogen binds with ERs in the target and control gene expression (Fig. 6.3). *AAS*, Anabolic-androgenic steroids.

Esters of testosterone and DHT: Various esterified variants of testosterone are used as intramuscular depot injection to treat low or absent testosterone that includes testosterone acetate, testosterone cypionate, testosterone enanthate, testosterone isobutyrate, testosterone isocaproate, testosterone propionate, testosterone undecanoate, testosterone phosphate, and many others. Testosterone esters are long-acting androgens, have different absorption rates and half-lives, but the mode of action is just like testosterone. The synthetic DHT is also known as stanolone or androstanolone. Similarly, DHT esters have been formed, including androstanolone benzoate, androstanolone enanthate, androstanolone propionate, androstanolone valerate, etc.[48] Methyltestosterone, a 1-methyl AAS, structurally resembles endogenous testosterone and acts at the molecular level just like testosterone (Figs. 6.5 and 6.6).

17α-alkylated AAS: Oxymetholone, a 17α-alkylated AAS and synthetic derivative of testosterone or DHT, is used to build muscle mass in HIV patients and

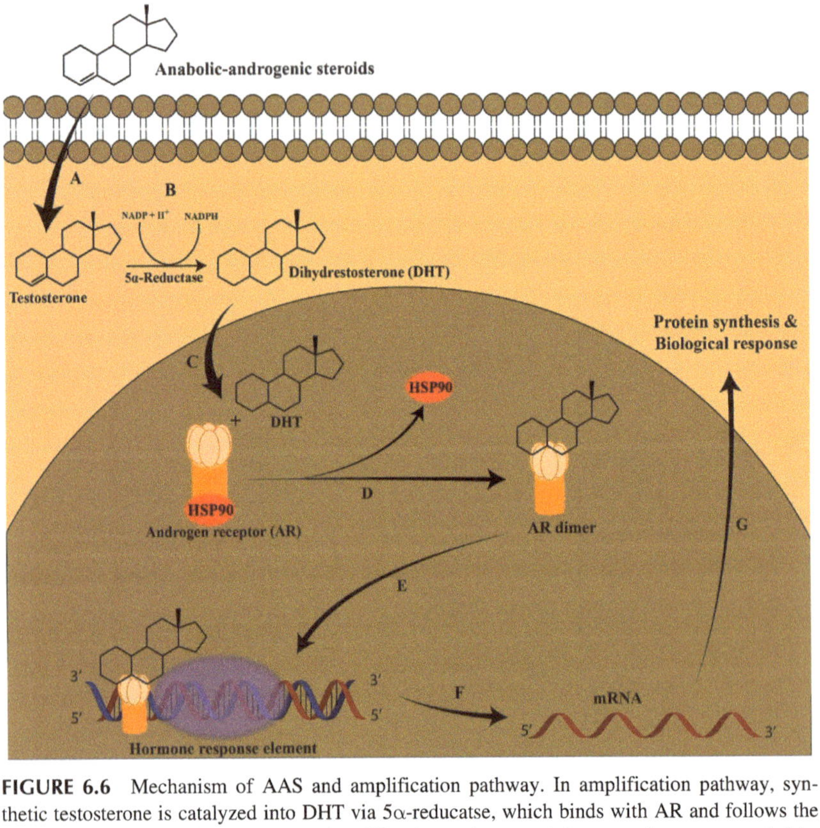

FIGURE 6.6 Mechanism of AAS and amplification pathway. In amplification pathway, synthetic testosterone is catalyzed into DHT via 5α-reducatse, which binds with AR and follows the similar pathway of AAS-testosterone. Amplification pathway mainly occurs in prostate and skin. *AAS*, Anabolic-androgenic steroids; *ARs*, androgen receptors; *DHT*, dihydrotestosterone.

treat different types of anemia.[49,50] It functions similarly to testosterone and exerts androgenic properties. Fluoxymesterone is a synthetic androgen and anabolic steroid similar to testosterone and DHT, which is used to treat hypogonadism, delayed puberty in boys, anemia, and breast cancer. Fluoxymesterone is a 17α-alkylated AAS, and like testosterone, it activates AR and enhances protein synthesis (Fig. 6.7). The anabolic activity of fluoxymesterone is associated with the retention of nitrogen, potassium, and phosphorus. Fluoxymesterone also exerts antitumor activity, especially against breast tumors,[51] by the competitive reduction of estrogens or prolactin receptors. Danazol is also a 17α-alkylated AAS and a modified form of testosterone that has antigonadotrophic and antiestrogenic effects, used for the treatment of endometriosis and benign fibrocystic breast.

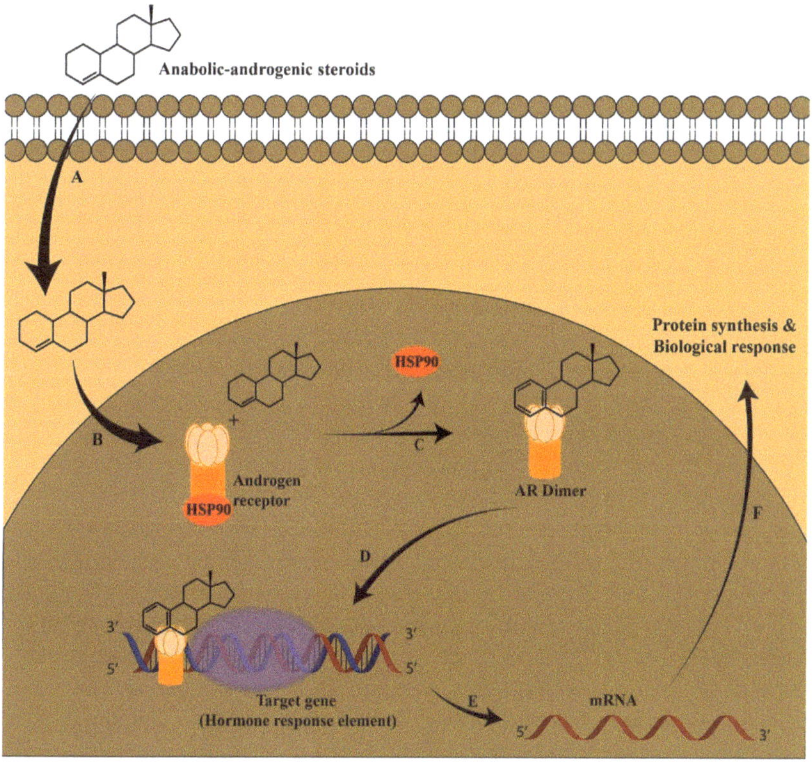

FIGURE 6.7 Mechanism of action of AAS or synthetic androgens. (A) AAS, being steroids (lipophilic), can pass through plasma membrane of the target cell via passive diffusion. (B) Inactive ARs, located in the nucleus, are bounded with the receptor-associated proteins, such as HSP90. AAS then enters the nucleus where it binds ARs, (C) and HSPs dissociates. The binding of ligand (AAS) with ARs forms androgen-receptor complex and causes dimerization, which (D) binds with hormone-response elements (HRE) and (E) regulates transcriptional program (F) and gene expression for required biological function. *AAS*, Anabolic-androgenic steroids; *ARs*, androgen receptors; *HSP*, heat-shock protein.

Danazol acts as a pituitary–ovarian axis suppressant that inhibits anterior pituitary output of gonadotrophins, suppresses mid-cycle FSH and LH surge, leading toward anovulation (Fig. 6.2). Danazol also has an affinity to bind estrogen, progesterone, and glucocorticoid receptors and SHBG and CBG.[52] By this, danazol depresses the biosynthesis of steroids from cholesterol (steroidogenesis) in the corpus luteum, as well as increases metabolic clearance of progesterone. In endometriosis treatment, danazol suppresses ovulation and causes the inactivation of the endometrium by lowering immunoglobulin (IgA, IgB, IgC) concentration. Another mechanism of action by which danazol treats hereditary angioedema is increasing serum C1 esterase inhibitor levels. The increase in C1 esterase inhibitors increases C4 synthesis that balances the biochemical deficiency in angioedema and improves the complement system. Danazol suppresses gonadal hormone secretion by inhibiting the CYP450 enzyme. Oxandrolone is also a 17α-alkylated AAS which also exerts anabolic and androgenic activity in target cells by interacting with PRs. Oxandrolone has been used to treat bone pain associated with osteoporosis and muscle loss due to catabolic effects of prolonged corticosteroid therapy. It also aids in gaining weight following extensive surgery or trauma. Various other synthetic 17α-alkylated AAS are also used as pharmacological agents, including Stanozolol, Ethylestrenol, Methandrostenolone, and Norethandrolone that exert their therapeutic anabolic and androgenic effects via interacting with ARs.[49]

Nandrolone and prodrugs: Another class of injectable AAS and derivate of testosterone is Nandrolone, also known as 19-nortestosterone or 19-norandrostenolone, which is used as a pharmacological agent in the form of aliphatic fatty esters.[49] Nandrolone is also an endogenous intermediate during testosterone conversion into estradiol, catalyzed by aromatase (Fig. 6.5). As compared to testosterone, nandrolone is demethylated at the C-19 position and esters (decanoate and phenylpropionate) at the C-17β. The ester salts of nandrolone include nandrolone decanoate and nandrolone phenylpropionate[53] that are used to treat senile and postmenopausal osteoporosis by increasing bone density and muscle mass, breast cancer, anemia, etc. Nandrolone decanoate is an alkylated anabolic steroid that, when administered via intramuscular injection, undergoes hydrolysis in the liver by phosphodiesterase 7B (PDE7B) and is converted into nandrolone. Nandrolone phenylpropionate is also a prodrug of nandrolone that is catalyzed into nandrolone, an active form of drug, in first-pass hepatic metabolism.[54] Nandrolone penetrates the target cell by receptor-mediated endocytosis and binds with the AR, causing a conformational change and a complex form. This complex enters the nucleus, where it interacts with the specific nucleotide sequence of DNA, androgen response element, regulating specific transcription signaling pathway and causing required change in function of the target cell. Nandrolone decanoate also suppresses LH and FSH secretion by the negative feedback mechanism[55] (Fig. 6.2). Similar to testosterone, nandrolone is also converted into 3-norandrosterone by 5α-reductase, which causes the low androgenic activity of nandrolone. When nandrolone is reduced via 5α-reductase, the resulting metabolite has a low affinity toward ARs. As estradiol is the metabolite of nandrolone, therefore it has low estrogenic activity.

References

1. Miller WL, Auchus RJ. The molecular biology, biochemistry, and physiology of human steroidogenesis and its disorders. *Endocr Rev*. 2011;32(1):81–151.
2. Schiffer L, et al. Human steroid biosynthesis, metabolism and excretion are differentially reflected by serum and urine steroid metabolomes: a comprehensive review. *J Steroid Biochem Mol Biol*. 2019;194:105439.
3. Gorski J, Gannon F. Current models of steroid hormone action: a critique. *Annu Rev Physiol*. 1976;38:425–450.
4. Chan L, O'Malley BW. Mechanism of action of the sex steroid hormones (first of three parts). *N Engl J Med*. 1976;294(24):1322–1328.
5. Chan L, O'Malley BW. Mechanism of action of the sex steroid hormones (second of three parts). *N Engl J Med*. 1976;294(25):1372–1381.
6. Chan L, O'Malley BW. Mechanism of action of the sex steroid hormones (third of three parts). *N Engl J Med*. 1976;294(26):1430–1437.
7. Bruce D, Rymer J. Symptoms of the menopause. *Best Pract Res Clin Obstet Gynaecol*. 2009;23(1):25–32.
8. Hale GE, Burger HG. Hormonal changes and biomarkers in late reproductive age, menopausal transition and menopause. *Best Pract Res Clin Obstet Gynaecol*. 2009;23(1):7–23.
9. Rohr UD. The impact of testosterone imbalance on depression and women's health. *Maturitas*. 2002;41:25–46.
10. Tyagi V, et al. Revisiting the role of testosterone: are we missing something? *Rev Urol*. 2017;19(1):16–24.
11. Meier RK. Polycystic ovary syndrome. *Nurs Clin North Am*. 2018;53(3):407–420.
12. Diamanti-Kandarakis E, Dunaif A. Insulin resistance and the polycystic ovary syndrome revisited: an update on mechanisms and implications. *Endocr Rev*. 2012;33(6):981–1030.
13. Khan MJ, Ullah A, Basit S. Genetic basis of polycystic ovary syndrome (PCOS): current perspectives. *Appl Clin Genet*. 2019;12:249–260.
14. Davidson JM, et al. Hormonal changes and sexual function in aging men*. *J Clin Endocrinol Metab*. 1983;57(1):71–77.
15. Basaria S. Male hypogonadism. *Lancet*. 2014;383(9924):1250–1263.
16. Hammes SR, Levin ER. Impact of estrogens in males and androgens in females. *J Clin Invest*. 2019;129(5):1818–1826.
17. Andersen ML, Tufik S. Does male sexual behavior require progesterone? *Brain Res Rev*. 2006;51(1):136–143.
18. Missmer SA, et al. Endogenous estrogen, androgen, and progesterone concentrations and breast cancer risk among postmenopausal women. *J Natl Cancer Inst*. 2004;96(24):1856–1865.
19. Ho SM. Estrogen, progesterone and epithelial ovarian cancer. *Reprod Biol Endocrinol*. 2003;1:73.
20. Olson SH, Bandera EV, Orlow I. Variants in estrogen biosynthesis genes, sex steroid hormone levels, and endometrial cancer: a HuGE review. *Am J Epidemiol*. 2007;165(3):235–245.

21. Sasaki M, et al. Methylation and inactivation of estrogen, progesterone, and androgen receptors in prostate cancer. *J Natl Cancer Inst*. 2002;94(5):384–390.
22. Yager JD, Davidson NE. Estrogen carcinogenesis in breast cancer. *N Engl J Med*. 2006;354(3):270–282.
23. Wen C, et al. Unifying mechanism in the initiation of breast cancer by metabolism of estrogen (Review). *Mol Med Rep*. 2017;16(2):1001–1006.
24. Trabert B, et al. Progesterone and breast cancer. *Endocr Rev*. 2019;41(2):320–344.
25. Diep CH, et al. Progesterone action in breast, uterine, and ovarian cancers. *J Mol Endocrinol*. 2015;54(2):R31–R53.
26. Fujita K, Nonomura N. Role of androgen receptor in prostate cancer: a review. *World J Men's Health*. 2019;37(3):288–295.
27. Pienta KJ, Bradley D. Mechanisms underlying the development of androgen-independent prostate cancer. *Clin Cancer Res*. 2006;12(6):1665.
28. Santoro N, et al. Compounded bioidentical hormones in endocrinology practice: an endocrine society scientific statement. *J Clin Endocrinol Metab*. 2016;101(4):1318–1343.
29. Fait T. Menopause hormone therapy: latest developments and clinical practice. *Drugs Context*. 2019;8:212551.
30. Arreguin-Arevalo JA, Nett TM. A nongenomic action of estradiol as the mechanism underlying the acute suppression of secretion of luteinizing hormone in ovariectomized ewes. *Biol Reprod*. 2006;74(1):202–208.
31. Temple JL, et al. Direct action of estradiol on gonadotropin-releasing hormone-1 neuronal activity via a transcription-dependent mechanism. *J Neurosci*. 2004;24(28):6326–6333.
32. Henríquez-Hernández LA, et al. Role of pituitary hormones on 17alpha-ethinylestradiol-induced cholestasis in rat. *J Pharmacol Exp Ther*. 2007;320(2):695–705.
33. Anderson GL, et al. Effects of conjugated equine estrogen in postmenopausal women with hysterectomy: the Women's Health Initiative randomized controlled trial. *JAMA*. 2004;291 (14):1701–1712.
34. Janocko L, Larner JM, Hochberg RB. The interaction of C-17 esters of estradiol with the estrogen receptor. *Endocrinology*. 1984;114(4):1180–1186.
35. DeMayo FJ, et al. Mechanisms of action of estrogen and progesterone. *Ann NY Acad Sci*. 2002;955:48–59. discussion 86–8, 396–406.
36. O'Malley BW, Strott CA. Mechanism of action of progesterone. In: Sartorelli AC, Johns DG, eds. *Antineoplast Immunosuppressive Agents: Part II*. Berlin, Heidelberg: Springer; 1975:158–169.
37. Apgar BS, Greenberg G. Using progestins in clinical practice. *Am Fam Phys*. 2000;62 (8):1839–1846. 1849–50.
38. Moghissi KS, Syner FN, McBride LC. Contraceptive mechanism of microdose norethindrone. *Obstet Gynecol*. 1973;41(4):585–594.
39. Pérez-Palacios G, et al. On the mechanism of action of progestins. *Acta Endocrinol*. 1981;97(3):320–328.
40. Kahlenborn C, Peck R, Severs WB. Mechanism of action of levonorgestrel emergency contraception. *Linacre Q*. 2015;82(1):18–33.
41. Hemrika DJ, et al. The effects of levonorgestrel, desogestrel and gestodene on the pulsatile release of luteinizing hormone in oral contraceptive users. *Gynecol Endocrinol*. 1993;7 (3):191–200.
42. Katsuki Y, et al. Effects of dienogest, a synthetic steroid, on experimental endometriosis in rats. *J Endocrinol Eur J Endocrinol*. 1998;138(2):216–226.

43. Sasagawa S, et al. Dienogest, a selective progestin, reduces plasma estradiol level through induction of apoptosis of granulosa cells in the ovarian dominant follicle without follicle-stimulating hormone suppression in monkeys. *J Endocrinol Invest.* 2008;31(7):636–641.
44. Sitruk-Ware R, et al. Nestorone: clinical applications for contraception and HRT. *Steroids.* 2003;68(10–13):907–913.
45. Basaria S, Wahlstrom JT, Dobs AS. Anabolic-androgenic steroid therapy in the treatment of chronic diseases. *J Clin Endocrinol Metab.* 2001;86(11):5108–5117.
46. Albano GD, et al. Adverse effects of anabolic-androgenic steroids: a literature review. *Healthcare (Basel).* 2021;9(1):97.
47. Joseph JF, Parr MK. Synthetic androgens as designer supplements. *Curr Neuropharmacol.* 2015;13(1):89–100.
48. El Osta R, et al. Anabolic steroids abuse and male infertility. *Basic Clin Androl.* 2016;26:2.
49. Tauchen J, et al. Medicinal use of testosterone and related steroids revisited. *Molecules (Basel, Switz).* 2021;26(4):1032.
50. Pavlatos A, et al. Review of oxymetholone: a 17 alpha-alkylated anabolic-androgenic steroid. *Clin Ther.* 2001;23:789–801. discussion 771.
51. Kennedy BJ. Fluoxymesterone therapy in advanced breast cancer. *N Engl J Med.* 1958;259 (14):673–675.
52. Jenkin G. Review: The mechanism of action of danazol, a novel steroid derivative. *Aust N Z J Obstet Gynaecol.* 1980;20(2):113–118.
53. Ayotte C. Significance of 19-norandrosterone in athletes' urine samples. *Br J Sports Med.* 2006;40(Suppl 1):i25–i29.
54. van der Vies J. On the mechanism of action of nandrolone phenylpropionate and nandrolone decanoate in rats. *J Acta Endocrinol.* 1965;49(2):271–282.
55. Patanè FG, et al. Nandrolone decanoate: use, abuse and side effects. *Medicina (Kaunas, Lithuania).* 2020;56(11):606.

Chapter 7

Mechanism of action of sedatives, hypnotics, and antianxiety drugs

Muhammad Azhar Nisar[1] and Muhammad Zubair Saleem[2]
[1]Department of Pathology and Laboratory Medicine, Tulane University School of Medicine, New Orleans, LA, United States, [2]Fujian Provincial Key Laboratory of Natural Medicine Pharmacology, Fujian Medical University, Fuzhou, P.R. China

Introduction

There has always been confusion regarding the categories used to classify sedatives, hypnotics, and antianxiety medications. The nomenclature of drugs in human medicine is primarily concerned with their clinical applications. Sedatives and hypnotics are considered sisters because they both induce drowsiness in patients. Hypnotics induce sleep that is electroencephalographically similar to natural sleep, whereas sedatives induce calmness in the recipient and moderate excitement to the point where the patient cannot be easily aroused. Antianxiety medications, also known as anxiolytic medications, are similar in that they inhibit central nervous system (CNS) activity to alleviate anxiety. Antipsychotic drugs are also occasionally used to refer to medications used to treat psychosis. Sedatives may also be used to alleviate anxiety, particularly in hyperactive patients who require gentle handling for examination positioning. Combining anxiolytics and sedatives is a common practice in the provision of anesthesia, as they induce calmness while also facilitating anxiolysis. Due to the tendency of sedative drugs to cause respiratory depression, dose administration must be carefully estimated in relation to standard cardiorespiratory monitoring. Here in this chapter, we will focus on the mode of action of the drugs in the discussion concerning the pathological conditions.

Generalized mode of action of anxiolytics, sedatives/hypnotics

The search for molecular and neurocircuit changes that cause anxiety has made significant progress. Animal models are used for the study of the effects

How Synthetic Drugs Work. DOI: https://doi.org/10.1016/B978-0-323-99855-0.00007-5

of chemicals on neurobiology. Despite this advancement, no mechanistically innovative antianxiety drugs have been approved in over two decades. The present animal models of human anxiety disorders still require significant improvements, making medication discovery difficult.[1] Current treatments are inadequate to address this major public health issue. For instance, the effectiveness of benzodiazepines (BZNs)[2] or azapirones (e.g., buspirone) for panic attacks has recently been questioned.[3] Similarly, treatments for Posttraumatic stress disorder (PTSD), generalized anxiety disorder (GAD), and seasonal affective disorder, serotonin-selective reuptake inhibitors (SSRIs), are only partially effective.[4,5] Developing innovative pharmacotherapeutic agents for anxiety addresses a significant unmet medical need. Over the last two decades, there has been a tremendous effort to better understand the complicated actions that involve neurochemical processes which govern anxiety in healthy and pathological states.[6] Clinical research has utilized neuroimaging, electrophysiological, and molecular study of postmortem brains, among other techniques, to deduce the mechanisms behind pathological anxiety and anxiety patients. While great progress has been achieved, the precise mechanisms underlying therapeutic interventions for the neurobiology of anxiety, particularly maladaptive anxiety, however remain unknown. Complementary techniques explore anxiety pathways in animal models, laying the groundwork for understanding the etiology and treatment of anxiety and its related problems in humans.[7] Given how strongly anxiety systems are preserved throughout species,[8] research involving animal models is of particular significance. However, there are serious shortcomings to this translation, including that of the distinctiveness of human brain structure and cognitive traits, as highlighted in numerous studies.[9,10] With these outcomes the fundamental processes related to anxiety are progressively being uncovered and effectively replicated in other animal models.[11]

The idea that sedatives/hypnotics act on lipid bilayers has long been disqualified. Evidence suggests that sedatives or hypnotics work via specific molecular mechanisms involving membrane-bounded protein components. According to current scientific findings, sedatives act through ion channels that are ligand-gated. The majority of hypnotic/sedative drugs in clinical usage are GABAA (γ-aminobutyric acid type A) receptor agonists, a G protein–coupled chloride channel composed of five subunits[12] (Fig. 7.1). When triggered, the receptor permits chloride ions to enter, hyperpolarizing the lipid bilayer (Fig. 7.2). It is not the GABA-binding region that is directly affected by sedatives, but rather other locations on GABA subunits that are affected.[13] The actions of various drugs are mediated by different isoforms of receptor subunits, as shown by knock-out and knock-in mice.[14] The notion that sedatives activate Kþ channels has been around for a long time, and evidence is suggesting that Kþ channels are involved in at least some of the effects of volatile drugs. When sedatives are used to stimulate Kþ channels, they decrease excitement by either increase the conductance or/and

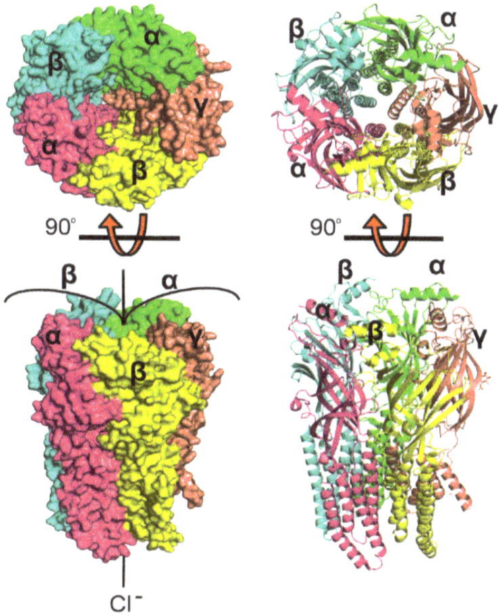

FIGURE 7.1 Illustration of GABA receptor with five subunits.

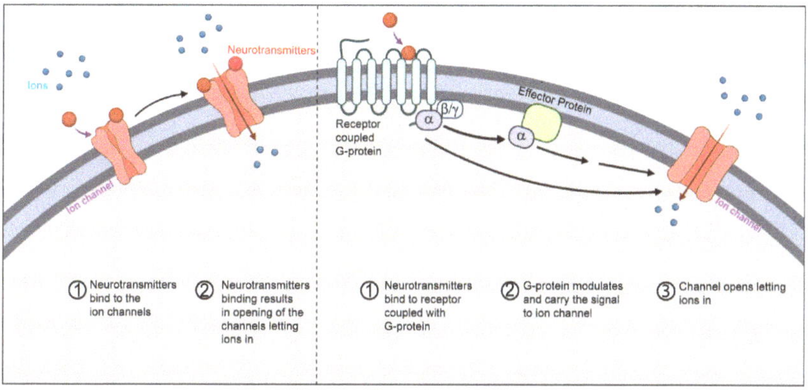

FIGURE 7.2 Generalized mode of action of ion channels in response to the binding of neurotransmitter.

polarization of the membrane (Fig. 7.2). Nitrous oxide, ketamine, and xenon, which reduce excitatory neurotransmission, are considered as agonist for NMDA (*N*-methyl-D-aspartate) receptor. The most essential prerequisites for consciousness are alertness and awareness, and it is considered that the thalamus plays a critical part in these processes. The perception of external and internal sensory information is insufficient to define awareness on its own terms. To be conscious of an object in the external environment, the many features of the entity must be "bonded" together until they are transported to working memory via several sensory paths. In various cortex regions the synchronization of gamma frequency (w40 Hz) oscillations is thought to be the mechanism by which the process of "binding" takes place.

Functional imaging methods have been used to show the dissociation of word and phrase perception from higher cognitive processes such as semantic ambiguity processing.[15] At (or near) loss of consciousness, sedatives or anesthetics have the most noticeable regional effect on the thalamus, with decreased metabolism and blood flow. All sedatives/anesthetics do not reduce thalamic activity. Ketamine stimulates the global metabolic rate, particularly in the thalamus. It is possible that anesthetic effects on the thalamus are primarily indirect. During the administration of sedatives, spontaneous thalamic activity is mostly regulated by signals from cortical neurons. In the vast majority of cases the mediodorsal nucleus, posterior cingulate cortex, and precuneus in the parietal lobe are suppressed while under the influence of a sedative. Sedatives might impact the integration of the brain's cortico-cortical regions, operating on the parts that promote long-range connectivity.[16]

Anxiety and antianxiety medications

Antianxiety medications have been used for centuries. Opium and ethanol are the first two anxiolytics having a documented history of widespread use dating back thousands of years. Ethanol is still extensively used in self-medication for anxiety. According to existing global clinical guidelines for anxiety and associated disorders, the recommended initial therapies are psychotherapy and medication (Table 7.1), with the decision between the two depending on availability and/or patient preference. Table 7.1 shows the approved drugs in the EU and United States currently under recommendation for various anxiety disorders.

Historically, more conventional pharmacotherapeutic approaches have focused on known neurochemical dysregulations. Numerous neurochemical systems, which display substantial system variation in expression, collaborate with their receptors to regulate anxiety in a highly sophisticated and precise manner. There is evidence that these systems are disrupted in various brain regions associated with a variety of anxiety-related diseases.[17] A deep understanding of the neurobiological disturbances associated with various anxiety disorders is critical for optimizing pharmacotherapeutic therapies. The endogenous cannabinoids (eCBs), glutamate system, neuropeptides, and neurosteroids are currently being examined in clinical trials.

Novel molecules with diverse pharmacological targets

Systems containing monoamines

Certain physiological and behavioral processes such as aggressiveness and stress responses are governed by monoamine neurotransmitters such as

TABLE 7.1 Medicines authorized in the United States or Europe for at least one anxiety, trauma-related, or obsessive–compulsive disorder (OCD) are mentioned.

	GAD	SAD	PTSD	OCD
SSRIs				
Citalopram	Europe	Europe	Off-label	Europe
Escitalopram	Europe, United States	Europe, United States	Off-label	Europe
Fluoxetine	Off-label	Off-label	Off-label	Europe, United States
Fluvoxamine	Europe, United States	Europe, United States	Off-label	Europe, United States
Paroxetine	Europe, United States	Europe, United States	Europe, United States	Europe, United States
Sertraline	Europe, United States	Europe, United States	Europe, United States	Europe, United States
SNRIs				
Desvenlafaxine		Off-label		
Venlafaxine	Europe, United States	Europe, United States	Off-label	Off-label
Duloxetine	Europe, United States	Off-label	Off-label	Off-label
TCAs				
Clomipramine	Off-label	Off-label	Off-label	Europe, United States
Imipramine				
Opipramol	Europe			

(*Continued*)

TABLE 7.1 (Continued)

	GAD	SAD	PTSD	OCD
MAOIs				
Moclobemide		Europe		
Phenelzine			Off-label	
Other antidepressants				
Mirtazapine	Off-label	Off-label	Off-label	Off-label
Trazodone			Off-label	
Benzodiazepines				
Alprazolam	Europe, United States	Off-label		
Bromazepam	Off-label			
Chlordiazepoxide	Europe, United States	Off-label		
Clonazepam	Off-label	Off-label		
Clorazepate	United States	Off-label		
Diazepam	Europe, United States	Off-label		
Lorazepam	Europe, United States	Off-label		
Oxazepam	Europe, United States	Off-label		
Prazepam	Off-label			

GAD, Generalized anxiety disorder; *PTSD*, posttraumatic stress disorder; *SAD*, seasonal affective disorder; *SSRI*, serotonin-selective reuptake inhibitor; *SNRI*, Serotonin and norepinephrine reuptake inhibitors; *TCAs*, tricyclic antidepressants; *MAOIs*, monoamine oxidase inhibitors.

selective serotonin (5-HT), dopamine, and noradrenaline. Numerous current drugs for anxiety-related diseases, including serotonin and noradrenaline reuptake inhibitors, SSRIs, monoamine oxidase inhibitors, and tricyclic antidepressants (Table 7.1), all affect 5-HT neurotransmission.

Vilazodone

Villazoledone (5-HT reuptake inhibitor and partial agonist of 5-HT1A receptor) has been shown to affect 5-HT levels significantly in comparison to pure SSRIs. The FDA authorized it in 2011 for serious adult depression. Vilazodone has not been demonstrated to effectively relieve the symptoms of PTSD and concomitant depression.[18]

AVN-101

In addition to 5-HT7 receptors, AVN-101 (2,8-dimethyl-5-penethyl-2,3,4,5-tetrahydro-1h-pyrido [4,3-B]indole hydrochloride) also has a significant affinity for the histaminergic H1 and adrenergic 2B receptors, making it a multimodal antagonist of the antihistamine latrepirdine. While preliminary study indicates that it has both anxiolytic and antidepressant qualities, further research is being done to look into it as a treatment for GAD and schizophrenia.[19] In 2018 a Phase 1b clinical trial of AVN-101 came to the conclusion that, although side effects were very minimal, the medication was safe and well-tolerated over a broad range of dosages and was recommended for further study.

Brexpiprazole

Brexpiprazole, an antipsychotic, a partial agonist at the dopamine D2 and D3 receptors and antagonist at the 5-HT2A, 5-HT2B, and 5-HT7, 1-adrenoceptor, 2-adrenoceptor, and histaminergic H1 receptor receptors.[20] In addition, despite being less affinitive to D1 receptor, an increase glutamatergic transmission in the medial prefrontal cortex have been demonstrated via brexpiprazole, which may contribute to its anxiety-reducing effects.[21] It obtained its global approval in 2015 for schizophrenia treatment and as adjunctive therapy for serious depression.

Cyclobenzaprine VLD (TNX-102)

VLD-cyclobenzaprine, commonly known as Tonmya and TNX-102 (sublingual), is a therapeutic drug manufactured by Vela Pharmaceuticals that works by blocking the 5-HT2A, 1, and H1 receptors. It is recommended in very low doses that allow for rapid absorption and is indicated for long-term use with a low risk. Cyclobenzaprine has been proposed to improve sleep quality by inhibiting 5-HT2A and H1 receptors and minimizing trauma-related nightmares and sleep disturbances by inhibiting 1-adrenoceptors.[22]

Glutamate system

Glutamate is one of the brain's primary and most important excitatory neurotransmitters, exerting its numerous biological processes via NMDA and kainate, α-amino-3-hydroxy-5-methyl-4-isoxazolepropionic acid (AMPA) receptors.[23] This system plays a vital role in the development of neuroplasticity-dependent memory formation, including fear extinction. The development of anxiolytic drugs that work via glutamatergic pathways has long been a focus of research. Despite these attempts, little is known about the role of glutamate systems in treating anxiety disorders.[17] Stress is a known factor for anxiety that affects glutamate contents in rodents, and indeed, humans with anxiety disorders also exhibit aberrant glutamate and glutamate receptor levels.[24]

Ketamine

In addition to having considerable pain-relieving properties, ketamine is also a dissociative anesthetic, hallucinogen, and psychotomimetic drug. Ketamine is a combination of (S)- and (R)-NMDA receptor antagonist that acts as a noncompetitive anti-NMDA receptor via clinging at the innermost region of the receptor. At subanesthetic doses, ketamine reaches brain concentrations sufficient to modulate certain NMDA receptor subpopulations.[25] This aspect appears to be essential, as anesthetic levels of ketamine do not appear to have antidepressant properties.[26] Over the past 20 years, researchers have conducted numerous studies into the mechanisms of action of ketamine, especially in connection to its antidepressant effects that are both immediate and long-lasting. Ketamine has a multifaceted effect on NMDA receptor blockage, exhibiting both direct and indirect actions as a result of its administration. The anxiolytic effects of ketamine are thought to be mediated through a number of different potential antidepressant pathways, some of which are not fully understood.

Xenon gas (NBTX-001)

NBTX-001 has the inert noble gas xenon as an active ingredient, which is a commonly used anesthetic that has the advantage of generating no metabolites and hence is nontoxic. From a pharmaceutical standpoint, it is a multi-targeted agent that inhibits several neurotransmitter receptors such as the 5-HT3 receptor, the AMPA receptor, the nicotinic acetylcholine receptor, the NMDA receptor, and the hyperpolarization-activated cyclic nucleotide-gated channel, in addition to causing neuronal hyperpolarization.[27] In addition, xenon treatment reduces pro-inflammatory cytokine levels, such as TNF and IL1, while increasing growth factors such as BDNF.[28] Fear-related behaviors were decreased in mice when subanesthetic doses of xenon (25% for an hour) were administered, indicating that xenon treatment have therapeutic potential for minimizing fear-memory reconsolidation.[29]

Endocannabinoid system

Anandamide (AEA) and 2-arachidonoylglycerol (2-AG) are broken down by three enzymes: fatty acid amide hydrolase (FAAH), monoacylglycerol lipase (MAG-L), and COX-2. This enzyme system creates the endocannabinoid (eCB) system. The main associated receptors are the presynaptic transient receptor potential (TRP1), vanilloid receptor cannabis 1 receptor (CB1), and the cannabinoid 2 receptor (CB2).[30] CB1 is highly expressed in areas of the brain associated with anxiety, facilitating eCB's numerous behavioral and cognitive effects. The eCB system modulates neuronal activity that is associated with stress and anxiety. As a consequence of suppressing serine hydrolase, the enhanced eCB signaling reduces anxiety and stress responses.[31]

Inhibitors of fatty acid amide hydrolase

As previously stated, the membrane-bound enzyme FAAH is responsible for the hydrolysis of the eCB and AEA. It has been reported that the AEA levels decreased in patients with PTSD.[32] The FAAH gene's destabilizing mutation also raised AEA levels, lowered trait anxiety indices, and improved the cortico-amygdala link with decreased amygdala activity in response to stress incentives.[30] In mice investigations the suppression FAAH genetically and pharmacologically resulted in antinociceptive effects, particularly when the environment was highly unpleasant or stressful. Sanofi has discontinued the production of SSR-411298, a FAAH inhibitor, which was being investigated to treat serious depression and anxiety, following a dismal Phase 2b trial in older adults.[33]

Additional targets for the eCB system

It's possible that modulators of the activity of 2-AG's degrading enzymes, MAG-L and COX-2, may potentially serve as anxiolytic therapeutic targets; given that preclinical research has demonstrated the anxiolytic-like properties. 2-AG has anxiolytic-like properties. 2-AG plasma levels were lower in individuals with PTSD or depression than in control subjects.[34] Animal model missing the enzyme diacylglycerol lipase, which produces 2-AG, exhibits more anxiety-related behavior.[35] Inhibiting MAG-L, the primary degrading enzyme of 2-AG increases central 2-AG concentrations and lowers anxiety-related behaviors in mice. COX-2, which degrades eCBs, could be an alternate eCB target. AEA and 2-AG accumulate when COX-2 is suppressed in the brain.[36] A substantial anxiolytic effect was seen in rats when COX-2 inhibitors were administered.[30] In addition, the COX-2 inhibitors have the potential to benefit from the suppression of pro-inflammatory cytokines and chemokines, which have been associated to increased anxiety.[37] However, despite the fact that Lumiracoxib and Celecoxib (COX-2 inhibitors) are approved as antiinflammatory drugs, no clinical investigation addressing the anxiolytic impact of COX-2 inhibitors has been done.

GABA system

GABA is synthesized from glutamate decarboxylase, released from vesicles, and reabsorbed into nerve terminals or glial cells. It is the brain's primary inhibitory neurotransmitter. Specifically, GABA activates postsynaptic, as well as pre- and extrasynaptic locations on GABA receptors. Rapid GABA's inhibitory effects are mediated by the expansion of ligand-gated ion channel's pore. This delays the chloride entry and causes the membrane to hyperpolarize. The substantial structural variability and heterogeneous expression of GABAA receptors in neural pathways and subcellular compartments in brain enables the complex and precise inhibition of anxiety-related brain circuits.[38] The progressive and sustainable inhibition of potassium or calcium channels is due to the coupling of inhibitory Gi proteins to the metabotropic receptor. Animal and human studies have linked anxiety disorders' etiology and pathology to GABAA and GABAB receptor.[17]

Sedatives and hypnotics

Minors under age 10, those with learning difficulties, and individuals who are violent enough to be a danger to medical professionals or to themselves should receive anxiolytic medications before being sedated. Presurgical visits by the anesthesiologist do not always relieve patient anxiety. For this reason, use of an anxiolytic medication may assist the patient, and this may aid the subsequent delivery of anesthesia. For day-case adult surgery, there is no evidence to suggest that anxiolytic drugs used during surgery cause delayed postoperative discharges.[39]

Sedation is frequently delivered by the technician or a nonmedical trainee under the specialist's guidance during small procedures such as endoscopy. General anesthesia doesn't have a fatality rate anywhere as high as that linked with these procedures. One aspect that is likely to contribute to this is the widespread use of medication combinations. Fentanyl and midazolam are widely used together in intravenous bolus dosages because they have a powerful but variable synergy regarding respiratory depression and sedation. Midazolam's pharmacokinetics is suboptimal if used alone, with the peak effect occurring around 13 min after an IV bolus dosage.

Benzodiazepines

BZNs are the most frequently utilized anxiolytic and sedative medicines before surgery. CNS 7056 and Mr04A3 are still in development and have not been approved for clinical use, although both of these have significant pharmacokinetic advantages over earlier drugs.[40] BZNs have a high therapeutic index and are particularly effective anxiolytics with anterograde amnesia. They do this via hypnotic pharmacodynamic interactions. The administration via intranasal and rectal routes is as effective as the oral delivery method. Altered consciousness and coma are among the adverse outcomes. Cardiorespiratory depression in the elderly or fragile may be exacerbated by BZNs pharmacokinetic and pharmacodynamic factors. Sedative medicines are also extremely toxic to patients with reduced consciousness. Sedatives are also exceedingly harmful, which is crucial in neurosurgery patients with space-occupying lesions because respiratory depression can increase intracranial pressure causing CNS and respiratory depression.

Additional agents

For its antisialogogue effects, hyoscine is sometimes used as a premedication. Barbiturates, due to the availability of safer alternatives and their limited therapeutic index, are rarely utilized as premedication. Anxiolytic and sedative effects of opioid premedication are often used in people with heart disease due to their usefulness. The drawback of premedication with opioids is that unpleasant symptoms like nausea, vomiting, impaired vision, skin rash, and respiratory distress are frequently encountered. Using transmucosal fentanyl citrate candy as oral administration to children, effective sedation can be achieved.

In addition, chloral hydrate and triclofos are utilized for pediatric premedication. Ketamine administered intramuscularly or rectally may be beneficial in uncooperative children. Intravenous propofol is a safe and beneficial technique for giving "immediate" anxiety relief and sedation during the pre−operative period when supplied via a patient-maintained sedation system which is beneficial for the management of patient.[41] In addition to its anxiolytic and analgesic characteristics, melatonin may be utilized as anesthetic supplement because of its ability to regulate sleep and wakefulness. Although there is limited knowledge of melatonin, current research indicates that it may play a role in therapeutic practice in the future.[42]

Hypnotics are used to induce and maintain anesthesia

Selection of a hypnotic agent

In adults, anesthesia is often induced through the administration of intravenous anesthetic drugs. Traditionally, inhalation anesthesia was used to induce sedation in babies and young children; however, since topical local anesthetic creams have been more widely available, intravenous anesthesia has seen a rise in popularity. A single breath of sevoflurane or a progressive inhalational induction of anesthesia is used to induce anesthesia in adults. The most often used method of maintaining anesthesia is through the delivery of a volatile sedative drug. This option is based on the efficacy of the pulmonary route of elimination and relatively poor clearance rates of certain intravenous medicines. Total intravenous sedatives are becoming more common for the maintenance of anesthesia due to medications with favorable pharmacological characteristics and improved delivery technologies. Individual medicines, whether intravenous or inhalational, are chosen based on personal preference and clinical indications. Table 7.2 highlights the most important features of the most frequently used intravenous sedatives/anesthetics in the medical field.

TABLE 7.2 A summary of the most essential aspects of the most regularly used sedative drugs.

Drug	Chemical group	Protein binding	Clearance (mL/kg/min)	Metabolism	Induction dose (mg/kg)
Propofol	Phenol derivative	0.97	18–4	Hepatic and extra-hepatic and inactive metabolites	1.5–2.5
Thiopentone	Barbiturate	0.8	2.7–4.1	Hepatic oxidation to inactive metabolites	3–7
Etomidate	Imidazole derivative	0.76	12.5–26	Hydrolysis by plasma esterase and liver microsomal enzymes and inactive metabolites	0.3
Ketamine	Phencyclidine derivative	20%–50%	17	Norketamine-active metabolite, hepatic enzyme induction, and hepatic extractionratio 0.9	1.2

Sedatives/anesthetics administered intravenously

Propofol is a drug that is frequently used to induce sedation due to its quick recovery characteristics. It is particularly useful in day cases due to its antiemetic and antipruritic characteristics. Propofol dramatically lowers myocardial contractility and vascular resistance by reducing arterial blood pressure. These consequences are more pronounced among the elderly and people having impaired cardiac output. Propofol induces apnea and also affects the reaction to hypercarbia following an inducing dosage.

In addition, when the mean arterial pressure is decreased, it leads to rapid drops in intracranial and intraocular pressures and decreases in cerebral perfusion pressure. Prescription of propofol has long been associated with injection discomfort, bacterial contamination, and unexpected excitatory effects. Individuals with uncontrolled epilepsy are mostly avoided for the administration of propofol.[43]

Thiopentone is the sole barbiturate for widespread usage, often reserved for quick sequence induction or hypersensitive to propofol or its components. Negative side effects such as fatigue, dizziness, prolonged recovery, accumulation, nausea, and vomiting have contributed to the drug's dwindling reputation. In mildly anesthetized patients, laryngospasm and bronchospasm are more common than propofol. Thiopentone has been linked to a greater ability to maintain cerebral perfusion pressure and reduce cerebral oxygen uptake (approximately 50%). The aforementioned adverse effects of large dosages of thiopentone commonly result in burst suppression, and experts believe that this symptom is advantageous in cases of focal brain injury.

Ketamine (phencyclidine derivative) causes analgesic effects, disruptive hypnosis, and undesirable psychomimetic symptoms like hallucinations after surgery. Although sympathetic stimulation may cause complications in individuals with ischemic heart disease, it is suitable for battlefield surgery. It increases cerebral metabolic rate by increasing the intracranial blood flow which makes it unsuitable for intracranial hypertension patients. Ketamine is most frequently used for sedation during localized procedures, burn dressing changes, and postoperative pain relief. Despite the fact that S-ketamine is much more potent and has minimal side effects as compared to R-ketamine, regrettably, the only version of the drug that is approved is the racemic combination.

Etomidate is typically used in emergency cases when substantial hypotension is caused by propofol and thiopentone. An abdominal aortic aneurysm repair procedure that uses fast sequence induction is a classic example. Reversible adrenocortical inhibition is caused by Etomidate's suppression of the 11b- and 17a-hydroxylases. Consistent doses have been shown to raise the risk of morbidity and death, while a single dose in critical patients can cause adrenal function impairment.[44,45]

Closing remarks

When evaluating the overall safety profile of a medicine, it is important to take the broad variety of pharmacological substances into account, in addition to their pharmacokinetic and pharmacodynamic characteristics, as well as the patient's co-morbidity and the clinician's knowledge of anxiolytic, sedative, and hypnotic drugs. All of these elements have a major influence on the outcome.

It's possible that the hunt for anxiolytic medicines is approaching its end. We now have a better grasp of fear-related behavior in cognitive neuroscience because of a boom in research over the past decade. On the other hand, these developments have not yet resulted in the discovery of more effective treatments for human fear and anxiety disorders that are mechanistically unique. As previously stated, studies on anxiety disorders and animal models of anxiety disorders both have persistent knowledge deficits of the biochemistry of depression and anxiety, and each poses a significant barrier in the development of novel anxiety medications and treatments. Because of the fluctuating diagnostic limits of anxiety disorders, the pharmaceutical development process has been further impeded by the lack of accurate biomarkers. It will be critical to undertake substantial cooperation among basic and clinical investigators to push the discipline toward therapy development.

Due to the possibility of severe respiratory depression with all sedative drugs, they should be administered in conjunction with standard physiological cardiorespiratory monitoring. Although the pharmacology of sedative/anesthetic agents varies, they all generally have comparable clinical effects. The majority of intravenous drugs are assumed to affect consciousness via an action on GABAA, NMDA, or both receptors. Our grasp of the mode of action of sedative/hypnotic agents is inadequate, in part due to the lack of awareness. Numerous hypotheses have been offered during the last century, but none have succeeded thoroughly in elucidating the processes at work. There is currently an expectation that by utilizing modern imaging techniques, the action of these drugs can be better understood, which will aid in our knowledge of consciousness and cognitive functioning.

References

1. Griebel G, Holmes A. 50 years of hurdles and hope in anxiolytic drug discovery. *Nat Rev Drug Discov*. 2013;12(9):667–687.
2. Watanabe N, Churchill R, Furukawa TA. Combined psychotherapy plus benzodiazepines for panic disorder. *Cochrane Database Syst Rev*. 2009;(1). p. CD005335.
3. Imai H, et al. Azapirones vs placebo for panic disorder in adults. *Cochrane Database Syst Rev*. 2014;(9). p. CD010828.
4. Stein DJ, Ipser JC, Seedat S. Pharmacotherapy for post traumatic stress disorder (PTSD). *Cochrane Database Syst Rev*. 2006;(1). p. CD002795.
5. Kapczinski F, et al. Antidepressants for generalized anxiety disorder. *Cochrane Database Syst Rev*. 2003;(2). p. CD003592.

6. Duval ER, Javanbakht A, Liberzon I. Neural circuits in anxiety and stress disorders: a focused review. *Ther Clin Risk Manag*. 2015;11:115–126.
7. Kas MJ, et al. *Translational neuroscience of schizophrenia: seeking a meeting of minds between mouse and man. Sci Transl Med*. 2011;3(102):102mr3.
8. Shi L, et al. Efficacy and tolerability of vilazodone for major depressive disorder: evidence from phase III/IV randomized controlled trials. *Drug Des Dev Ther*. 2016;10:3899–3907.
9. Cryan JF, Sweeney FF. The age of anxiety: role of animal models of anxiolytic action in drug discovery. *Br J Pharmacol*. 2011;164(4):1129–1161.
10. Flores A, et al. Lost in translation: how to upgrade fear memory research. *Mol Psychiatry*. 2018;23(11):2122–2132.
11. Stewart AM, Kalueff AV. Anxiolytic drug discovery: what are the novel approaches and how can we improve them? *Expert Opin Drug Discov*. 2014;9(1):15–26.
12. Zhu S, et al. Structure of a human synaptic GABAA receptor. *Nature*. 2018;559 (7712):67–72.
13. Garcia PS, Kolesky SE, Jenkins A. General anesthetic actions on GABA(A) receptors. *Curr Neuropharmacol*. 2010;8(1):2–9.
14. Weir C, Mitchell S, Lambert JJBBJOA. Role of GABAA receptor subtypes in the behavioural effects of intravenous general anaesthetics. *Br J Anaesth*. 2017;119(suppl_1): i167–i175.
15. Davis MH, et al. Dissociating speech perception and comprehension at reduced levels of awareness. *Proc Natl Acad Sci USA*. 2007;104(41):16032–16037.
16. Alkire MT, Hudetz AG, Tononi G. Consciousness and anesthesia. *Science*. 2008;322 (5903):876–880.
17. Bandelow B, et al. Biological markers for anxiety disorders, OCD and PTSD: a consensus statement. Part II: neurochemistry, neurophysiology and neurocognition. *World J Biol Psychiatry*. 2017;18(3):162–214.
18. Ramaswamy S, et al. A double-blind, placebo-controlled randomized trial of vilazodone in the treatment of posttraumatic stress disorder and comorbid depression. *Prim Care Companion CNS Disord*. 2017;19(4).
19. Ivachtchenko AV, Lavrovsky Y, Okun I. AVN-101: a multi-target drug candidate for the treatment of CNS disorders. *J Alzheimers Dis*. 2016;53(2):583–620.
20. Maeda K, et al. Brexpiprazole I: in vitro and in vivo characterization of a novel serotonin-dopamine activity modulator. *J Pharmacol Exp Ther*. 2014;350(3):589–604.
21. Bjorkholm C, et al. The novel antipsychotic drug brexpiprazole, alone and in combination with escitalopram, facilitates prefrontal glutamatergic transmission via a dopamine D1 receptor-dependent mechanism. *Eur Neuropsychopharmacol*. 2017;27(4):411–417.
22. Krystal AD, Richelson E, Roth T. Review of the histamine system and the clinical effects of H1 antagonists: basis for a new model for understanding the effects of insomnia medications. *Sleep Med Rev*. 2013;17(4):263–272.
23. Reiner A, Levitz J. Glutamatergic signaling in the central nervous system: ionotropic and metabotropic receptors in concert. *Neuron*. 2018;98(6):1080–1098.
24. Krystal JH, et al. It is time to address the crisis in the pharmacotherapy of posttraumatic stress disorder: a consensus statement of the PTSD Psychopharmacology Working Group. *Biol Psychiatry*. 2017;82(7):e51–e59.
25. Dravid SM, et al. Subunit-specific mechanisms and proton sensitivity of NMDA receptor channel block. *J Physiol*. 2007;581(Pt 1):107–128.
26. Zorumski CF, Izumi Y, Mennerick S. Ketamine: NMDA receptors and beyond. *J Neurosci*. 2016;36(44):11158–11164.

27. Zhou C, Liu J, Chen XD. General anesthesia mediated by effects on ion channels. *World J Crit Care Med*. 2012;1(3):80–93.
28. Dobrovolsky A, et al. Xenon in the treatment of panic disorder: an open label study. *J Transl Med*. 2017;15(1):137.
29. Meloni EG, et al. Xenon impairs reconsolidation of fear memories in a rat model of post-traumatic stress disorder (PTSD). *PLoS One*. 2014;9(8):e106189.
30. Patel S, et al. The endocannabinoid system as a target for novel anxiolytic drugs. *Neurosci Biobehav Rev*. 2017;76(Pt A):56–66.
31. Gunduz-Cinar O, et al. Amygdala FAAH and anandamide: mediating protection and recovery from stress. *Trends Pharmacol Sci*. 2013;34(11):637–644.
32. Hill MN, et al. Reductions in circulating endocannabinoid levels in individuals with post-traumatic stress disorder following exposure to the World Trade Center attacks. *Psychoneuroendocrinology*. 2013;38(12):2952–2961.
33. Mandrioli R, Mercolini L. Discontinued anxiolytic drugs (2009 - 2014). *Expert Opin Investig Drugs*. 2015;24(4):557–573.
34. Hauer D, et al. Plasma concentrations of endocannabinoids and related primary fatty acid amides in patients with post-traumatic stress disorder. *PLoS One*. 2013;8(5):e62741.
35. Jenniches I, et al. Anxiety, stress, and fear response in mice with reduced endocannabinoid levels. *Biol Psychiatry*. 2016;79(10):858–868.
36. Hermanson DJ, et al. Substrate-selective COX-2 inhibition decreases anxiety via endocannabinoid activation. *Nat Neurosci*. 2013;16(9):1291–1298.
37. Felger JC. Imaging the role of inflammation in mood and anxiety-related disorders. *Curr Neuropharmacol*. 2018;16(5):533–558.
38. Engin E, Benham RS, Rudolph U. An emerging circuit pharmacology of GABAA receptors. *Trends Pharmacol Sci*. 2018;39(8):710–732.
39. Walker KJ, Smith AF. Pre-medication for anxiety in adult day surgery. *Cochrane Database Syst Rev*. 2009;(4). p. CD002192.
40. Kilpatrick GJ, et al. CNS 7056: a novel ultra-short-acting Benzodiazepine. *Anesthesiology*. 2007;107(1):60–66.
41. Murdoch JA, Kenny GN. Patient-maintained propofol sedation as pre-medication in day-case surgery: assessment of a target-controlled system. *Br J Anaesth*. 1999;82(3):429–431.
42. Ismail SA, Mowafi HA. Melatonin provides anxiolysis, enhances analgesia, decreases intraocular pressure, and promotes better operating conditions during cataract surgery under topical anesthesia. *Anesth Analg*. 2009;108(4):1146–1151.
43. Sneyd JR. Propofol and epilepsy. *Br J Anaesth*. 1999;82(2):168–169.
44. Absalom A, Pledger D, Kong A. Adrenocortical function in critically ill patients 24 h after a single dose of etomidate. *Anaesthesia*. 1999;54(9):861–867.
45. Ledingham IM, Watt I. Influence of sedation on mortality in critically ill multiple trauma patients. *Lancet*. 1983;1(8336):1270.

Chapter 8

Mechanism of action of antiepileptic drugs

Haider Ali[1], Naushad Ahmad Khan[1], Mirza Masroor Ali Beg[1], Mohammed Zahed Sarwar[1], Nurida Kemelbek Kyzy[1], Tilekeeva Ulankul Muktarovna[2], Kudaibergen Osmonaliev[1], Faez Iqbal Khan[3] and Muhammed Burak Ay[1]

[1]Faculty of Medicine, Ala-Too International University, Bishkek, Kyrgyzstan, [2]Department of Basic and Clinical Pharmacology, Kyrgyz State Medical Academy, Bishkek, Kyrgyzstan, [3]Department of Biological Sciences, School of Science, Xi'an Jiaotong-Liverpool University, Suzhou, Jiangsu, China

Introduction

It has been recognized as a very difficult problem over the centuries. Epilepsy has its origins in the Greek term "to seize" or "take hold of" since it indicates the seizure is usually results in being taken out of control. Epilepsy is one of the most common brain diseases or neurological disorders. The word epilepsy refers to a category of chronic CNS disorders marked by the incidence of recurrent seizures, which are normally followed by lack of awareness and motion (convulsion). Epilepsy is traditionally characterized as being at least two unprovoked seizures divided by at least 24 h, but the most recent international consensus concept allowed a sole epileptic seizure whether there is an inherent predisposition to have epileptic seizures. Although some causes of an initial seizure in the aged lead to recurrent seizures, several others prolong the issue.[1,2]

Several numbers of herbs have been extensively used in Ayurvedic medicinal practice for the treatment of epilepsy, asthma, cramps, diabetes, microbial infection, inflammation, tumor, wound healing, and rheumatism. Experimentally drugs with a potential antiepileptic activity are assessed by injecting medullary stimulants or by applying a maximal electrical shock.[3–5] Drugs that antagonize chemically induced seizures are effective in petit mal epilepsy and which protect against electrically induced seizures in grand mal epilepsy. A plant containing phytoconstituents, namely, flavonoids shows CNS activity as well as atropine also possesses antiepileptic activity. Atropine is one of the important alkaloids,

How Synthetic Drugs Work. DOI: https://doi.org/10.1016/B978-0-323-99855-0.00008-7

which acts as active constituents. Extract of herbs that contain the atropine could be demonstrated significant antiepileptic activity on animal models. Traditionally several herbs were used for treating asthma, epilepsy, and other ailments. However, antiepileptic activity of some herbs has not been documented in the scientific literature. So in this view, the option is open to investigate the possible antiepileptic properties of the herb.[6,7]

Pathophysiology and pathogenesis of epilepsy

Individuals vary in their vulnerability to having an epileptic seizure. Any individuals could have a smaller resistance to epileptic seizures, making them highly vulnerable to the disease. Every brain, when excessively stimulated, can cause seizures. The phenomenology of seizures differs from one individual to another individual and multiple seizure types can appear in the same person. Epilepsy is a disease that may be influenced by several intracranial structural,[8] cellular, or molecular factors and presents in several forms. The irregular hypersynchronous electrical behavior of nerves in epileptic seizures[9] is often triggered by an inconsistency of excitation and inhibition in the brain[10]; originally, only a limited fraction of nerves fire anomalously. Too much stimulation or suppression of a huge number of cortical neurons causes seizures. Medical symptoms are determined by the direction of the focus, the magnitude of irritability in the adjacent brain region, and the frequency of the impulse.[11,12]

Since synapses play such an important role in mediating contact between neurons in the human brain, a seizure may result from poor synaptic performance.[13] A seizure could be caused by a decline in inhibitory synaptic function or an increase in excitatory synaptic function. A significant depolarization of the nerve cell membranes is correlated with a spurt of electrical impulses in the depolarization change. The capacity of sodium channels to rebound from inactivation is believed to be reduced, which inhibits high-frequency shooting. The popping event that occurs when the nerve cell membrane is depolarized for a longer period is caused by an influx of extracellular calcium, which causes the opening of voltage-dependent sodium channels, entry of Na + , and emission of repeated action potentials. Based on the type of cell, gamma-aminobutyric acid (GABA) receptors and chloride entry or potassium efflux mediate the resulting hyperpolarizing after potential.[14,15]

Synced hyperexcitability may be caused by a variety of mechanisms, such as:

1. Changes in ion channel dispersion, quantity, form, and biophysical characteristics in nerve cell membranes.
2. Alterations to receptor biochemistry.
3. Mechanism differentiation in genetic expression and secondary messenger.
4. Alteration in Ion concentrations outside of the cell.

5. Glial cell variations in neurotransmitter uptake and metabolism.[16]
6. Alterations in inhibitory circuit proportion and process information. However, transitory inequalities in the major neurotransmitters glutamate (excitatory), GABA (inhibitory), and several other neuromodulators like noradrenaline, acetylcholine, and 5-hydroxytryptamine can take a part in causing seizures in prone patients.[17–19]

   Throughout a seizure, hypersynchronous discharges can originate in a small, isolated area of the cortex, but then propagate to the surrounding areas.[20] The onset of a seizure is marked by two occurrences that happen at the same time:

   1. Nerve impulse pulses with a strong intensity
   2. A neural network hyper synchronization

   Seizures involve three constraints which from a huge physiologic standpoint:

   1. A group of neurons that are excitable in a pathological way.
   2. To disperse the discharge, there are several pathologically overexcited neurons and a raise in excitatory glutaminergic function via repetitive contacts.
   3. A decrease in the expression of GABAergic projections that is usually inhibitory.

Once there is enough activity to attract nearby neurons, seizure proliferation happens, that's when a partial seizure extends across the brain. It often causes a lack of surround inhibition, allowing seizure activity to extend into nearby regions via specific cortical associations and farther out via long association pathways like the corpus callosum.[21] Hyperpolarization and an area of adjacent repression produced by inhibitory nerves usually avoid the expansion of exploding activity.

Following are the consequences of repeated discharges:

1. a rise in outer membrane K + that depolarizes adjacent nerves and blunts hyperpolarization.
2. Ca+ + aggregation in presynaptic terminals contributes to increased neurotransmitter production.
3. Ca+ + increase in the number and neural induction is caused by depolarization-induced activation of the N-methyl-D-aspartate (NMDA), an excitatory amino acid receptor.[22–24]

It is hypothesized that the expansion of excitation to the subcortical, thalamic, and brainstem centers is accompanied by the tonic phase and the loss of consciousness by an increase in the overactive signals of autonomic function. In states of convulsions, the brain may assist in ending seizures and postrelated anxiety may occur. This deed helps to control the convulsions by affecting adenosine A1 receptors.[25] The emergence of astrogliosis as a marker in epileptics' brains,[26] as well as the detection of astrocytes as essential effectors of neural development, indicates that astrocyte impairment may serve a significant purpose in epilepsy pathogenesis.[27]

Role of GABA

The excitatory postsynaptic potential (EPSP) is the major symbol of stimulation in the brain,[28] while the inhibitory postsynaptic potential (IPSP) is the major symbol of inhibition.[29] A precise equilibrium between EPSP and IPSP regulates the neural membrane potential.[30] An epileptic seizure will occur if this equilibrium is disrupted. GABAergic induction may be presynaptic or postsynaptic, depending on whether it is released from GABAergic neuronal endings and GABA is catabolized by GABA-transaminase postsynaptically. GABA receptors are known as GABAA, GABAB, or GABAC. The GABAA receptor is the very well GABA receptor subclass.[31] It is indeed ligand-gated chloride ion channels and "ionotropic receptor" that opens after GABA is released via presynaptic neurons and mediates rapid postsynaptic inhibition.[32] Numerous neuromodulator medications, including benzodiazepines and barbiturates, work on this receptor. Abnormalities in synapses GABA discharge or the postsynaptic GABA receptor may induce GABA process impairment. Throughout the cerebrospinal fluids of epileptic patients, decreased GABA and elevated glutamate levels were detected.[33] When excitatory pathways prevail, whether, by enhanced stimulation or reduced inhibition, neural hyper synchronization arises. Many neurons will also be stimulated (high-frequency depolarization or repolarization) as the pathological neuronal hypersynchronous activation occurs, resulting in the epileptic seizure (Fig. 8.1).[34,35]

Role of glutamate

Because neurons in a certain region of the brain fire under an unexpectedly synchronous pattern, a seizure occurs. Within that mechanism of neuronal excitation, upwards of 100 neurotransmitters or neuromodulators are being discovered to perform a function. Synaptic impulses produced by the excitatory neurotransmitters glutamate and aspartate are responsible for action potentials in particular. Excitability amino acids, particularly L-glutamate,[36] function on even more than 50% of the brain's nerve terminals, contributing significantly to seizure propagation. For epileptogenic disorder, there is indeed a spike in glutamate production throughout the brain. Stimulation is caused by neurotransmitter amino acids produced from the nerve terminals and acting on postsynaptic NMDA and non-NMDA receptors.[37] By regulating excess neural potassium levels and suppressing excitatory neurotransmitters including glutamate, glial cells serve an essential homeostatic function throughout the regulation of neuroexcitation. Ions like magnesium can indeed affect neuronal excitability (Fig. 8.2).[38–40]

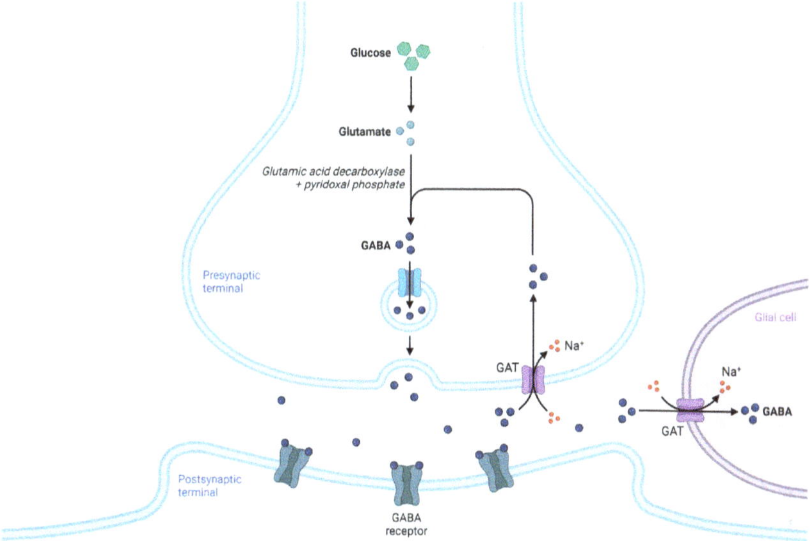

FIGURE 8.1 GABA synthesis and mechanism of action.

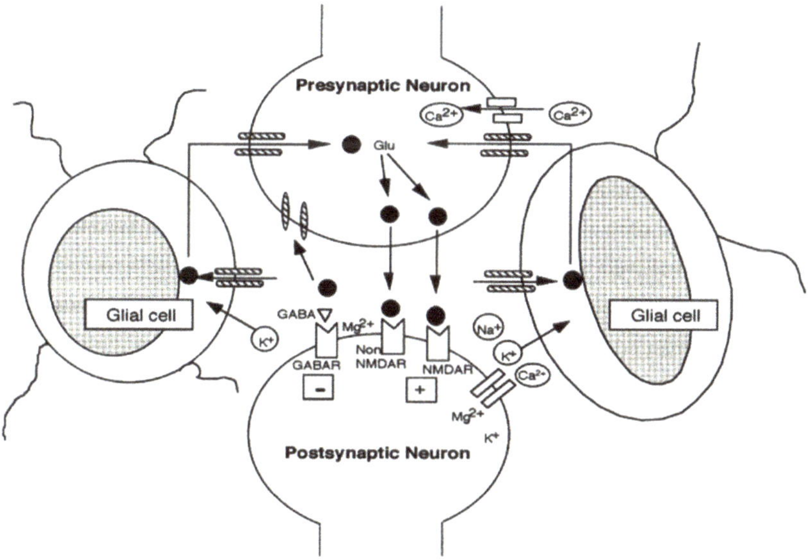

FIGURE 8.2 Glutamate action.

Remote stimulation of excitatory circuits causes neural synchronization. Contraction happens after NMDA receptors are activated, allowing more calcium to reach the cells and increasing stimulation. Perhaps, there is a decrease only in the operation of inhibitory circuits that are downward controlled throughout high-frequency stimulation as most of these excitatory mechanisms improve.

General treatment

Drugs never eradicate seizures, but they do assist in seizure prevention. Epilepsy also has a societal stigma attached to it, and being diagnosed with it will lead to community isolation a lower standard of life, stress, and the deterioration of preexisting mental illnesses.[41] Whenever a drug is abruptly discontinued, the individual can have further epilepsy which is quite difficult to control. Brain surgery can be recommended if pharmaceutical services were unable to prevent seizures. Earlier drugs including phenytoin, valproic acid, carbamazepine, and ethosuximide are commonly prescribed as first-line treatments to many seizure problems around the globe because they are usually as efficient as newer therapies and are far more affordable. While several of the current medications are already being implemented as first-line monotherapy, the majority of the modern medications can be utilized as an add-on or replacement treatment (Fig. 8.3).[42,43]

Commonly used antiepileptic drugs:

1. Barbiturate (e.g., phenobarbitone)[44]
2. Deoxybarbiturate (e.g., primidone)[45]

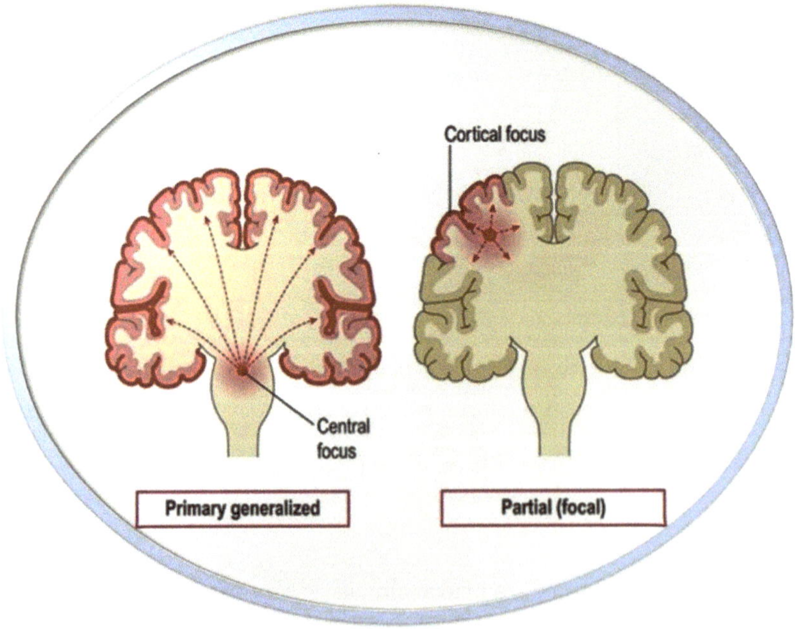

FIGURE 8.3 Origin of generalized and partial seizure.

3. Hydantoin (e.g., phenytoin)[46]
4. Iminostilbene (e.g., carbamazepine)[47]
5. Succinimide (e.g., ethosuximide)[48]
6. Aliphatic carboxylic acid (e.g., valproic acid)[49]
7. Benzodiazepines (e.g., clonazepam)[50]
8. Phenyltriazine (e.g., lamotrigine)[51]
9. Cyclic GABA analog (e.g., gabapentin)[52]
10. Newer drugs (e.g., vigabatrin and topiramate)[53–56]

Phenobarbital mechanism of action

Potentiation of synapses repression by an act just on GABAA receptor is most probably the process by which phenobarbital prevents seizures. Phenobarbital stimulates exposures to iontophoretically implemented GABA, according to intracellular studies of mice cortical or spinal cord nerve cells. Such results were identified at therapeutically important phenobarbital levels. Phenobarbital enhanced the GABAA receptor–mediated activity by increasing the duration of spikes of GABAA receptor–mediated currents without altering the intensity of spikes, according to studies of single channels in outside-out patches differentiated from mice spinal cord nerve cells. Phenobarbital restricts repeated regular firing at levels above clinical doses, which may explain a few of the anticonvulsant benefits of elevated phenobarbital concentrations obtained through status epilepticus treatment.[57,58]

Bromide (potassium bromide/sodium bromide)

Bromide is also a viable first-line treatment option (in patients with hepatic dysfunction). The antiepileptic properties of bromide are unknown. Hyperpolarization of the postsynaptic membrane is thought to be how the treatment works. Oral delivery of bromide salts helps in fast absorption. Since these are not attached to plasma proteins, they may easily move across membranes. Bromide's elimination half-life is extremely large (about 28 days). Thus, after taking 16 weeks of treatment, the patient might be in a stable condition. Renal efflux is based on the presence of concurrent chloride ingestion.[59]

Phenytoin mechanism of action

It is indeed a safe and efficient anticonvulsant that has been recognized as diphenylhydantoin for years.[60] Phenytoin reduces the frequency at which electrical signals are elicited by repeated depolarization of neurons. The whole result is induced by a lowering of the level at which voltage-activated $Na+$ channels recover from inactivation, which is based on both voltage and usage. Phenytoin seems to have a stabilizing effect on neural membranes that further prohibits regular brain cells from detonating repeatedly throughout epileptic depolarization transitions, which are characterized by asynchronous and extremely high depolarization over which action potentials are transposed. These were accomplished by extending the inactive condition of voltage-sensitive neuronal $Na+$ channels, which controls the neuron's refractory duration. Such results can be seen at doses within the therapeutic drug spectrum.[61]

Benzodiazepines mechanism of action

Because of its fast removal half-life and quick (5–7 days) emergence of resistance to their antiepileptic activity, benzodiazepines are unsuccessful in the long therapy of canine epilepsy. The tendency of benzodiazepines to promote GABA-mediated neural suppression accounts for a substantial part of their anticonvulsant efficacy, and other nonsedating benefits. The benzodiazepine receptor is an essential component of the GABAA receptor, according to molecular cloning and recombinant receptor research. Benzodiazepines operate on subtypes of receptor site and enhance the rate, but never the length, of openings at GABA-activated $Cl-$ channels at pharmacologically appropriate doses.[62] Diazepam and several other benzodiazepines, along with phenytoin, carbamazepine, and valproate, can suppress prolonged increased stimulation of nerves at larger doses.[63] All such doses are far greater than those linked with antiseizure or antianxiety symptoms in ambulatory individuals because they correlate to doses reached in patients following diazepam therapy with status epilepticus.[64–66]

Carbamazepine mechanism of action

It is prescribed as first-line therapy for intermittent and tonic–clonic seizures. The pathways that cause carbamazepine's health effects are not well known. Carbamazepine, like phenytoin, inhibits the repeated discharge of electrical impulses elicited by prolonged depolarization. It tends to be driven by just a slower rate of voltage-activated $Na+$ channel reactivation after downregulation. Carbamazepine does have actions in cerebrospinal fluid (CSF) of patients at doses in the therapeutic drug scale. In those doses, carbamazepine has a specific impact without any influence on random action or reactions to iontophoretically applied GABA or glutamate. In pharmacologically impactful doses the carbamazepine metabolite 10,11-epoxycarbamazepine also restricts persistent recurrent shooting,[67] indicating how this metabolite can contribute to carbamazepine's antiseizure efficiency.[68–70]

Ethosuximide mechanism of action

It is used to treat absence epilepsy as first-line therapy. In neuronal cells, ethosuximide lowers low-threshold $Ca2+$ currents (T currents). The thalamus is involved in the production of 3-Hz spike-and-wave patterns, which are common in absence seizures. A huge T pulse in the thalamus underpins blasts of electrical impulses and is thought to perform a part in thalamic oscillatory operation including 3-Hz spike-and-wave activity. Ethosuximide blocks the T current at therapeutically appropriate doses. Ethosuximide decreases this current without affecting the voltage dependency of steady-state downregulation or the recovery period.[71] At therapeutically significant doses, ethosuximide may not suppress repeated repetitive shooting or improve GABA reactions. The latest research supports the hypothesis that ethosuximide acts by inhibiting T currents to suppress absence seizures.[72–74]

Valproic acid mechanism of action

Valproic acid has phenytoin and ethosuximide-like actions on separated nerve cells. Valproate prevents persistently repeated discharge caused by depolarization of mouse cortical or spinal cord neurons at clinically appropriate doses. The activity tends to be driven by a delayed regeneration of voltage-activated $Na+$ channels from downregulation, close to that of phenytoin and carbamazepine. Valproic acid has little effect on neural reactions to GABA applied iontophoretically. Valproate causes minor decreases in the low-threshold (T) $Ca2+$ current in nerve cells derived from the nodose ganglion at medically significant but considerably larger amounts than others who restrict repeated firing; this action on T currents is close to that of ethosuximide in thalamic neurons. These acts of restricting persistent frequent shooting and decreasing T currents can come together to make valproic acid more efficient toward partial and tonic–clonic seizures, as well as absence seizures. One more pathway that could lead to valproate's antiseizure effects is GABA metabolism.[75] About the fact that valproate has little influence on GABA reactions, it does improve the volume of GABA which can be retrieved from the brain after the drug has been given to animals.[76]

Gabapentin mechanism of action

A GABA compound is chemically conjugated to a lipid-soluble cyclohexane ring, making it an anticonvulsant drug. Gabapentin was created to be a centrally acting GABA agonist with greater lipid solubilization that would enable it to pass through the blood–brain barrier more easily. With the electroshock seizure model, gabapentin prevents tonic hind limb expansion. Gabapentin even prevents pentylenetetrazol-induced clonic epilepsy. In each of these studies, its effectiveness is comparable to that of valproic acid, although it differs from phenytoin and carbamazepine. Gabapentin's antiepileptic mode of action remains unclear. Gabapentin can encourage nonvesicular GABA discharge via a pathway that is currently unknown.[77–81]

Newer antiepileptic drugs

Mechanism of action of eslicarbazepine acetate

It is available in prodrug form. S-licarbazepine is its active metabolite, also referred to as eslicarbazepine. It is the active enantiomer of the monohydroxy derivative of oxcarbazepine. Eslicarbazepine exerts its mechanism of action by blocking the sodium channels and giving stability to the inactivated state of the voltage-gated sodium channel. A 2015 scientific study pointed out that it differs from carbamazepine, in enhancing the slow inactivation of voltage-gated sodium channels.[82] Eslicarbazepine acetate is found to be efficacious as a first-line monotherapy in focal seizures. Eslicarbazepine acetate is not accompanied by a spike in CSF while this CSF spike occurs in oxacarbazapine which further explains the reason behind its adverse effect.[83]

Levetiracetam

Levetiracetam acts by attaching to the SV2A (synaptic vesicle protein) eventually causing nonspecific decrease in the release of neurotransmitter during hyperactivation of neurons.[84] It is successfully used as a first-line treatment in cases of focal and generalized tonic–clonic seizures (GTCS) and its IV formulation is popularly employed as second-line treatment for status epilepticus.[85–87]

Brivaracetam

Its mechanism of action is similar to Levetiracetam (attachment to SV2A). Its efficacy and selectivity is 20 times higher than Levetiracetam and was approved by the USFDA for the management of partial-onset seizures in case of 16 years and older patients.[88]

Lacosamide

Lacosamide acts by blocking sodium channels, causing enhancement of slow inactivation thereby differing from most of the drugs which act as sodium channel blockers (enhancer of fast sodium channel inactivation). It is employed for the management (as mono and adjunctive therapy) of focal seizures.[89]

Perampanel

Perampanel is a selective noncompetitive antagonist of α-amino-3-hydroxy-5-methyl-4-isoxazolepropionic acid (AMPA) glutamate receptor. Perampanel is used in patients with focal seizures (both as adjunctive and monotherapy) and as adjunctive in the management of primary GTCS.[90–93]

Cannabidiol

In 2018 cannabidiol was first introduced in the booming pharmaceutical market of the United States. It neither possesses the affinity for cannabinoid receptor CB1 nor psychoactive properties typical of tetrahydrocannabinol. It causes an enhancement of the activity of GABA mediated through the GABA-A receptor allosteric modulation and an increase in currents produced by low GABA level. The USFDA approved this drug in the management of Lennox–Gastaut syndrome or Dravet syndrome–associated seizures in patients of 2 years or more of age.[94–96]

Stiripentol

This drug was approved by the USFDA in 2018. It was used to manage the Dravet syndrome–associated seizures in patients taking clobazam. It acts directly on GABA-A receptor and CYP enzyme inhibition causing augmentation in the level of clobazam and its metabolite.[97]

Conclusion

Antiepileptic medications generally used can successfully manage epileptic seizures in around 50% of people, another 25% may demonstrate progress, and the rest 25% of anticonvulsant medications have little substantial advantage. Besides that, unpleasant side effects from widely prescribed medications make recovery complicated and would need the development of newer antiepileptics. Investigating naturally existing molecules that could relate to different molecular groups is one path to finding new antiepileptic treatments. In the traditional medicine system, many plants and herbs claimed to have antiepileptic activity without any scientific evidence. So it is my opinion that we should try to extract active pharmaceutical ingredients from the herb that will be responsible for the treatment of epilepsy.

References

1. Armijo JA, Adín-Ibarra J, Sánchez-Baglietto N, Vega-Gil N. [Monitoring serum levels of new antiepileptics]. *Rev Neurol.* 2002;35(Suppl 1):S116–S134.
2. Bagnato F, Good J. The use of antiepileptics in migraine prophylaxis. *Headache.* 2016;56 (3):603–615.
3. Castel-Branco MM, Alves GL, Figueiredo IV, Falcão AC, Caramona MM. The maximal electroshock seizure (MES) model in the preclinical assessment of potential new antiepileptic drugs. *Methods Find Exp Clin Pharmacol.* 2009;31(2):101–106. Available from: https://doi.org/10.1358/mf.2009.31.2.1338414. PMID: 19455265.
4. Socała K, Wyska E, Szafarz M, Nieoczym D, Wlaź P. Acute effect of cannabidiol on the activity of various novel antiepileptic drugs in the maximal electroshock- and 6 Hz-induced seizures in mice: Pharmacodynamic and pharmacokinetic studies. *Neuropharmacology.* 2019;158:107733. Available from: https://doi.org/10.1016/j.neuropharm.2019.107733. Epub 2019 Aug 1. PMID: 31377197.

5. Balachandran P, Elsohly M, Hill KP. Cannabidiol interactions with medications, illicit substances, and alcohol: a comprehensive review. *J Gen Intern Med.* 2021. Available from: https://doi.org/10.1007/s11606-020-06504-8. Epub ahead of print. PMID: 33515191.
6. Banach M, Miziak B, Borowicz-Reutt KK, Czuczwar SJ. Advances with extended and controlled release formulations of antiepileptics in the elderly. *Expert Opin pharmacotherapy.* 2019;20(3):333–341.
7. Baum L, Kwan P. Antiepileptic drug delivery. *Adv Drug Delivery Rev.* 2012;64 (10):885–886.
8. Baumgartner C, Koren JP, Britto-Arias M, Zoche L, Pirker S. Presurgical epilepsy evaluation and epilepsy surgery. *F1000Res.* 2019;8. Available from: https://doi.org/10.12688/f1000research.17714.1. F1000 Faculty Rev-1818. PMID: 31700611; PMCID: PMC6820825.
9. Bartolomei F, Lagarde S, Lambert I, et al. Brain connectivity changes during ictal aggression (a strangulation attempt). *Epileptic Disord.* 2017;19(3):367–373. Available from: https://doi.org/10.1684/epd.2017.0925. PMID: 28830845.
10. Zanoci C, Dehghani N, Tegmark M. Ensemble inhibition and excitation in the human cortex: an Ising-model analysis with uncertainties. *Phys Rev E.* 2019;99(3-1):032408. Available from: https://doi.org/10.1103/PhysRevE.99.032408. PMID: 30999501.
11. Bialer M, Johannessen SI, Koepp MJ, et al. Progress report on new antiepileptic drugs: A summary of the Fourteenth Eilat Conference on New Antiepileptic Drugs and Devices (EILAT XIV). I. Drugs in preclinical and early clinical development. *Epilepsia.* 2018;59 (10):1811–1841.
12. Błaszczyk B, Czuczwar SJ. Epilepsy coexisting with depression. *Pharmacol Rep: PR.* 2016;68(5):1084–1092.
13. Fernández-Marmiesse A, Roca I, Díaz-Flores F, et al. Rare variants in 48 genes account for 42% of cases of epilepsy with or without neurodevelopmental delay in 246 pediatric patients. *Front Neurosci.* 2019;13:1135. Available from: https://doi.org/10.3389/fnins.2019.01135. PMID: 31780880; PMCID: PMC6856296.
14. Brodtkorb E, Spigset O. [Interactions with antiepileptics]. *Tidsskr den Norske laegeforening: Tidsskr praktisk medicin, ny raekke.* 2002;122(20):2002–2004.
15. Burstein AH. Lamotrigine. *Pharmacotherapy.* 1995;15(2):129–143.
16. Gadea A, López-Colomé AM. Glial transporters for glutamate, glycine, and GABA: II. GABA transporters. *J Neurosci Res.* 2001;63(6):461–468. Available from: https://doi.org/10.1002/jnr.1040. PMID: 11241581.
17. Akyuz E, Polat AK, Eroglu E, Kullu I, Angelopoulou E, Paudel YN. Revisiting the role of neurotransmitters in epilepsy: an updated review. *Life Sci.* 2021;265:118826. Available from: https://doi.org/10.1016/j.lfs.2020.118826. Epub 2020 Nov 28. PMID: 33259863.
18. Donovan MD, Boylan GB, Murray DM, Cryan JF, Griffin BT. Treating disorders of the neonatal central nervous system: pharmacokinetic and pharmacodynamic considerations with a focus on antiepileptics. *Br J Clin Pharmacol.* 2016;81(1):62–77.
19. Eadie MJ. Antiepileptics. *Contemp Issues Clin Biochem.* 1985;3:135–153.
20. McWilliam M, Al Khalili Y. *Idiopathic Generalized Epilepsy.* 2021. Treasure Island, FL: StatPearls Publishing; 2021. PMID: 31536218.
21. Cissé Y, Crochet S, Timofeev I, Steriade M. Synaptic responsiveness of neocortical neurons to callosal volleys during paroxysmal depolarizing shifts. *Neuroscience.* 2004;124(1):231–239. Available from: https://doi.org/10.1016/j.neuroscience.2003.11.003. PMID: 14960354.
22. Martínez M. Características clínicas y diagnóstico de los estados epilépticos [Clinical and diagnostic characteristics in status epilepticus]. *Neurologia.* 1997;12(Suppl 6):25–30. Spanish. PMID: 9470434.

23. Farrokh S, Bon J, Erdman M, Tesoro E. Use of newer anticonvulsants for the treatment of status epilepticus. *Pharmacotherapy*. 2019;39(3):297–316.
24. Farrokh S, Tahsili-Fahadan P, Ritzl EK, Lewin 3rd JJ, Mirski MA. Antiepileptic drugs in critically ill patients. *Crit Care (London, Engl)*. 2018;22(1):153.
25. Weltha L, Reemmer J, Boison D. The role of adenosine in epilepsy. *Brain Res Bull*. 2019;151:46–54. Available from: https://doi.org/10.1016/j.brainresbull.2018.11.008. Epub 2018 Nov 20. PMID: 30468847; PMCID: PMC6527499.
26. Hanin A, Lambrecq V, Denis JA, et al. Cerebrospinal fluid and blood biomarkers of status epilepticus. *Epilepsia*. 2020;61(1):6–18. Available from: https://doi.org/10.1111/epi.16405. Epub 2019 Dec 11. PMID: 31828792.
27. Goswami JN, Vaidya PC, Saini AG, De D, Radotra BD, Singhi PD. Drug reaction with eosinophilia and systemic symptoms in a child on multiple antiepileptics. *Turk J Pediatr*. 2017;59(2):197–199.
28. Schiller Y, Bankirer Y. Cellular mechanisms underlying antiepileptic effects of low- and high-frequency electrical stimulation in acute epilepsy in neocortical brain slices in vitro. *J Neurophysiol*. 2007;97(3):1887–1902. Available from: https://doi.org/10.1152/jn.00514.2006. Epub 2006 Dec 6. PMID: 17151229.
29. Garland SJ, Gallina A, Pollock CL, Ivanova TD. Effect of standing posture on inhibitory postsynaptic potentials in gastrocnemius motoneurons. *J Neurophysiol*. 2018;120(1):263–271. Available from: https://doi.org/10.1152/jn.00555.2017. Epub 2018 Apr 4. PMID: 29617216; PMCID: PMC6093953.
30. Danober L, Pape HC. Mechanisms and functional significance of a slow inhibitory potential in neurons of the lateral amygdala. *Eur J Neurosci*. 1998;10(3):853–867. Available from: https://doi.org/10.1046/j.1460-9568.1998.00092.x. PMID: 9753153.
31. Karpova MN, Kuznetzova LV, Klishina NY. [GABA and its receptors in pathogenesis of epilepsy]. *Usp Fiziol Nauk*. 2015;46(3):46–59. Russian. PMID: 26506642.
32. Barbara GS, Zube C, Rybak J, Gauthier M, Grünewald B. Acetylcholine, GABA and glutamate induce ionic currents in cultured antennal lobe neurons of the honeybee, *Apis mellifera*. *J Comp Physiol A Neuroethol Sens Neural Behav Physiol*. 2005;191(9):823–836. Available from: https://doi.org/10.1007/s00359-005-0007-3. Epub 2005 Sep 13. PMID: 16044331.
33. Kälviäinen R, Halonen T, Pitkänen A, Riekkinen PJ. Amino acid levels in the cerebrospinal fluid of newly diagnosed epileptic patients: effect of vigabatrin and carbamazepine monotherapies. *J Neurochem*. 1993;60(4):1244–1250. Available from: https://doi.org/10.1111/j.1471-4159.1993.tb03283.x. PMID: 8095971.
34. Holzgrabe U. [New antiepileptics in review]. *Pharmazie unserer Zeit*. 1997;26(3):152–156.
35. Huband N, Ferriter M, Nathan R, Jones H. Antiepileptics for aggression and associated impulsivity. *Cochrane Database Syst Rev*. 2010;2010(2):Cd003499.
36. Krnjević K. When and why amino acids? *J Physiol*. 2010;588(Pt 1):33–44. Available from: https://doi.org/10.1113/jphysiol.2009.176990. Epub 2009 Oct 12. PMID: 19822549; PMCID: PMC2821545.
37. Hanada T. Ionotropic glutamate receptors in epilepsy: a review focusing on AMPA and NMDA receptors. *Biomolecules*. 2020;10(3):464. Available from: https://doi.org/10.3390/biom10030464. PMID: 32197322; PMCID: PMC7175173.
38. Tangvoraphonkchai K, Davenport A. Magnesium and Cardiovascular Disease. *Adv Chronic Kidney Dis*. 2018;25(3):251–260. Available from: https://doi.org/10.1053/j.ackd.2018.02.010. PMID: 29793664.

39. Italiano D, Spina E, de Leon J. Pharmacokinetic and pharmacodynamic interactions between antiepileptics and antidepressants. *Expert Opin Drug Metab Toxicol.* 2014;10 (11):1457–1489.
40. Jacob S, Nair AB. An updated overview on therapeutic drug monitoring of recent antiepileptic drugs. *Drugs R&D.* 2016;16(4):303–316.
41. Ostendorf AP, Gedela S. Effect of epilepsy on families, communities, and society. *Semin Pediatr Neurol.* 2017;24(4):340–347. Available from: https://doi.org/10.1016/j.spen.2017.10.007. Epub 2017 Oct 7. PMID: 29249514.
42. Johannessen Landmark C, Patsalos PN. Drug interactions involving the new second- and third-generation antiepileptic drugs. *Expert Rev Neurother.* 2010;10(1):119–140.
43. Kennedy R, Burnett DM, Greenwald BD. Use of antiepileptics in traumatic brain injury: a review for psychiatrists. *Ann Clin Psychiatry: Off J Am Acad Clin Psychiatrists.* 2001;13 (3):163–171.
44. Alvarez N. Barbiturates in the treatment of epilepsy in people with intellectual disability. *J Intellect Disabil Res.* 1998;42(Suppl 1):16–23. PMID: 10030427.
45. Gallagher BB, Baumel Irwin P, Mattson RH. *Neurology.* 1972;22(11):1186. Available from: https://doi.org/10.1212/WNL.22.11.1186.
46. Gupta M, Tripp J. *Phenytoin.* Treasure Island, FL: StatPearls Publishing; 2021. Available from: https://www.ncbi.nlm.nih.gov/books/NBK551520/.
47. Lee HM, Graudins A. Iminostilbene anticonvulsants: carbamazepine and oxcarbazine. In: Brent J, et al., eds. *Critical Care Toxicology.* Cham: Springer; 2017. Available from: https://doi.org/10.1007/978-3-319-17900-1_37.
48. Teschendorf HJ, Kretzschmar R. Succinimides. In: Frey HH, Janz D, eds. *Antiepileptic Drugs. Handbook of Experimental Pharmacology (Continuation of Handbuch der experimentellen Pharmakologie).* 74. Berlin, Heidelberg: Springer; 1985. Available from: https://doi.org/10.1007/978-3-642-69518-6_19.
49. National Library of Medicine. *Compound Summary for Valproic Acid.* Bethesda, MD: National Center for Biotechnology Information; 2021. Available from: https://pubchem.ncbi.nlm.nih.gov/compound/Valproic-acid.
50. Ochoa JG, Kilgo WA. The role of benzodiazepines in the treatment of epilepsy. *Curr Treat Options Neurol.* 2016;18(4):18. Available from: https://doi.org/10.1007/s11940-016-0401-x. PMID: 26923608.
51. Lamotrigine. In: Aronson JK, ed. *Meyler's Side Effects of Drugs.* 16th ed. Elsevier; 2016:451–468. ISBN 9780444537164. Available from: https://doi.org/10.1016/B978-0-444-53717-1.00954-9. Available from: https://www.sciencedirect.com/science/article/pii/B9780444537171009549.
52. Czuczwar SJ, Patsalos PN. The new generation of GABA enhancers. Potential in the treatment of epilepsy. *CNS Drugs.* 2001;15(5):339–350. Available from: https://doi.org/10.2165/00023210-200115050-00001. PMID: 11475940.
53. French JA, Gazzola DM. New generation antiepileptic drugs: what do they offer in terms of improved tolerability and safety? *Ther Adv Drug Saf.* 2011;2(4):141–158. Available from: https://doi.org/10.1177/2042098611411127. PMID: 25083209; PMCID: PMC4110862.
54. O'Callaghan FJ, Edwards SW, Alber FD, et al.Participating investigators Safety and effectiveness of hormonal treatment vs hormonal treatment with vigabatrin for infantile spasms (ICISS): a randomised, multicentre, open-label trial. *Lancet Neurol.* 2017;16(1):33–42. Available from: https://doi.org/10.1016/S1474-4422(16)30294-0. Epub 2016 Nov 10. PMID: 27838190.

55. Khalil NY, AlRabiah HK, Al Rashoud SS, Bari A, Wani TA. Topiramate: Comprehensive profile. *Profiles Drug Subst Excip Relat Methodol.* 2019;44:333–378. Available from: https://doi.org/10.1016/bs.podrm.2018.11.005. Epub 2019 Jan 14. PMID: 31029222.
56. Hansen CC, Ljung H, Brodtkorb E, Reimers A. Mechanisms underlying aggressive behavior induced by antiepileptic drugs: focus on topiramate, levetiracetam, and perampanel. *Behav Neurol.* 2018;2018:2064027. Available from: https://doi.org/10.1155/2018/2064027. PMID: 30581496; PMCID: PMC6276511.
57. Löscher W. Animal models of seizures and epilepsy: past, present, and future role for the discovery of antiseizure drugs. *Neurochem Res.* 2017;42(7):1873–1888. Available from: https://doi.org/10.1007/s11064-017-2222-z. Epub 2017 Mar 13. PMID: 28290134.
58. Rai S, Drislane FW. Treatment of refractory and super-refractory status epilepticus. *Neurotherapeutics.* 2018;15(3):697–712. Available from: https://doi.org/10.1007/s13311-018-0640-5. PMID: 29922905; PMCID: PMC6095773.
59. Martinez CS, Feas DA, Siri M, et al. In vivo study of teratogenic and anticonvulsant effects of antiepileptics drugs in zebrafish embryo and larvae. *Neurotoxicol Teratol.* 2018;66:17–24.
60. Keppel Hesselink JM, Kopsky DJ. Phenytoin: 80 years young, from epilepsy to breast cancer, a remarkable molecule with multiple modes of action. *J Neurol.* 2017;264(8):1617–1621. Available from: https://doi.org/10.1007/s00415-017-8391-5. Epub 2017 Jan 12. PMID: 28083647.
61. Tunnicliff G. Basis of the antiseizure action of phenytoin. *Gen Pharmacol.* 1996;27(7):1091–1097. Available from: https://doi.org/10.1016/s0306-3623(96)00062-6. PMID: 8981053.
62. MacVicar BA, Tse FW, Crichton SA, Kettenmann H. GABA-activated Cl- channels in astrocytes of hippocampal slices. *J Neurosci.* 1989;9(10):3577–3583. Available from: https://doi.org/10.1523/JNEUROSCI.09-10-03577.1989. PMID: 2477511; PMCID: PMC6569885.
63. Erkola O, Salmenperä M, Tammisto T. Does diazepam pretreatment prevent succinylcholine-induced fasciculations? – a double-blind comparison of diazepam and tubocurarine pretreatments. *Anesth Analg.* 1980;59(12):932–934. PMID: 7004273.
64. Meinardi H. [Antiepileptics]. *Ned Tijdschr voor geneeskunde.* 1987;131(30):1292–1296.
65. Haut SR, Seinfeld S, Pellock J. Benzodiazepine use in seizure emergencies: a systematic review. *Epilepsy Behav.* 2016;63:109–117. Available from: https://doi.org/10.1016/j.yebeh.2016.07.018. Epub 2016 Sep 6. PMID: 27611828.
66. Mula M. Emerging drugs for focal epilepsy. *Expert Opin Emerg Drugs.* 2018;23(3):243–249.
67. Tomson T, Almkvist O, Nilsson BY, Svensson JO, Bertilsson L. Carbamazepine-10,11-epoxide in epilepsy. A pilot study. *Arch Neurol.* 1990;47(8):888–892. Available from: https://doi.org/10.1001/archneur.1990.00530080072013. PMID: 2375696.
68. Beydoun A, DuPont S, Zhou D, Matta M, Nagire V, Lagae L. Current role of carbamazepine and oxcarbazepine in the management of epilepsy. *Seizure.* 2020;83:251–263. Available from: https://doi.org/10.1016/j.seizure.2020.10.018. Epub 2020 Dec 14. PMID: 33334546.
69. Djordjevic N, Jankovic SM, Milovanovic JR. Pharmacokinetics and pharmacogenetics of carbamazepine in children. *Eur J Drug Metab Pharmacokinet.* 2017;42(5):729–744. Available from: https://doi.org/10.1007/s13318-016-0397-3. PMID: 28064419.
70. Gierbolini J, Giarratano M, Benbadis SR. Carbamazepine-related antiepileptic drugs for the treatment of epilepsy – a comparative review. *Expert Opin Pharmacother.* 2016;17(7):885–888. Available from: https://doi.org/10.1517/14656566.2016.1168399. PMID: 26999402.

71. Brigo F, Igwe SC. Ethosuximide, sodium valproate or lamotrigine for absence seizures in children and adolescents. *Cochrane Database Syst Rev*. 2017;2(2):CD003032. Available from: https://doi.org/10.1002/14651858.CD003032.pub3. Update in: Cochrane Database Syst Rev. 2019 Feb 08;2:CD003032. PMID: 28195639; PMCID: PMC6464603.
72. Gören MZ, Onat F. Ethosuximide: from bench to bedside. *CNS Drug Rev*. 2007;13 (2):224–239. Available from: https://doi.org/10.1111/j.1527-3458.2007.00009.x. PMID: 17627674; PMCID: PMC6528725.
73. Mulleners WM, McCrory DC, Linde M. Antiepileptics in migraine prophylaxis: an updated Cochrane review. *Cephalalgia*. 2015;35(1):51–62.
74. Ouchi K. The number and kind of antiepileptics affect propofol dose requirement for anesthesia: observational study. *Odontology*. 2020;108(1):102–108.
75. Sztajnkrycer MD. Valproic acid toxicity: overview and management. *J Toxicol Clin Toxicol*. 2002;40(6):789–801. Available from: https://doi.org/10.1081/clt-120014645. Erratum in: *J Toxicol Clin Toxicol*. 2003;41(4):215. PMID: 12475192.
76. Piskorska B, Miziak B, Czuczwar SJ, Borowicz KK. Safety issues around misuse of antiepileptics. *Expert Opin Drug Saf*. 2013;12(5):647–657.
77. Sankaraneni R, Lachhwani D. Antiepileptic drugs – a review. *Pediatr Ann*. 2015;44(2): e36–e42.
78. Satzinger G. Antiepileptics from gamma-aminobutyric acid. *Arzneimittel-Forschung*. 1994;44(3):261–266.
79. Reinert JP, Dunn RL. Management of overdoses of loperamide, gabapentin, and modafinil: a literature review. *Expert Rev Clin Pharmacol*. 2019;12(9):901–908.
80. Seretny M, Murray SR, Whitaker L, et al. The use of brain functional magnetic resonance imaging to determine the mechanism of action of gabapentin in managing chronic pelvic pain in women: a pilot study. *BMJ Open*. 2019;9(6):e026152.
81. Eller-Smith OC, Nicol AL, Christianson JA. Potential mechanisms underlying centralized pain and emerging therapeutic interventions. *Front Cell Neurosci*. 2018;12:35.
82. Hebeisen S, Pires N, Loureiro AI, et al. Eslicarbazepine and the enhancement of slow inactivation of voltage-gated sodium channels: a comparison with carbamazepine, oxcarbazepine and lacosamide. *Neuropharmacology*. 2015;89:122–135. Available from: https://doi.org/10.1016/j.neuropharm.2014.09.008.
83. Nunes T, Rocha JF, Falcão A, et al. Steadystate plasma and cerebrospinal fluid pharmacokinetics and tolerability of eslicarbazepine acetate and oxcarbazepine in healthy volunteers. *Epilepsia*. 2013;54(1):108–116. Available from: https://doi.org/10.1111/j.1528-1167.2012.03595.x.
84. Fukuyama K, Tanahashi S, Nakagawa M, et al. Levetiracetam inhibits neurotransmitter release associated with CICR. *Neurosci Lett*. 2012;518(2):69–74. Available from: https://doi.org/10.1016/j.neulet.2012.03.056.
85. Gujjar AR, Nandhagopal R, Jacob PC, et al. Intravenous levetiracetam vs phenytoin for status epilepticus and cluster seizures: a prospective, randomized study. *Seizure*. 2017;49:8–12. Available from: https://doi.org/10.1016/j.seizure.2017.05.001.
86. Beuchat I, Novy J, Rossetti AO. Newer antiepileptic drugs for status epilepticus in adults: what's the evidence? *CNS Drugs*. 2018;32(3):259–267. Available from: https://doi.org/10.1007/s40263-018-0509-5.
87. Brigo F, Bragazzi N, Nardone R, Trinka E. Direct and indirect comparison *meta*-analysis of levetiracetam vs phenytoin or valproate for convulsive status epilepticus. *Epilepsy Behav*. 2016;64(pt A):110–115. Available from: https://doi.org/10.1016/j.yebeh.2016.09.030.

88. Ben-Menachem E, Mameniškienė R, Quarato PP, et al. Efficacy and safety of brivaracetam for partial-onset seizures in 3 pooled clinical studies. *Neurology*. 2016;87(3):314–323. Available from: https://doi.org/10.1212/WNL.0000000000002864.
89. Sake JK, Hebert D, Isojärvi J, et al. A pooled analysis of lacosamide clinical trial data grouped by mechanism of action of concomitant antiepileptic drugs. *CNS Drugs*. 2010;24 (12):1055–1068. Available from: https://doi.org/10.2165/11587550-000000000-00000.
90. Crespel A, Gelisse P, Tang NP, Genton P. Perampanel in 12 patients with Unverricht-Lundborg disease. *Epilepsia*. 2017;58(4):543–547. Available from: https://doi.org/10.1111/epi.13662.
91. Dirani M, Nasreddine W, Abdulla F, Beydoun A. Seizure control and improvement of neurological dysfunction in Lafora disease with perampanel. *Epilepsy Behav Case Rep*. 2014;2:164–166. Available from: https://doi.org/10.1016/j.ebcr.2014.09.003.
92. Goldsmith D, Minassian BA. Efficacy and tolerability of perampanel in ten patients with Lafora disease. *Epilepsy Behav*. 2016;62:132–135. Available from: https://doi.org/10.1016/j.yebeh.2016.06.041.
93. Schorlemmer K, Bauer S, Belke M, et al. Sustained seizure remission on perampanel in progressive myoclonic epilepsy (Lafora disease). *Epilepsy Behav Case Rep*. 2013;1:118–121. Available from: https://doi.org/10.1016/j.ebcr.2013.07.003.
94. Devinsky O, Cross JH, Laux L, et al. Trial of cannabidiol for drug-resistant seizures in the Dravet syndrome. *N Engl J Med*. 2017;376(21):2011–2020. Available from: https://doi.org/10.1056/NEJMoa1611618.
95. Devinsky O, Patel AD, Cross JH, et al. Effect of cannabidiol on drop seizures in the Lennox-Gastaut syndrome. *N Engl J Med*. 2018;378(20):1888–1897. Available from: https://doi.org/10.1056/NEJMoa1714631.
96. Thiele EA, Marsh ED, French JA, et al. Cannabidiol in patients with seizures associated with Lennox-Gastaut syndrome (GWPCARE4): a randomised, double-blind, placebo-controlled phase 3 trial. *Lancet*. 2018;391(10125):1085–1096. Available from: https://doi.org/10.1016/S0140-6736(18)30136-3.
97. Nickels KC, Wirrell EC. Stiripentol in the management of epilepsy. *CNS Drugs*. 2017;31 (5):405–416. Available from: https://doi.org/10.1007/s40263-017-0432-1. PMID: 28434133.
98. Karmakar S, Biswas S, Bera R, et al. Beverage-induced enhanced bioavailability of carbamazepine and its consequent effect on antiepileptic activity and toxicity. *J Food Drug Anal*. 2015;23(2):327–334. Available from: https://doi.org/10.1016/j.jfda.2014.07.012.

Chapter 9

Mechanism of action of anti-Parkinson's drugs

Muhammad Shahid Nadeem[1], Salman Bakr I. Hosawi[1], Bibi Nazia Murtaza[2] and Imran Kazmi[1]

[1]*Department of Biochemistry, Faculty of Science, King Abdulaziz University, Jeddah, Saudi Arabia,* [2]*Department of Zoology, Abbottabad University of Science and Technology (AUST), Abbottabad, Pakistan*

Introduction to Parkinson's disease

Parkinson's disease (PD) is a neurodegenerative disorder with approximately 10 million victims worldwide. Mostly, people above 60 years of age are affected by PD. Bradykinesia, tremor, loss of postural reflexes, and rigidity are cardinal signs and symptoms of PD.[1] The disorder is represented by familial and sporadic types, and the former, with genetic basis, accounts for only less than 10% of total PD cases.[2] Many genes have been associated with the onset of PD, *PARK1* gene, coding for alpha-synuclein (α-Syn). (a presynaptic protein), was the first gene identified for its association with the disorder.[3,4] Etiologically, it is a slow-processing, multifactorial condition involving several genetic and environmental factors.[5] Age is the most important risk factor for the onset of PD; this disease is more common among women as compared to men with an estimated ration of 3:2. Many environmental pollutants including pesticides and insecticides have also been associated with the progression of PD.[6] Recently, dysregulation of gut–brain axis by alteration in gut microbiota has also been linked with the onset of PD.[7] However, PD continues to be an enigmatic disorder with no available cure or preventive therapy.[6] Owing to about 70% loss of dopamine-producing neurons at the stage of visible symptoms and overlapping clinical features with other neurodegenerative disorders, the early diagnosis of disease has always been a topic of research and debate.[8] The identification of subtypes of PD during diagnosis is also an important consideration to select and start therapies. There is no established diagnostic marker for the early diagnosis of PD.[9] The International Parkinson and Movement Disorder Society has proposed a diagnosis system based on the Queen's Square Brain Bank Criteria,

How Synthetic Drugs Work. DOI: https://doi.org/10.1016/B978-0-323-99855-0.00009-9

which has been used since last few decades.[10] These criteria have shown very good specificity (95%) and sensitivity (96%) for the diagnosis of PD. Pathophysiologically, PD is caused by the degeneration and dysfunctioning of substantia nigra (SN) neurons resulting the deficiency of neurotransmitter dopamine and by accumulation of α-Syn in Lewy bodies (LBs).[11] Recently, the expression pattern of calcium-binding protein S100B, responsible for the regulation of dopamine metabolism and neuroinflammation, has been associated with the pathophysiology of PD and also considered as an important biomarker for the early diagnosis of disease.[12] In addition to the accumulation of LBs by the aggregation of α-Syn, the accumulation of Tau aggregates has also been linked with the progression of PD.[13] Dysregulation of long noncoding RNAs and microRNAs in brain tissues has been linked with the onset of PD in the animal models.[14] PD has been managed by Levo-DOPA (L-DOPA) supplementation to compensate for the deficiency of dopamine in the patients since the 1970s. The disease has been treated by the application of inhibitors of any of the following enzymes: catechol-O-methyltransferase (COMT), peripheral L-amino acid decarboxylase, or monoamine oxidase B (MAO B).[15] These medicines have their specific mechanisms of action, merits, and disadvantages. The present chapter describes the subtypes of PD, genes, genetic and environmental factors responsible for the disorder, pathophysiology of disease, and mechanism of action of different drugs used to treat PD.

Parkinson's disease symptoms, and its subtypes

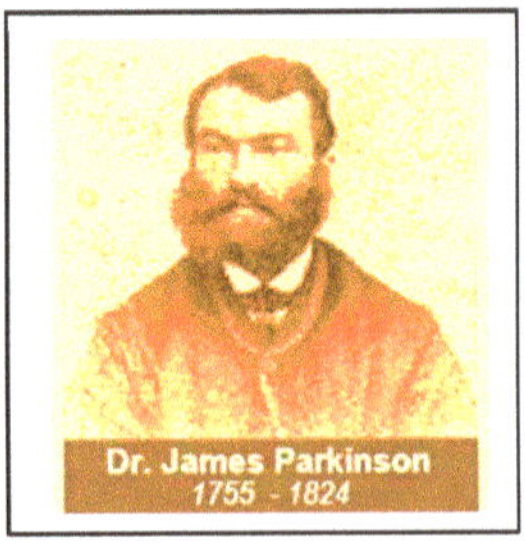

PD was first described by James Parkinson, who was a political activist, as well as an expert in geology, paleontology, and medicine. In his book *An Essay on the Shaking Palsy*, published in 1817, he described the disease with prominent characteristics, including festinant gait, classic Parkinsonian posture, and tremor.[16] At present, the disease has features including mood disturbance, dementia, cognitive dysfunction, sleep–wake dysregulation, dysautonomia, and pain. James Parkinson described the disease on the basis of the nonmotor symptoms encapsulated in Table 9.1.

TABLE 9.1 Parkinson's description of nonmotor symptoms.[16]

Sr. no.	Nonmotor symptom	Parkinson's original description
1	Sleep disturbances	Sleep disturbance with tremulous motion of hands and limbs during sleep, frequently with agitation and alarm.
2	Speech problems	The words of patient are often scarcely intelligible.
3	Constipation	The bowels are commonly torpid, require stimulating medicines. Sometimes, the expulsion of feces from the lower area of large intestine needs mechanical aid.
4	Sialorrhea	The patients fail to direct saliva to the back part of the fauces; hence, it is continually draining out via mouth.
5	Dysphagia	The patient is no longer able to feed himself/herself, and once the food is inside his/her mouth, the muscles of mouth cavity, tongue, and pharynx cannot perform their role properly to retain food inside the mouth cavity and while swallowing.
6	Incontinence	The patient loses control, and urine or feces pass out involuntarily.

PD is divided into subtypes on the basis of Lewis study principle,[17] after the evaluation of medical record of first 5 years after disease diagnosis. According to the above criteria, the subtypes are defined as follows:

1. *Earlier disease onset (EDO):* when disease onset and diagnosis occur at an age below 55 years.
2. *Tremor dominant (TD):* tremor is the sole, initially sustained or dominant symptom that dominates over bradykinesia and rigidity. It can occur at an age of 55 years or above.
3. *Non-TD:* predominant motor feature being bradykinetic with mild or no rest tremor. Onset at an age of 55 or above.
4. *Rapid disease progression without dementia:* unusually rapid progression, no dementia, irrespective of age; death within 10 years from the first PD symptoms.

The subtypes of PD are not distinct entities but have overlapping features that collectively represent the multidimensional spectrum of disorder.[18] Currently, there are no well-established biomarkers for the early diagnosis of PD. Several neuropsychological and neuroimaging tools and procedures have been applied for the diagnosis of disease. Computerized axial tomography and magnetic resonance imaging are useful methods for the efficient diagnosis of PD.

Epidemiology and risk factors for Parkinson's disease

PD is the second most common neurodegenerative disease worldwide.[19] Age is the most important factor for the onset of PD; it is gender-biased disorder.[20,21] Application of certain pesticides in the rural areas also contributes to promote PD, whereas smoking has inverse association with the onset of disease.[22] Family history has a positive association with the incidence of PD; it has been estimated that first-degree relatives of PD patients have up to threefold increased chances to have the disease.[23] Familial forms of PD are found among 5%–15% cases. There are several genes associated with PD, a few important have been tabulated in Table 9.2.

Mutation of LRRK-2 (leucine-rich repeat kinase-2)

- When a mutation occurs in LRRK-2 gene, downregulation of endosome lysosome pathway occurs, due to which α-Syn amount increases and they form clumps called LBs, which cause death of dopaminergic neuron.
- It can also lead to decrease in RAS and MAP-K, which ultimately leads to decrease in the dopaminergic transmission.

TABLE 9.2 Genes associated with the onset of Parkinson's disease.

Name of gene	Gene locus	Protein name	Chromosome	References
PINK1	PARK6	PTEN-induced putative kinase I	1p35–37	24,25
PRKN	PARK2	Parkin	6q25–27	26
UCHL1	PARK5	UCHL-1	4p14	27
DJ-1	PARK7	Protein DJ-1	1p36	28
LRRK2	PARK8	Leucine-rich repeat serine/threonine-protein kinase-2	12p11–q13	29
SNCA	PARK1/4	α-Syn	4q21–23	30
VPS35	PARK17	Vacuolar protein sorting-associated protein 35	16q11	31
PLA2G6	PARK14	A2 phospholipase	22q13	32
FOXB7	PARK15	F-box protein 7	22q12–13	33

- When a mutation occurs there, it can form a protein called "Tau," which forms neurofibrillary tangles and affects dopaminergic neuron.

Mutation in PARK-2

- It causes the downregulation of E_3 ubiquitin ligase, whose function is to fragment the α-Syn peptide. When it is disturbed so that concentration of α-Syn peptide increases, clumps called LBs will occur and ultimately result in the death of dopaminergic neuron.

Mutation on DJ-1 gene

- Also called Parkinson-7 protein, with neuroprotective function from oxidative stress by forming protein, which has antioxidant as well as mitochondrial-regulating property but when mutated can reduce the number of proteins, and thus, reactive oxygen species (ROS) increases as well as mitochondrial function is disturbed as result cell death of dopaminergic neuron occurs.

Contamination of synthetic opioids:

- MPPP (1-methyl-4-phenyl-4-propionoxypiperidine) was developed for its analgesic activity because it a synthetic opioid, but when contaminated, it got converted to MPTP (1-methyl 4-phenyl 1,2,3,6-tetrahydropyridine), which has neurotoxin effect, thus leading to PD.

Substantia nigra and its association with neuronal components

This history of investigations on pathophysiology begins in 1952 when Irving Cooper implicated the role of the thalamus and the basal ganglia in movement disorder. Treatment or changes of basal ganglion were further established by Albin and colleagues in the 1980s. Anatomical connections between the basal ganglia and thalamocortical circuits provide the links by which deep brain stimulation is applied for the treatment of PD. The work by Albin, Alexander, and Delong in the mid-1980s has described the details of anatomical links between different parts of brain and their related functions. The basal ganglion is a component of nervous system constituting of cerebellum, thalamus, and frontal lobes.[34] Its role in the cognitive and motor functions has been well established.[35] Basal ganglion consists of five subcortical components: putamen, caudate, globus pallidus, the subthalamic nucleus of Luys, and SN.

The SN is found directly below the thalamus and is divided into two zones: a ventral pole zone known as pars reticulata and a dorsal darkly pigmented zone known as pars compacta. The internum's dopaminergic neurons are located in the pars compacta. The putamen's pars reticulata globus and pallidus internum are the major output nuclei of the basal ganglia. The basal ganglia receive afferent input from the cerebral cortex and frontal lobes; most afferent information to the basal ganglia terminates in the caudate and putamen; the caudate controls eye movements and cognitive processes, while the putamen controls motor processes. The SN produces the majority of its output through the globus pallidus and the pars reticulata. In collaboration with the prefrontal cortex, the basal ganglia and cerebellum coordinate higher cognitive tasks. It causes cortico-striato-cerebello-thalamocortical (CSPTC) loops, which may have cognitive rather than motor function (Fig. 9.1).

- *Direct pathway*

  Here, due to the death of D_1 (inhibitory neuron), impulse for globus pallidus interna is downregulated by producing less GABA (gamma-Aminobutyric acid), where the subsequent GABAergic neuron will get activated by producing more GABA, and ultimately the neuron moving from cortical region will get inhibitory impulse as more GABA is produced in previous neuron. This inhibitory impulse will be transferred through primary cortical region to muscles.

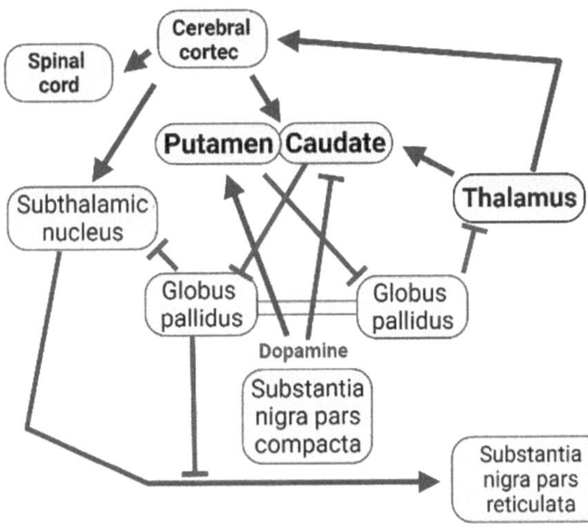

FIGURE 9.1 A description of the many components of the CSPTC loop. The cerebral projects to the striatum, which also gets dopaminergic projections from the pars compacta of the substantia nigra (SNc). The striatum inhibits both the GP and the substantia nigra's pars reticulata (SN pr). The STN transmits exciting projections to the GPi, GPe, and SNpr. The thalamus is inhibited (GABAergic) by GPi or SN pr. The thalamus sends signals to the cortex (also excitatory). The direct channel results in reduced thalamic inhibition [i.e., the striatum suppresses GPi, which in turn reduces its usual (inhibitory) impact on the thalamus, resulting in more excitation from the thalamus to the cortex]. This enables activities to be sustained or initiated. The indirect approach stimulates the GPi, enhancing its inhibition of the thalamus and, as a result, suppressing undesired movements.

- *Indirect pathway*

Due to the death of D_2 (inhibitory neuron), impulse for globus pallidus externa from putamen will be excitatory, and as a result, it will increase the release of more GABA at neuron in globus interna. Now due to more GABA release, the impulse for subthalamus will be inhibitory due to which less GABA will be released, which will ultimately increase the excitatory impulse for globus pallidus interna by eliciting glutamate release. Globus interna will then send excitatory impulse by releasing more GABA at thalamus due to which inhibitory impulse will be generated, finally transferred to muscles.

Because of both inhibitory impulse from brain due to cell death of D_1 and D_2 to muscles, the subject will face hard time in contracting muscles, that is, akinesia and bradykinesia. Due to imbalance of neurotransmitter dopamine, their will be a rise in acetylcholine level, which will impart excitatory effects on muscles causing tremors and rigidity.

CSPTC loops are engaged in projections from unique cortical regions to distinct locations within subcortical structures. The motor circuit is the most important loop in the development of PD. Dopamine has a substantial influence on the flow activity in the basal ganglia circuit outlined above. The primary symptoms of PD are bradykinesia, stiffness, and tremor, which are caused by a decrease or full loss of dopaminergic input to the striatum. According to the most widely accepted hypotheses, dopamine deficiency causes an increase in information via the indirect pathway rather than the direct channel, resulting in suppression of target thalamocortical processes and hyperactivation of the GPi/SNr pathway.

Pathophysiology and pathoanatomy of Parkinson's disease

PD is caused by the degradation of "pigmented" nuclei in SN brain cells. The pigmentation of the dopaminergic cells of the SN is due to the presence of a protein known as melanin. When these cells die, the processing and execution of voluntary actions and movements ceases. After a diagnosis, PD symptoms develop and worsen over time. A protein called -synuclein is normally present in nerve cells. Mutations in -synuclein coding genes, such as PARK1 and PARK4, cause the creation and accumulation of misfolded -synuclein variations known as LBs inside the substantia nigral neurons. The mechanism of cell death due to an accumulation of such misfolded proteins resulting in the cell death needs further investigations. Death or damage to the nigral cells of SN results in the absence of deficiency of neurotransmitter dopamine, hinders the signaling through neurons, and impairs cognitive functions (Fig. 9.2).

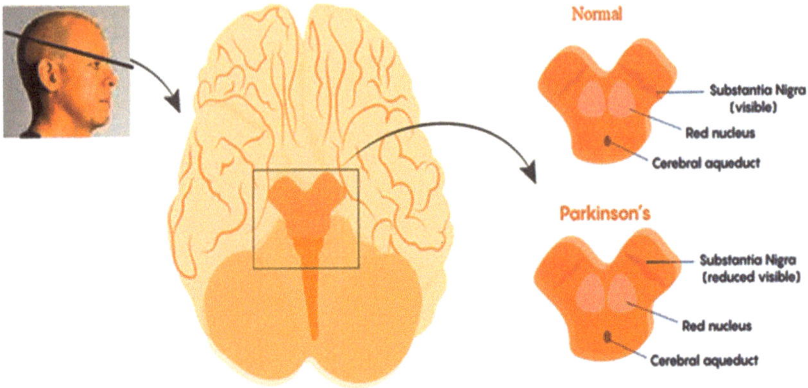

FIGURE 9.2 During Parkinson's disease, dopaminergic neurons in the substantia nigra degenerate. The picture depicts the position of the substantia nigra in the midbrain. The normal substantia nigra is on the right-hand side above, while the reduced substantia nigra is at the bottom.

Anti-Parkinson's disease drugs

> Most of the PD management drugs are either aimed to increase the level of dopamine, dopamine antagonists or to retain the level of dopamine for long time

At present, there is no cure for PD or neuroprotective measures against the disease, and only therapies for the management of symptoms are available. The medicines and therapies are often decided on the basis of patient's age, level of cognitive impairments, and general medical conditions of the patient. Initially, the treatment is targeted to alleviate the common disease symptoms, and to maintain the normal life activities, the medication is matched with the patient's tolerance levels. A wide range of anti-PD drugs are available, and a few of them have been described here:

Levo-DOPA

Torquato Torquati discovered L-DOPA from the bean of Vicia Faba in 1911 as the L-isomer of dihydroxyphenylalanine.[36,37] Peter Holtz identified the enzyme that converts inert L-DOPA to an active molecule known as catecholamine dopamine (DA) in 1938.[38] Later investigations on the brains of dogs and humans revealed the presence of DA in the putamen and caudate nuclei, indicating a role for DA in reserpine-induced Parkinsonism.[39] The next year, research revealed that the caudate nucleus and putamen of PD patients showed a substantial decrease in DA.[40] Currently, L-DOPA has been considered to be the best suited medicine to manage the early stage symptoms of PD. Once in the human body, L-DOPA is converted to dopamine by an enzyme known as decarboxylase. As dopamine cannot cross the blood–brain barrier (BBB), L-DOPA is applied to the PD patients. It is converted to dopamine in the brain cells and improves the dopamine levels to control the PD symptoms mainly caused by the deficiency of dopamine. An average half-life of L-DOPA in the human body is about one hour, and the half-life increases significantly by the use of carbidopa to slow down the conversion of L-DOPA to dopamine.

Long-term application of L-DOPA results in the progression of PD and loss of the dopaminergic nerve terminals. L-DOPA starts losing its impact to manage the disease symptoms. How the long term application of L-DOPA promotes dyskinesia is not very clear.

Dopamine agonists

These are molecules similar in structure with dopamine and directly act on the dopamine receptors. The dopamine agonists are often used with L-DOPA or prescribed before the use of L-DOPA to delay the "wearing off" effect and other complications caused by the long-term use of L-DOPA. Bromocriptine was the first dopamine agonist identified in the 1970s. Since that time, a number of such molecules have been approved and prescribed for the management of PD.[41] Bromocriptine, ropinirole, dihydroergocriptine, pergolide, pramipexole, apomorphine, cabergoline, lisuride, and piribedil are the most commonly used agonists[42] (Fig. 9.3).

Catechol-o-methyltransferase

Axelrod and Tomchick first described COMT (EC 2.1.1.6) in 1958. It is the enzyme that catalyzes the transfer of a methyl group to a catechol. Mg2 + ions are required for enzyme activity, while S-adenosyl-l-methionine (SAM) serves as a methyl group donor. COMT's primary substrates are catecholamines, particularly dopamine. The enzyme is involved in the elimination of physiologically active or poisonous catechols, including neurotransmitters such as dopamine, from the body through modification and removal. The following is the total reaction catalyzed by COMT.

The human soluble COMT is a nonglycosylated 221 amino acid protein with a molecular weight of 24.7 kDa.[43] The membrane-bound COMT has an

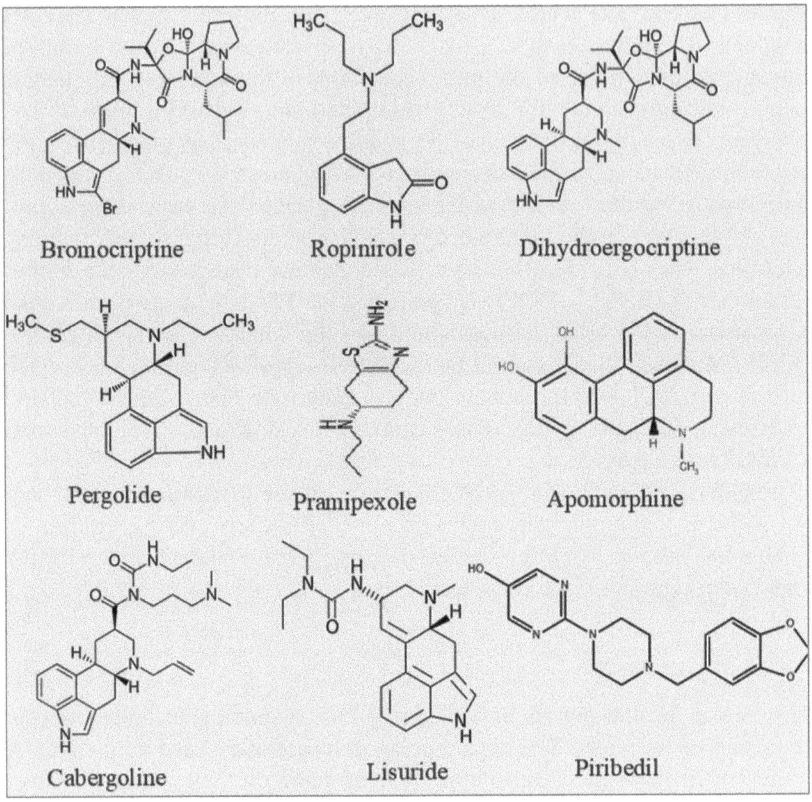

FIGURE 9.3 Some selected dopamine agonists and their structural formulae.

extra peptide of 50 amino acids and a molecular weight of 30 kDa. The majority of this extra peptide is made up of hydrophobic amino acids. MB-COMT is a membrane protein with a catalytic domain directed toward the cytoplasm. Both isozymes exhibit a comparable need on SAM, Mg^{2+}, and Ca^{2+} ions, as well as similar pH and temperature requirements. However, the two isoenzymes have highly variable affinities for different substrates. The affinities of these to isozymes from different sources are tabulated in Table 9.3.

Catechol-O-methyltransferase inhibitors and Parkinson's disease

Most of the inhibitors are competitive substrates of COMT with catechol structure; typically, these include the derivatives of catechols and pyrogallol. The examples include caffeic acid, gallic acid, rutin, and 2-hydroxyoestrogens. Some other compounds may not have catecholic structures like tropolones,

TABLE 9.3 Affinities of S- and MB-COMT, from different sources, for several substrates.

Enzyme source		Substrate	S-COMT/MB-COMT km (μM)		References
Human	Brain	Dopamine	280	3.3	44
	Recombinant Sf9 cells	DBA	39*	30*	45
		Norepinephrine	369*	24*	45
		L-DOPA	613*	266*	45
		Dopamine	207*	15*	45
Recombinant *E. coli*	Catechol	108	10	Malherbe et al.[46]	47
	Liver, brain, and kidney	Norepinephrine	304–464	5.5–11	48
Rabbit	Aorta	2-Hydroxyestradiol	0.27	0.15	49
Mouse	Liver	Epinephrine	242	12	50
Pig	Brain	R-Salsolinol	156	43	51

* *indicates significant figures.*

ascorbic acid, 3-hydroxylated pyrones or pyridones, etc. Some typical COMT inhibitors described initially as first-generation inhibitors.

In the late 1980s, a new class of nitrocatecholic COMT inhibitors, known as second-generation inhibitors, was identified. These had nitro group in the structure and were found more effective in their efficacy, but soon there appeared some concerns of toxicity and of unfavorable pharmacokinetics of these inhibitors.

During the early 1990s, another class of COMT inhibitors was identified and introduced. A pyridine compound known as CGP 28014 was identified as COMT inhibitor. interestingly, it lacked the typical catechol structure.

Substitution of dopamine to compensate its deficiency in PD is the most important target of all kinds of medicinal therapies. Physiologically, COMT is used to inactivate dopamine after the signaling process across two neurons. Hence, the COMT inhibitors are used to slow down the inactivation of dopamine to make available the ample amounts of neurotransmitter and subsequent inhibition of PD symptoms. Dyskinesia, somnolence, orthostatic hypotension, anorexia, dizziness, nausea, vomiting, diarrhea, headache, and sleep disorders are common adverse effects of COMT inhibitor therapies.

Monoamine oxidase

MAO (EC 1.4.3.4.) catalyzes the oxidative deamination of a large number of monoamines. This enzyme is an ubiquitous mitochondrial enzyme that has higher expression levels in the liver, neuronal cells, and gastrointestinal tract. Physiologically, MAO has a role to metabolize the neurotransmitters after the completion of their function in the synaptic cleft and detoxification of a variety of amines. In a typical reaction, MAO oxidizes dopamine and reduced FAD. Production of an aldehyde along with hydrogen peroxide (H_2O_2) in the MAO catalyzed reaction that can result in the production of ROS suggests that the MAO reaction can be neurotoxic[52,53].

However, in the normal conditions the ROS produced by the MAO reaction are detoxified by the activity of scavenger enzymes, for example, catalase. In case of SN pars compacta (SNpc) this increase in the oxidative stress results in the complete or partial loss of neuronal cells or their subsequent dopamine production ability.

Monoamine oxidase-A and monoamine oxidase-B

Two isoenzymes of MAO are found in the human body, that is, MAO-A and MAO-B. Both isoforms of the enzyme are encoded by the genes located on X-chromosome, both have more than 70% homology. Both isoenzymes can be differentiated on the basis of their substrate and inhibitor specificities. MAO-A has greater affinities with hydroxylated amines, for example, serotonin (5-hydroxytryptamine, 5-HT) and noradrenaline, whereas MAOB exhibits better affinities with nonhydroxylated amines including beta-phenylethylamine and benzylamine. Some amines such as tyramine and dopamine exhibit comparable affinities for both isoenzymes. MAO-B is localized in glial cells and serotonergic neurons exposed toward the intermembrane space, whereas MAO-A is found on the cytoplasmic face of the outer mitochondrial membrane in catecholaminergic neurons[54]. According to the old school of thought, MAO-B was responsible for the regulation of dopamine. However, according the recent reports MAO-B controls tonic GABA levels and MAO-A regulates dopamine levels[55].

Inhibitors of monoamine oxidase-A and monoamine oxidase-B

Both irreversible and reversible inhibitors of both isoenzymes have been discovered and tested for their potential use in the treatment of neurological diseases. Cyclopropylamines, hydrazines, and propargylamines are basic irreversible inhibitors that bind covalently with the flavin residue at the N5 atom and dissociate at varying speeds. Following the identification of the enzyme target site, the inhibitor molecule is metabolized as a reactive intermediate after covalently joining with the N5 atom of FAD, resulting in the creation of a drug-receptor adduct. The term "suicide inhibitor" refers to this sort of pharmacological activity.[56] By these inhibitors, the enzyme will be inactivated irreversibly, and the enzyme activity may be retained only when new enzyme molecules are synthesized by the cells, the process may require days or even weeks. In normal routine, the drugs are administered that can inhibit about 90% or more enzymes.

Monoamine oxidase-B inhibitor selegiline and Parkinson's disease

MAO-B is an enzyme of dopamine metabolism; rasagiline and selegiline (N-Propargyl-methamphetamine) are MAO-B inhibitors widely used for the management of PD symptoms. Selegiline is an irreversible MAO-B inhibitor, its application has been used to prolong the L-DOPA therapy and to prevent the adverse effects of L-DOPA. [57,58] Long-term application of selegiline also reduced the requirement of L-DOPA.[59] In the nutshell, application of selegiline preserved the reabsorbed dopamine and conserved to be reused in the next signaling cascade in the synaptic cleft (Fig. 9.4).

Monoamine oxidase-B inhibitor lazabemide in Parkinson's disease

Lazabemide (N-(2-aminoethyl)-5-chloro-2-pyridinecarboxamide) has a shorter "wash out" time, and it has better efficacy than selegiline and mild adverse effects[60,61] (Table 9.4).

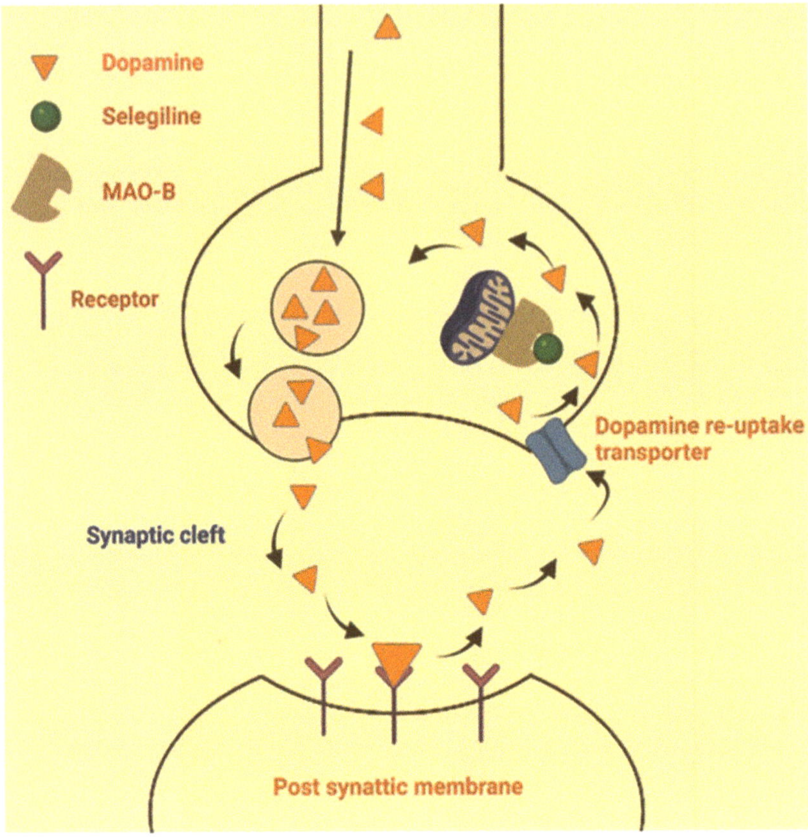

FIGURE 9.4 Mechanism of action of selegiline illustrated as an irreversible MAO inhibitor.

Summary

PD symptoms are largely produced by the loss of dopaminergic neurons in the basal ganglia's nigrostriatal pathway. Dopamine, a neurotransmitter, is used by neurons in this route to regulate the activity of the basal ganglia, which are in charge of initiation and motor regulation. The degeneration of dopaminergic neurons results in a reduction in dopamine concentration, poor control of the circuits involved, and the development of PD symptoms. Many techniques were then created within the scope of this pathology's management. The therapies available today are primarily symptomatic; they seek to lessen the intensity of the symptoms but do not halt or stop the course of the disease. L-DOPA is the most commonly prescribed chemical for the treatment of PD. It crosses the BBB and is converted to dopamine centrally by DOPA-decarboxylase. Dopamine, unlike L-DOPA, is not able to cross the BBB. As a result, it remains in the circulation and is unavailable at the brain

TABLE 9.4 Illustration of some selected MAO inhibitors.

Compound	Activity	Status	Chemical structure
Phenelzine	Irreversible MAO-A + MAO-B	Used as antidepressant Hepatotoxicity Needs dietary control for restriction of tyramine intake	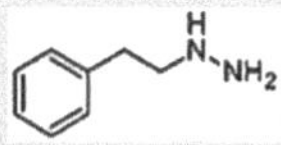
Tranylcypromine	Irreversible MAO-A + MAO-B	Used as antidepressant with dietary control	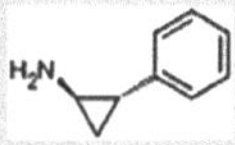
Pargyline	Irreversible MAO-A and MAO-B	Antidepressant and antihypertensive Currently not in clinical use	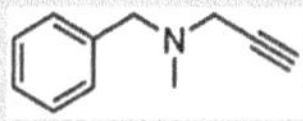
Selegiline	Irreversible MAO-B selective (R-enantiomer) Selectivity is dose dependent in vivo	Metabolism to amphetamines	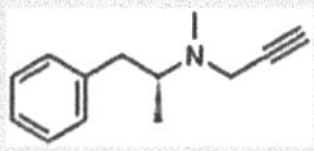
Clorgyline	Irreversible highly MAO-A selective	Antidepressant effect demonstrated in humans but not in clinical use	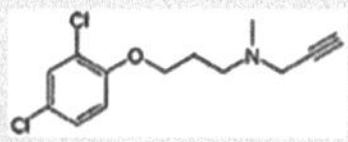
Moclobemide	Reversible highly MAO-A selective	Moderately effective antidepressant drug	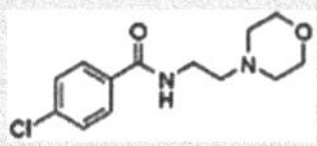
Rasagiline	Irreversible MAO-B selective (R + enantiomer Selectivity) is dose dependent in vivo	Neuroprotective in vivo, anti-Parkinson drug, metabolism to 1-aminoindan	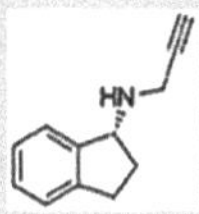
Safinamide	Reversible highly MAO-B selective	Anti-Parkinson drug, glutamate receptor antagonistic and Na + channel blocking properties	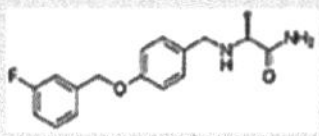

(*Continued*)

TABLE 9.4 (Continued)

Compound	Activity	Status	Chemical structure
Ladostigil	MAO-A + MAO-B Relative brain selectivity, minimal tyramine potentiation	Cholinesterase and MAO inhibition	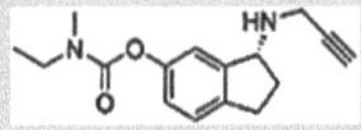
VAR 10303	MAO-A + MAO-B Relative brain selectivity, minimal tyramine potentiation	Fe chelation and MAO inhibition	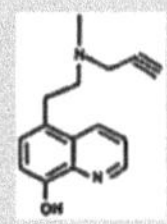
M30	MAO-A and MAO-B Relative brain selectivity	Fe chelation and MAO inhibition	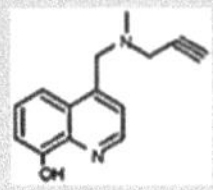

level. In addition to L-DOPA, carbidopa and benserazide are utilized. They aid in limiting L-DOPA breakdown at the peripheral level (that is to say at the blood level, before passing to the brain). Their goal is to enhance the concentration of L-DOPA that penetrates the central nervous system by reducing its degradation at the peripheral level. Dopamine is processed by specific enzymes at the physiological level. Treatments based on inhibiting these enzymes to prevent its breakdown are used to enhance the accessible concentration of dopamine. COMT blocker. Dopamine is metabolized by this enzyme to 3-methoxy-tyramine. This family contains two molecules: entacapone and tolcapone. Entacapone is the most often used and is present in the medication. Dopamine is metabolized by MAO-B producing dihydroxyphenylacetic acid. Rasagiline, selegiline, and sulfonamide are MAO-B inhibitors that can assist to protect accessible dopamine for extended periods of time. All currently known medicines' mechanisms of action, including L-DOPA, COMT inhibitors, and MAO-B inhibitors, have been well documented in the literature.

References

1. Jankovic J. Parkinson's disease: clinical features and diagnosis. *J Neurol Neurosurg Psychiatry*. 2008;79(4):368–376.
2. Gasser T. Genetics of Parkinson's disease. *J Neurol*. 2001;248(10):833–840.
3. Polymeropoulos MH, Higgins JJ, Golbe LI, et al. Mapping of a gene for Parkinson's disease to chromosome 4q21-q23. *Science*. 1996;274(5290):1197–1199.

4. Polymeropoulos MH, Lavedan C, Leroy E, et al. Mutation in the α-synuclein gene identified in families with Parkinson's disease. *Science*. 1997;276(5321):2045–2047.
5. Lichter DG, Benedict RH, Hershey LA. Freezing of gait in Parkinson's disease: risk factors, their interactions, and associated nonmotor symptoms. *Parkinson's Dis*. 2021;.
6. Tolosa E, Garrido A, Scholz SW, Poewe W. Challenges in the diagnosis of Parkinson's disease. *Lancet Neurol*. 2021;20(5):385–397.
7. Kaur G, Behl T, Bungau S, et al. Dysregulation of the gut-brain axis, dysbiosis and influence of numerous factors on gut microbiota associated Parkinson's disease. *Curr Neuropharmacol*. 2021;19(2):233–247.
8. Jakubowski JL, Labrie V. Epigenetic biomarkers for Parkinson's disease: from diagnostics to therapeutics. *J Parkinson's Dis*. 2017;7(1):1–2.
9. Marras C, Lang A. Parkinson's disease subtypes: lost in translation? *J Neurol Neurosurg Psychiatry*. 2013;84(4):409–415.
10. Postuma RB, Berg D, Stern M, et al. MDS clinical diagnostic criteria for Parkinson's disease. *Mov Disord*. 2015;30(12):1591–1601.
11. Vázquez-Vélez GE, Zoghbi HY. Parkinson's disease genetics and pathophysiology. *Annu Rev Neurosci*. 2021;44:87–108.
12. Angelopoulou E, Paudel YN, Piperi C. Emerging role of S100B protein implication in Parkinson's disease pathogenesis. *Cell Mol Life Sci*. 2021;78(4):1445–1453.
13. Pan L, Meng L, He M, Zhang Z. Tau in the pathophysiology of Parkinson's disease. *J Mol Neurosci*. 2021;1–3.
14. Rezaei O, Nateghinia S, Estiar MA, Taheri M, Ghafouri-Fard S. Assessment of the role of non-coding RNAs in the pathophysiology of Parkinson's disease. *Eur J Pharmacology*. 2021;173914.
15. Nagatsu T, Sawada M. L-dopa therapy for Parkinson's disease: past, present, and future. *Parkinsonism Relat Disord*. 2009;15:S3–S8.
16. Parkinson J. An essay on the shaking palsy. 1817. *J Neuropsychiatry Clin Neurosci*. 2002;14:223–236. discussion 2.
17. Lewis SJG, Foltynie T, Blackwell AD, Robbins TW, Owen AM, Barker RA. Heterogeneity of Parkinson's disease in the early clinical stages using a data driven approach. *J Neurol Neurosurg Psychiatry*. 2005;76(3):343–348.
18. McMillan CT, Wolk DA. Presence of cerebral amyloid modulates phenotype and pattern of neurodegeneration in early Parkinson's disease. *J Neurol Neurosurg Psychiatry*. 2016;87 (10):1112–1122.
19. Schapira AH, Chaudhuri KR, Jenner P. Non-motor features of Parkinson disease. *Nat Rev Neurosci*. 2017;18(7):435–450.
20. Gillies GE, Pienaar IS, Vohra S, Qamhawi Z. Sex differences in Parkinson's disease. *Front Neuroendocrinol*. 2014;35(3):370–384.
21. Lee A, Gilbert RM. Epidemiology of Parkinson disease. *Neurologic Clin*. 2016;34 (4):955–965.
22. Breckenridge CB, Berry C, Chang ET, Sielken Jr RL, Mandel JS. Association between Parkinson's disease and cigarette smoking, rural living, well-water consumption, farming and pesticide use: systematic review and *meta*-analysis. *PLoS One*. 2016;11(4):e0151841.
23. Gasser T. Genetics of Parkinson's disease. *Clin Genet*. 1998;54(4):259–265.
24. Ibánez P, Lesage S, Lohmann E, et al. Mutational analysis of the PINK1 gene in early-onset parkinsonism in Europe and North Africa. *Brain*. 2006;129(3):686–694.
25. Wang D, Qian L, Xiong H, et al. Antioxidants protect PINK1-dependent dopaminergic neurons in Drosophila. *Proc Natl Acad Sci*. 2006;103(36):13520–13525.

26. Oczkowska A, Kozubski W, Lianeri M, Dorszewska J. Mutations in PRKN and SNCA genes important for the progress of Parkinson's disease. *Curr Genomics*. 2013;14(8):502–517.
27. Saini P, Runako U, Yu E, et al. Association study of DNAJC13, UCHL1, HTRA2, GIGYF2, and EIF4G1 with Parkinson's disease. *Neurobiol Aging*. 2021;100. 119-e7.
28. Mencken P, Boussac I, Romano CD, Kitami T, Linkster CL, Kruger R. The role of DJ-1 in cellular metabolism and pathophysiological implications for Parkinson's disease. *Cells*. 2021;10(2):347.
29. Lai D, Ali Panahi B, Fontanilla P, et al. Genome wide Association Studies of LRRK2 modifiers of Parkinson's disease. *Ann Neurol*. 2021;90(1):76–88.
30. Ramazani M, Mooches P, Yoon E, et al. Investigating the relationship between the SNCA gene and cognitive abilities in idiopathic Parkinson's disease using machine learning. *Sci Rep*. 2021;11(1). 1-0.
31. Sassine J, Realer C, Data G, Region M, Pollachi MT, Aravalli B. The role of VPS35 in the pathobiology of Parkinson's disease. *Cell Mol Neurobiol*. 2021;41(2):199–227.
32. Liu H, Wang Y, Pan H, et al. Association of rare heterozygous PLA2G6 variants with the risk of Parkinson's disease. *Neurobiol Aging*. 2021;101. 297-e5.
33. Balestrino R, Schapiro AH. Parkinson disease. *Eur J Neurol*. 2020;27(1):27–42.
34. Thatch Jr. WT. The cerebellum. In: Mount Casgle DD, ed. *Medical Physiology*. 14th Mosby: St. Louis; 1980:837–858.
35. Middleton FA, Strick PL. Basal ganglia and cerebellar loops: motor and cognitive circuits. *Brain Res Rev*. 2000;31(2–3):236–250.
36. Leisman G, Melillo R. The basal ganglia: motor and cognitive relationships in a clinical neurobehavioral context. *Rev Neurosci*. 2013;24(1):9–25.
37. Torquate T. Sulla pretense di una so stanza azotea nei gemelli del semi di "vici faba.". *Arch Pharmacal Sper*. 1913;15:213–223.
38. Holtz P. Dopa decarboxylase. *Naturwissenschaften*. 1939;27:724–725.
39. Bertler Å, Rosengren E. Occurrence and distribution of dopamine in brain and other tissues. *Experiential*. 1959;15:10–11.
40. Behringer H, Gronkiewicz O. Overtoiling von Noradrenalin und Dopamine (3-Hydroxytyramin) mi Gehring des Menschen und hire Verhaegen bee Reranking des extrapyramidal Systems. *Linisher Wochenschr*. 1960;38(24):1236–1239.
41. Tan E-K, Jankovic J. Choosing dopamine agonists in Parkinson's disease. *Clin Neuropharmacol*. 2002;24:247–253.
42. Antonina A, Tools E, Mizuno Y, Yamamoto M, Power WH. A reassessment of risks and benefits of dopamine agonists in Parkinson's disease. *Lancet Neurol*. 2009;8(10):929–937.
43. Lundström K, Salinan M, Jaakko A, Savolainen R, Ullmann I. Cloning and characterization of human placental catechol-*O*-methyltransferase cDNA. *DNA Cell Biol*. 1991;10:181–189.
44. Jeffery DR, Roth JA. Kinetic reaction mechanism for magnesium binding to membrane-bound and soluble catechol O-methyltransferase. *Biochemistry*. 1987;26(10):2955–2958.
45. Lotta T, Vidgren J, Tilgmann C, et al. Kinetics of human soluble and membrane-bound catechol-*O*-methyltransferase: a revised mechanism and description of the thermolabile variant of the enzyme. *Biochemistry*. 1995;34:4202–4210.
46. Malherbe P, Bertocci B, Caspers P, Zurcher G, Da Prada M. Expression of functional membrane-bound and soluble catechol-*O*-methyltransferase in *Escherichia coli* and a mammalian cell line. *J Neurochem*. 1992;58:1782–1789.
47. Bonifácio MJ, Vieira-Coelho MA, Borges N, Soares-da-Silva P. Kinetics of rat brain and liver solubilized membrane-bound catechol-*O*-methyltransferase. *Arch Biochem Biophys*. 2000;384:361–367.

48. Masuda M, Tsunoda M, Imai K. High-performance liquid chromatography-fluorescent assay of catechol-*O*-methyltransferase activity in rat brain. *Anal Bioanal Chem.* 2003;376:1069–1073.
49. Reid JJ, Stitzel RE, Head RJ. Characterization of the *O*-methylation of catechol oestrogens by intact rabbit thoracic aorta and subcellular fractions thereof. *Naunyn Schmiedebergs Arch Pharmacol.* 1986;334:17–28.
50. Bonifácio MJ, Palma PN, Almeida L, Soares-da-Silva P. Catechol-O-methyltransferase and its inhibitors in Parkinson's disease. *CNS drug Rev.* 2007;13(3):352–379.
51. Hotzl BK, Thomas H. *O*-methylation of (+)-(R)- and (−)-(S)-6,7-dihydroxy-1-methyl-1,2,3,4-tetrahydroisoquinoline (salsolinol) in the presence of pig brain catechol-*O*-methyltransferase. *Chirality.* 1997;9:367–372.
52. Jenner P. Oxidative stress in Parkinson's disease. *Ann Neurol.* 2003;53(S3):S26–S38.
53. Westfall TC, Westfall DP. Neurotransmission: the autonomic and somatic motor nervous systems. In: Brunton LL, ed. *The Pharmacological Basis of Therapeutics.* 12th ed. New York: McGraw Hill; 2011:171–218.
54. Naoi M, Maruyama W, Inaba-Hasegawa K. Revelation in the neuroprotective functions of rasagiline and selegiline: the induction of distinct genes by different mechanisms. *Expert Rev Neurotherap.* 2013;13(6):671–684.
55. Cho HU, Kim S, Sim J, et al. Redefining differential roles of MAO-A in dopamine degradation and MAO-B in tonic GABA synthesis. *Exp Mol Med.* 2021;53(7):1148–1158.
56. Finberg JP. Update on the pharmacology of selective inhibitors of MAO-A and MAO-B: focus on modulation of CNS monoamine neurotransmitter release. *Pharmacol Ther.* 2014;143(2):133–152.
57. Parkinson Study Group. Effects of tocopherol and deprenyl on the progression of disability in early Parkinson's disease. *N Engl J Med.* 1993;328:176–183.
58. Turnbull K, Caslake R, Macleod A. Monoamine oxidase B inhibitor for early Parkinson's disease. *Cochrane Database Syst Rev.* 2005;(3)). Available from: https://doi.org/10.1002/14651858.
59. Palhagen S, Heinonen E, Hagglund JSwedish Parkinson's Study Group. Selegiline slows the progression of the symptoms of Parkinson's disease. *Neurology.* 2006;25(66):8.
60. LeWitt PA, Taylor DC. Protection against Parkinson's disease progression: clinical experience. *Neurotherapeutics.* 2008;5(2):210–225.
61. Werner P, Seppi K, Tanner CM, et al. Parkinson disease. *Nat Rev Dis Prim.* 2017;3 (17013).

Chapter 10

Mechanism of action of antipsychotics and antimanics

Muhammad Shahid Nadeem[1], Muhammad Naeem Riaz[2], Salman Bakr I. Hosawi[1], Hisham N. Altayb[1], Aziz Ud-din[3] and Tanzeela Fazal[4]

[1]Department of Biochemistry, Faculty of Science, King Abdulaziz University, Jeddah, Saudi Arabia, [2]Department of Pharmacy, COMSATS University, Abbottabad, Pakistan, [3]Department of Genetic Engineering and Biotechnology, Hazara University, Mansehra, Pakistan, [4]Department of Chemistry, Abbottabad University of Science and Technology (AUST), Abbottabad, Pakistan

Introduction

Mental disorders, also known as psychological disorders, are a group of psychological and behavioral symptoms that impact one's quality of life. This group of behavioral issues causes suffering and poor functioning in daily life. Some of the most common mental illnesses affecting people include bipolar disorder, which includes generalized anxiety disorder, persistent depressive disorder, obsessive–compulsive disorder, major depressive disorder, schizophrenia, posttraumatic stress disorder, and social anxiety disorder.

Psychosis is not an illness but a symptom of illness. It can be initiated and promoted by a physical injury, substance abuse, mental illness, extreme stress, and trauma. Schizophrenia-like disorders include psychosis, which often disturbs the life of a patient during the early adulthood or during late teen ages. In addition to other mental health issues, psychosis can be caused by substance abuse such as alcoholism, drugs of abuse, and several disease conditions. Multiple roots of psychosis suggest the involvement of many similar or different pathological mechanisms in the brain of affected individuals. For example, Brain tumors, HIV, traumatic brain injuries, strokes, and some brain diseases such as dementia, Alzheimer's, and Parkinson's, can also cause psychosis. Therefore, psychosis is sometimes a symptom of schizoaffective disorder, bipolar disorder, schizophrenia, and long-term depression. Psychosis is often predicted by high levels of depression, long duration of symptoms, poor functioning, and reduced attention.

Neuroleptic drugs are mostly used for the management of psychotic symptoms associated with neuropsychiatric disorders. The majority of

How Synthetic Drugs Work. DOI: https://doi.org/10.1016/B978-0-323-99855-0.00010-5

neuroleptics reduce or block the dopamine (DA) neurotransmission; the cell types mediating their actions need further investigations. Antipsychotics includes a class of psychotropic medication basically applied to manage psychosis, which includes delusions, hallucinations, and in some selected cases, disorders like schizophrenia but also in a range of other psychotic disorders. These drugs work as a major tranquilizer and help with sleeping difficulties. They are also used as a supportive treatment for bipolar disorder, reactive disorders, and as mood stabilizers. Recently, a study has demonstrated a shrinkage of brain tissue or decrease in the brain volume by the application of antipsychotic drugs.

Many adverse effects have been associated with the long-term application of antipsychotic drugs. These adverse effects include gynecomastia, involuntary movement disorders, impotence, metabolic syndrome tardive dyskinesia, and weight gain. All antipsychotics have a specific dopamine D_2 receptor blocking action except for clozapine. Phenothiazine and thioxanthene classes also block D_1, D_3, and D_4 receptors. In this action, their potency for the psychotic action is controversial to treat psychotic patients. For antipsychotic effect, blockade of dopaminergic and preferentially temporal and prefrontal region is responsible. Drugs that increase dopaminergic activity like amphetamines, levodopa and bromocriptine have been observed to induce schizophrenia-like syndromes in particular patients. As an adaptive change to the blockade of D_2 receptors, the firing of dopaminergic neurons and dopamine turnover increase initially. However, over a period of time, this subsides and give away to diminish activity, especially in basal ganglia, corresponds to emergence of Parkinson-like effect. Clozapine is a group of atypical antipsychotics responsible to weakly block D_2 receptor and have significant $alpha_{1,}$ and D4 blocking action. The antipsychotic abilities of such drugs may depend on specific and variable properties of a drug on different neurotransmitter-associated receptors.

Extrapyramidal symptoms associated with dopaminergic blockade in the basal ganglia appear to be responsible for antiemetic effect. The therapeutic efficacy of quetiapine and clozapine for the D2 receptor is moderately low (up to 40%). The particular activities of these medicines are determined by their rate of release and binding affinity for the D2 receptor. Quetiapine, despite its short biological half-life, has been proposed to have transiently high occupancy, which is sufficient for therapeutic activity. Several additional theories, on the other hand, suggest that quetiapine differs from other antipsychotic medications in ways that suggest a different method of action (Fig. 10.1).

Psychological disorders at a glance

A psychological disease clearly shows changes in behaviors and thoughts. Although reaching an agreement on what types of thoughts, feelings, and

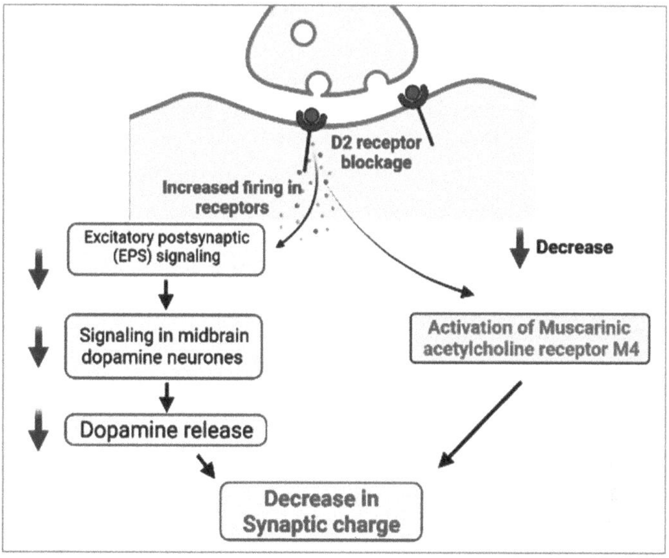

FIGURE 10.1 Alternative hypotheses for dopamine D2-receptor-blocking antipsychotic medications' indirect action. Both hypotheses propose that antipsychotic medications inhibit the production of cyclic adenosine monophosphate (cAMP) by causing greater firing of striatal cholinergic interneurons.

behaviors are truly aberrant in the sense that they legitimately signal the presence of psychopathology is difficult, it is critical for mental health practitioners to agree. Certain patterns of conduct and inner experience are easily identified as aberrant and definitively indicate psychological distress.

A person who washes his/her hands 30 times a day, or the one who claims to hear devils speak may have habits and inner experiences that most people would consider abnormal: beliefs and behaviors that point to the presence of a mental illness.

Behaviors represented by a psychological disorder

Psychologists try to separate psychological diseases from situational, unique, or unusual interior sensations and actions.

Definition of physiological disorders

The simplest way to think about psychological disorders is to define abnormal, distressing, dysfunctional, and often even dangerous behaviors, thoughts, and interior sensations as indications of a condition.

One would undoubtedly be disappointed if they asked a classmate out on a date and were turned down. Such emotions would be understandable. If they were depressed to the point where they lost interest in activities, had trouble eating or sleeping, felt completely useless, and considered suicide, their sensations would be abnormal, out of the ordinary, and could indicate the presence of a psychiatric disease. However, just because something is uncommon does not indicate it is disordered.

Because red hair is seen in just around 4% of persons in the United States, it is considered an uncommon trait, but it is not disordered; it is simply rare. In Scotland, where around 13% of the population has red hair ("DNA Project Aims," 2012), it is less uncommon. Some illnesses, while not precisely normal, are far from atypical, and their prevalence in the general population is astonishing. Is it reasonable to view conduct or interior experiences that deviate from generally recognized cultural standards or expectations as disordered if we believe that being atypical is insufficient criterion for having a psychiatric disorder?

A woman who goes around a subway station in July wearing a bulky winter coat while screaming obscenities at strangers may be regarded to be exhibiting symptoms of a psychological condition in accordance with this criterion. Her conduct and clothing go against socially acceptable dress and behavior norms; these features are unusual.

Common symptoms of psychological disorders

- Although the symptoms of psychological disorders differ depending on the disorder, mood and behavioral symptoms are similar.
- Symptoms can be long-term and recurrent.
- They can make it difficult for one to interact with others in society. Physical symptoms can occur as a result of several psychiatric diseases.
- Panic episodes associated with anxiety disorders, for example, might mimic the symptoms of a heart attack. Pain and achiness are common symptoms of somatoform illnesses, which are syndromes in which symptoms suggest a medical reason but none can be determined.
- Psychological disorders – common symptoms include:
- Angry, hostile, or aggressive behavior.
- Abuse of alcohol or drugs.
- Changes in energy levels.
- Anxiety.
- Perplexity or a sense of disconnection.
- Behavior that is erratic.
- Mood swings and irritability.
- Psychoses, such as hallucinations and delusions, affect perception or thinking processes.
- Persistent or sudden mood swings that might cause problems in daily life.
- Denial of the problem.
- Isolation from others.

Physical symptoms of psychological disorders

Physical symptoms may be linked to psychological diseases, such as:
- Inexplicable physical difficulties.

- Fatigue or malaise;
- Sleep disruptions;
- Changes in weight and appetite.

Some serious symptoms that might indicate a life-threatening condition

Psychological problems can be life-threatening in some instances. If you or someone you are with has any of these life-threatening symptoms, seek medical help right once.

- Posing a threat to oneself or others, including threatening, illogical, or suicidal behavior.
- Trauma, including deformities of the bones, burns, eye injuries, and other ailments.

Causes psychological disorders

Psychological disorders have no known causes, but they are assumed to be influenced by a number of circumstances. Neurotransmitters in the brain, childhood experiences, inheritance, severe illnesses, prenatal exposures, and stress are some of these causes. Some, but not all, psychological diseases are influenced by gender.

Risk factors for psychological disorders

- A variety of factors contribute to the development of psychiatric diseases. Psychological problems do not affect everyone who has risk factors. Abuse or neglect as a youngster are risk factors for psychological problems.
- Temperament issues in childhood.
- Mental illness or substance misuse in the family or personal history. Intelligence below normal.
- Low birth weight is associated with a lower socioeconomic level.
- Absence of one or both parents, criminal activities, and substance abuse.
- Prenatal exposures to alcohol or drugs, for example.
- Serious medical issues like cancer, persistent pain, and hypothyroidism.
- Social exclusion.
- Life events that are stressful or distressing.
- Abuse of drugs and alcohol.

Treatment of psychological disorders

Recognizing that a problem exists is the first step in treating psychological problems. People with psychological problems frequently deny they have a problem and do not seek medical treatment for their symptoms. Regular medical treatment is beneficial because it permits a healthcare provider to perform early screening tests. Regular medical care also allows one's healthcare provider to quickly assess their symptoms and their risk of developing psychiatric illnesses. Psychotherapy is widely used in treatment to address behaviors, skill development, and thinking processes. Coexisting medical problems, serious complications, severe disorders, or substance dependence may need an initial hospitalization. Some personality problems can benefit from medication. With the right treatment, one can see significant improvements.

Common treatments for psychological disorders

- Anti-anxiety drugs are a common treatment for psychiatric illnesses.
- Mood enhancers such as antidepressants.
- Antipsychotic drugs are used to address abnormal mental processes and perceptions.
- Cognitive behavioral therapy to work on thought patterns and behavior.
- Family therapy to help develop support and understanding.
- Identification and treatment of coexisting issues
- Hospitalization for coexisting medical problems, serious complications, severe disorders, and substance abuse
- Individual counseling.
- Medications that help one stay in a good mood.
- Psychodynamic treatment, which focuses on identifying and comprehending previous difficulties, as well as their connections to contemporary beliefs and behaviors.
- Self-help groups.
- Cognitive behavioral treatment.

Ways to improve your psychological disorders

One may be able to alleviate their symptoms and reduce their chance of recurrence in addition to seeking and receiving treatment by:

- Avoiding alcohol or illegal drug usage.
- Avoiding caffeine or other stimulants.

- Maintaining a consistent eating schedule.
- Exercising on a regular basis.
- Getting adequate rest.
- Scheduling visits and according to medication instructions.

Potential complications of psychological disorders

Untreated or poorly controlled psychiatric diseases can have serious consequences, even posing a threat to one's life in some situations. Following the treatment plan one and their healthcare expert devised specifically for them can help reduce their chances of significant problems.

• Difficulties with the law, at work, in social contexts, with relationships, and with finances are only a few of the complications of psychiatric disorders.

- There is a higher chance of getting hurt.
- Self-harm.
- Isolation from others.
- Relationships within the family are strained.
- Abuse of drugs and alcohol.
- Suicide or acts of violence

Etiology of schizophrenia

Schizophrenia is an illness brought on by biopsychosocial factors such as genetic, perinatal, neuroanatomic, neurochemical, and other biological problems. Furthermore, psychological and socio-environmental factors may raise the incidence of schizophrenia in foreign migrants or ethnic minority urban populations. Increased paternal age is linked to a higher likelihood of developing schizophrenia.

Genetic factors

According to studies, schizophrenia runs in families. Adopted relatives of people with schizophrenia have a higher risk of developing schizophrenia than biological relatives. In first-degree relatives of people with schizophrenia, the risk of developing schizophrenia is 10%. If both parents have schizophrenia, their child has a 40% chance of developing it as well. For schizophrenia, dizygotic twins have a 10% concordance rate, while monozygotic twins have a 40–50% concordance rate. Researchers have discovered additional genetic loci previously unknown to be linked to schizophrenia in a recent study. The study found 108 genetic loci connected to schizophrenia, but just one of them was linked to schizophrenia, 83 had never been discovered before. Other genetic variations affect the gene's structure. As can be seen, determining the specifics of these genetic elements is challenging. Interactions with the rest of the genome and the environment will very certainly play a role. Despite this, a meta-analysis of twin studies found that genetic factors account for roughly four-fifths of schizophrenia risk.

Neurotransmitters

Multiple metabolic pathways are thought to play a role in schizophrenia, which makes finding a single aberration difficult. Patients' responses to psychoactive drugs have been used to relate a variety of neurotransmitters to this illness. Common neurotransmitters involved in the etiology of schizophrenia include dopamine, serotonin, norepinephrine, gamma aminobutyric acid (GABA), and glutamate. The dopamine hypothesis, which arose from two observations, explains the function of dopamine in schizophrenia.

First, phenothiazines, a class of drugs that disrupt dopamine action, may help alleviate psychotic symptoms. Second, amphetamines, which boost dopamine release, can cause paranoia and exacerbate schizophrenia, while disulfiram inhibits dopamine hydroxylase, causing schizophrenia to worsen. GABA is another neurotransmitter implicated in the pathophysiology of schizophrenia. It has a regulating function.

Pregnancy and birth complications

According to the findings, pregnancy and birth problems may have a minor impact on the likelihood of developing schizophrenia later in life. Women who are underweight or have certain viral infections during their pregnancy are more likely to have children who develop schizophrenia later in life. Children born to malnourished Dutch women during WWII, for example, have a high risk of schizophrenia. An increased risk of schizophrenia may be linked to obstetric difficulties. A study of Finnish women found that hereditary and environmental factors both play a role in the development of schizophrenia.[1] A review of 9596 women in Helsinki who received hospital treatment for an upper urinary tract infection during pregnancy between 1947 and 1990 found no overall significant increase in the risk of schizophrenia in their offspring, but there was a fivefold increased risk in the offspring of women who also had a family history of psychosis.

Season of birth

Children born during the cold months may be more susceptible to schizophrenia. Winter birth is a strong epidemiological finding in those who acquire schizophrenia later in life, at least in the northern hemisphere. It is more than likely a proxy signal for some seasonal environmental component. Seasonal variations in exposure to intrauterine viral infections around the time of birth, as well as variations in light, temperature/weather, or exogenous toxins, are among the most prevalent explanations.

Cannabis use

According to various studies, excessive marijuana use in teenagers aged 15–17 years may speed the onset of psychosis in those who are at high risk of developing a psychotic condition. The Allied Cohort on the Early Course of Schizophrenia (ACES)-II project looked at 247 hospitalized patients who had experienced first-episode psychosis and found that the onset of psychosis in those who used cannabis between the ages of 15 and 17 years occurred at a mean age of 21.07 years, compared to a mean age of 23.86 years in those who did not use cannabis during those same teenage years. However, the researchers were unable to determine if marijuana use causes early onset psychosis or whether those who have a proclivity for early onset psychosis are also more likely to use marijuana because of a variety of variables (Table 10.1).

Genetic factors for psychological diseases

Genetics of schizophrenia

Because there is no well-defined, focused, and unique microscopic neuropathology in schizophrenia, it is particularly resistant to molecular advancement. Our understanding of schizophrenia is changing from oligogenic to polygenic models, but its genetic architecture remains mostly unknown. According to current evidence, the mutation frequency spectrum contains a mixture of common and unusual mutations.

Familial clustering

Schizophrenia is characterized by familial clustering. The child of a parent with schizophrenia has a 10-fold increase in empirical risk compared to the general population (for a review, see below). Amelio-specific(s) is a term used to describe the risk of a disease in a certain type of relative compared to the general population.

Genetic changes

NRG1

Although there exists considerable evidence that NRG1 genetic variation increases the risk of schizophrenia, specific susceptibility and protection variations have yet to be discovered. One study found considerable evidence of a link between the core Icelandic risk haplotype and bipolar illness vulnerability, with an effect size equivalent to that seen in schizophrenia.[2]

TABLE 10.1 Indicating diseases with symptoms.

S. No	DISEASE	DESCRIPTION	SYMPTOMS
1.	*Schizophrenia*	Severe disorder marked by a full loss of one's capacity to operate in daily life; it frequently necessitates hospitalization. Hallucinations and delusions are common in people with schizophrenia, and they have a hard time controlling their emotions and behavior.	*Positive symptoms*: (Hearing voices or seeing things that do not exist, paranoia, and exaggerated or distorted perceptions, beliefs, and behaviors are all symptoms of schizophrenia. Negative symptoms include a loss or reduction in one's capacity to plan ahead, speak, convey emotion, or find pleasure, those who are unusually present) *Disorganized symptoms*: Confused and disordered thinking and speech, trouble with logical thinking and sometimes bizarre behavior or abnormal movements.
2.	*Bipolar disorder*	Bipolar disorder, formerly known as manic depression, is a mental health illness that involves emotional highs (mania or hypomania) and lows (depression).	*Bipolar I disorder*. At least one manic episode has occurred, maybe preceded or followed by hypomanic or significant depressive episodes. Mania can sometimes lead to a disconnection from reality (psychosis). *Bipolar II disorder*. One has experienced at least one severe depressive episode and at least one hypomanic episode but no manic episode. *Cyclothymic disorder*. One has had frequent times of hypomania symptoms and periods of depressive symptoms for at least two years – or one year in children and teenagers (though less severe than major depression). Other types: Bipolar and associated illnesses, for example, might be caused by particular drugs or alcohol, or by a medical condition such as Cushing's syndrome, multiple sclerosis, or stroke.

3.	*Anorexia nervosa*	Anorexia nervosa is an eating disorder characterized by an abnormally low body weight, an intense fear of gaining weight, and a distorted perception of weight. People with anorexia place a high value on controlling their weight and shape, using extreme efforts that tend to significantly interfere with their lives.	*Physical symptoms*
			Extreme weight loss or not making expected developmental weight gains, Thin appearance, abnormal blood counts, fatigue, insomnia, dizziness or fainting, bluish discoloration of the fingers, hair that thins, breaks or falls out, Soft, downy hair covering the body, Absence of menstruation, Constipation and abdominal pain, dry or yellowish skin, intolerance of cold, irregular heart rhythms, low blood pressure, dehydration, swelling of arms or legs, eroded teeth and calluses on the knuckles from induced vomiting
4.	*Obsessive–compulsive disorder (OCD)*	OCD features a pattern of unwanted thoughts and fears (obsessions) that lead you to do repetitive behaviors (compulsions). These obsessions and compulsions interfere with daily activities and cause significant distress.	*Obsession symptoms*
			OCD obsessions are repeated, persistent, and unwanted thoughts, urges or images that are intrusive and cause distress or anxiety. One might try to ignore them or get rid of them by performing a compulsive behavior or ritual. These obsessions typically intrude when one is trying to think of or do other things. Obsessions often have themes to them, such as: fear of contamination or dirt, doubting and having difficulty tolerating uncertainty, needing things orderly and symmetrical, aggressive or horrific thoughts about losing control and harming oneself or others, unwanted thoughts, including aggression, or sexual or religious subjects *Compulsion symptoms* Washing and cleaning, checking, counting
			orderliness, following a strict routine, demanding reassurance.

(*Continued*)

TABLE 10.1 (Continued)

S. No	DISEASE	DESCRIPTION	SYMPTOMS
5.	*Autism*	Autism spectrum disorder is a condition related to brain development that impacts how a person perceives and socializes with others, causing problems in social interaction and communication. The disorder also includes limited and repetitive patterns of behavior. The term "spectrum" in autism spectrum disorder refers to the wide range of symptoms and severity.	Fails to respond to his or her name or appears not to hear you at times. Resists cuddling and holding, and seems to prefer playing alone, retreating into his or her own world. Has poor eye contact and lacks facial expression. Does not speak or has delayed speech, or loses previous ability to say words or sentences. Cannot start a conversation or keep one going, or only starts one to make requests or label items. Speaks with an abnormal tone or rhythm and may use a singsong voice or robot-like speech. Repeats words or phrases verbatim but does not understand how to use them. Does not appear to understand simple questions or directions. Does not express emotions or feelings and appears unaware of others' feelings. Does not point at or bring objects to share interest. Inappropriately approaches a social interaction by being passive, aggressive or disruptive. Has difficulty recognizing nonverbal cues, such as interpreting other people's facial expressions, body postures or tone of voice.
6.	*Tourette syndrome*	Tourette syndrome is a disorder that involves repetitive movements or unwanted sounds (tics) that cannot be easily controlled. For instance, one might repeatedly blink their eyes, shrug their shoulders, or blurt out unusual sounds or offensive words.	Tics are classified as: *Simple tics.* These sudden, brief and repetitive tics involve a limited number of muscle groups. *Complex tics.* These distinct, coordinated patterns of movements involve several muscle groups.

Dysbindin (DTNBP1)

Straub et al. were the first to disclose evidence linking dysbindin to schizophrenia. In a subset of bipolar patients having primarily psychotic episodes of mood disorder, there is marginally significant evidence for an association. Although replication is essential, the actual susceptibility variations have yet to be found.

G72(DAOA)/G30

The best-supported locus for bipolar disorder is the DAOA locus on chromosome 13q22–34. Chumakov and colleagues were the first to link this locus to schizophrenia research. There has yet to be identified a pathologically significant variation, and the biological mechanism is yet unknown.

Disrupted in schizophrenia 1 (DISC1)

A balanced chromosomal translocation (1;11)(q42;q14.3) showed high evidence for relation to schizophrenia, bipolar illness, and recurrent depression, according to studies of an extensive pedigree. Two genes on chromosome 1 were revealed to be disrupted by the translocation: DISC1 and DISC2.

COMT

COMT is found in the 22q11 region of the chromosome, which has been linked to schizophrenia, bipolar disorder, and schizoaffective disorder bipolar type. Because of its importance in dopamine catabolism, it has been extensively researched. In schizophrenia, the results have been inconsistent, with recent meta-analyses reporting no general evidence of a link between the valine allele and the disorder.

Brain-derived neurotrophic factor

The brain-derived neurotrophic factor (BDNF) gene is found on chromosome 11p13 and encodes a precursor peptide (proBDNF) that is proteolytically broken to produce the mature protein. At codon 66, a single-nucleotide polymorphism (SNP) causes valine to be replaced by methionine (Val66Met). To confirm (or dispute) the significance of BDNF in determining susceptibility to mood and mental disease, more genetic and biological research is needed. A systematic examination of variance across the entire gene, as well as research in additional independent samples, is necessary.

Meta-analysis of genome-wide association study data and the major histocompatibility complex Locus

A combined examination of schizophrenia genome-wide association study (GWAS) data revealed evidence of the involvement of major histocompatibility complex (MHC) in schizophrenia. The MHC region on chromosome 6 produced a genome-wide significant association as a result of this study. Near a cluster of histone genes and many immune-related genes, the best evidence for connection (rs13194053, p = 9.54109) was found. Although many of them may indicate a genic area signal due to LD, 50% of the top 1000 highest scoring GWAS SNPs were intergenic, positioned outside the 10-kb region on each side of a gene. The causal variation's position is unknown; however, it could be in one or more genes or a nongenic area of the MHC. Many of these areas feature highly conserved sequences that are thought to play a regulatory role.

Significance of non-MHC loci

In a combined examination of schizophrenia GWAS samples, researchers discovered relationships with neurogranin (NRGN) and transcription factor 4 (TCF4) that were later found to be genome-wide significant. N-methyl-d-aspartate (NMDA) receptor signaling is critical for learning and memory, and NRGN encodes a postsynaptic protein kinase substrate that binds calmodulin. Pitt–Hopkins syndrome is a neurodevelopmental condition marked by delayed language development, microcephaly, epilepsy, and facial dysmorphisms caused by TCF4 mutations.

Conclusion

There are genetic loci that contribute to schizophrenia, bipolar disorder, and schizoaffective disorders susceptibility across the Kraepelinian split. DISC1/2 and NRG1 mutations tend to predispose to both prototypical and prototypical psychiatric diseases. The hormones DAOA/G30 and BDNF appear to be the most strongly linked to mood disorders (Tables 10.2 and 10.3).

Environmental factors

Pollution

Introduction

Pollutants are dangerous chemicals in form of solids, liquids, or gases that are created in larger concentrations than usual, lowering environmental quality. Human actions pollute the water, air, and soil in which they grow plants, which has a negative impact on the ecosystem. The industrial revolution was a big success in terms of society, technology, and the supply of a wide range of services, but it also released massive amounts of pollutants, which is harmful to human health. Environmental pollution is regarded as a global public health concern because of a number of factors. This issue is also linked to legislative, social, and economic considerations. In this era, globalization and urbanization have reached unsettling proportions.

TABLE 10.2 Gene involvement in different psychiatric disorders.

Chromosomal location	Evidence in schizophrenia	Evidence in cases with mixed bipolar-psychosis features	Evidence in bipolar disorder
6p22		++++ +	+
8p12	++++	+	+
1q42	++ +	++	+
22q11	+		+
13q33	++		++
11p13	+		++

TABLE 10.3 Gene involvement in the psychic disorders.

Psychic disorder	Gene involved
In bipolar disorder	Ank3 and cacna1c, a relatively specific association between common variation in GABA-A receptor genes.
In schizophrenia	F804a, a relatively specific association between common variation in GABAA receptor genes.
Velocardiofacial disorder (VCFS)	Emerging from cancellation on chromosome 22q119,10.
Prader–Willi condition	Emerging from maternal uniparental disomy on chromosome 15q11–q13.11.
Alzheimer's disease	AD + Preplication (e.g., APOE)
Pitt–Hopkins syndrome	Mutations in TCF4
Autism	Contactin-associated protein-2 (CNTNAP2)

Toxicology of pollution

Pollution's effects on living things is not confined to human and animal health but also has a negative impact on the entire environment. The health of living beings and the environment, especially animal life, is affected by global climate change, varied geographical conditions, and environmental variation.

Environmental damages

Pollution has the potential to harm the environment by contaminating the land, water, and air. It also poses a serious threat to life's diversity. The link between reduced species diversity and air pollution demonstrates how environmental contaminants have a negative impact on the extinction of plant and animal species. Animals' reproductive consequences are caused by toxicants. Temperature fluctuations, acid rain, and global climate changes caused by greenhouse gas emissions have significant ecological consequences.

The link between pollution exposure and the nervous system has long been debated. These hazardous compounds, on the other hand, are thought to have negative effects on the nervous system. Psychiatric illnesses and neurological difficulties are among the harmful effects of pollution on the nervous system. Neurological disability causes disastrous repercussions, especially in children, whereas psychiatric issues promote antisocial behaviors and violence. Pollution has been linked to neurological hyperactivity, age-inappropriate behaviors, and criminal activities in recent studies.

Pathophysiology of psychotic disease

Psychotropic or psychopharmacological agents are medications that have a primary effect on the central nervous system (CNS) and are commonly used to treat a variety of mental disorders. Psychiatric treatment has seen significant modifications in recent years as a result of the development of new medications that may have negative effects on mental health. The focus has shifted to reuniting the individual patient with his or her community. Before 1952, the only thing that could be done was to deal with and calm down the hostile, agitated, and violent patients. The discovery of chlorpromazine (CPZ) in that year changed the lives of schizophrenic patients, allowing the majority of them to return to a productive life. Reserpine was found not long after. Despite being a very potent pharmacological tool for studying monoaminergic systems in the brain and peripheral system, reserpine has only been used in clinical trials for a few years. In 1957–58, antidepressants with tricyclic and monoamine oxidase inhibitors were introduced. In the 1980s, many novel antidepressants including atypical selective serotonin reuptake inhibitors (SSRIs) were developed. The discovery of meprobamate (1954) raised hopes that anxiety could be treated without sedation. Buspirone is a crucial component of the later inclusion. Furthermore, Cade's 1949 report, which revealed that lithium might be utilized for mania and excitation and was largely employed in psychiatry, received little attention. In bipolar disorders and mania, antiepileptics such as valproate, carbamazepine, and lamotrigine, as well as some atypical antipsychotics, have showed promise.

Psychoses

Hallucinations and delusions are serious psychiatric disorders that cause fatal distortions in thought, capacity to perceive, behavior, reality, and perceptions. There is an irrational belief that the patient is incapable of coping with everyday tasks.

1. Cognitive disorders

   Cognitive disorders include organic brain syndromes, both acute and chronic. Some of the toxic or pathogenic foundation can often be defined in conditions like dementia and delirium with psychotic characteristics. Disorientation, disorganized mind, faulty memory, and behavior are the most common symptoms.
2. Functional disorders

There is no underlying cause of the condition in functional disorders. The majority of one's orientation and memory remain kept, but one's behavior, emotion, thought, and reasoning are transformed.

Schizophrenia—split mind

There is a splitting of vision, thoughts, and interpretation from reality in schizophrenia (divided mind), such as inability to think rationally, hallucination, false beliefs, fixed delusions, paranoid states, and loss of understanding into the abnormality are all examples of false beliefs. Mood (affective) disorders: The first symptom is a mood swing, which might take the form of mania. Irritable mood, hyperactivity, unrestrained thought, and poor sleep and speech are all symptoms of mania, which can be accompanied by reckless or violent behavior. Depression manifests itself as a loss of interest and pleasure, a lack of sleep, and self-destructive thoughts. Remorse, melancholy, and physical and mental slowness are all symptoms of worthlessness. Bipolar disorder, which involves numerous depressed and mania stages, is a frequent type of mood disease.

In neuroses, the ability to comprehend the reality is not lost, although the patient may be undergoing severe suffering. Depending on the dominant symptoms, it may manifest as:

In neuroses ability to comprehend the reality is not lost, although the patient may undergo severe suffering. Depending on the dominant symptoms, it may manifest as:

- Anxiety: An unfavorable emotional state that is commonly associated with fear uneasiness, tension and worry of the future.
- Phobic states: Fear without any logical cause or some particular person, object or situations.
- Obsessive compulsive disorder (OCD): A very limited abnormality of behavior and thought recurrent intrusive thoughts that the patient may realize as abnormal or stupid but is unable to overcome
- Depression: It may be caused by physical illness, blow to self-esteem, loss or bereavement, but is extreme.

- Posttraumatic stress disorders: They have various symptoms following disturbing experiences like riots, earthquakes, war, etc.
- Hysterical dramatic symptoms: They resemble serious physical illness but situational patient does not feign but undergoes the symptoms, though the basis is only psychic and not physical (Table 10.4)

Chlorpromazine

Chlorpromazine is an individual from the category antipsychotic or neuroleptic drug class, which are also known as first-generation antipsychotics (FGAs). It delivers its antipsychotic activity by blocking postsynaptic activity at D2 receptors in the mesolimbic pathway. Chlorpromazine is used for the treatment of schizophrenia, manic-depressive illness, controls nausea and vomiting, for chronic hiccups, for relieving anxiety before surgery (Figs. 10.2 and 10.3).

Trifluoperazine

Trifluoperazine is also an antipsychotic medication. It is the only medicine that can be purchased as a generic. This medication is prescribed for the treatment of mental illnesses such as schizophrenia and psychotic disorders. Trifluoperazine improves one's ability to think clearly, lowers anxiety, and keeps them active and cheerful. It has the potential to lessen aggressive behavior. It is also used to treat hallucinations. It helps the brain to rebalance various natural molecules. This medication has also been used to relieve anxiety in the short term. It is not, however, the first line of treatment for anxiety.

Fluphenazine

Fluphenazine is a common antipsychotic used to treat the symptoms of psychosis in schizophrenia patients. This medication is used to treat the symptoms of various mental illnesses such as schizophrenia. It has an impact on the brain's natural chemical equilibrium (neurotransmitters). Reduced instances of hallucinations, delusions, or unusual behaviors in people with schizophrenia are among the diseases it helps.

Pimozide

Pimozide is a diphenylbutylpiperidine-based antipsychotic medication with a high potency. It operates by inhibiting D1–D2 receptors and calcium channels selectively. Pimozide is a type of antipsychotic drug known as a conventional antipsychotic. It works by reducing excessive brain excitation. Pimozide is used to treat Tourette syndrome, which is characterized by motor or verbal tics (an uncontrollable compulsion to repeat certain motions or

TABLE 10.4 Aliphatic antipsychotics.

S. N	Drugs	Molecular formulae	Structural formulae	Application of drugs
01	Chlorpromazine	$C_{17}H_{19}ClN_2S$	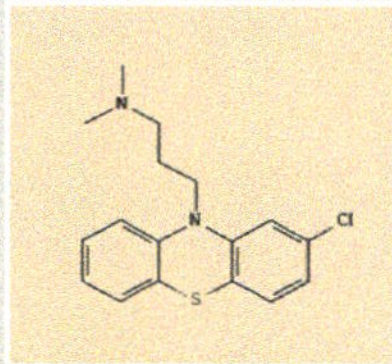	Schizophrenia Psychotic disorders Manic phase of bipolar disorder Severe behavioral problems in children
02	Trifluoperazine	$C_{21}H_{24}F_3N_3S$	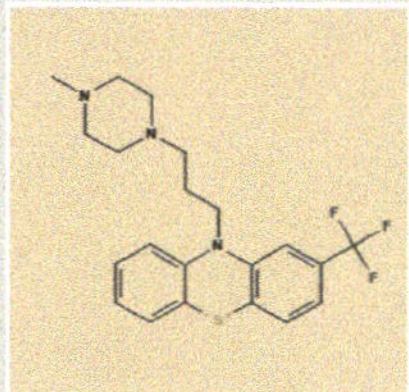	Neuroleptic malignant syndrome (NMS) Dementia Tardive dyskinesia Infections
03	Fluphenazine	$C_{22}H_{28}Cl_2F_3N_3OS$	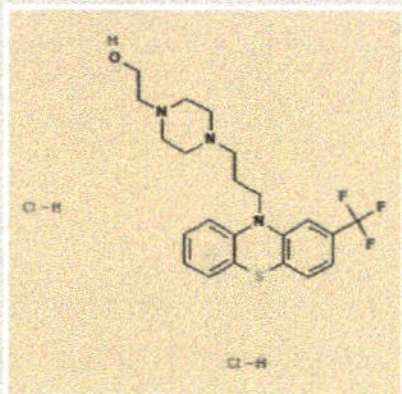	Psychotic disorders

(*Continued*)

TABLE 10.4 (Continued)

S. N	Drugs	Molecular formulae	Structural formulae	Application of drugs
04	Pimozide	$C_{28}H_{29}F_2N_3O$	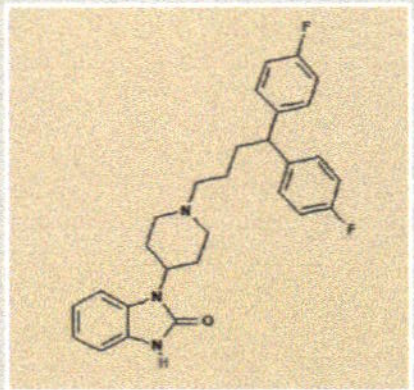	Control motor or verbal tics caused by Tourette syndrome Disbelieves.
05	Mesoridazine	$C_{21}H_{26}N_2OS_2$	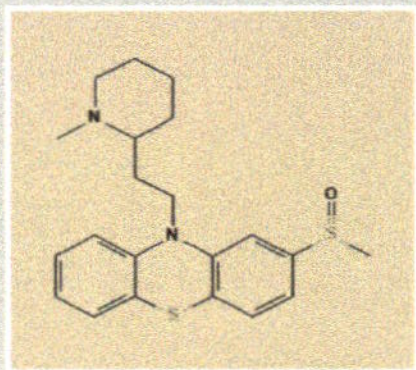	Schizophrenia Reduce restlessness, anxiety, and tension. It can also reduce hyperactivity and uncooperativeness.
06	Haloperidol	$C_{21}H_{23}ClFNO_2$	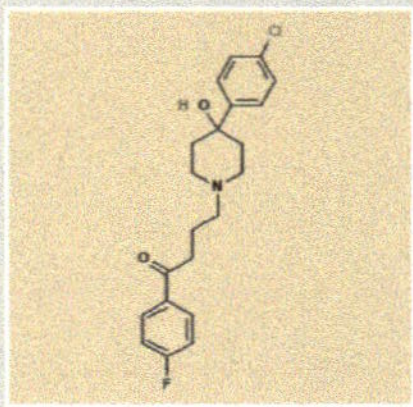	Symptoms of schizophrenia, such as hallucinations and delusions.

07	Droperidol	$C_{22}H_{22}FN_3O_2$	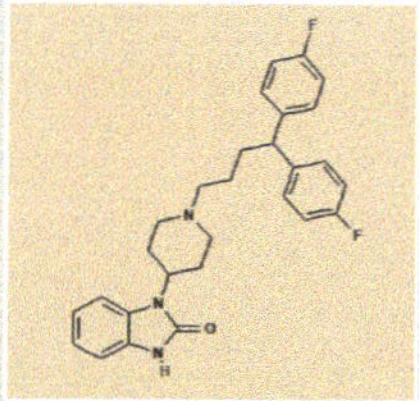	Reduce nausea and vomiting caused by surgery or other medical procedures.
08	Penfluridol	$C_{28}H_{27}ClF_5NO$	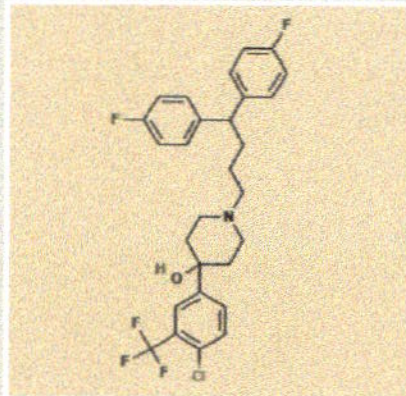	Chronic schizophrenia Similar psychotic disorders.
09	Benperidol	$C_{22}H_{24}FN_3O_2$	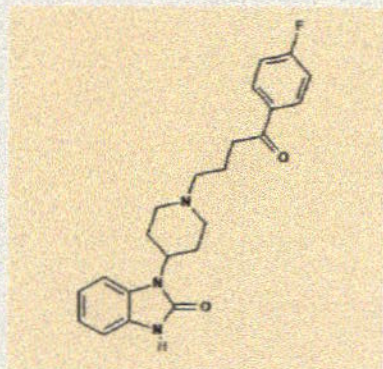	Psychoses Manic episodes Psychomotor agitation.
10	Benzhexol	$C_{20}H_{31}NO$	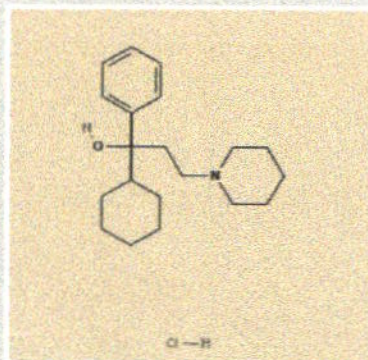	Parkinson's disease Depression To control extrapyramidal symptoms (tremor, slurred speech) caused by certain medications.

(*Continued*)

TABLE 10.4 (Continued)

S. N	Drugs	Molecular formulae	Structural formulae	Application of drugs
11	Thioridazine	$C_{21}H_{27}N_2S_2Cl$	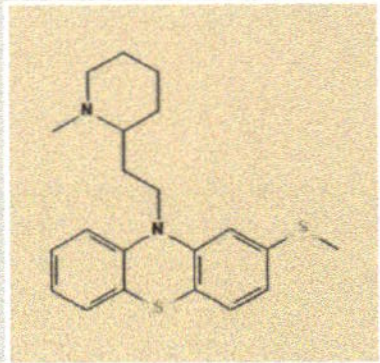	Schizophrenia, control of severely disturbed or agitated behavior. It has little antiemetic activity.
12	Triflupromazine	$C_{18}H_{19}F_3N_2S$	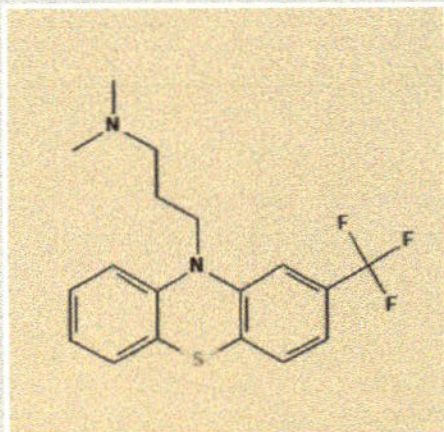	Antiemetic Psychotic disorders

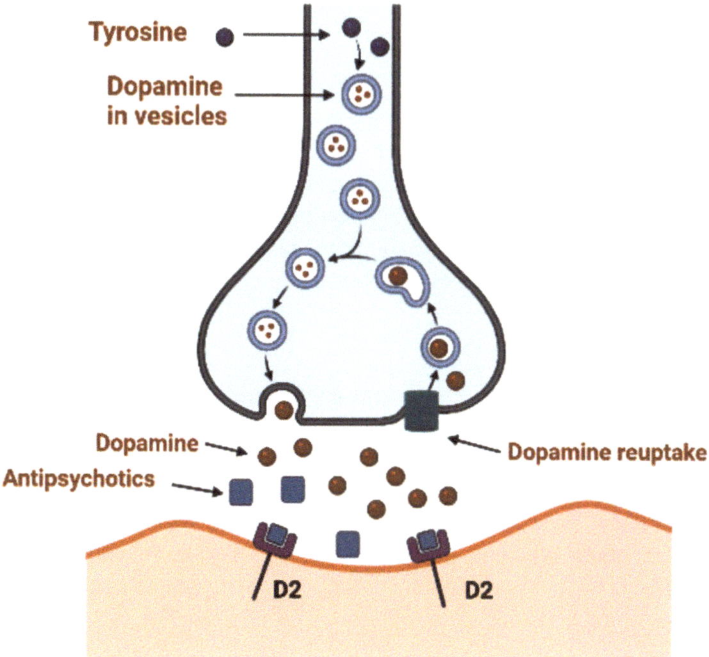

FIGURE 10.2 Diagram showing dopamine (DA) blockade by aliphatic compounds at postsynaptic level of neurons.

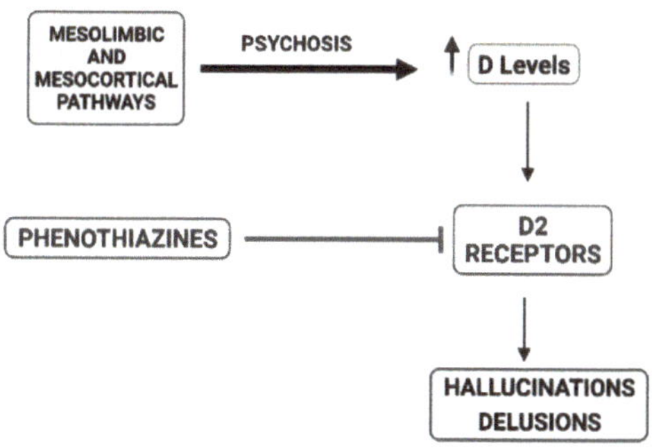

FIGURE 10.3 Effect of phenothiazines on the dopamine (DA) levels.

sounds). Pimozide is only prescribed to those who are unable to take other medications or who have failed to respond to previous medications.

Mesoridazine

Mesoridazine is a phenothiazine with an extremely short half-life that belongs to the phenothiazine class. It has the potential to be used as a hypnotic. It is a medication that is used to treat illnesses such as schizophrenia, as well as restlessness, anxiety, and tension. It can also help with hyperactivity and a lack of cooperation.

Haloperidol

Haloperidol is an FGA medication that is widely prescribed around the world. It is used to treat hallucinations and delusions associated with schizophrenia. Tourette syndrome, severe behavioral issues in children, hyperactivity, acute mania, chemotherapy-induced nausea and vomiting, agitation linked with psychiatric diseases, and obstinate hiccups are all treated with it.

Droperidol

Droperidol, like haloperidol, is a short-acting medication that belongs to the butyrophenone family. It acts as a 2-adrenoceptor agonist, 5HT3 serotonin antagonist, and H1 histamine antagonist in addition to being a strong dopamine D2 antagonist. Droperidol is an anti-nausea, sedative, and tranquilizer. It is also used to treat problems such as nausea and vomiting brought on by surgery or other medical procedures. It is also an excellent migraine treatment.

Penfluridole

Penfluridole is an FGA medication that belongs to the diphenylbutylpiperidine family. Its effects continue for many days after a single oral dose, and it can be given once a week for improved symptom management and compliance. It is a long-acting antipsychotic medication that is used to treat schizophrenia and other psychotic illnesses.

Benperidol

Benperidol is a neuroleptic butyrophenone derivative that is used to treat psychosis, manic episodes, and psychomotor agitation. It is an antipsychotic medication that can be used to treat schizophrenia. However, it is primarily used to treat hypersexuality disorders, and it is occasionally administered to sex offenders as a condition of parole as an alternative to anti-androgen medications like cyproterone acetate.

Benzhexol

It is an antimuscarinic drug that has a direct parasympathetic nerve system inhibitory action. In mono and combination therapy, it is used to treat the symptoms of Parkinson's disease. postencephalitic, arteriosclerotic, and idiopathic types are all active. The medication is also often used to alleviate adverse effects associated with antipsychotic therapy. It may help with psychotic sadness and mental lethargy, which are common symptoms of

Parkinson's disease, as well as symptomatic issues induced by antipsychotic medication (Table 10.5).

Mechanism of action of antipsychotics

Lithium

Lithium has a variety of pharmacological effects, biological pathways, and cell measurements. This creates an unusual situation in which a drug with such complicated effects has the explicit clinical effects in all of psychiatry. Lithium's effects are difficult to categorize in a linear, progressive fashion; it appears to balance complex administrative organizations through several critical hubs. Individual (and frequently deeply linked) consequences are occasionally overlooked when our profession moves on to more current hypotheses while rejecting previous ones. For those who are interested, point-by-point surveys are available, with the most recent ones focusing heavily on neuroprotective equipment. Nonetheless, the historical background of lithium pharmacology is dense with recent facts – views formed at various times and never compared to more recent findings. As a result, how may clinical views inform the search for better medications, such as those that provide the core benefits of lithium without the side effects? Investigations of lithium activity are also linked to those of Behcet's disease (BD) pathophysiology; frequently, fresh alterations were studied in terms of lithium's influence, and alternatively, lithium-interceded impacts were considered as a possible cause for BD neurobiology. However, this method, which is common in most psychopharmacological research, is not without flaws.

Mechanisms of action of lithium

- The response to preventive therapy runs in families
- Most patients require plasma levels between 0.6 and 1.0 mmol/L for a full clinical impact
- Lithium is beneficial for preventing recurrences of BD and lowering risk of suicide.
- Lithium is most effective in people with classic (typical) BD symptoms.
- It has been shown to be neuroprotective in vitro and in vivo.

Assume

- Lithium's effects may be independent of one another.
- Early in the course of the disease, lithium may function better; rapid cessation of lithium may raise the chance of recurrence.
- Lithium responders differ from those who react to other stabilizers.

TABLE 10.5 Nonaliphatic antipsychotics.

	Drugs	Molecular formulae	Structural formulae	Application of drugs
12	Clozapine	$C_{18}H_{19}ClN_4$	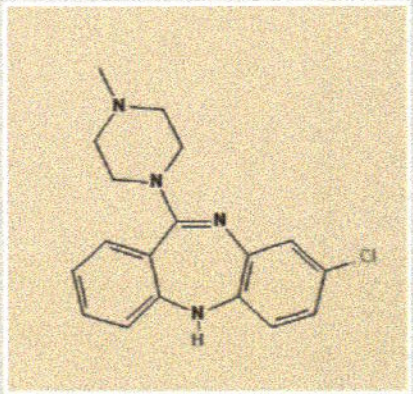	Schizophrenia, schizoaffective disorders.
13	Loxapine	$C_{22}H_{24}ClN_3O_5$	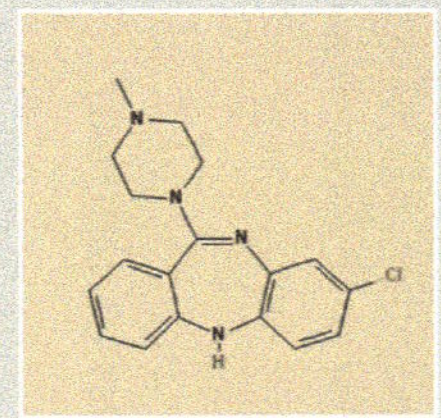	Psychosis Helps to decrease hallucinations.
14	Quetiapine	$C_{21}H_{25}N_3O_2S$	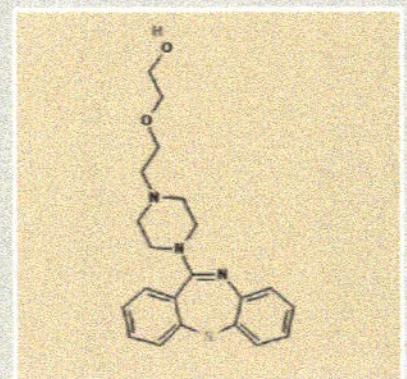	Bipolar disorder Sudden episodes of mania or depression associated with bipolar disorder.

15	Risperidone	$C_{23}H_{27}FN_4O_2$	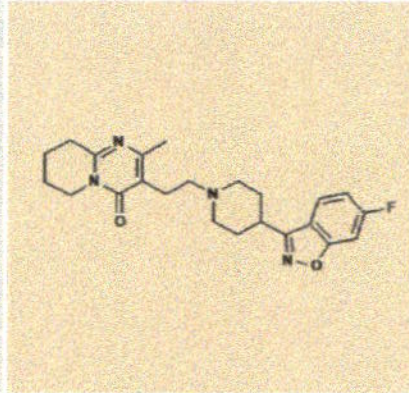	Schizophrenia bipolar disorder Irritability associated with autistic disorder.
16	Olanzapine	$C_{17}H_{20}N_4S$	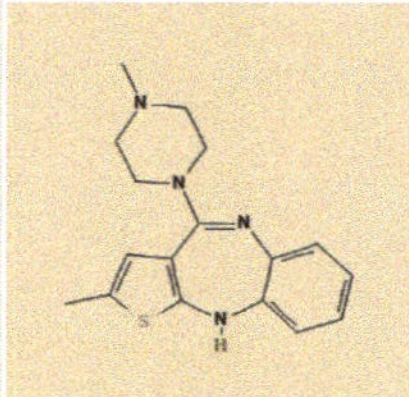	Schizophrenia Bipolar disorder
17	Aripiprazole	$C_{23}H_{27}Cl_2N_3O_2$	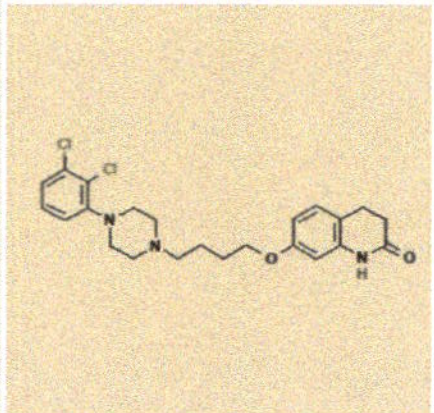	Bipolar I disorder (manic depression) Major depressive disorder.
18	Zotepine	$C_{18}H_{18}ClNOS$	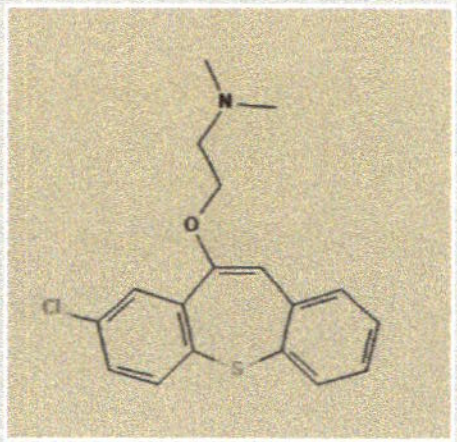	Schizophrenia in adults. This medicine is not recommended for use in children and adolescents below 18 years of age.

(*Continued*)

TABLE 10.5 (Continued)

	Drugs	Molecular formulae	Structural formulae	Application of drugs
19	Paliperidone	$C_{23}H_{27}FN_4O_3$	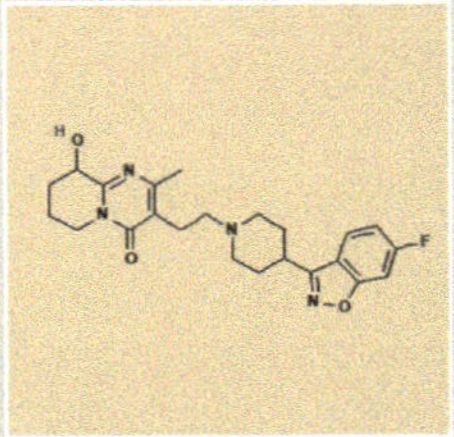	Schizophrenia Schizoaffective disorder.

Unclear

- Do all patients have the same mechanism of action?
- Does the neuroprotective have a role in mood regulation?
- Is there a difference between partial responders and "great" responders?

A perfect opportunity to react is another essential element. The general consensus is that dreariness on lithium may in any event be elevated in individuals who react fully in the long run during the first year of therapy. This distinction might cause heterogeneity in components of activity in quick and slow responders, yet it could likewise reflect mental elements, consistence issues, time expected to accomplish viable yet okay blood levels, communication with the normal flow of the sickness, and different variables. Furthermore, the opportunity to reaction contrasts broadly between hostile to hyper or energizer increasing impacts on the one hand, and disposition balancing out or against self-destructive consequences on the other. Some of the impacts depicted in this text trail intense organization, while others grow just during ongoing therapy (cf. inverse impacts of present moment and long-haul medicines on glutamate flagging or adenylate cyclase).

Because lithium has so many pharmacologic effects, determining which ones are responsible for its mind-set balancing characteristics is challenging. This would not be surprising if separate components played role in a variety of discrete clinical effects or even comparative different patients. Many effects are circular, as seen below, although it is not difficult to decipher what may be puzzling administrative organizations with multiple critique rings, in which activity at various hubs might have similar consequences.

Electrolytes, membrane transport, membrane potential

Dynamic investigation of electrolyte balance in BD and intermittent wretchedness became probably the most punctual theories of the component of lithium activity. Studies of BD revealed increased lingering sodium amid scenes of sadness and lunacy, as well as its consistency across the course of lithium therapy. Later investigations also discovered increased intracellular NA (sodium) levels. Furthermore, it was shown that lithium is not evenly distributed throughout the brain, raising questions about the validity of the lithium percentage, particularly when measured in fringe cells. Lithium transfer is important in each scenario, depending on the system. A few cycles maintain the balance of intra- and extra-cell lithium focuses. Bicarbonate-sensitive vehicle also plays an important role in other types of cells, such as erythrocytes. During lithium therapy, the Lithium + sodium + counter vehicle is suppressed. Despite the fact that the ouabain-sensitive Na + −K + siphon does not reflect lithium transport under physiological in vivo settings, it is critical for the electrochemical Na + inclination, and the Na + −K + ATPase is a major source of energy for maintaining the resting layer potential. As a result, the energy required to keep up with the siphon action originates from glycolysis, although mitochondrial adenosine triphosphate plays a considerably larger role. Mitochondrial function in BD has received piqued attention, with evidence of severe impairment. The role of sodium K + ATPase in signal transduction, cAMP response element-binding protein (CREB) movement adjustment, apoptotic cycles, and calcium homeostasis regulation has recently been highlighted. It appears as one of a few important cross streets in cell motioning in edgy tissues in this fashion. One of the pathophysiological systems of BD has been proposed as its brokenness (reduced movement). Research indicating that lithium activates the Na + −K + ATPase are consistent with this; however, not all studies agree. Lithium appears to reduce intracellular sodium (and calcium) via voltage-gated sodium channels (VGSC), notably in hyperactive neurons.

Monoaminergic signaling

Lithium has a strong influence on a number of neurotransmitters. It has been shown in animal studies to increase serotonin transmission through a variety of mechanisms, including increased serotonin synthesis, increased tryptophan uptake, increased serotonin release, activation of postsynaptic 5HT1A receptors, and downregulation of 5HT2 receptors. Lithium's anti-suicidal and anti-aggressive properties, as well as its antidepressant enhancement, have been attributed to its serotonergic effects. However, two-week research on healthy volunteers revealed modest alterations in noradrenergic signaling, consistent with enhanced norepinephrine release, but no evidence of a significant effect on serotonergic function. Lithium does not appear to decrease baseline dopaminergic tone, but it does impede enhanced dopaminergic activity, perhaps through its impact on arrestin complexes. This has been suggested as a possible contributor to antimanic and antipsychotic effects, but the latter is debatable.

Second messenger system

Lithium has well-known influence on many intracellular signaling cascade components. G proteins and PKA signaling pathway were studied in the beginning, as well as the influence of lithium ion adenylate cyclase (AC). G proteins, which are generically classified as stimulatory (Gs) or inhibitory (I), regulate AC (Gi). The effects of lithium on AC/PKA signaling changes in BD have been studied. Young et al. were the first to notice an increase in the Gs subunit in bipolar patients' postmortem brains, as well as an increase in the second messenger cAMP, after forskolin stimulation. Lithium has been shown to inhibit both Gi and Gs, lowering the signaling amplitude. The arrestin complex stops the activation of G protein-coupled receptor signaling by uncoupling G proteins from receptors. AC produces cAMP, which activates PKA, causing a number of cellular processes to be regulated, including transcription factors like CREB. With little or no influence on baseline activity, lithium inhibits AC and PKA, especially their calmodulin and forskolin induced activities. Acute effects may be mediated (and reversed) by Mg^{2+} competition, but chronic effects are not. The activation of phospholipase B by G proteins – or phospholipase C by tyrosine kinase receptors (try) receptors – and subsequent hydrolysis of phosphatidylinositol 5-bisphosphate begins the phosphoinositide (PI) cycle, which is another key signal transduction cascade. Lithium inhibits inositol monophosphates (IMPase) and inositol polyphosphate-1-phosphatase (IPPase), lowering accessible inositol and the cycle's downstream targets, inositol trisphosphate (IP3), which reduces calcium release, diacylglycerol activation, and protein kinase C activity. Alterations in PI signaling in BD have been described in tandem with lithium effects, and the inositol transporter has been discovered to be overexpressed in BD and downregulated by lithium. Lithium therapy decreases myo-inositol in magnetic resonance spectroscopy, according to in vivo investigations. To date, the inositol depletion theory remains one of the most viable lithium mechanisms of action possibilities. Lithium affects numerous structurally related enzymes, including glycogen synthase kinase and the -arrestin-2-Akt complex, in addition to inhibiting IMPase. Mg^{2+} is a co-factor in almost all of these enzymes. Lithium is also known to inhibit guanylate cyclase [and cyclic guanosine monophosphate (cGMP)] and reduce nitric oxide generation (NO). The action of lithium on the cGMP/NO pathway, like other regulatory systems, does not function in isolation, and it is likely to alter monoaminergic signaling, adding to its neuroprotective role. Lithium's effects were inconsistent in various trials (increase in NO and cGMP production under chronic treatment). However, if one considers that lithium reduces excessive route activity while increasing underactive signaling, the contradicting data may be reconciled.

Transcription factors

Activator protein 1 (a combination of transcription factors) and CREB are widely used to regulate transcription activity as a result of signal transduction effects. The gene expression of multiple pathways is altered as a result of their regulation. For example, CREB promotes the production of (BDNF) and anti-apoptotic b-cell lymphoma 2 (bcl-2) while suppressing the expression of tumor proteins p53 (p53) and bcl-2-associated X protein (BAX), both of which are pro-apoptotic. GSK3 and PKA/cAMP are two of the many elements that control CREB. Chronic lithium treatment causes a reduction in CREB-directed gene expression and phosphorylation of CREB. Stress has also been found to enhance CREB-mediated transcription, which is inhibited by lithium.

Regulation of intracellular calcium

Calcium has a variety of functions in neurons. It serves as a second messenger in cell bodies, triggering neurotransmitter release in presynaptic terminals, maintaining neuronal periodicity, and contributing to synaptogenesis, plasticity, and cell death. Calcium enters cells via numerous distinct pathways during membrane depolarization, including voltage-gated, ligand-gated, receptor-operated, and store-operated channels, from both external and intracellular (endoplasmic reticulum) locations. Lithium regulates them, for example, through NMDA receptors or IP3 downstream effects. Calcium anomalies in BD have been thoroughly documented, as they have the function of mood stabilizers in calcium homeostasis regulation.

Glycogen synthase kinase

GSK3 is a crucial enzyme that connects many signaling systems. Ionotropic glutamate signaling, numerous transcription factors, and the Wingless-related integration site catenin pathway are only a few of its downstream targets. Wnt signaling is involved in neural development, synapse formation, and neuronal plasticity, among other structural brain functions. The possibility of GSK3 and endothelin cross-regulation is little understood. One suggested method includes serum- and glucocorticoid-inducible-kinase-1 regulation (SGK1). SGK1 is thought to be involved in glucocorticoid-mediated neurogenesis inhibition, and new evidence suggests it may also play a role in depression and stress response. GSK3 activity is inhibited by protein kinase B (Akt), which is triggered by lithium; however, it is unclear whether lithium has a direct or indirect impact on GSK. Lithium, for example, has been hypothesized to inhibit GSK3 by competing with $Mg2+$, although this action would necessitate higher than therapeutic Li levels. As a result, an indirect inhibition through increasing phosphorylation of GSK3 N-terminal serine residues is more likely. GSK3 function is also linked to CREB activity, which GSK3 inhibits (and the inhibition is attenuated by lithium). Activation of Akt causes a decrease in apoptotic processes, which is mediated via -arrestin. Furthermore, dopamine and serotonin modulate the GSK3/Akt pathway, and part of these effects are presumably mediated via -arrestin complexes (Fig. 10.4).

Carbamazepine

Carbamazepine inhibits action potentials and reduces synaptic transmission via modulating VGSC. Carbamazepine is thought to bind to the alpha subunit of VGSC, specifically at a binding pocket created by the exterior pore loop and the pore-lining portion of the domain, similar to other anticonvulsant. Carbamazepine, according to the researchers, keeps sodium channels

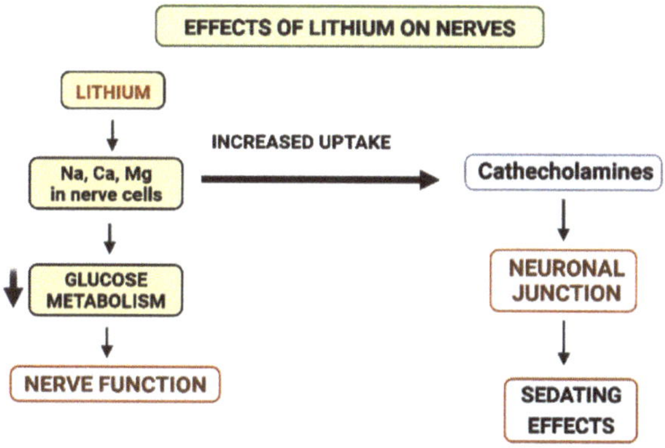

FIGURE 10.4 Effect of lithium on nerves.

inactive, causing fewer channels to open and therefore inhibiting the production of action potentials. Other voltage-gated ion channels, including as voltage-gated calcium channels, are similarly bound by carbamazepine.

Valproic acid

Valproic acid has pharmacologic effects through affecting GABA levels in the CNS, blocking voltage-gated ion channels, and inhibiting histone deacetylase, among other things. Because regulating this route is a potential target for antiepileptic medicines, impaired GABAergic inhibitory function is a well-established pathophysiology of seizure onset and propagation. Through the tricarboxylic acid cycle, GABA is produced from -ketoglutarate and converted into succinate semialdehyde and subsequently succinate by GABA transaminase and succinate semialdehyde dehydrogenase, respectively.

Valproic acid may also have antiepileptic effects by blocking voltage-gated sodium, potassium, and calcium channels, which reduces high-frequency firing of neurons. Valproic acid influences nociception and alters the physiological phenomena of aura by altering GABA and/or glutamate-mediated neurotransmission. Valproic acid has been shown to reduce neurogenic inflammation in neuropathic pain via GABA-A receptor inhibition. Valproic acid has recently been discovered to inhibit histone deacetylase (HDAC), notably HDAC1, as well as other HDAC. Inhibition of histone deacetylase may increase the expression of genes.

Mechanism

The specific processes by which valproate works to treat epilepsy, migraine headaches, and bipolar disorder are unknown, however there are numerous routes that might be involved. Valproate has been shown to block succinic semialdehyde dehydrogenase. This inhibition causes a rise in succinic semialdehyde, which serves as a GABA transaminase inhibitor, lowering GABA metabolism and boosting GABAergic neurotransmission. This increase in inhibitory activity is due to the fact that GABA is an inhibitory neurotransmitter. A possible secondary contributor to cortical inhibition is a direct suppression of voltage gated sodium channel activity and indirect suppression through effects on GABA.

Valproate may potentially have an effect on the extracellular signal-related kinase pathway (ERK). These effects appear to be mediated by the mitogen-activated protein kinase, which phosphorylates ERK1/2. This activation raises the expression of several downstream targets, including ELK-1, which increases c-fops, growth cone-associated protein-43, which contributes to neural plasticity, B-cell lymphoma/leukemia-2, an anti-apoptotic protein, and BDNF, which is also involved in neural plasticity and growth. The effects of valproate on neurogenesis and neurite development are linked to this route. An increase in GABAA receptors appears to be another downstream consequence of enhanced BDNF expression, which contributes to higher GABAergic activity. Valproate inhibits myo-inosital-1-phophate synthase in a non-competitive indirect manner. As a result, de novo production of inositol monophosphates is decreased, resulting in inositol depletion. It's unclear how this influenced valproate's impact on bipolar illness, but lithium is known to deplete inositol in a similar way. Valproate appears to cause downregulation of protein kinase C proteins (PKC)- and -, which might be linked to bipolar illness because PKC is uncontrolled in bipolar patients' frontal brain. This is backed up by a comparable decrease in PKC when lithium is used. Inhibition of the PKC pathway may potentially have a role in migraine prevention. Valproate also inhibits reisolated alanine-rich C kinase substrate, a PKC substrate, which may contribute to synaptic remodeling by affecting the cytoskeleton. Valproate appears to have an effect on fatty acid metabolism as well. Less fatty acid substrate incorporation in sterols and glycolipids is considered to affect membrane fluidity and result in a higher action potential threshold, perhaps contributing to valproate's antiepileptic effect. Valproate has been discovered to be a non-competitive direct inhibitor of long-chain fatty acyl-CoA synthetase in brain microsomes. The availability of arachidonoyl-CoA, a substrate for the synthesis of inflammatory prostaglandins, is reduced when this enzyme is inhibited. Because migraines are commonly treated with non-steroidal anti-inflammatory medications, which also suppress prostaglandin synthesis, this is considered to be a reason underlying valproate's effectiveness in migraine prophylaxis.

Finally, valproate inhibits HDAC directly. DNA relaxing was aided by hyper acetylation of lysine residues on histones, which allowed for more gene transcription. The genomic effects of valproate are extensive, with 461 genes up- or downregulated. Although the relationship between these genetic changes and therapeutic efficacy is not fully understood, H3 and H4 hyper acetylation has been linked to improved symptoms in bipolar patients. Histone hyper acetylation at the BDNF gene, which increases BDNF production and is considered to be a neuroprotective mechanism that valproate may augment or extend, is known to occur post-seizure. The decrease in glyceraldehyde-3-phosphate dehydrogenase, a pro-apoptotic enzyme, is linked to H3 hyper acetylation, adding to valproate's neuroprotective benefits.

Olanzapine

Olanzapine is a second-generation atypical antipsychotic that predominantly affects dopamine and serotonin receptors. It acts as an antagonist on dopamine D2 receptors in the mesolimbic pathway, preventing dopamine from acting at the postsynaptic receptor. It binds to the receptor loosely and dissociates quickly, enabling normal dopamine neurotransmission to occur. Positive symptoms in patients, such as hallucinations, delusions, and disordered speech, cognition, and behavior, are reduced as a result of the impact on D2 receptors. Olanzapine acts as an antagonist on serotonin 5HT2A receptors in the frontal brain. Negative symptoms such as anhedonia, flat affect, alogia, avolition, and poor attention are reduced by olanzapine's impact on serotonin.

Risperidone

D2 receptors are antagonized by all antipsychotics to some extent. At 60 to 80 percent D2 occupancy, FGAs exhibit antipsychotic effects. Second-generation antipsychotics (SGAs) like risperidone work by blocking certain D2 receptors but mostly serotonin receptors like 5HT2A. SGAs bind to D2 receptors loosely and quickly dissociate from them, which might explain why they are less likely to cause extrapyramidal symptoms. SGAs also cause agonism at the 5HT1A receptor. Risperidone is thought to work by inhibiting serotonin and norepinephrine reuptake, which might explain its antidepressant properties. The inhibition of D2 receptors, especially in the mesolimbic pathway, is considered to be responsible for the alleviation of positive symptoms. Antipsychotics' capacity to inhibit D2 receptors in the prefrontal cortex and nucleus accumbent is critical for alleviating some psychiatric symptoms. It's worth noting that risperidone has no anticholinergic effects, which may be beneficial to patients in some groups, such as the elderly with dementia.

Thioridazine

Thioridazine is a member of the phenothiazine medication class, which has been widely utilized for antipsychotic purposes because of the danger of extrapyramidal side effects. This medication is used to treat schizophrenia and other mental and emotional problems. This medicine allows you to think more clearly, feel less anxious, and participate more fully in daily activities. It can also aid in the prevention of suicide in individuals who are at risk of harming themselves, as well as the reduction of aggressiveness and the desire to harm others. It can assist one in reducing unpleasant thoughts and hallucinations.

Triflupromazine

Triflupromazine is a psychiatric medication that is used to treat psychomotor excitation in individuals with schizophrenia, paranoid and manic-depressive disorders, and neurosis. Vespine is the most frequent synonym.

Clozapine

Clozapine is atypical antipsychotic medication for the treatment of schizophrenia that is resistant to other treatments. Treatment-resistant schizophrenia is defined as persistent or moderate delusions or hallucinations after two antipsychotic drug treatments have failed. Even though it has a wide variety of adverse effects, it has been the medication of choice for treatment-resistant schizophrenia since its inception. Clozapine is not the medication of choice because of its wide range of side effects, which makes compliance difficult for many patients.

Loxapine

Loxapine is a tricyclic chemical that belongs to the dibenzoazepine medication family and is used to treat acute and chronic schizophrenia, a mental disorder characterized by abnormal or odd thinking and intense or inappropriate emotions. It belongs to a class of drugs known as conventional antipsychotics. It works by reducing excessive brain excitation.

Quetiapine

Quetiapine is a prescription-only medication. It is available as an oral tablet. Two variants of the tablet available. The immediate-release form is immediately absorbed into the circulation. The extended-release version enters your bloodstream gradually over time. The oral quetiapine is used to treat the symptoms of schizophrenia, bipolar disorder, and depression. Quetiapine is a medication that can be used to alleviate symptoms in individuals with depressive disorders. Quetiapine can be used to treat manic episodes induced by bipolar I disorder in children aged 10 to 17 years.

Risperidone

Risperidone is an antipsychotic medication that acts by inhibiting dopamine and serotonin activity in the brain. It binds to serotonergic 5-HT2 receptors with more affinity than dopamine D2 receptors. Risperidone is used for schizophrenia, bipolar I acute manic or mixed episodes as monotherapy, Bipolar I acute manic or mixed episodes in combination with lithium or valproate, and autism-associated irritability. When psychotic symptoms are present, it is also helpful in treating them. Tourette syndrome, trichotillomania, stuttering, movement problems, and developmental impairments are all examples of Lesch–Nyhan syndrome.

Olanzapine

Olanzapine is a thienobenzodiazepine antipsychotic that belongs to the thienobenzodiazepine family of drugs. It is used to treat Schizophrenia; however, the patient must be at least 13 years old. Olanzapine is a selective serotonin reuptake inhibitor (SSRI) that can be used in conjunction with fluoxetine to treat depression and bipolar disorder type 1 in patients. It can also be used to treat treatment-resistant depression.

Aripiprazole

Aripiprazole is a dopamine D2 receptor agonist with partial agonist action at serotonin 5HT1A receptors and a 5HT2A receptor antagonist. It is an antipsychotic medication of the second generation. It is a drug that is used to treat schizophrenia, bipolar I disorder mania, autistic spectrum disorder irritability, major depressive disorder disjunctive treatment, and Tourette syndrome.

Zotepine

It belongs to the family of antipsychotics known as atypical antipsychotics. It is used in individuals who are experiencing intolerable adverse effects from traditional antipsychotics or who have relapsed after being mismanaged.

Paliperidone

Paliperidone is an antipsychotic medication. It works by altering the activity of a variety of natural chemicals in the brain. It is a drug that is used to treat schizophrenia and schizo-affective disorder. It's also a mood stabilizer and antidepressant (Table 10.6).

Lithium carbonate

Lithium is a monovalent cation with a modest size. It was shown to act as a sedative for animals and to have beneficial effects on manic patients in 1949. The importance of maintaining a limited range of blood lithium concentration was understood in the 1960s and 1970s, and convincing confirmation of its medicinal effectiveness was obtained. At dosages that have no overt CNS effects, lithium is a one-of-a-kind medication that reduces mania and acts as a preventive in bipolar (manic depressive) illness. Lithium is well-known as an antimanic and mood-stabilizing medication.

TABLE 10.6 Antimanic drugs.

S. No.	Drugs	Molecular formula	Structural formula	Application of drugs
01	Lithium carbonate	Li_2CO_3	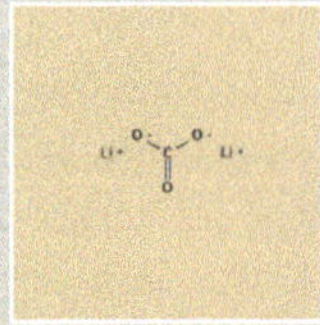	Standard antimanic Mood stabilizing drug.
02	Carbamazepine	$C_{15}H_{12}N_2O$	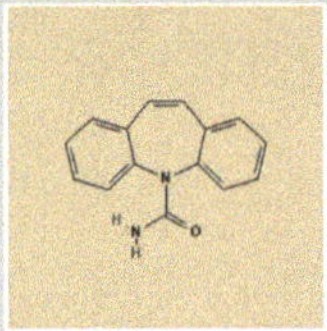	Antiepileptic Mania Bipolar disorders Epilepsy
03	Sodium valproate	$C_8H_{15}NaO_2$	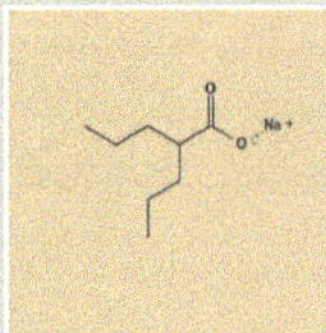	Bipolar disorders First line treatment of acute mania in which high dose valproate acts faster than lithium.
04	Lamotrigine	$C_9H_7Cl_2N_5$	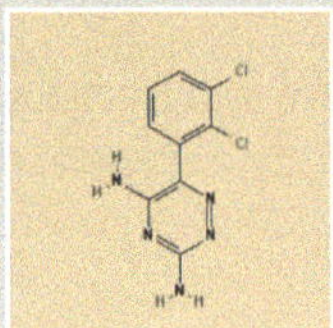	Anticonvulsant for prophylaxis of depression in bipolar disorder.

Carbamazepine

Carbamazepine was thought to extend remission in bipolar illness after its discovery as an antileptic. It has also been shown to help with mania and bipolar disorder. However, it is not as well-known as valproate as a lithium substitute. Carbamazepine is less effective than lithium or valproate in treating acute mania. Furthermore, acute mania necessitates a fast-acting medication, whereas therapeutic dosages of carbamazepine are long-acting and have a delayed beginning of action.

Sodium valproate

When valproate is used to treat bipolar disorder, it suppresses manic episodes. It is currently a preferred treatment for acute mania, as high-dose valproate acts quicker than lithium and is a viable alternative to antipsychotic and benzodiazepine medications. It may be beneficial for people who are allergic to lithium or who are unable to tolerate it. Valproate treatment is very helpful for individuals who have a fast-cycling pattern.

Lamotrigine

Lamotrigine is a newer anticonvulsant used to prevent depression in people with bipolar illness. It is ineffective in both the treatment and prevention of mania. It is currently widely used in the maintenance treatment of type II bipolar illness, as the risk of causing mania is low in this setting. To increase the effectiveness of lamotrigine, it can be taken with lithium. Lamotrigine has an excellent tolerability profile.

References

1. Howes OD, McCutcheon R, Owen MJ, Murray RM. The role of genes, stress, and dopamine in the development of schizophrenia. *Biol Psychiatry*. 2017;81(1):9–20.
2. Thomson PA, Christoforou A, Morris SW, et al. Association of Neuregulin 1 with schizophrenia and bipolar disorder in a second cohort from the Scottish population. *Mol Psychiatry*. 2007;12(1):94–104.

Chapter 11

Mechanism of action of antidepressants

Kuldeepak Sharma[1], Ankush Sundriyal[2], Aanchal Loshali[2], Mohit Agrawal[3], Chinnabonia Gopala Krishna[4] and Yogendra Singh[5]
[1]Institute of Pharmacology and Toxicology, Faculty of Medicine, University of Ljubljana, Slovenia, [2]Department of Pharmaceutical Sciences and Technology, Sardar Bhagwan Singh University, Dehradun, Uttarakhand, India, [3]School of Medical & Allied Sciences, K.R. Mangalam University, Gurgaon, Haryana, India, [4]A.M. Reddy Memorial College of Pharmacy, Narasaraopet, Andhra Pradesh, India, [5]Department of Pharmacology, Maharishi Arvind College of Pharmacy, Jaipur, Rajasthan, India

Introduction

Major depressive disorder (MDD) is more prevalent in individuals that lack close intimate relationships, are unmarried, separating, or widowed. There has been no discernible variation in the occurrence of MDD across races or socioeconomic classes. MDD in most behaviors is distinguished for at least 2 weeks by poor mood or by lack of appetite or enjoyment. Depression is also marked by sleep and eating disorders and memory and energy deficiencies. Guilt, loss of interest, and suicidal tendency are popular. In stressed patients, coronary heart disease, diabetes, and strokes tend to be more likely, and depression could make the estimate for patients with a variety of medical conditions considerably worse.

Depression incidence varies widely across societies and continents. Previous studies have shown a 12-month incidence of depression of 0.3% in Czech Republic, 10% in the United States, 4.5% in Mexico, 5.2% in West Germany, and a lifetime of depression in Czech Republic of 1.0%, 16.9% in the United States, 8.3% in Canada, and 9.0% in Chile.[1,2]

Pathophysiology of major depression

We have understood the pathophysiology of major depression substantially in the last decade. MDD is thought to have a multifactorial etiology that includes biological, genetic, environmental, and psychosocial causes. Besides, the older

How Synthetic Drugs Work. DOI: https://doi.org/10.1016/B978-0-323-99855-0.00011-7

theory that depression genetics has a deficiency of activity or volume of monoamines (a monoamine hypothesis), neurotrophic, and endocrine influences play an important part (the neurotrophic hypothesis).[3] Histological experiments, literature on structural and functional brain imagery, genomic discoveries, and steroid research all show complicated MDD pathophysiology with significant opioid therapy consequences. As alternative pathways have been suggested for understanding brain volume reduction in depression glucocorticoid neurotoxicity, glutamatergic toxicity, declined neurotrophic factor, and lower neurogenesis.[4]

Monoamines and other neurotransmitters hypotheses

The past 50 years have seen the dominance of "monoamine theory," which indicates that the pathogenesis and maintenance of depressive symptoms are motivated by a reduction in essential serotonin level, noradrenalin and likely dopamine levels.[5] Depression seems to be associated with major downstream consequences of changes in the signals of serotonin or norepinephrine in the brain (or both). The majority of antidepressants induce amine signaling changes. DAG (diacylglycerol); 5-hydroxytryptamine (5-HT), serotonin; IP3, tri-phosphate inositol; maoamine oxidase; NET (norepinephrine transporter); PKC (protein kinase C); PLc, phospholipase C; serotonin-transporter (SERT), AC, adenylyl cyclase, cREB, cAMP reaction element-binding (protein).[6,7] For several years it has been known to be linked with depression in a group of patients with reserpine medication and is known to deplete monoamines. Depressed patients reacting to serotonergic antidepressants, including fluoxetine, are often rapidly recovering from tryptophan-free diets that constitute a precursor to serotonin synthesis. Genetic experiments provide more data to support the monoamine hypothesis. For the promoter area of the serotonin carrier gene, a functional polymorphism occurs that controls the sum of the transporter protein. Subjects that are homozygous to the (short) allele may be most vulnerable to major depression and suicidal behavior. Furthermore, homozygotes for the allele will less often respond to serotonergic antidepressants and withstand them. By contrast, l-Allel subjects appear to be more stress tolerant and are more likely to respond to serotonergic antidepressants. To date, first-line antidepressant products are only selective serotonin reuptake inhibitors (SSRIs) and norepinephrine reuptake inhibitors. Finally, the perhaps most compelling evidence supporting the theory is that monoamine is shown to be having a major impact on monoamine systems with all the available antidepressants. The synaptic availability of 5-HT, norapinephrine, or dopamine tends to improve all groups of antidepressants. Tentative attempts have not been successful to date in designing antidepressants that function on other neurotransmitter systems. However, the lack of universal effectiveness and a 2–3 weeks clinical latency associated with antidepressants potentiating monoamine, however, contributed to the assumption that monoamine defects are a consequence of synaptic impairment but may not be a fundamental characteristic of depression.[8,9] This hypothesis emphasizes studies outside of monoamines and on the suspected function of growth factors, such as brain-derived neurotrophic factors (BDNFs), which are believed to play a crucial role in adult brain control[10,11] (Fig. 11.1).

Neurotrophic hypotheses

There is significant evidence that neuronal plasticity, durability, and neurogenesis are crucial for the regulation of nerve growth factors such as the BDNF. The research has shown that the lack of neurotrophic reinforcement is correlated with depression and that efficient antidepressant therapy increases neurogenesis and synaptic connectivity in cortical areas like the hippocampus. BDNF has its impact on neuronal survival and growth effects by neuronal neurons and glia activation via the tyrosine kinase receptor B.[12] The neurotrophic hypothesis is supported with many lines of evidence. Animal and human research suggest that stress and pain are linked to a decrease in BDNF levels, which help atrophically alter structures in the hippocampus and possibly other areas such as the medial frontal cortex and anterior cingulate. It is understood that hippocampus is essential for both contextual memory and the regulation for the HPA (Human Protein Atlas) axis. The study of BDNF's causal impact on the emotional control also promoted the neurotrophic theory of depression. Direct BDNF injection into the

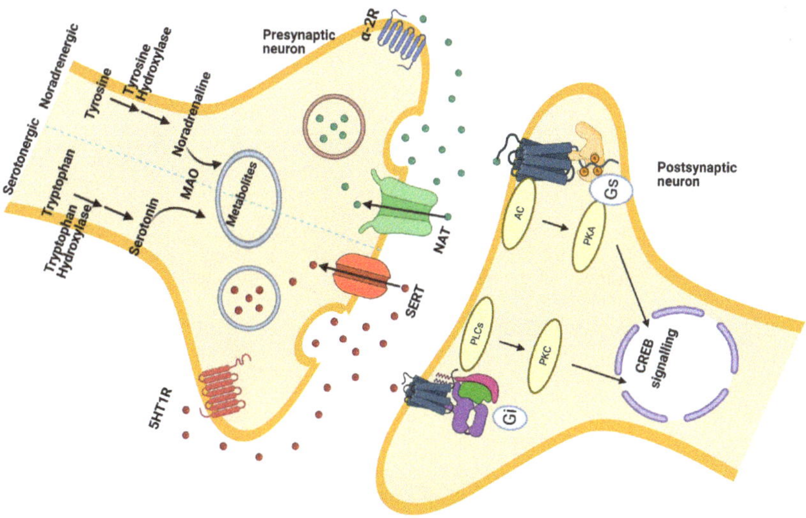

FIGURE 11.1 Pathophysiology of depression mediated changes in norepinephrine or serotonin signaling in the brain with significant downstream effects.

midbrain, hippocampus, and lateral ventricles of rodents induces animal models with an antidepressant function with an increase in tyrosine kinase receptor B activity. Moreover, in animal models of chronic (but not acute) administration, all known types of antidepressants are associated with increased levels of BDNF.[13–16] This rise in BDNF levels in these animal models is consistent with increased hippocampal neurogenesis. In addition, the amount of BDNF in peripheral blood and postmortem has been reduced in depressing patients and others have indicated that antidepressant therapy normalizes the patient's condition.[17,18] In addition, there was some evidence that BDNF and its receptor gene associations are related to treatment-resistant depression.[19] Recent studies have stated that the BDNF (BDNF pro-peptide) pro-domain is lower than the controls in suicidal patients. This is a presynaptic long-term depression on the hippocampus, which suggests that it is a promising synaptic regulator.[20] A proposal to explain the discrepancy of neurotrophic factors in depression is that polymorphisms for BDNF may have quite different consequences. In either animal or human research, mutations in the BDNF gene were shown to be linked to altered anxiety and depression (Fig. 11.2).

Stress-responsive/HPA axis hypotheses

Stress causes or contributes to depression. Long-term or persistent stress can particularly contribute to HPA axis dysfunction and promote hormone discharge including cortisol, adrenocorticotropic hormone, corticotropin-releasing hormone, vasopressin arginine, and vasopressin. Roughly 40%–60% of

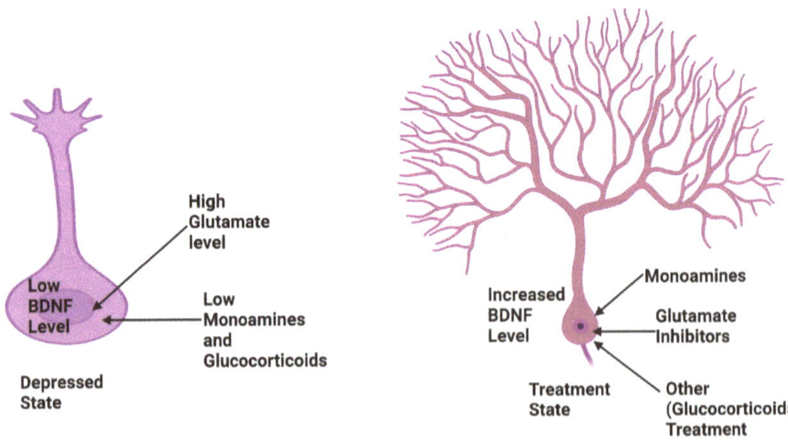

FIGURE 11.2 Low level of BDNF and monoamines in depressed state mediated changes in dendritic growth in neurons. *BDNF*, Brain-derived neurotrophic factor.

patients with depression have a disordered HPA, including hypercortisol, reduced rhythm, and increased cortisol concentrations.[21,22] The defects of the HPA axis in MDD patients are among the most reported of the findings. More extreme depressive types such as bipolar depression tend to be more frequently diagnosed with HPA than milder symptoms of major depression. It is well-known that both exogenous and endogenous cortisol elevations have identical mood signs and cognitive deficiencies as in MDD. Despite these encouraging findings, past literature has shown that medications controlling the HPA axis, such as glucocorticoid receptor antagonists, do not alleviate depressed patients' symptoms.[23,24]

Thyroid dysregulation has also been found in people who are stressed. Thyroid dysfunction is estimated to affect up to 25% of depressive patients. This includes a shutdown of thyrotropin reactivity to thyrotropin-releasing hormone and increases in circulating thyroxine under depressive conditions. Clinical hypothyroidism sometimes manifests as depressive symptoms that improve with thyroid hormone replacement. Thyroid hormones are also widely used in combination with conventional antidepressants to improve their therapeutic effects.[25–28]

Finally, the pathophysiology of depression often involves sex steroids. Estrogen deficiency states that occur in postpartum and postmenopausal cycles are suspected to play a role in some women's etiology of depression. Similarly, extreme male deficiency of testosterone often involves depressive symptoms. The hypogonadal men and women's hormone replacement therapy can include improved mood and depressive symptoms.[29–31]

Dysbiosis/gut/brain axis hypotheses

Recently, due to his capacity to control brain activities, the microbiota–gut–brain axis has gained greater interest. Many experiments have demonstrated a significant role for the microbiota–gut–brain axis in the control of mood, behavior and synaptic transmission in the brain.[32] For instance, many mood disorders including anxiety, depression, or autism have also developed similarities to functional GI disorders, while GI illness (e.g., irritable bowel syndrome and irritable bowel disease) also involves psychiatric comorbidities related to stress associated gut microbiome disorders (dysbiosis).[33–36] Some cytokines, such as IL-6 and IL-1 β formed during stress associated dysbiosis, can leak into the brain via the blood–brain barrier. The periphery and central immune systems communicate in a complex way. Previous evidence indicated that peripheral inflammation/infection can spread in a certain way and provoke neuroimmune reaction to the central nervous system (CNS).[37,38] Interestingly, there is evidence that rats are depressed following fecal transplants in depressed patients.[39] In animal experiments, on the other hand, certain probiotics have mitigated depressive behavior.[40]

Glutamate hypotheses

In depression pathophysiology, glutamate, the excitatory neurotransmitter tends to be essential. Several experiments of depressive patients have shown a high glutamate level and reduced glutamine/glutamate levels in plasma in cerebrospinal fluids of depressed patients. Glutamate is the primary excitatory brain-released neurotransmitter; it involves plasticity, neural functions, reward, and emotional processes. Neuronal stress can cause presynaptic glutamate release and glutamate strongly links to ionotropic glutamate receptors like NMDARs (N-methyl D-aspartic acid (NMDA) receptors)/AMPARs (AMPA receptors)/KRs (kainate receptors).[41] Furthermore, postmortem findings show that the prefrontal dorsal and frontal cortex in depressive patients have increased significantly. Likewise, in the brain regions of depressive patients with glutamate neurons and their associations most abundantly including amygdala and hippocampus, systemic neuroimaging experiments also repeatedly found volumetric shifts.[42–44] NMDARs have an antidepressant effect and defend hippocampal neurons against stress-induced morphological abnormalities, while antidepressants decrease the glutamate Secretion and NMDARs activity.[45] Most interestingly, the effects of antagonists such as ketamine on both animal models, as well as key depressive disorders, were stated to be profound and rapid.[46] Ketamine and esketamine (S) + ketamine enantiomers are both active, noncompetitive NMDAR antagonists, but they have various other pharmacodynamic properties. For major therapeutic depression in 2019, esketamine has been approved. In addition, many other antagonists of NMDA receptors, partial antagonists, and glutamate metabotropic receptor modulators as possible antidepressants have been studied (Fig. 11.3).

Assimilation of hypotheses on depression pathophysiology

Monoamine, neuroendocrine, and neurotrophic mechanisms are clearly interrelated. For example, the suppression of the transcription of the gene BDNF can lead to HPA and steroid abnormalities. Higher density glucocorticoid receptors in the hippocampus are observed. The chronic stimulation by antidepressants of monoamine receptors seems to have the reverse influence of depression and outcomes like hippocampus. The chronic stimulation of monoamine receptors by antidepressants seems to be having a downward impact on stress. In addition, monoamine receptor activation tends to downgrade the HPA axis and can equalize the activity of HPA.

One of the drawbacks of the monoamine theory is that amine levels rise with antidepressant use instantly but maximum positive effects are not observed for several weeks with most antidepressants. To understand this delay in antidepressant effect, the time needed to synthesize neurotrophic factors has been suggested. It is usually 2 weeks or longer to get an

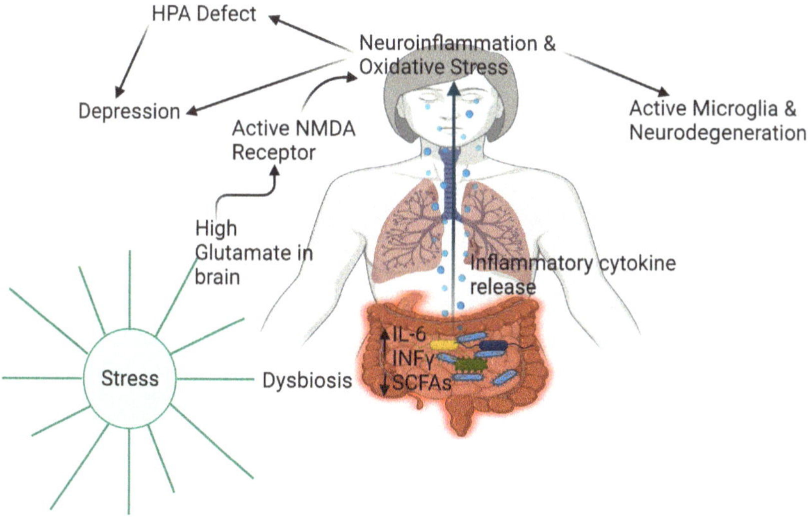

FIGURE 11.3 Represent stressed patients with high glutamate and gut/brain axis defect aggravate consequence of depression.

appreciable protein synthesis in drugs like BDNF and to coincide with an antidepressant therapy in the medicine.

Fundamental pharmacology of antidepressants

A remarkable range of chemical forms is the commercially active antidepressants. The variations in molecular key targets and their differences provide the basis for the classification between many subgroups.

Selective serotonin reuptake inhibitors

Medications called SSRIs are usually the first-line treatment for depression in children and young people because most patients experience only minor (or no) side effects, and the medication is generally administered once a day.[47,48] Fluoxetine, sertraline, and citalopram occur as isomers and have racemic formulation, whereas optically, paroxetine and fluvoxamine are not involved. Escitalopram is the citalopram enantiomer (S). In the United States, fluoxetine was launched in 1988, which soon became one of the most used drugs.[49] Fluoxetine was developed in the study for chemicals that were very similar to monoamine receptors but which lacked the affinity for histamine, acetylcholine, and α-adrenoceptors seen with tricyclic antidepressants (TCAs). The role of serotonin or 5-HT in the CNS is best known to control a range of functions, including mood, behavior, and appetite. 5-HT impairment is associated with mental conditions including depression. On synthesis, 5-HT is secreted across circulation, where platelets are taken up by the serotonin reuptake transporter (SERT) directly and deposited in its thick granules. Platelets release the granule material, like 5-HT after activation.[50] SERT is a glycoprotein with 12 transmembrane regions that are found in the membranes of serotonergic neurons' axon terminals and cell bodies. When extracellular serotonin attaches to receptors on the transporter, the transporter undergoes conformational changes, allowing serotonin, Na + , and Cl to enter the cell. As intracellular K + binds to the transporter, serotonin is released into the cell and the transporter reverts to its original conformation. The SSRIs can affect the concentration of important brain neurotransmitters and are therefore thought to have effects on the symptoms of depression. SSRIs block the transporter allosterically by binding to the SERT receptor in a location other than the serotonin binding site.[51] At therapeutic doses, nearly 80% of the transporter's activity is blocked. SERT has functional polymorphisms that affect the transporter's behavior.[52] Fluoxetine has been metabolized to an active substance, norfluoxetine, that may be higher than fluoxetine plasma concentrations. Norfluoxetine has a nearly threefold elimination half-life of fluoxetine and corresponds to the longest half-life of SSRIs. To reduce the risk of serotonin syndrome, fluoxetine must be halted 4 weeks or later before monoamine oxidase inhibitor (MAOI) is administered.

Serotonin-norepinephrine reuptake inhibitors

Many antidepressants have a mixed inhibition effect on all transporters of serotonin and norepinephrine. The newest agents (venlafaxine and duloxetine) in this class are called serotonin-norepinephrine reuptake inhibitors (SNRIs); they are called TCAs depending on the structure of the older class.

Selective serotonin-norepinephrine reuptake inhibitors

Venlafaxine and its metabolite desvenlafaxine, levomilnacipran, and duloxetine are often used in SNRIs. Levomilnacipran is the active SNRI enantiomer milnacipran. Milnacipran was approved for fibromyalgia treatment in the United States and was used for several years in Europe for depression treatment.[53] All the SNRIs are binding to transporters like serotonin (SERT) and norepinephrine (NET). In contrast to the TCAs, though, the SNRIs have a little affinity toward several other receptors. SNRIs bind both the transporters of serotonin and of norepinephrine. Venlafaxine is a poor glycoprotein inhibitor of NET, whereas both SERT and NET are more sustainable inhibitors for desvenlafaxine, duloxetine, milnacipran and levomilnacipran.[54,55] Fortunately, SERT appears to be much more closely related to most SNRIs than NET. Additionally, apart from depression, it was initially suggested that the SERT polymorphism accounted for 7%–9% of the genetic variation of anxiety-related disorders.[56] The SNRIs are different from TCAs because of the powerful antihistamines, α-adrenergic blockages, and anticholinergic effects of TCAs. The SNRIs, therefore, appear to be favored against TCAs for their increased tolerability in the treatment of MDD and pain syndromes.[53,57–59] Venlafaxine is widely metabolized to O-desmethylvenlafaxine in the liver via the CYP2D6 isoenzyme. Both are around 8–11 h long and have identical half-lives. In spite of their comparatively short half-lives, the two medications can be dosed once a day in formulations. The lowest protein binding of all antidepressants is venlafaxine and desvenlafaxine (27%–30%). Duloxetine is well tolerated and has a half-life of 12–15 h; however, it is only administered once daily. It is extremely protein-bound (97%) and undergoes substantial oxidative metabolism through the enzymes CYP2D6 and CYP1A2.[53]

Tricyclic antidepressants

Until SSRIs were introduced in the 1980s and 1990s, the TCAs were the main class of antidepressants. There are nine TCAs in the United States and they all have a tricyclic configuration. The FDA has approved amoxapine, desipramine, amitriptyline, nortriptyline, trimipramine, protriptyline, imipramine, and doxepin for the treatment of MDD.[60–63] The TCAs are currently mostly used in depressive conditions that do not respond to more widely used antidepressants like SSRIs or SNRIs. Owing to the substantial heterogeneity in TCAs' affinity for SERT versus NET, clomipramine has a low affinity for NET but a strong affinity for SERT. This SERT selectivity leads to clomipramine's well-documented advantages in the treatment of OCD.[64] On the other hand, the TCAs, desipramine, and nortriptyline secondary amine, for NET, are comparatively more selective. While the TCA imipramine tertiary amine initially has a stronger impact on serotonin, its metabolite desipramine balances this with further NET inhibition.[65] TCAs exert their effects via distinct neurotransmitter pathways. They inhibit serotonin and norepinephrine reuptake in presynaptic terminals, resulting in an increase in their concentration in the synaptic cleft. Increased norepinephrine and serotonin concentrations in the synaptic cleft possibly lead to its antidepressant impact. Additionally, they function as antagonists against postsynaptic cholinergic muscarinic, and histaminergic receptors.[66,67]

5-Hydroxytryptamine receptor modulators

Both nefazodone and trazodone tend to exert their effects primarily by inhibition of the 5-HT2A receptor. Inhibition of this pathway has been linked to significant antianxiety, antipsychotic, and antidepressant activity in both animal and human research.[68] By comparison, 5-HT2A receptor agonists such as lysergic acid (LSD) and mescaline are often hallucinogenic and anxiogenic.[69] The 5-HT2A receptor is a G protein–coupled receptor that is found in the neocortical structure.[69] Nefazodone, like its metabolites, is a weak inhibitor of SERT and NET but a powerful antagonist of the postsynaptic 5-HT2A receptor.[70] Trazodone is also a weak but selective SERT inhibitor with a marginal effect on NET.[71] Its primary metabolite, m-cpp, is a powerful 5-HT2 antagonist, and this effect can account for a significant proportion of trazodone's antidepressant benefits.[72,73] Trazodone also has poor to moderate presynaptic α-adrenergic–blocking properties and is a mild H1 receptor antagonist.[74] Trazodone and nefazodone are absorbed quickly and metabolized in the liver. Both drugs are protein-bound and have a low bioavailability due to extensive metabolic degradation.[75] Nefazodone is a powerful CYP3A4 pathway inhibitor that can interact with medication that has been metabolized by this enzyme.[76] Vortioxetine does not have a potent CYP isoenzyme inhibitor. However, oxidation by CYP2D6 and other isoenzymes is thoroughly metabolized and is eventually conjugated by glucuronic acid.[77,78]

Monoamine oxidase inhibitors

In the 1950s the first introduction of MAOIs was made.[79,80] MAOIs mitigate the effects of MAO in the neuron and increase the amount of monoamine. MAO has two forms. The dominant substrate of MAO-A is norepinephrine, epinephrine, serotonin, and neurons of both dopamine and norepinephrine and is located mainly in the brain and intestines, placenta, and liver. MAO-B is predominantly present in serotonergic and histaminergic neurons and scattered through the cortex, liver, and platelet. MAO-B mostly affects benzylamine, dopamine, tyramine, and phenylethylamine. The metabolizing of tryptamine in MAO-A and -B is almost the same.[81,82]

MAOIs are categorized according to their MAO-A or -B specificity and whether their results are reversible or permanent. Examples of irreversible, nonspecific MAOIs are phenelzine and tranylcypromine. Moclobemide is a reversible and potent MAO-A receptor that is not available in the United States.[83]

Moclobemide may be substituted by tyramine from MAO-A, which decreases the possibility of food interactions. Selegiline is, by contrast, an irreversible, low-dose MAO-B-specific agent. Selegiline is effective at these low doses for the treatment of Parkinson's disease, although at larger dosages it is comparable to other agents to a nonselective MAOI.[81,83,84] The multiple MAOIs are metabolized by various mechanisms but appear to have a significant influence of first pass, which can greatly minimize bioavailability. The hydroxylated and N-acetylated rings are tranylcypromine, while acetylation seems to be a minor mechanism in phenelzine. N-demethylated selegiline is hydroxylated and consequently. MAOIs from gastrointestinal tract are well absorbed[85,86] (Fig. 11.4).

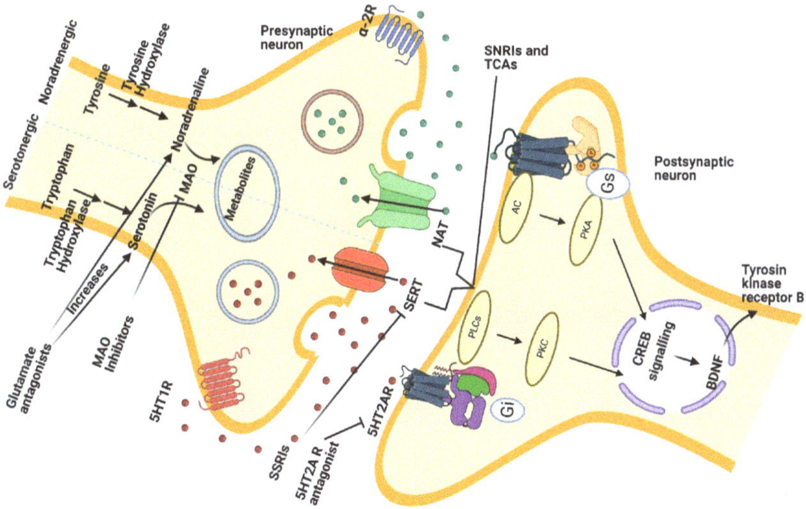

FIGURE 11.4 Explore various target sites for antidepressant drugs.

Glutamate signaling antagonist

Although ketamine and esketamine are considered to be mainly noncompetitive NMDA receptor antagonists, these medications have several other pharmacodynamic activities that can lead to depressive and other disorders' efficacy. Interactions with opium receptors, monoaminergic receptors, colinergic receptors, and Ca2 + channels are all part of this. Ketamine appears to have little effect on GABA receptors despite its use as an anesthetic. Ketamine and esketamine have no well-defined effects on monoamines, as are NMDA effects.[87] Most but not all research show ketamines can enhance levels of dopamine dramatically by inhibiting the reuptake of dopamine. The dopaminergic reaction is associated with the drug's euphoric and psychotomimetic impact.[88] Ketamine is often assumed to improve the function of decreasing serotonergic receptors that may be significant for antidepressant and analgesic characteristics of the medication.[89] Racemic ketamine (normally given IV) and esketamine (intranasal) pharmacokinetics are identical but are partially distinct due to different administration pathways. It is 48% bioavailable intranasally esketamine, while IV ketamine is completely bioavailable.[90] Esketamine is 7–12 h long, while the primary metabolite, namely, noresketamine, is about 8 h long. The ketamine is thoroughly metabolized by N-demethylation to norketamine in the body by CYP2B6 and CYP3A4. The half-life of IV ketamine is around 3 h. The median plasma concentration is 20–40 min from the last nasal spray for intranasal esketamine. With 78% of metabolites in urine and 2% in feces, less than 1% of esketamine was excreted unchanged[91,92] (Table 11.1).

TABLE 11.1 Blocking/antagonistic property of some antidepressant drugs on several receptors and transporters.

Antidepressant	SERT	ACh M	5-HT2	α1	H1	N E T
Amitriptyline	++	+++	+	+++	++	+
Citalopram	+++	NA	NA	NA	NA	NA
Amoxapine	+	+	+++	++	+	++
Desipramine	+	+	+	+	+	+++
Clomipramine	+++	+	+	++	+	+
Fluoxetine	+++	NA	+	NA	NA	NA
Doxepin	+	++	+	+++	+++	+
Sertraline	+++	NA	NA	NA	NA	NA
Imipramine	++	++	+	+	+	+
Trazodone	+	NA	++	++	+	NA
Nefazodone	+	NA	++	+	NA	+
Venlafaxine	++	NA	NA	NA	NA	+

NA, No activity or minimal affinity; +, mild affinity; ++, moderate affinity; +++, high affinity.

Adverse effect and interaction of antidepressant drugs

While all antidepressants have such possible adverse reactions, most of the adverse reactions are unique to a subclass of the agents and their pharmacodynamic impact. The chance of elevated suicidality in patients younger than 25 years is an FDA alert used by any antidepressant. The warnings say that the use of antidepressants in up to 4% of patients under 25 who were prescribed antidepressants in clinical trials is linked to suicidal ideation and movements, but not completed suicides.

SSRIs increase the serotonergic signal of the body and increasing serotonergic activity in the intestines is often caused by nausea, gastrointestinal disturbance, diarrhea, and other gastric symptoms.[49] The FDA teratogenic classification scheme most antidepressants are group C agents. In the first trimester exposures, paroxetine is associated with septal heart defects. Paroxetine is also an agent in Group D. SNRIs have several SSRI-related adverse serotonergic effects. Moreover, SNRIs may have noradrenergic effects, including elevated heart and blood pressure and stimulation by CNS, such as insomnia, anxiety, or frustration. TCAs are probably the most prevalent anticholinergic symptoms. This includes dry mouth, constipation, urine retention, vision blurred, and confusion. Tertiary amine TCAs, including amitriptyline and imipramine, are more common than the secondary amine

TCAs, desipramine, and nortriptyline.[93] The most frequent adverse consequences of the MAOIs are orthostatic hypotension and weight gain that contribute to the discontinuation of these medications. Additionally, of all antidepressants, permanent nonselective MAOIs are correlated with the greatest risk of sexual side effects. Certain MAOIs have amphetamine-like effects, which can cause activation, insomnia, and restlessness in some patients. Phenelzine has a sedative effect comparable to selegiline or tranylcypromine. Confusion is often occasionally associated with higher MAOI doses. MAOIs can cause harmful interactions with certain foods and serotonergic medications because they inhibit the metabolism of tyramine and related ingested amines. Finally, MAOIs have been related to a condition of rapid discontinuation that presents as a delirium-like state of psychosis, excitement, and uncertainty.[94] Furthermore, ketamine and esketamine have a variety of side effects that are consistent with their pharmacologic profile. Sedation, disorientation, hypertension, vomiting, tachycardia, and cognitive dysfunction are all short-term side effects of these medications.[92,95]

Conclusion

Based on the proof of the effectiveness of each approved antidepressant, it is obvious that acceptability should be the main criterion when considering a treatment. Numerous mechanisms have been identified that may contribute to the discovery of novel therapeutic targets for a sizable proportion of the treatment population.

Depression's immense heterogeneity has been widely recognized throughout previous research. Around one-third of patients on existing antidepressants are remitters, but the same percentage is nonresponders. Nonresponders to standard antidepressants are a diverse population, as almost every trial of novel antidepressants demonstrates. Though preclinical and early clinical data is encouraging for many of the targets mentioned, the effectiveness of targeting these mechanisms remains unknown in the absence of large-scale double-blind, placebo-controlled randomized trials. While these new types of drugs usually have increased tolerability and safety in earlier therapies, no uniformly successful pharmacological treatments are available for mood problems and diligent medical treatment for such medicines also warrants them.

References

1. Andrade L, Caraveo-Anduaga JJ, Berglund P, et al. The epidemiology of major depressive episodes: results from the International Consortium of Psychiatric Epidemiology (ICPE) surveys. *Int J Methods Psychiatr Res*. 2003;12:3–21. Available from: https://doi.org/10.1002/mpr.138.
2. Kessler RC, Bromet EJ. The epidemiology of depression across cultures. *Annu Rev Public Health*. 2013;34:119–138. Available from: https://doi.org/10.1146/annurev-publhealth-031912-114409.

3. Shao X, Zhu G. Associations among monoamine neurotransmitter pathways, personality traits, and major depressive disorder. *Front Psychiatry*. 2020;11. Available from: https://doi.org/10.3389/fpsyt.2020.00381.
4. Hasler G. Pathophysiology of depression: do we have any solid evidence of interest to clinicians? *World Psychiatry*. 2010;9:155–161. Available from: https://doi.org/10.1002/j.2051-5545.2010.tb00298.x.
5. Hindmarch I. Beyond the monoamine hypothesis: mechanisms, molecules and methods. *Eur Psychiatry*. 2002;17(Suppl 3):294–299. Available from: https://doi.org/10.1016/s0924-9338(02)00653-3.
6. Delgado PL. Aminergic hypotheses for depression. In: Stolerman IP, ed. *Encyclopedia of Psychopharmacology*. Berlin, Heidelberg: Springer; 2010:70–73.
7. Meyer JH, Ginovart N, Boovariwala A, et al. Elevated monoamine oxidase A levels in the brain: an explanation for the monoamine imbalance of major depression. *Arch Gen Psychiatry*. 2006;63:1209–1216. Available from: https://doi.org/10.1001/archpsyc.63.11.1209.
8. Nestler EJ, Barrot M, DiLeone RJ, Eisch AJ, Gold SJ, Monteggia LM. Neurobiology of depression. *Neuron*. 2002;34:13–25. Available from: https://doi.org/10.1016/s0896-6273(02)00653-0.
9. Duman RS, Heninger GR, Nestler EJ. A molecular and cellular theory of depression. *Arch Gen Psychiatry*. 1997;54:597–606. Available from: https://doi.org/10.1001/archpsyc.1997.01830190015002.
10. Thoenen H. Neurotrophins and neuronal plasticity. *Science*. 1995;270:593–598. Available from: https://doi.org/10.1126/science.270.5236.593.
11. Kafitz KW, Rose CR, Thoenen H, Konnerth A. Neurotrophin-evoked rapid excitation through TrkB receptors. *Nature*. 1999;401:918–921. Available from: https://doi.org/10.1038/44847.
12. Groves JO. Is it time to reassess the BDNF hypothesis of depression? *Mol Psychiatry*. 2007;12:1079–1088. Available from: https://doi.org/10.1038/sj.mp.4002075.
13. Wang JQ, Mao L. The ERK pathway: molecular mechanisms and treatment of depression. *Mol Neurobiol*. 2019;56:6197–6205. Available from: https://doi.org/10.1007/s12035-019-1524-3.
14. Li K, Shen S, Ji YT, Li XY, Zhang LS, Wang XD. Melatonin augments the effects of fluoxetine on depression-like behavior and hippocampal BDNF-TrkB signaling. *Neurosci Bull*. 2018;34:303–311. Available from: https://doi.org/10.1007/s12264-017-0189-z.
15. Zhang JJ, Gao TT, Wang Y, et al. Andrographolide exerts significant antidepressant-like effects involving the hippocampal BDNF system in mice. *Int J Neuropsychopharmacol*. 2019;22:585–600. Available from: https://doi.org/10.1093/ijnp/pyz032.
16. Albert PR, Benkelfat C, Descarries L. The neurobiology of depression—revisiting the serotonin hypothesis. I. Cellular and molecular mechanisms. *Philos Trans R Soc Lond B Biol Sci*. 2012;367:2378–2381. Available from: https://doi.org/10.1098/rstb.2012.0190.
17. Youssef MM, Underwood MD, Huang YY, et al. Association of BDNF Val66Met polymorphism and brain BDNF levels with major depression and suicide. *Int J Neuropsychopharmacol*. 2018;21:528–538. Available from: https://doi.org/10.1093/ijnp/pyy008.
18. Chiou YJ, Huang TL. Serum brain-derived neurotrophic factors in Taiwanese patients with drug-naïve first-episode major depressive disorder: effects of antidepressants. *Int J Neuropsychopharmacol*. 2017;20:213–218. Available from: https://doi.org/10.1093/ijnp/pyw096.
19. Li Z, Zhang Y, Wang Z, et al. The role of BDNF, NTRK2 gene and their interaction in development of treatment-resistant depression: data from multicenter, prospective, longitudinal clinic practice. *J Psychiatr Res*. 2013;47:8–14. Available from: https://doi.org/10.1016/j.jpsychires.2012.10.003.

20. Kojima M, Matsui K, Mizui T. BDNF pro-peptide: physiological mechanisms and implications for depression. *Cell Tissue Res.* 2019;377:73–79. Available from: https://doi.org/10.1007/s00441-019-03034-6.
21. Pariante CM, Lightman SL. The HPA axis in major depression: classical theories and new developments. *Trends Neurosci.* 2008;31:464–468. Available from: https://doi.org/10.1016/j.tins.2008.06.006.
22. Murphy BE. Steroids and depression. *J Steroid Biochem Mol Biol.* 1991;38:537–559. Available from: https://doi.org/10.1016/0960-0760(91)90312-s.
23. Stetler C, Miller GE. Depression and hypothalamic-pituitary-adrenal activation: a quantitative summary of four decades of research. *Psychosom Med.* 2011;73:114–126. Available from: https://doi.org/10.1097/PSY.0b013e31820ad12b.
24. Aubry JM. CRF system and mood disorders. *J Chem Neuroanat.* 2013;54:20–24. Available from: https://doi.org/10.1016/j.jchemneu.2013.09.003.
25. Wu X, Zhang K, Xing Y, et al. Dysregulated thyroid hormones correlate with anxiety and depression risk in patients with autoimmune disease. *J Clin Lab Anal.* 2021;35:e23573. Available from: https://doi.org/10.1002/jcla.23573.
26. Hage MP, Azar ST. The link between thyroid function and depression. *J Thyroid Res.* 2012;2012:590648. Available from: https://doi.org/10.1155/2012/590648.
27. Du F-M, Kuang H-Y, Duan B-H, Liu D-N, Yu X-Y. Effects of thyroid hormone and depression on common components of central obesity. *J Int Med Res.* 2019;47:3040–3049. Available from: https://doi.org/10.1177/0300060519851624.
28. Li C, Lai J, Huang T, et al. Thyroid functions in patients with bipolar disorder and the impact of quetiapine monotherapy: a retrospective, naturalistic study. *Neuropsychiatr Dis Treat.* 2019;15:2285–2290. Available from: https://doi.org/10.2147/ndt.S196661.
29. Soares CN, Zitek B. Reproductive hormone sensitivity and risk for depression across the female life cycle: a continuum of vulnerability? *J Psychiatry Neurosci: JPN.* 2008;33:331–343.
30. Thériault R-K, Perreault ML. Hormonal regulation of circuit function: sex, systems and depression. *Biol Sex Differences.* 2019;10:12. Available from: https://doi.org/10.1186/s13293-019-0226-x.
31. Daniell HW. Sex hormone deficiency in depressed patients receiving opioids. *Arch Intern Med.* 2004;164:804. Available from: https://doi.org/10.1001/archinte.164.7.804-a.
32. Clapp M, Aurora N, Herrera L, Bhatia M, Wilen E, Wakefield S. Gut microbiota's effect on mental health: the gut-brain axis. *Clin Pract.* 2017;7:987. Available from: https://doi.org/10.4081/cp.2017.987.
33. Kennedy PJ, Clarke G, Quigley EM, Groeger JA, Dinan TG, Cryan JF. Gut memories: towards a cognitive neurobiology of irritable bowel syndrome. *Neurosci Biobehav Rev.* 2012;36:310–340. Available from: https://doi.org/10.1016/j.neubiorev.2011.07.001.
34. Whitehead WE, Palsson O, Jones KR. Systematic review of the comorbidity of irritable bowel syndrome with other disorders: what are the causes and implications? *Gastroenterology.* 2002;122:1140–1156. Available from: https://doi.org/10.1053/gast.2002.32392.
35. Kennedy PJ, Cryan JF, Dinan TG, Clarke G. Irritable bowel syndrome: a microbiome-gut-brain axis disorder? *World J Gastroenterol.* 2014;20:14105–14125. Available from: https://doi.org/10.3748/wjg.v20.i39.14105.
36. Ruepert L, Quartero AO, de Wit NJ, van der Heijden GJ, Rubin G, Muris JW. Bulking agents, antispasmodics and antidepressants for the treatment of irritable bowel syndrome. *Cochrane Database Syst Rev.* 2011;Cd003460. Available from: https://doi.org/10.1002/14651858.CD003460.pub3.
37. Miller AH, Raison CL. The role of inflammation in depression: from evolutionary imperative to modern treatment target. *Nat Rev Immunol.* 2016;16:22–34. Available from: https://doi.org/10.1038/nri.2015.5.

38. Li Z, Wang Z, Zhang C, et al. Reduced ENA78 levels as novel biomarker for major depressive disorder and venlafaxine efficiency: result from a prospective longitudinal study. *Psychoneuroendocrinology*. 2017;81:113–121. Available from: https://doi.org/10.1016/j.psyneuen.2017.03.015.
39. Zheng P, Zeng B, Zhou C, et al. Gut microbiome remodeling induces depressive-like behaviors through a pathway mediated by the host's metabolism. *Mol Psychiatry*. 2016;21:786–796. Available from: https://doi.org/10.1038/mp.2016.44.
40. Hao Z, Wang W, Guo R, Liu H. *Faecalibacterium prausnitzii* (ATCC 27766) has preventive and therapeutic effects on chronic unpredictable mild stress-induced depression-like and anxiety-like behavior in rats. *Psychoneuroendocrinology*. 2019;104:132–142. Available from: https://doi.org/10.1016/j.psyneuen.2019.02.025.
41. Correia-Melo FS, Leal GC, Vieira F, et al. Efficacy and safety of adjunctive therapy using esketamine or racemic ketamine for adult treatment-resistant depression: a randomized, double-blind, non-inferiority study. *J Affect Disord*. 2020;264:527–534. Available from: https://doi.org/10.1016/j.jad.2019.11.086.
42. Hashimoto K. The role of glutamate on the action of antidepressants. *Prog Neuropsychopharmacol Biol Psychiatry*. 2011;35:1558–1568. Available from: https://doi.org/10.1016/j.pnpbp.2010.06.013.
43. Sanacora G, Zarate CA, Krystal JH, Manji HK. Targeting the glutamatergic system to develop novel, improved therapeutics for mood disorders. *Nat Rev Drug Discov*. 2008;7:426–437. Available from: https://doi.org/10.1038/nrd2462.
44. Duman RS, Voleti B. Signaling pathways underlying the pathophysiology and treatment of depression: novel mechanisms for rapid-acting agents. *Trends Neurosci*. 2012;35:47–56. Available from: https://doi.org/10.1016/j.tins.2011.11.004.
45. Musazzi L, Treccani G, Mallei A, Popoli M. The action of antidepressants on the glutamate system: regulation of glutamate release and glutamate receptors. *Biol Psychiatry*. 2013;73:1180–1188. Available from: https://doi.org/10.1016/j.biopsych.2012.11.009.
46. Kadriu B, Musazzi L, Henter ID, Graves M, Popoli M, Zarate Jr CA. Glutamatergic neurotransmission: pathway to developing novel rapid-acting antidepressant treatments. *Int J Neuropsychopharmacol*. 2019;22:119–135. Available from: https://doi.org/10.1093/ijnp/pyy094.
47. Wise J. GPs in England prescribed 2.7 million extra antidepressants during 2012 recession. *BMJ*. 2014;348:g3607. Available from: https://doi.org/10.1136/bmj.g3607.
48. Gualano MR, Bert F, Mannocci A, La Torre G, Zeppegno P, Siliquini R. Consumption of antidepressants in Italy: recent trends and their significance for public health. *Psychiatr Serv*. 2014;65:1226–1231. Available from: https://doi.org/10.1176/appi.ps.201300510.
49. Ferguson JM. SSRI antidepressant medications: adverse effects and tolerability. *Prim Care Companion J Clin Psychiatry*. 2001;3:22–27. Available from: https://doi.org/10.4088/pcc.v03n0105.
50. El-Merahbi R, Löffler M, Mayer A, Sumara G. The roles of peripheral serotonin in metabolic homeostasis. *FEBS Lett*. 2015;589:1728–1734. Available from: https://doi.org/10.1016/j.febslet.2015.05.054.
51. Hirschfeld RM. Antidepressants in long-term therapy: a review of tricyclic antidepressants and selective serotonin reuptake inhibitors. *Acta Psychiatr Scand Suppl*. 2000;403:35–38. Available from: https://doi.org/10.1111/j.1600-0447.2000.tb10946.x.
52. Serretti A, Kato M. The serotonin transporter gene and effectiveness of SSRIs. *Expert Rev Neurother*. 2008;8:111–120. Available from: https://doi.org/10.1586/14737175.8.1.111.
53. Sansone RA, Sansone LA. Serotonin norepinephrine reuptake inhibitors: a pharmacological comparison. *Innov Clin Neurosci*. 2014;11:37–42.

54. Raouf M, Glogowski AJ, Bettinger JJ, Fudin J. Serotonin-norepinephrine reuptake inhibitors and the influence of binding affinity (Ki) on analgesia. *J Clin Pharm Ther.* 2017;42:513–517. Available from: https://doi.org/10.1111/jcpt.12534.
55. Banzi R, Cusi C, Randazzo C, Sterzi R, Tedesco D, Moja L. Selective serotonin reuptake inhibitors (SSRIs) and serotonin-norepinephrine reuptake inhibitors (SNRIs) for the prevention of migraine in adults. *Cochrane Database Syst Rev.* 2015;. Available from: https://doi.org/10.1002/14651858.CD002919.pub3.
56. Lesch KP, Bengel D, Heils A, et al. Association of anxiety-related traits with a polymorphism in the serotonin transporter gene regulatory region. *Science.* 1996;274:1527–1531. Available from: https://doi.org/10.1126/science.274.5292.1527.
57. Haller E, Geier M, Finley P. Antidepressants, pharmacology of. In: Aminoff MJ, Daroff RB, eds. *Encyclopedia of the Neurological Sciences.* 2nd ed. Oxford: Academic Press; 2014:219–223.
58. Wasan AD, Gallagher RM. Chapter 14 - Psychopharmacology for pain medicine. In: Benzon HT, Raja SN, Molloy RE, Liu SS, Fishman SM, eds. *Essentials of Pain Medicine and Regional Anesthesia.* 2nd ed. Philadelphia, PA: Churchill Livingstone; 2005:124–133.
59. Shah BJ, Janata JW. Pain; psychiatric and psychological interventions. In: Aminoff MJ, Daroff RB, eds. *Encyclopedia of the Neurological Sciences.* 2nd ed. Oxford: Academic Press; 2014:757–760.
60. National Institute of Diabetes and Digestive and Kidney Diseases. *Antidepressant Agents. LiverTox: Clinical and Research Information on Drug-Induced Liver Injury.* Bethesda, MD: National Institute of Diabetes and Digestive and Kidney Diseases; 2012.
61. Dopheide JA. Recognizing and treating depression in children and adolescents. *Am J Health Syst Pharm.* 2006;63:233–243. Available from: https://doi.org/10.2146/ajhp050264.
62. Boafo A, Greenham S, Sullivan M, et al. Medications for sleep disturbance in children and adolescents with depression: a survey of Canadian child and adolescent psychiatrists. *Child Adolesc Psychiatry Ment Health.* 2020;14:10. Available from: https://doi.org/10.1186/s13034-020-00316-8.
63. Stokes PRA, Jokinen T, Amawi S, et al. Pharmacological treatment of mood disorders and comorbid addictions: a systematic review and *meta*-analysis: Traitement Pharmacologique des Troubles de L'humeur et des Dépendances Comorbides: Une Revue Systématique et une Méta-Analyse. *Can J Psychiatry.* 2020;65:749–769. Available from: https://doi.org/10.1177/0706743720915420.
64. Del Casale A, Sorice S, Padovano A, et al. Psychopharmacological treatment of obsessive-compulsive disorder (OCD). *Curr Neuropharmacol.* 2019;17:710–736. Available from: https://doi.org/10.2174/1570159x16666180813155017.
65. Gillman PK. Tricyclic antidepressant pharmacology and therapeutic drug interactions updated. *Br J Pharmacol.* 2007;151:737–748. Available from: https://doi.org/10.1038/sj.bjp.0707253.
66. Hillhouse TM, Porter JH. A brief history of the development of antidepressant drugs: from monoamines to glutamate. *Exp Clin Psychopharmacol.* 2015;23:1–21. Available from: https://doi.org/10.1037/a0038550.
67. Richelson E. Antimuscarinic and other receptor-blocking properties of antidepressants. *Mayo Clin Proc.* 1983;58:40–46.
68. Celada P, Puig M, Amargós-Bosch M, Adell A, Artigas F. The therapeutic role of 5-HT1A and 5-HT2A receptors in depression. *J Psychiatry Neurosci: JPN.* 2004;29:252–265.

69. Kim K, Che T, Panova O, et al. Structure of a hallucinogen-activated Gq-coupled 5-HT2A serotonin receptor. *Cell*. 2020;182:1574–1588. Available from: https://doi.org/10.1016/j.cell.2020.08.024. e19.
70. Horst WD, Preskorn SH. Mechanisms of action and clinical characteristics of three atypical antidepressants: venlafaxine, nefazodone, bupropion. *J Affect Disord*. 1998;51:237–254. Available from: https://doi.org/10.1016/s0165-0327(98)00222-5.
71. Stein DJ, Hemmings S, Moolman-Smook H, Audenaert K. 5-HT2A: its role in frontally mediated executive function and related psychopathology. *CNS Spectr*. 2007;12:512–516. Available from: https://doi.org/10.1017/S1092852900021246.
72. Stahl SM. Mechanism of action of trazodone: a multifunctional drug. *CNS Spectr*. 2009;14:536–546. Available from: https://doi.org/10.1017/S1092852900024020.
73. Werneck ALDS, Rosso AL, Vincent MB. The use of an antagonist 5-HT2a/c for depression and motor function in Parkinson' disease. *Arq Neuropsiquiatr*. 2009;67:407–412.
74. Lin OA, Karim ZA, Vemana HP, Espinosa EVP, Khasawneh FT. The antidepressant 5-HT2A receptor antagonists pizotifen and cyproheptadine inhibit serotonin-enhanced platelet function. *PLoS One*. 2014;9:e87026. Available from: https://doi.org/10.1371/journal.pone.0087026.
75. Fiorentini A, Rovera C, Caldiroli A, et al. Efficacy of oral trazodone slow release following intravenous administration in depressed patients: a naturalistic study. *Riv Psichiatr*. 2018;53:261–266. Available from: https://doi.org/10.1708/3000.30005.
76. Kaul S, Shukla UA, Barbhaiya RH. Nonlinear pharmacokinetics of nefazodone after escalating single and multiple oral doses. *J Clin Pharmacol*. 1995;35:830–839. Available from: https://doi.org/10.1002/j.1552-4604.1995.tb04127.x.
77. Chen G, Højer AM, Areberg J, Nomikos G. Vortioxetine: clinical pharmacokinetics and drug interactions. *Clin Pharmacokinet*. 2018;57:673–686. Available from: https://doi.org/10.1007/s40262-017-0612-7.
78. Fagiolini A, Comandini A, Dell'Osso MC, Kasper S. Rediscovering trazodone for the treatment of major depressive disorder. *CNS Drugs*. 2012;26:1033–1049. Available from: https://doi.org/10.1007/s40263-012-0010-5.
79. Culpepper L. Reducing the burden of difficult-to-treat major depressive disorder: revisiting monoamine oxidase inhibitor therapy. *Prim Care Companion CNS Disord*. 2013;15. Available from: https://doi.org/10.4088/PCC.13r01515.
80. Rapaport MH. Dietary restrictions and drug interactions with monoamine oxidase inhibitors: the state of the art. *J Clin Psychiatry*. 2007;68(Suppl 8):42–46.
81. Müller T, Riederer P, Grünblatt E. Determination of monoamine oxidase A and B activity in long-term treated patients with Parkinson disease. *Clin Neuropharmacol*. 2017;40:208–211. Available from: https://doi.org/10.1097/wnf.0000000000000233.
82. Sandler M. Monoamine oxidase inhibitors in depression: history and mythology. *J Psychopharmacol*. 1990;4:136–139. Available from: https://doi.org/10.1177/026988119000400307.
83. Thomas SJ, Shin M, McInnis MG, Bostwick JR. Combination therapy with monoamine oxidase inhibitors and other antidepressants or stimulants: strategies for the management of treatment-resistant depression. *Pharmacotherapy*. 2015;35:433–449. Available from: https://doi.org/10.1002/phar.1576.
84. Thase ME. The role of monoamine oxidase inhibitors in depression treatment guidelines. *J Clin Psychiatry*. 2012;73(Suppl 1):10–16. Available from: https://doi.org/10.4088/JCP.11096su1c.02.

85. Quitkin F, Rifkin A, Klein DF. Monoamine oxidase inhibitors: a review of antidepressant effectiveness. *Arch Gen Psychiatry*. 1979;36:749–760. Available from: https://doi.org/10.1001/archpsyc.1979.01780070027003.
86. Finberg JPM, Rabey JM. Inhibitors of MAO-A and MAO-B in psychiatry and neurology. *Front Pharmacol*. 2016;7. Available from: https://doi.org/10.3389/fphar.2016.00340.
87. Kamp J, Van Velzen M, Olofsen E, Boon M, Dahan A, Niesters M. Pharmacokinetic and pharmacodynamic considerations for NMDA-receptor antagonist ketamine in the treatment of chronic neuropathic pain: an update of the most recent literature. *Expert Opin Drug Metab Toxicol*. 2019;15:1033–1041. Available from: https://doi.org/10.1080/17425255.2019.1689958.
88. Kokkinou M, Ashok AH, Howes OD. The effects of ketamine on dopaminergic function: *meta*-analysis and review of the implications for neuropsychiatric disorders. *Mol Psychiatry*. 2018;23:59–69. Available from: https://doi.org/10.1038/mp.2017.190.
89. Zanos P, Gould TD. Mechanisms of ketamine action as an antidepressant. *Mol Psychiatry*. 2018;23:801–811. Available from: https://doi.org/10.1038/mp.2017.255.
90. Bahji A, Vazquez GH, Zarate Jr CA. Comparative efficacy of racemic ketamine and esketamine for depression: a systematic review and *meta*-analysis. *J Affect Disord*. 2021;278:542–555. Available from: https://doi.org/10.1016/j.jad.2020.09.071.
91. Smith-Apeldoorn SY, Veraart JKE, Kamphuis J, et al. Oral esketamine for treatment-resistant depression: rationale and design of a randomized controlled trial. *BMC Psychiatry*. 2019;19:375. Available from: https://doi.org/10.1186/s12888-019-2359-1.
92. Matveychuk D, Thomas RK, Swainson J, et al. Ketamine as an antidepressant: overview of its mechanisms of action and potential predictive biomarkers. *Ther Adv Psychopharmacol*. 2020;10. Available from: https://doi.org/10.1177/2045125320916657. 2045125320916657.
93. Wang S-M, Han C, Bahk W-M, et al. Addressing the side effects of contemporary antidepressant drugs: a comprehensive review. *Chonnam Med J*. 2018;54:101–112. Available from: https://doi.org/10.4068/cmj.2018.54.2.101.
94. Danielson TJ. Monoamine oxidase inhibitors and tricyclic antidepressants. In: Mozayani A, Raymon LP, eds. *Handbook of Drug Interactions: A Clinical and Forensic Guide*. Totowa, NJ: Humana Press; 2004:149–173.
95. Szarmach J, Cubała WJ, Włodarczyk A, Wiglusz MS. Short-term ketamine administration in treatment-resistant depression: focus on cardiovascular safety. *Psychiatr Danub*. 2019;31:585–590.

Chapter 12

Mechanism on the action of drugs for heart failure

Waleed Hassan Almalki
Department of Pharmacology and Toxicology, College of Pharmacy, Umm Al-Qura University, Makkah, Saudi Arabia

Introduction

The pathology of heart failure (HF) is marked by the presence of impaired anatomy and mechanical capabilities that prevent the heart from filling or ejecting blood and by decreased ventricular compliance. The much more major reason for HF was drastically decreased left ventricular (LV) function. HF can be related to dysfunction of the different heart muscle layers like pericardium, myocardium, and endocardium which typically manifests with cardiac valvular disease or a combination of both. Enhanced hemodynamic pressure, ischemia-related impairment, ventricular remodeling, inappropriate biochemical stimuli, asymmetrical calcium pedaling in myocardial cells, high or insufficient noncellular component differentiation, rapid programmed cell death, and gene abnormalities are some of the main pathogenic pathways that contribute to HF.[1,2] Numerous cardiac failure pathways result in poor pump operation of the heart, which contributes to obstruction caused by mucus in the lungs and peripheral tissues. HF affects over 3 million US citizens, with over 400,000 new cases recorded each year. The symptoms and indices of HF vary greatly reliant on how rapidly it progresses and whether it affects the left, right, or both ventricles in a given individual.[3]

Classification of heart failure

Biventricular heart disease depends on location: it may be characterized as left or right ventricular or combined. The type of HF is determined by whether it occurs often or infrequently. Relying on the functioning state of the heart which usually divided into two main categories: HF type Iwhich retained the small volume of ejection and another is the HF type II which decreased the volume of ejection fraction. The LV cavity volume is normally

How Synthetic Drugs Work. DOI: https://doi.org/10.1016/B978-0-323-99855-0.00012-9

average, despite the thicker and robust LV wall, thus the fraction of LV mass end-diastolic volume is significant. HFpEF is defined as marginal HF if the EF stays between 41% and 49%, and increasing HF if the EF is more than 40%.[4] In those with HFrEF, the LV chamber is generally dilated, and the fraction of LV mass or end-diastolic volume is either normal or reduced. At the tissue level, HFpEF has a greater cardiomyocyte diameter and a greater myofibril size than HFrEF. Persons with HFrEF respond well to the standard pharmacological treatment regimen and have a positive impact when it comes to care and therapy. Patients with HFpEF, on the other hand, did not respond to typical pharmacological therapy, with the exception of nitrates, and hence had poor outcomes, especially during the decompensated phase of HF. Depending on cardiac output, HF is referred to as high- or low-output failures.[5] High-output loss is an uncommon syndrome characterized by an ambient cardiac index of 2.5–4.0 L/min/m^2 and poor systemic vascular tolerance. High production loss may also be caused by anemia, vascular propelling, thyroid illness, and vitamin B1 deficiency. Inadequate blood supply and stimulation stimulate the autonomic nervous system and the RAAS, causing ADH to be secreted, which leads to ventricular enlargement, negative ventricular remodeling, and HF. Failure usually results from the decreased output of blood at times of intense activity or inactivity, or excess metabolic request. Low-production loss is caused by LV impairment; right ventricle is heavily burdened with an acute pulmonary thromboembolism. Exercise intolerance in HFpEF is now believed to be caused by a loss in oxygen supply to or decreased oxygen consumption by exercising skeletal muscles. The arterial–venous oxygen content gap is used to measure oxygen utilization instead of decreased cardiac activity (CO).[6–8] Exercise therapy tends to be a rational and important factor in enhancing the inflammatory disturbance, discharging higher cardiac filling compressions, restoring exercise ability, increasing standard of living, and lowering disease burden and death correlated with HF, considering the slowed oxygen absorption kinetics and peripheral muscle function dysfunction in HF. As a consequence, exercise activity, often high intensity rather than low, was shown to increase the level of oxygen utilization or VO2 in HFpEF individuals without influencing endothelial activity.[9,10]

The practical grouping of the New York Heart Association (NYHA) is divided into four classes:

Class I: HF does not regulate physical exercise and does not induce problems when regular exercise activity is done.

Class II: HF limits physical exercise slightly; patients are relaxed at resting, but frequent regular exercise triggers HF symptoms.

Class III: HF induces severe physical limitations; individuals are relaxed at resting, but also less than normal exercise triggers HF symptoms.

Class IV: People with HF are unlikely to engage in any physical exercise without experiencing HF symptoms or have symptoms even though they are at ease.

When evaluating coronary risk, researcher uses the ACC/AHA staging scheme, which describes the four stages of HF.

Stage A: Higher chance of HF with no underlying cardiovascular disease or signs of HF.

Stage B: Structural heart attack, which doesn't have the typical signs of cardiac disease or failure of the function of heart.

Stage C: Acute structural heart attack with prominent signs and symptoms of cardiac dysfunction failure the function of heart.

Stage D: Structural heart attack with prominent signs and symptoms of cardiac dysfunction failure the function of heart that necessitates specialized treatment.[11,12]

Etiology

HF is a pathophysiologic complex linked to heart impairment and a typical end state for several cardiac problems. There are numerous reasons for heart problems, and the exact cause of each particular individual must still be determined. In particular, excessive workloads put mostly on heart may lead to HF, like pulmonary congestion or pressure overload, restricted heart loading, myocyte depletion, or reduced myocyte smooth muscle contraction. Most of these triggers will set in motion a chain of events that will be discussed later.[13–15] Each one of these triggers may be caused by a variety of pathways. In developing nations, for example, cell death due to an obstructed artery seems to be the most frequent cause of myocyte failure. Genetic abnormalities, on the other hand, may cause myocyte depletion.[16]

Pathophysiology

The pathophysiology of heart disease is complicated and needs many layers of understanding. Conventionally, study has concentrated on the hemodynamic modifications of a weakened heart, treating the heart as though it were a separate entity. Even so, research into the dying heart has highlighted the significance of recognizing molecular modifications and neurohormonal connections between the heart as well as different organ systems.[17–19]

Changes in hemodynamics

HF may be triggered by deteriorating systolic or diastolic activity, or a mixture of both, from a hemodynamic viewpoint. The isovolumic systolic pressure curve of the pressure–volume relationship is moved downhill in systolic dysfunction. This lowers the heart's stroke volume and, as a result, lowers myocardial contractility. The heart will use three compensatory pathways to preserve cardiac output: Initially, raised preload (blood return to the heart) can result in enhanced sarcomere contraction. The heart beats at rather than at in the pressure–volume relationship, and stroke improves slightly at the expense of elevated end-diastolic pressure. Second, increased catecholamine production increases cardiac performance by raising heart rate and moving the systolic isovolumetric curve to the left[20,21] (Fig. 12.1).

Finally, heart muscle hypertrophy and ventricular volume will also rise, allowing the diastolic curve to move to the right. While each of those compensatory mechanisms will sustain cardiac activity momentarily, their effectiveness is minimal, and if the underlying cause of systolic dysfunction is not addressed, the heart will eventually fail. The location of the systolic isovolumic curve persists intact in diastolic impairment (myocyte contractility is preserved). The diastolic pressure–volume curve, on the other hand, is moved to the left, resulting in a rise in LV end-diastolic pressure and HF symptoms. Any condition that induces reduced tension, reduced elastic recoil, or enhanced ventricle stiffness may cause diastolic disturbance. By altering all three dimensions, hypertension also causes compensatory rises in LV wall thickness which may induce diastolic malfunction. Ischemia, or a shortage of blood to the myocardial cells, may also induce diastolic impairment by reducing relaxation.[22] If the ischemic stroke is serious, as in an atrial fibrillation, long-term destruction to the myocardium can arise, with fibrosis replacing contractile cells, resulting in systolic impairment. HF signs are caused by a fusion of systolic and diastolic malfunction in the majority of cases.[23–25]

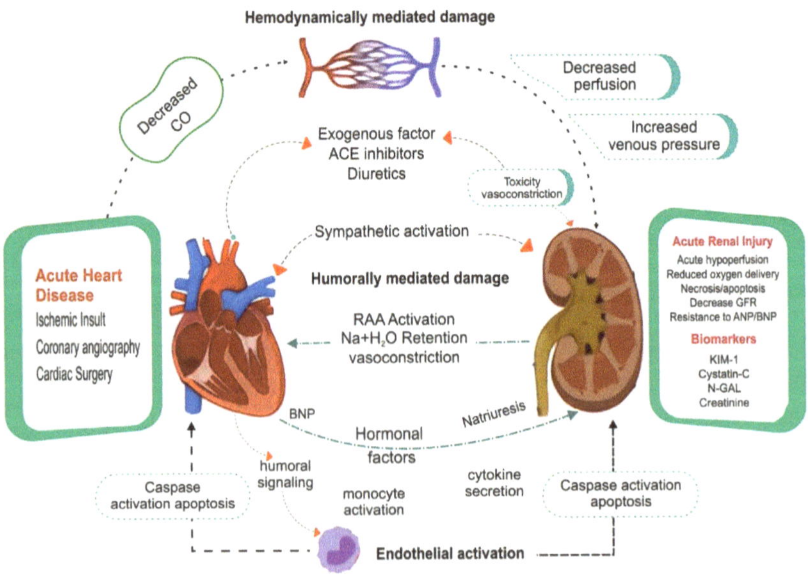

FIGURE 12.1 Changes in hemodynamics leading HF. *HF*, Heart failure.

Changes of neurohormones

Enhanced release of endogenous neurohormones and cytokines is found during a cardiac attack. At first, a rise in adrenergic and renin–angiotensin system activation produces a compensatory reaction that keeps vital organs perfused. These improvements, nevertheless, will lead to a gradual degradation in cardiac performance over time. Early on in the course of heart disease, there is an improvement in sympathetic function. Increased cardiac contraction and heart rate are caused by excessive plasma norepinephrine concentrations, which momentarily help regulate cardiac activity. Continued changes, on the other hand, result in elevated preload (due to venous vasoconstriction) and afterload (due to arterial vasoconstriction), which can exacerbate HF. Furthermore, sympathetic impulsiveness results in dangerous cellular events, which will be addressed in the next segment.[26,27] Reduced kidney blood pressure raises the synthesis of angiotensin II and promotes the secretion of renin. Both angiotensin II and sympathetic stimulation induce efferent renal arteriolar vascular constriction, which helps keep the glomerular filtration rate up despite a lower cardiac performance. Angiotensin II causes sodium resorption and potassium excretion by the kidneys by stimulating aldosterone production. Even so, persistent impulsiveness of the renin–angiotensin system causes extreme vascular constriction, elevated afterload, with a subsequent decrease in cardiac production and glomerular filtration volume, resulting in a vicious cycle. A rise in the secretion of vasopressin from the posterior pituitary gland is linked to HF. One other strong vasoconstrictor is vasopressin, which facilitates water reabsorption in the renal tubules. The production of cytokines, as well as other circulating peptides, is linked to HF. In response, to damage macrophages, lymphocytes, monocytes, and endothelial cells secrete a complex group of proteins known as cytokines. The two main classes of cytokines that can play a pathophysiologic function in heart problems are interleukins (ILs) and tumor necrosis factor (TNF).[28] Upregulation of the TNF gene was discovered, along with a rise in circulating TNF plasma concentration in the patient of HF. TNF seems to play an important part in the next section's discussion of myocyte hypertrophy and cell death (apoptosis). In vitro evidence suggests that IL-1 can hasten myocyte hypertrophy. The potent vasoconstrictor endothelin, which is produced by endothelial cells, is another peptide essential for facilitating a few of the pathophysiologic symptoms seen in HF. Too much endothelin secretion may be to blame for hypertension in the pulmonary arteries seen in patients with LVHF, according to initial findings. Endothelin is also related to interstitial myocyte development and collagen deposition[29,30] (Fig. 12.2).

Changes in the cell

Alterations in Ca2 + processing, adrenergic receptors, the contractile apparatus, and myocyte composition are also part of the pathophysiologic alterations at the cellular stage. Both Ca2 + delivery to the contractile apparatus and Ca2 + reuptake by the sarcoplasmic reticulum are reduced in HF. Some researchers have observed lower rates of messenger ribonucleic acid (mRNA) for the advanced Ca2 + release channels. Likewise, myocytes from weakening hearts have lower concentrations of mRNA for phospholamban and Ca2 + -ATPase, two sarcoplasmic reticulum proteins. In the human heart, there are two types of adrenergic receptors. Cardiomyocytes hypertrophy is caused by alpha1-adrenergic receptors, and the levels of these receptors are significantly elevated in HF. As a consequence of chronic sympathetic activation, cardiac failure is related to severe adrenergic receptor desensitization. Reduced expression of β1-adrenergic receptors, uncoupling of the signal transduction pathway downstream, and upregulation of inhibitory G proteins are all involved in this impact. Both of these modifications result in a decline in myocardium contractility.[31,32]

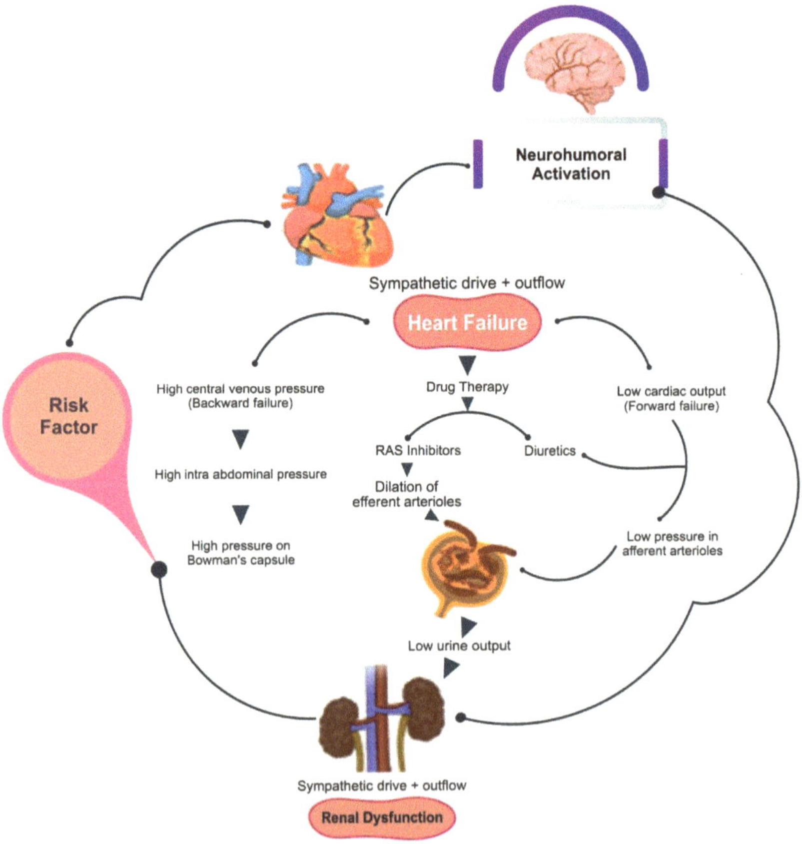

FIGURE 12.2 Role of RAS and diuretics in HF. *RAS*, Renin angiotensin system; *HF*, Heart failure.

Management of heart failure

Treatment for HF focuses on improving prognosis and lowering longevity, as well as relieving complications and overturning or reducing heart and peripheral dysfunction to reduce the risk of mortality. Other targets of treatment for in-hospital patients include reducing the duration of stay and eventual readmission to minimize organ system disruption and properly managing comorbidities that can lead to poor prognosis.

ACC/AHA revised recommendations from 2013, HFSA guidelines from 2010, and the 2008 ESC guidelines, all prescribe the following for various types of HF patients, based on differing levels of evidence[33] (Table 12.1).

Diuretics

Loop or high ceiling diuretics such as torsemide, bumetanide, and furosemide reversibly block the Na + K + 2Cl symporter in the thick ascending limb of the loop of Henle. Ethacrynic acid, for example, belongs to a second useful class of these chemicals that works exclusively in the tubule lumen and has a sluggish beginning of action and only limited reversibility. Loop diuretics work by preventing chloride, sodium, potassium, and hydrogen ions from being reabsorbed in the ascending Henle loop. Thiazides have a more distal effect on sodium and chloride reabsorption. Loop diuretics have no effect on this cotransporter.[34] When the renin–angiotensin–aldosterone pathway is active, more sodium enters the distal tubules, promoting

TABLE 12.1 List of various classes of drugs for management of heart failure.

Sr. No.	Category	Examples
1.	ACE inhibitors	Enalapril, lisinopril, quinapril, captopril
2.	Angiotensin-receptor blockers	Losartan, candesartan, valsartan
3.	Diuretics	Furosemide, chlorothiazide, bumetanide, amiloride
4.	Angiotensin-receptor neprilysin inhibitors	Valsartan, sacubitril
5.	If channel blocker	Ivabradine
6.	Beta-blockers	Carvedilol, metoprolol, bisoprolol
7.	Aldosterone antagonists	Eplerenone, spironolactone
8.	Others	Cholesterol-lowering drugs, anticoagulants

potassium exchange. In the distal renal tubule, thiazides may promote potassium active excretion. For symptomatic chronic HF, diuretics were originally the mainstay of therapy, but they are currently only used alone. They reduce symptoms and, in most cases, effort resistance when taken with angiotensin-converting enzyme inhibitors, blockers, and digoxin.[35]

Vasodilators

Vasodilators dilate or inhibit blood channel constriction, enabling more blood to flow to the body's various organs. Several vasodilators work by attaching to receptors on blood vessel endothelial cells to cause calcium release. The enzyme nitric oxide synthase (NO synthase), which converts L-arginine to NO, is activated by calcium. It may exit the endothelial cell and reach the smooth muscle cells[36] of the vascular system by diffusion. GTP is activated by NO and converted to cGMP. The myosin-light chain phosphatase enzyme is then activated, and one phosphate is removed from myosin and actin filaments. Vascular smooth muscle relaxes when myosin and actin filaments are dephosphorylated.[37,38]

Digoxin

In the two major ways that digoxin is used, it affects the two distinct systems of the body.

Positive ionotropic

It raises the force of heart contraction by blocking the Na^{+}-K^{+} ATPase pump in the myocardium, an enzyme that controls ion movement through the heart, in a reversible manner. Digoxin raises intracellular sodium levels, resulting in a calcium influx in the heart and enhanced contractility. Cardiac function increases as ventricular filling pressures are reduced.

Atrioventricular node inhibition

On AV node of heart digoxin will produce the vagomimetic action. The parasympathetic nervous system is activated, which reduces heart rate by slowing the conduction of electrical impulses in the atrioventricular (AV) node. As calcium levels rise, the AV node's refractory period increases, lengthening phase 4 and phase 0 of the cardiac action potential. Slower AV node conduction is linked to a lower ventricular response.[39,40]

Angiotensin-converting enzyme inhibitors

ACE inhibitors block vasoconstriction by inhibiting the conversion of angiotensin I to angiotensin II by blocking the angiotensin-converting enzyme. The angiotensin conversion enzyme is in charge of converting angiotensin I into angiotensin II, which causes vasoconstriction. Angiotensin II is a potent vasoconstrictor that is also accountable for vascular tissue hypertrophy and aldosterone production. The narrowing of arteries caused by hypertrophy of vascular tissues places further pressure on the heart. Water retention is mainly caused by aldosterone secretion, which can increase vascular fluid volume and thereby enhance the workload on the heart. As a result, inhibiting angiotensin II lowers blood pressure in the heart, reducing the workload on the heart. Another advantage of ACE inhibitors is that they increase blood bradykinin levels by reducing their degradation. Bradykinin is the hormone that causes vasodilation.[41,42]

Angiotensin-II blockers (AT1 antagonists)

Angiotensin II interacts with a subset of cell-bound angiotensin receptors. Angiotensin-II antagonists work by blocking the AT1 receptor, which has been shown to cause angiotensin II's negative effects in HF patients. Kininase 2, an enzyme that produces the inflammatory mediator bradykinin, is similar to ACE. ARBs are thought to minimize adverse effects and maybe improve treatment effectiveness by inhibiting angiotensin II selectively via competitive antagonism of the angiotensin-II receptors. ARBs work by antagonizing and inhibiting aldosterone production, catecholamine discharge, and arginine. Vasopressin discharge, hypertrophic water intake, and lowered blood pressure reactivity are caused by angiotensin II-induced vasoconstriction.[43,44]

Beta-blockers

The effects of excessive sympathetic activation are counteracted by beta-blockers. In patients with chronic heart disease, beta-blocker treatment improves LV systolic and diastolic activity, reverse remodeling, heart rate modulation, successful reduction of malignant arrhythmias, and lowering of both cardiac afterload and preload. Prolonged neurohormonal activation has negative impacts on the weakening heart's hemodynamics, as well as apoptosis, arrhythmia, and decreased myocardial blood supply. Beta-blocker therapy for a long period can relieve complications, boost health status, and lower the likelihood of mortality, as well as the overall risk of death and hospitalization.[45] Metoprolol is a sympathomimetic antagonist of the second generation with no inherent sympathomimetic operation. It has been shown to increase cardiac function, LV remodeling, and exercise capability in congestive heart failure (CHF) patients, as well as reduce HF symptoms.

Carvedilol is a nonspecific β-adrenoreceptor antagonist that also inhibits α1-receptors. It has novel antioxidant and antiproliferative properties, unlike other blockers, which may lead to its protective effects in HF patients.[46]

Calcium channel blockers

It is yet to be shown that these agents can be used for the treatment of CHF, but the nonrate-limiting/unrestrict rate-adverse calcium antagonists may be administered to patients with heart disease. Calcium channel blockers bind to the L-type voltage-gated calcium channels in vascular smooth muscle, blocking calcium from flowing inward. A wide range of antagonists, or important physiologic effects: endogenous calcium channel agents can be grouped into two classes based on their primary activities and channel binding. Nondihydropyridines block the sinoatrial and AV nodes, decreasing cardiac conduction and contractility. Hypertension, as well as oxygen consumption and tachydysrhythmia rates, may be addressed.[47] Dihydropyridines are largely peripheral vasodilators with no direct action on the heart at therapeutic doses, which explains why they are beneficial for hypertension, postintracranial hemorrhage–induced vasospasm, and migraines. When taken orally, calcium channel antagonists are quickly absorbed, although many have limited bioavailability owing to hepatic first-pass metabolism, particularly through CYP3A4. Calcium channel antagonists are highly protein-bound and have a wide delivery range[48] (Fig. 12.3).

Newer agents

Heart disease may be managed in the early development by a variety of agents. Neurohormonal imbalance is the main problem in patients with heart

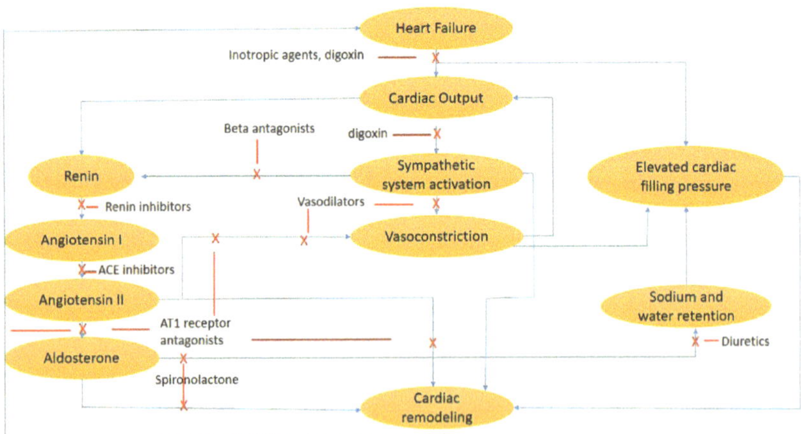

FIGURE 12.3 Mechanism of action of drugs on HF. *HF*, Heart failure.

disease. The atrial natriuretic peptide (ANP) and BNP work on the vasodilator, diuretic, and RAAS (renin and atrial natriuretic peptide) levels while suppressing renin–angiotensin system. The enzyme neutral endopeptidase (NEP or neparlysin) degraded the ANP and brain-type natriuretic peptide (BNP).[49] If inhibitors of this enzyme can be found, then studies may explore their use in treating the HF. An initial positive research report on NEP inhibitors found significant hemodynamic and neurohormonal results as well as increases in exercise tolerance. These findings have also been seen elsewhere. While the ecadotril problem that occurred along with these agents ended the further study of these agents, it was in itself very toxic. Uses of drugs that prevent both Angiotensin-converting enzyme (ACE) and NEP, such as omapatrilat are shown to be both cardio and neurovascular beneficial in the cases of HF.[49,50]

Conclusion

Preventative steps treating the root cause of the condition should be used in the pharmacological care of patients with CHF. In patients who have pulmonary or peripheral congestion, loop diuretics are needed. ACE inhibitors and beta-blockers will decrease death rates and avoid the worsening of symptoms and the need for hospitalization in HF patients if they are well tolerated. Spironolactone at a low dosage improves recovery in patients with serious heart disease who continue to have complications despite routine treatment. Before the function of angiotensin-II antagonists can be proven, more research is required. Patients with heart disease should see a significant improvement in their outcomes if these procedures are implemented effectively on an individual basis.

References

1. Ahmad FA, Petrie MC, McMurray JJV, Lang NN. Personalized medicine and hospitalization for heart failure: if we understand it, we may be successful in treating it. *Eur J Heart Fail.* 2019;21:699–702. Available from: https://doi.org/10.1002/ejhf.1463.
2. Alpert CM, Smith MA, Hummel SL, Hummel EK. Symptom burden in heart failure: assessment, impact on outcomes, and management. *Heart Fail Rev.* 2017;22:25–39. Available from: https://doi.org/10.1007/s10741-016-9581-4.
3. Andrès E, Zulfiqar AA, Talha S, et al. Telemedicine in elderly patients with heart failure. *Geriatr Psychol Neuropsychiatr Vieil.* 2018;16:341–348. Available from: https://doi.org/10.1684/pnv.2018.0758.
4. Anguita M. Heart failure and evidence-based medicine: not everything is in the guidelines. *Rev Esp Cardiol (Engl Ed).* 2020;73:802–803. Available from: https://doi.org/10.1016/j.rec.2020.03.025.
5. Ashraf H, Rosenthal JL. Right heart failure: causes and clinical epidemiology. *Cardiol Clin.* 2020;38:175–183. Available from: https://doi.org/10.1016/j.ccl.2020.01.008.

6. Bordoni B, Marelli F, Morabito B, Sacconi B. Depression and anxiety in patients with chronic heart failure. *Future Cardiol.* 2018;14:115–119. Available from: https://doi.org/10.2217/fca-2017-0073.
7. Rawat S, Gupta G, Pathak S, et al. Current biological and pharmacological updates on wogonin. *EXCLI J.* 2020;19:635–640.
8. Samuel VP, Dahiya R, Singh Y, et al. Metformin: a salutary candidate for colorectal cancer treatment in patients with diabetes. *J Environ Pathol Toxicol Oncol.* 2019;38.
9. Samuel VP, Gupta G, Dahiya R, Jain DA, Mishra A, Dua K. Current update on preclinical and clinical studies of resveratrol, a naturally occurring phenolic compound. *Crit Rev Eukaryotic Gene Expression.* 2019;29.
10. Singh Y, Gupta G, Shrivastava B, et al. Calcitonin gene-related peptide (CGRP): a novel target for Alzheimer's disease. *CNS Neurosci Ther.* 2017;23:457–461.
11. Coniglio AC, Mentz RJ. Sleep breathing disorders in heart failure. *Heart Fail Clin.* 2020;16:45–51. Available from: https://doi.org/10.1016/j.hfc.2019.08.009.
12. Corrà U, Agostoni PG, Anker SD, et al. Role of cardiopulmonary exercise testing in clinical stratification in heart failure. A position paper from the Committee on Exercise Physiology and Training of the Heart Failure Association of the European Society of Cardiology. *Eur J Heart Fail.* 2018;20:3–15. Available from: https://doi.org/10.1002/ejhf.979.
13. Cresci S, Pereira NL, Ahmad F, et al. Heart failure in the era of precision medicine: a scientific statement from the American Heart Association. *Circ Genom Precis Med.* 2019;12:458–485. Available from: https://doi.org/10.1161/hcg.0000000000000058.
14. Singhvi G, Girdhar V, Patil S, Gupta G, Hansbro PM, Dua K. Microbiome as therapeutics in vesicular delivery. *Biomed Pharmacother.* 2018;104:738–741.
15. Tiwari J, Gupta G, Dahiya R, et al. Recent update on biological activities and pharmacological actions of liraglutide. *EXCLI J.* 2017.
16. Crespo-Leiro MG, Metra M, Lund LH, et al. Advanced heart failure: a position statement of the Heart Failure Association of the European Society of Cardiology. *Eur J Heart Fail.* 2018;20:1505–1535. Available from: https://doi.org/10.1002/ejhf.1236.
17. de Gregorio C. Physical training and cardiac rehabilitation in heart failure patients. *Adv Exp Med Biol.* 2018;1067:161–181. Available from: https://doi.org/10.1007/5584_2018_144.
18. Gupta G, Kazmi I, Afzal M, et al. Sedative, antiepileptic and antipsychotic effects of *Viscum album* L. (Loranthaceae) in mice and rats. *J Ethnopharmacol.* 2012;141:810–816.
19. Verma RK, Sriramaneni R, Pandey M, Chaudhury H, Gorain B, Gupta G. Current updates on pharmacological roles of glucagon-like peptide 1 in obesity. *Panminerva Med.* 2018;60:224–225.
20. DeVore AD, Wosik J, Hernandez AF. The future of wearables in heart failure patients. *JACC Heart Fail.* 2019;7:922–932. Available from: https://doi.org/10.1016/j.jchf.2019.08.008.
21. Dewan P, Rørth R, Raparelli V, et al. Sex-related differences in heart failure with preserved ejection fraction. *Circ Heart Fail.* 2019;12:e006539. Available from: https://doi.org/10.1161/circheartfailure.119.006539.
22. Eisenberg E, Di Palo KE, Piña IL. Sex differences in heart failure. *Clin Cardiol.* 2018;41:211–216. Available from: https://doi.org/10.1002/clc.22917.
23. Emani S. Remote monitoring to reduce heart failure readmissions. *Curr Heart Fail Rep.* 2017;14:40–47. Available from: https://doi.org/10.1007/s11897-017-0315-2.

24. Gupta G, Jia Jia T, Yee Woon L, Kumar Chellappan D, Candasamy M, Dua K. Pharmacological evaluation of antidepressant-like effect of genistein and its combination with amitriptyline: an acute and chronic study. *Adv Pharm Sci*. 2015;2015.
25. Gupta G, Tiwari J, Dahiya R, Sharma RK, Mishra A, Dua K. Recent updates on neuro-pharmacological effects of luteolin. *EXCLI J*. 2018.
26. Ewen S, Nikolovska A, Zivanovic I, Kindermann I, Böhm M. [Chronic heart failure – new insights]. *Dtsch Med Wochenschr*. 2016;141:1560–1564. Available from: https://doi.org/10.1055/s-0042-102706.
27. Feldman AM, Kontos CD, McClung JM, Gerhard GS, Khalili K, Cheung JY. Precision medicine for heart failure: lessons from oncology. *Circ Heart Fail*. 2017;10. Available from: https://doi.org/10.1161/circheartfailure.117.004202.
28. Frederix I, Vanderlinden L, Verboven AS, et al. Long-term impact of a six-month telemedical care programme on mortality, heart failure readmissions and healthcare costs in patients with chronic heart failure. *J Telemed Telecare*. 2019;25:286–293. Available from: https://doi.org/10.1177/1357633x18774632.
29. Fridman MD, Mital S. Perspective on precision medicine in paediatric heart failure. *Clin Sci (Lond)*. 2017;131:439–448. Available from: https://doi.org/10.1042/cs20160414.
30. Galinier M, Cariou E, Lairez O, et al. [Place of natriuretic peptides in the early diagnosis of heart failure in community medicine]. *Presse Med*. 2018;47:804–810. Available from: https://doi.org/10.1016/j.lpm.2018.09.003.
31. Gorter TM, van Veldhuisen DJ, Bauersachs J, et al. Right heart dysfunction and failure in heart failure with preserved ejection fraction: mechanisms and management. Position statement on behalf of the Heart Failure Association of the European Society of Cardiology. *Eur J Heart Fail*. 2018;20:16–37. Available from: https://doi.org/10.1002/ejhf.1029.
32. Harjola VP, Mullens W, Banaszewski M, et al. Organ dysfunction, injury and failure in acute heart failure: from pathophysiology to diagnosis and management. A review on behalf of the Acute Heart Failure Committee of the Heart Failure Association (HFA) of the European Society of Cardiology (ESC). *Eur J Heart Fail*. 2017;19:821–836. Available from: https://doi.org/10.1002/ejhf.872.
33. Koehler F, Koehler K, Deckwart O, et al. Efficacy of telemedical interventional management in patients with heart failure (TIM-HF2): a randomised, controlled, parallel-group, unmasked trial. *Lancet*. 2018;392:1047–1057. Available from: https://doi.org/10.1016/s0140-6736(18)31880-4.
34. Kurmani S, Squire I. Acute heart failure: definition, classification and epidemiology. *Curr Heart Fail Rep*. 2017;14:385–392. Available from: https://doi.org/10.1007/s11897-017-0351-y.
35. Long B, Koyfman A, Gottlieb M. Management of heart failure in the emergency department setting: an evidence-based review of the literature. *J Emerg Med*. 2018;55:635–646. Available from: https://doi.org/10.1016/j.jemermed.2018.08.002.
36. Banerjee A, Roy D, Mazumdar H, Karmakar S, Bhowmik R, Biswas N, Roy A, Dey S, & Manna K, MicroRNA 155:145 ratio as a marker of atherogenic tilt manifested across different age groups and risk factor profiles. *Eur. Heart J*. 2022;43(Supplement_1): ehab849.063. Available from: https://doi.org/10.1093/eurheartj/ehab849.063.
37. Long B, Koyfman A, Gottlieb M. Diagnosis of acute heart failure in the emergency department: an evidence-based review. *West J Emerg Med*. 2019;20:875–884. Available from: https://doi.org/10.5811/westjem.2019.9.43732.
38. Maeder MT, Buser M, Brenner R, Rickli H. [Heart failure with preserved ejection fraction (HFpEF)]. *Ther Umsch*. 2018;75:161–169. Available from: https://doi.org/10.1024/0040-5930/a000983.

39. Martínez F, Martínez-Ibañez L, Pichler G, Ruiz A, Redon J. Multimorbidity and acute heart failure in internal medicine. *Int J Cardiol.* 2017;232:208–215. Available from: https://doi.org/10.1016/j.ijcard.2017.01.020.
40. Mazurek JA, Jessup M. Understanding heart failure. *Heart Fail Clin.* 2017;13:1–19. Available from: https://doi.org/10.1016/j.hfc.2016.07.001.
41. Menachem JN, Schlendorf KH, Mazurek JA, et al. Advanced heart failure in adults with congenital heart disease. *JACC Heart Fail.* 2020;8:87–99. Available from: https://doi.org/10.1016/j.jchf.2019.08.012.
42. Metra M, Teerlink JR. Heart failure. *Lancet.* 2017;390:1981–1995. Available from: https://doi.org/10.1016/s0140-6736(17)31071-1.
43. Mullens W, Damman K, Harjola VP, et al. The use of diuretics in heart failure with congestion – a position statement from the Heart Failure Association of the European Society of Cardiology. *Eur J Heart Fail.* 2019;21:137–155. Available from: https://doi.org/10.1002/ejhf.1369.
44. Mullens W, Damman K, Testani JM, et al. Evaluation of kidney function throughout the heart failure trajectory – a position statement from the Heart Failure Association of the European Society of Cardiology. *Eur J Heart Fail.* 2020;22:584–603. Available from: https://doi.org/10.1002/ejhf.1697.
45. Murphy SP, Ibrahim NE, Januzzi Jr JL. Heart failure with reduced ejection fraction: a review. *JAMA.* 2020;324:488–504. Available from: https://doi.org/10.1001/jama.2020.10262.
46. Napoli C, Benincasa G, Donatelli F, Ambrosio G. Precision medicine in distinct heart failure phenotypes: focus on clinical epigenetics. *Am Heart J.* 2020;224:113–128. Available from: https://doi.org/10.1016/j.ahj.2020.03.007.
47. Parikh KS, Sharma K, Fiuzat M, et al. Heart failure with preserved ejection fraction expert panel report: current controversies and implications for clinical trials. *JACC Heart Fail.* 2018;6:619–632. Available from: https://doi.org/10.1016/j.jchf.2018.06.008.
48. Piotrowicz E, Piepoli MF, Jaarsma T, et al. Telerehabilitation in heart failure patients: the evidence and the pitfalls. *Int J Cardiol.* 2016;220:408–413. Available from: https://doi.org/10.1016/j.ijcard.2016.06.277.
49. Prabhu S, Voskoboinik A, Kaye DM, Kistler PM. Atrial fibrillation and heart failure – cause or effect? *Heart Lung Circ.* 2017;26:967–974. Available from: https://doi.org/10.1016/j.hlc.2017.05.117.
50. Seferović PM, Fragasso G, Petrie M, et al. Sodium-glucose co-transporter 2 inhibitors in heart failure: beyond glycaemic control. A position paper of the Heart Failure Association of the European Society of Cardiology. *Eur J Heart Fail.* 2020;22:1495–1503. Available from: https://doi.org/10.1002/ejhf.1954.

Chapter 13

Mechanism of action of antiarrhythmic drugs

Hindol Mazumdar[1], Rudranil Bhowmik[1], Md. Adil Shaharyar[1], Avishek Mandal[1], Kumar Anand[1], Susmita Patra[2], Reshma Kumari[1], Sandipan Jana[1], Pallab Kanti Haldar[1] and Sanmoy Karmakar[1]

[1]Bioeuivalence Study Centre, Department of Pharmaceutical Technology, Jadavpur University, Kolkata, West Bengal, India, [2]Department of Pharmaceutical Technology, Adamas University, Barasat, Kolkata, West Bengal, India

Introduction

Cardiac electrophysiology as a scientific field began when Einthoven discovered the electrocardiogram (ECG) at the beginning of the 20th century. It was revealed by recording of cellular membrane currents that the body surface ECG is the total of the various cellular action potentials in both the atria and ventricles of the heart.[1] In the late 1960s, development of the intracavitary recordings marked the beginning of modern clinical electrophysiology. The process of adoption of various technologies to ablate cardiac tissue within the 1990s marked the birth of interventional cardiac electrophysiology.

The evaluation of patients with possible arrhythmias is extremely individualized. However, two key features—the patient's history and ECG records—are important in giving direction to the diagnostic evaluation and following treatment.[2] The clinical examination is always focused on determining whether there is cardiopulmonary disease that is related to some specific cardiac arrhythmias. The absence of significant markers often suggests a nonlethal cause of an arrhythmia. An important part in the diagnosis of patients with arrhythmias is the principled use of various noninvasive diagnostic tests, the most important factor still being the ECG records, especially if it is recorded at the time of symptoms.

In the last 20 years, various heritable arrhythmias' genetic basis has been explained, giving us important insights into the mechanisms not only of those rare arrhythmias but also of various other rhythm disturbances seen in additional common sorts of heart condition.[3]

Pharmacological therapy was the main treatment for cardiac arrhythmias for decades, including supraventricular and ventricular tachyarrhythmias.

How Synthetic Drugs Work. DOI: https://doi.org/10.1016/B978-0-323-99855-0.00013-0

However, increasing knowledge about the potential adverse effects of the antiarrhythmic agents, together with the emergence of new and more effective nonpharmacological approaches of good safety profile to the treatment of cardiac arrhythmias, has led to a considerable decline of antiarrhythmic drug therapy in the last few decades.[4]

However, some of the antiarrhythmic drugs when used appropriately are still effective options for the management of various cardiac arrhythmic conditions. This chapter discusses the pathophysiology of arrhythmia, followed by the molecular pharmacology of the classical antiarrhythmic drugs with a focus on those whose efficacy is supported by recent research.

Signs and symptoms of cardiac arrhythmia

General approach

Patients who have cardiac arrhythmias show a good spectrum of clinical signs, starting from various asymptomatic incidental ECG abnormalities to survival from sudden cardiac arrest (SCA). The features that are present may vary with circumstances, and arrhythmias are common within the setting of cardiovascular (CV) and medical diseases, resulting in overlap of symptoms and signs. The history is vital to directing the evaluation of patients. Generally, the more dangerous symptoms present, the more aggressive are the evaluation and treatment for those symptoms.[5] When a patient's loss of consciousness is believed to be of cardiac origin, it typically requires an exhaustive search for the etiology and might require invasive, device-based diagnostic evaluation and treatment. If structural heart disease and myocardial infarct (MI) is there, it often warrants a change in the approach to the management of syncope or ventricular arrhythmias.[6]

A case history of a big arrhythmia might not directly inform the prognosis of a patient, but it should alert the practitioner to the likelihood of a heritable trait which will increase susceptibility to development of an arrhythmia.[7]

Palpitations

Palpitation is the phenomenon which is caused by a rapidly increased pulse rate, irregularities in cardiac rhythm, or a rise within the force of cardiac contraction, as occurs with a post–extrasystolic beat; however, this phenomenon also can exist within the setting of a totally normal heart rhythm. Patients who complain of palpitations describe the sensation as an unpleasant awareness of a forceful, irregular, or rapid beating of the guts. Many patients are extremely conscious of any irregularity of cardiac type, whereas others are not, even to long continuation of a rapid ventricular tachycardia (VT) or fibrillation with rapid rates. The latter is especially noteworthy because if untreated, it may lead to stroke or may produce a cardiomyopathy induced by tachycardia.[8]

Those atrial or ventricular complexes which are premature in nature constitute the biggest common causes of palpitations. If they are frequent, or particularly if a sustained tachycardia is present, patients will likely possess additional symptoms, like light-headedness, syncope or near-syncope, chest discomfort, fatigue, or shortness of breath. The context and symptoms related to palpitations can be diagnostically and prognostically informative. Low-risk features include isolated palpitations not induced by exercise, the absence of heart conditions of structural nature or symptoms like syncope or pain, no case history of sudden cardiac death (SCD), and a traditional 12-lead ECG. Associated symptoms, like syncope or pain, the presence of structural heart condition, or a documented arrhythmia, and family history of SCD could also be related to a more ominous explanation for palpitations.[9]

The onset and offset of palpitations can suggest the etiology of the arrhythmia. A sudden, abrupt, onset, "like a light-weight switch turning on," is according to a paroxysmal tachycardia like atrioventricular (AV) nodal reentrant tachycardia, whereas gradual speeding and slowing are more according to atrial or sinus tachycardia. However, even tachycardias that start abruptly can begin and end with extra beats appearing to possess a more gradual onset and offset.[6]

Patients with bradyarrhythmias may have symptoms of low cardiac output, including fatigue, weakness, dizziness, dyspnea, and syncope. Palpitations may result from an increased force of contraction related to longer ventricular filling times and should be prominent symptoms in bradycardias.[10]

Syncope and presyncope

Syncope, commonly mentioned as "fainting" or "passing out," is a transient, self-limited loss of consciousness and posture resulting from a drop by vital sign with cerebral hypoperfusion and will always prompt an enquiry for a cause. It is important to distinguish syncope from other causes of transient loss of consciousness, such as seizures, metabolic disorders [hypoglycemia, hypoxia (e.g., airline decompression)], intoxication, cataplexy, and pseudosyncope.[11]

The etiologies of true syncope are varied with similarly diverse prognoses. The unheralded loss of consciousness in any patient, even if benign from the cardiac perspective, is often dangerous depending on the circumstances (e.g., while driving a vehicle, at the highest of a flight of stairs). However, because syncope is often a harbinger of SCD, it is important to spot cardiac from more benign causes of syncope (Table 13.1).[12]

The onset of syncope is rapid when it is caused by an arrhythmia, and therefore the duration of the same majorly remains brief and is not typically followed by a postictal state of confusion. Bodily injury can occur if the patient falls while unconscious.[13]

TABLE 13.1 Criteria for immediate evaluation—syncope.

Presence of structural heart disease	Heart failure
	Significant left ventricular dysfunction of hypertrophy
	Prior myocardial infarction
Clinical features	External syncope
	Syncope while supine
	Palpitations associated with syncope
	Family history of sudden death
Electrocardiographic features	Ventricular tachycardia
	Bifascicular block
	Intraventricular conduction delay
	Sinus bradycardia, sinoatrial block
	Preexcited QRS complex
	Prolonged or short-QT interval
	Brugada pattern on ECG
	T wave inversion and late potentials in right precordial leads
Significant comorbidities	Anemia
	Electrolyte disturbance

Palpitations preceding syncope may support an arrhythmic explanation for syncope but are often absent if the loss of consciousness is rapid. The history of syncope of the patient should be explained and interpreted carefully, because older ones, those who have fallen, might not admit to loss of consciousness during the event because of persisting amnesia.[14] Bradyarrhythmias caused by sinus node dysfunction (SND) or AV block and tachyarrhythmia are the common arrhythmic causes of syncope, mainly ventricular but also supraventricular at times. Bradycardia can follow tachycardia in patients with the bradycardia–tachycardia syndrome, and treatment of both may be necessary.[15]

Sudden cardiac arrest and aborted sudden cardiac death

SCD is common, although estimates of the incidence are confounded by inadequate case identification and secular trends that have influenced both the rates and therefore the etiologies of overtime. SCD caused by cardiac arrhythmias is most frequently the result of VT or fibrillation but may result from profound bradycardia, as could be observed in Adams–Stokes syndrome, or asystole. A variety of noncardiac conditions could also be related to life-threatening arrhythmias, including neurologic disorders, diabetes, obesity, cirrhosis, anorexia, and bulimia. Around 80% of cases of SCD occur in patients with some sort of structural heart disease, like coronary heart diseases, cardiomyopathy, or congenital heart condition.[16] Other cardiac causes of SCD, mentioned as "autopsy negative," include electrical diseases like long-QT syndrome (LQTS), Brugada syndrome (BrS), catecholaminergic polymorphic VT (CPVT), idiopathic ventricular fibrillation (IVF), and, under some circumstances, Wolff–Parkinson–White (WPW) syndrome.[17]

For the need of evaluation, SCA should be considered as SCD that someone has survived. It is essential that patients who have SCA undergo a comprehensive evaluation to spot the cause and proper treatment. A history of cardiac disease is critically important in directing the evaluation and management, as may be a case history of SCD or significant cardiac arrhythmias. The circumstances at the time of SCA are often informative. Cardiac symptoms that predate the SCD suggest preexisting structural heart condition. A spread of precipitating factors can provide clues to the etiology of SCA. Exercise, emotional upset, or stress may precipitate asystole within the setting of a spread of structural heart diseases, arrhythmogenic cardiomyopathy (arrhythmogenic right ventricular cardiomyopathy/dysplasia), and primary electrical diseases like LQTS (types 1 and 2) and CPVT. SCD in LQTS3 or BrS is more likely to occur at rest or with sleep.[18]

Physical findings

The physical examination is concentrated on determining whether CV disease is present. Benignity of a rhythm disturbance can often be suggested by the absence of serious cardiopulmonary diseases; however, it is not the case always. In contrast, a more ominous prognosis exists for other indications like palpitations, syncope, or near-syncope within the premise of significant heart or lung disease. In addition, physical examinations may reveal presence of a persistent arrhythmia like atrial fibrillation (AF).[19] If a tachycardia is present, the priority is to get a 12-lead ECG if the patient is hemodynamically stable. If it is impossible to get an ECG, several clues on the physical examination can help to form a diagnosis. The presence of normal cannon A waves within the jugular venous pulse would be according to a 1:1 retrograde ventriculoatrial activation, as in tachycardias like AV reentrant tachycardia (AVRT), atrioventricular nodal reentrant tachycardia (AVNRT), and a few junctional tachycardias and VTs.[20]

Genetics of cardiac arrhythmias

Inheritable arrhythmia syndromes that are potentially lethal involve electrical disturbances with the possibility to supply fatal arrhythmias inside a structurally normal heart. Collectively these—called the "cardiac channelopathies"—often unassuming electrical abnormalities have the capacity to develop a potentially lethal arrhythmia, resulting in the sudden and early demise of an otherwise healthy individual.[21] In fact, it is now recognized that nearly one-third of autopsy-negative sudden unexplained death (SUD) in young persons and approximately 10% of sudden infant death syndrome (SIDS) stem from these genetically inherited cardiac channelopathies.[22]

Molecular advances within the field of CV genetics have uncovered the underlying genetic basis liable for many inherited cardiac arrhythmia syndromes, and for others, their underlying genetic substrates are on the cusp of discovery. Over the past decade, a specific set of themes, including extreme genetic heterogeneity, reduced or incomplete penetrance, and variable expressivity, have proved to be common among the cardiac channelopathies. For a few disorders, however, important genotype–phenotype correlates are recognized and have provided diagnostic, prognostic, and therapeutic impact[23] (Table 13.2).

The QT-opathies

Long-QT syndrome

Clinical description and manifestations

A definite group of cardiac channelopathies known as congenital LQTS is characterized by delayed repolarization of the myocardium, QT prolongation (QTc >480 ms), and increased risk of syncope, seizures, and SCD for a healthy individual with an otherwise normally functioning heart.[24] The incidence of LQTS may exceed 1 in 2500 persons. Individuals who have LQTS may or might not manifest QT prolongation on a resting 12-lead surface ECG. This abnormality almost always is without consequence; rarely, however, internal and external triggers can produce potentially life-threatening arrhythmias.[25] Although the heart rhythm most frequently spontaneously returns to normal, leading to only a transient episode of syncope, 5% of LQTS patients without treatment might succumb to a fatal arrhythmia.[26] However, it is estimated that nearly half of the individuals with SCD experience, stemming from this treatable disorder, may have exhibited prior warning signs that went unrecognized. LQTS may explain approximately 20% of autopsy-negative SUD in young persons and 10% of SIDS cases.[27]

Genetic basis

LQTS may be a genetically heterogeneous disorder largely inherited in an autosomal dominant pattern, previously referred to as "Romano–Ward syndrome."[28] Rarely, LQTS is inherited because the recessive trait was first described by Jervell and Lange-Nielsen and is characterized by a severe cardiac phenotype and sensorineural deafness.[29] Spontaneous or sporadic

TABLE 13.2 Summary of heritable arrhythmia syndrome susceptible diseases.

Gene	Locus	Protein
Long-QT syndrome		
Major LQT genes		
KCNQ1 (LQT1)	11p19.5	I_{Ks} potassium channel alpha subunit (KVLQT1, K_V7.1)
KCNH2 (LQT2)	7q35–36	I_{Kr} potassium channel alpha subunit (HERG, K_V11.1)
SCN5A (LQT3)	3p21-p24	Cardiac sodium channel alpha subunit (Na_V1.5)
Minor LQT genes		
CALM1	14q32.11	Calmodulin 1
CALM 2	2p21	Calmodulin 2
CALM3	19q13.2-q13.3	Calmodulin 3
KCNE1	21q22.1	Potassium channel beta subunit (MinK)
KCNE2	21q22.1	Potassium channel beta subunit (MiRP1)
KCNJ5	11q24.3	Kir3.4 subunit of I_{KACH} channel
SCN4B	11q23.3	Sodium channel $beta_4$ subunit
Short-QT syndrome		
KCNH2 (SQT1)	7q35–36	I_{Kr} potassium channel alpha subunit (HERG, K_V11.1)
KCNQ1 (SQT2)	11p15.5	I_{Ks} potassium channel alpha subunit (KVLQT1, K_V7.1)
KCNJ2 (SQT3)	17q23	I_{K1} potassium channel (Kir2.1)
CACNA1C (SQT4)	12p13.3	Voltage-gated L-type calcium channel (Ca_V1.2)
CACNB2 (SQT5)	10p12	Voltage-gated L-type calcium channel $beta_2$ subunit
CACN2D1 (SQT6)	7q21-q22	Voltage-gated L-type calcium channel 2 delta subunit
Catecholaminergic polymorphic ventricular tachycardia (CPVT)		
RYR2 (CPVT1)	1q42.1-q43	Ryanodine receptor 2
CASQ2 (CPVT2)	1p13.3	Calsequestrin 2
KCNJ2 (CPVT3)	17q23	I_{K1} potassium channel, Kir2.1

(Continued)

TABLE 13.2 (Continued)

Gene	Locus	Protein
CALM1	14q32.11	Calmodulin 1
CALM3	19q13.2-q13.3	Calmodulin 3
TRDN	6q22.31	Cardiac triadin
Brugada syndrome (BrS)		
SCN5A (BrS1)	3p21-p24	Cardiac sodium channel alpha subunit ($NA_v1.5$)
Sick sinus syndrome		
ANK2	4q25-q27	Ankyrin B
HCN4	15q24-q25	Hyperpolarization-activated cyclic nucleotide-gated channel 4

germline mutations can account for about 5%–10% of LQTS cases. To date, many mutations have now been identified in 14 LQTS susceptibility genes liable for a nonsyndromic "classic" LQTS phenotype.[30] In addition, two extremely rare, multisystem disorders related to marked QT prolongation (Timothy syndrome, formerly annotated as LQT8) and prolonged QU intervals (Andersen–Tawil syndrome, formerly annotated as LQT7), also as LQT4, which is best classified as "ankyrin-B syndrome," have also been described.[31, 32]

Phenotypic correlates for the three canonical long-QT syndrome genotypes

Specific genotype–phenotype associations in LQTS have emerged, suggesting relatively gene-specific triggers, ECG patterns, and response to therapy.[33] Swimming- and exertion-induced cardiac events are strongly related to mutations in KCNQ1 (LQT1) gene, whereas in patients with LQT2, auditory triggers and events occurring during the postpartum period most frequently occur. Physical or emotional stress–induced events are mostly found in LQT1, and events that occur during periods of sleep or rest are commonest in LQT3. Employing a study population of 721 LQT1 and 634 LQT2 genetically confirmed patients from the US portion of the international LQTS registry, a multivariate analysis was conducted to assess the independent contribution of clinical and mutation-specific factors to the occurrence of a primary triggered event related to exercise, arousal, or sleep/rest.[34,35] Among the 221 symptomatic LQT1 patients, their first cardiac event was most frequently associated with exercise (55%), followed by sleep/rest (21%), arousal (14%), and nonspecific (10%) triggers, whereas the 204 symptomatic

LQT2 patients most frequently had their first event related to either arousal triggers (44%) or nonexercise/nonarousal triggers (43%), and only 13% of the symptomatic LQT2 patients had an exercise-induced first event.[36]

Short-QT syndrome

Clinical description and manifestations

Short-QT syndrome (SQTS), first noted in 2000 by Gussak et al., is related to a brief QT interval (usually $\leq$320 ms) on a 12-lead ECG, paroxysmal fibrillation, syncope, and an increased risk for SCD.[37]

Genetic basis

SQTS is most frequently inherited in an autosomal dominant manner; however, some de novo sporadic cases are described. To date, mutations in six genes are implicated within the pathogenesis of SQTS, including gain-of-function mutations within the potassium-channel encoding genes KCNH2 (SQT1), KCNQ1 (SQT2), and KCNJ2 (SQT3) and loss-of-function mutations in CACNA1C (SQT4), CACNB2b (SQT5), and CACNA2D1 (SQT6) encoding for LTCC alpha, beta, and delta subunits, respectively.[38]

Genotype–phenotype correlates

Insufficient data exist to define genotype–phenotype correlations clearly in SQTS. Although not more than 60 cases have been described within the literature so far, certain gene-specific ECG patterns have emerged. The standard ECG pattern consists of a QT interval of 320 ms or less (QTc $\leq$340 ms) and tall, peaked T waves in the precordial leads with either no or a brief ST segment present. The T waves tend to be symmetric in SQT1 but asymmetric in SQT2 to SQT4. In SQT2, inverted T waves are often observed. In SQT5, a BrS-like ST elevation within the right precordial lead may be seen (Fig. 13.1).[39]

Drug-induced torsade de pointes

Clinical description and manifestations

Drug-induced torsades de pointes (DI-TdP) might be a chronic concern for physicians prescribing particular drugs with the capacity for producing such unwanted and potentially life-threatening side effects. The estimated incidence of antiarrhythmic drug–induced TdP has ranged from 1% to 8% counting on the drug and dose.[40]

DI-TdP and subsequent sudden death are rare events, but the list of potential "QT liability" or "torsadegenic" drugs is extensive and includes not only antiarrhythmic drugs like quinidine, sotalol, and dofetilide but also many noncardiac medications, like antipsychotics, methadone, antimicrobials, antihistamines, and

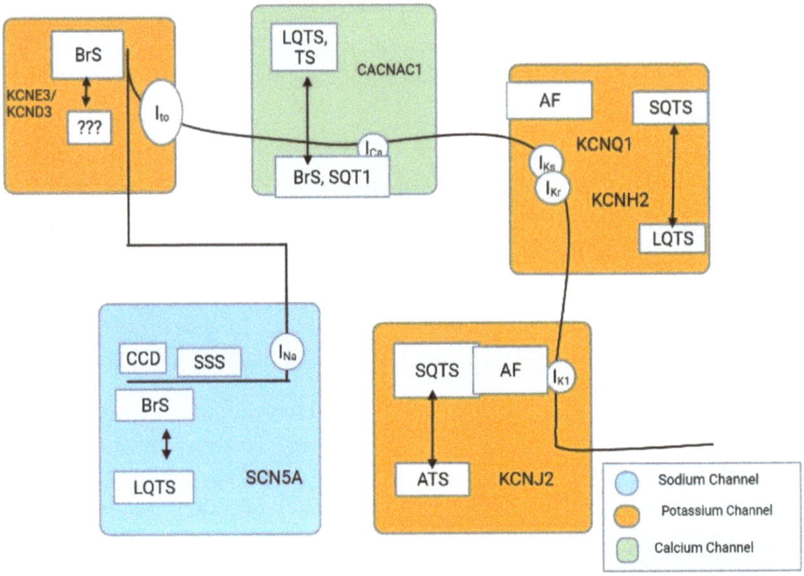

FIGURE 13.1 Cardiac nerve impulse disorders. Illustrated are the key ion currents (white circles) along with the ventricular cardiocyte's nerve impulse that are associated with potentially lethal arrhythmia disorders. Disorders leading to gain-of-function mutations are shown in green rectangles and people with loss-of-function mutations in blue rectangles. for instance, gain-of-function mutations within the SCN5A encoding cardiac sodium channel liable for INa cause long-QT syndrome (LQTS), and loss-of-function SCN5A mutations end in Brugada syndrome (BrS), cardiac conduction disorder (CCD), and sick sinus syndrome (SSS). *AF*, Atrial fibrillation; *ATS*, Andersen–Tawil syndrome; *SQTS*, short-QT syndrome.

therefore the gastrointestinal stimulant cisapride[41] (see www.qtdrugs.org for a comprehensive list).

IKr channel blockers and therefore the "repolarization reserve"

Besides their intended function and their intended target of action, the overwhelming majority of medicines with a possible unwanted TdP predisposing side effect is IKr/Kv11.1 channel blockers (also referred to as HERG channel blockers). In effect, QT-prolonging drugs create an "LQT2-like" phenotype through reduced repolarization efficiency and subsequent lengthening of the cardiac nerve impulse.[42] However, IKr drug blockade alone doesn't appear sufficient to supply the potentially lethal TdP substrate. One particular thesis centers on the observation that cardiac repolarization relies on the interaction of several ion currents that provide some level of redundancy so as to protect against extreme QT prolongation by "QT liability" drugs.[43]

This "repolarization reserve" could also be reduced through anomalies in the repolarization machinery, as a result of common or rare genetic variants in critical ion channels that produce a subclinical loss of the repolarizing currents IKs and IKr.[44] Actually, studies revealed that 10%–15% of patients with DI-TdP hosted rare ion channel mutations.[45] A recent smaller study found potential LQTS susceptibility mutations in 40% of cases of seemingly isolated, drug-induced LQTS.[46] It has been shown that in clarithromycin treated rat heart, hypokalemia can come out as a potent risk factor for QTc prolongation.[147] Lately it was also found out in rat heart with depleted repolarisation reserve provoked by hypokalemia and arrhythmogen administration, ranitidine, which is known to be safe, can precipitate QTc prolongation.[148]

The other channelopathies

Catecholaminergic polymorphic ventricular tachycardia

Clinical description and manifestations

CPVT may be a heritable arrhythmia syndrome that classically manifests with exercise-induced syncope or overtime, is predominantly expressed in young persons, and closely mimics the phenotypic byline of LQT1 but appears to be far more lethal.[47] Similar LQT1, a potentially lethal trigger that precipitates arrhythmia in CPVT, is swimming. In fact, LQT1 and CPVT are shown to underlie several cases of unexplained drowning or near-drowning in young, healthy swimmers. However, CPVT is related to a totally normal resting ECG (perhaps bradycardia and mild U waves) and is suspected on ECG after exercise or catecholamine stress testing that demonstrates significant ventricular ectopy, occasionally with CPVT's pathognomonic arrhythmia of bidirectional VT.[48]

Brugada syndrome

Clinical description and manifestations

BrS is a heritable arrhythmia syndrome which is characterized by an ECG pattern consisting of coved-type ST-segment elevation ($\geq$2 mm) followed by a negative T wave within the right precordial leads V1 through V3 (often mentioned as type 1 Brugada ECG pattern) and an increased risk for SCD resulting from episodes of polymorphic ventricular tachyarrhythmias.[49]

Genetic basis

BrS is inherited as an autosomal dominant trait, although quite half of BrS cases could also be sporadic. Approximately 20%–30% of BrS cases result from loss-of-function mutations within the SCN5A-encoded cardiac sodium channel and are classified as BrS1. In 2009 an international compendium of SCN5A mutations in patients referred for BrS genetic testing reported almost 300 distinct mutations in 438 of 2111 (21%) unrelated patients, and therefore the mutation detection yield ranged from 11% to 28% across nine centers.[50]

Phenotypic correlates of SCN5A-mediated Brugada syndrome (BrS1)

Because the bulk of BrS cases is elusive genetically, genotype–phenotype correlations in BrS haven't been analyzed to an equivalent degree as in LQTS. SCN5A mutations are related to a better incidence of conduction abnormalities in BrS patients, and therefore the presence of an extended PQ interval could also be indicative of SCN5A-mediated BrS1, whereas the presence of a brief QT interval (QTc < 350 ms) may be indicative of LTCC-mediated BrS pathology.[51]

Sick sinus syndrome

Clinical description and manifestations

SND or sick sinus syndrome (SSS), manifesting as inappropriate sinus bradycardia, sinus arrest, atrial standstill, tachycardia-bradycardia syndrome, or chronotropic incompetence, is the leading reason for pacemaker implantation and has been attributed to dysfunction of the sinoatrial (SA) node. SSS usually occurs in the elderly population (1 in 600 cardiac patients over age 65) with acquired cardiac conditions, including cardiomyopathy, congestive heart failure, ischemic heart condition, and metabolic disease. However, a significant number of patients show no identifiable cardiac anomalies or cardiac conditions underlying SND ("idiopathic" SND), which can occur at any age, including in utero. In addition, familial sorts of idiopathic SND according to autosomal dominant inheritance with reduced penetrance and recessive forms with complete penetrance have been reported.[52]

Genetic basis

Mutational analysis of small cohorts and case reports of patients with idiopathic SSS have so far implicated four genes: SCN5A, HCN4, ANK2, and MYH6. To date, 15 SSS-associated mutations are reported in SCN5A.[53] The mutations either produced nonfunctional sodium channels through loss of expression or channels with mild to severe loss of function through an altered biophysical mechanism of the channel.[54]

Principles of electrophysiology

Descriptive physiology

Pacemaker cells, which are situated within the SA node, at the junction of the proper atrium and therefore the superior vena cava, generate the normal cardiac impulse. Slowly, it is conducted through the nodal tissues, to the anatomically complex atria, after which the impulse is conducted more rapidly to the cardiac muscle, shown in the P wave of the ECG. There's a delay in conduction through the AVN. The PR interval of the ECG is nothing but the time needed for the atrial activation and the AVN delay. The electrical impulse emerges from the AVN and is transmitted to the His-Purkinje system, then the left and right bundle branches, then to the Purkinje network. Normally, the ventricles are activated rapidly and this shows in the QRS complex. The time of activation and duration of various regional action potentials govern recovery of electrical excitability which occurs more slowly. The relatively short life of epicardial action potentials in the ventricle leads to repolarization that happens first on the epicardial surface then proceeds to the endocardium, which produces a T wave. Ventricular activation and recovery duration is showcased by the atrial premature depolarization (APD) and is represented on the ECG by the QT interval.[55]

The regional variability in action potentials is probably a result of quantitative and qualitative differences between ion channel proteins expressed by different cell types within the heart. Unique sets of ionic currents are also active in pacemaker and cardiac muscle cells, and therefore the relative contributions of those currents may vary substantially (Fig. 13.2).

Ion channels are transmembrane glycoproteins with multiple subunits which open and shut responding to various biologic stimuli, including a change in membrane voltage, ligand binding, and mechanical deformation. Ion pumps are the motive forces behind the ionic gradients across the cell membrane that maintain the current flow through ion channels. Electrogenic

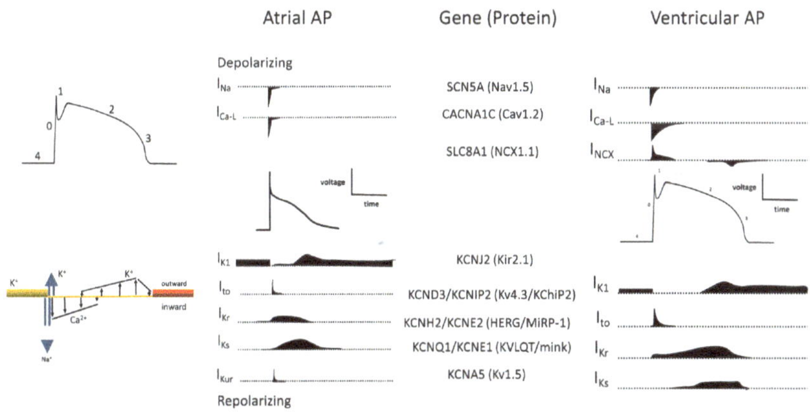

FIGURE 13.2 (A) Cellular atrial and ventricular action potentials. Phases 0–4 are the rapid upstroke, early repolarization, plateau, late repolarization, and diastole, respectively. The ionic currents and their respective genes are shown above and below the action potentials. The currents that underlie the action potentials vary in atrial and ventricular myocytes. (B) A ventricular nerve impulse with a schematic of the ionic currents flowing during the phases of the nerve impulse. Potassium current (IK1) is the principal current during phase 4 and determines the resting membrane potential of the myocyte. Sodium current generates the upstroke of the nerve impulse (phase 0); activation of Ito with inactivation of the Na current inscribes early repolarization (phase 1). The plateau (phase 2) is generated by a balance of repolarizing potassium currents and depolarizing calcium current. Inactivation of the calcium current with persistent activation of potassium currents (predominantly IKr and IKs) causes phase 3 repolarization.

transporters or exchangers are those that don't move ions in an electrically neutral manner and contribute directly to the nerve impulse profile.[56]

Voltage-gated ion channels are the most abundant ion channels present within the heart. There are many structural themes that are common to all voltage-dependent ion channels. To begin with, the architecture is modular, consisting either of four homologous subunits (e.g., K channels) or of four internally homologous domains (e.g., Na and Ca channels). Second, the proteins fold around a central pore lined by amino acids which showcase exquisite conservation within a given channel family of similar type. Third, the general strategy for activation gating (opening and closing in response to changes in membrane voltage) is very conserved: the fourth transmembrane segment lies within the membrane field and moves in response to depolarization, as a result opening the channel. Fourth, most of the ion channel complexes consist of the pore-forming proteins (α subunits) as well as auxiliary subunits (e.g., β subunits) that modify channel function.[57]

Mechanisms of cardiac arrhythmias

Abnormalities of electrical impulse generation and/or conduction are the main reasons behind cardiac arrhythmia generation. Bradyarrhythmias generally arise from disturbances in impulse formation at the extent of the pacemaker or from disturbances in impulse propagation at any level. Tachycardias can be classified according to their various mechanisms, including enhanced automaticity, triggered arrhythmias, or reentry (Table 13.3).

Alterations in impulse initiation: automaticity

Spontaneous (fourth phase) diastolic depolarization underlies the property of automaticity characteristic of pacemaker cells within the SA and AV nodes, His-Purkinje system, sinus coronarius, and pulmonary veins. Phase 4 depolarization generally results from the coordinated action of a number of ionic currents, including K^+ currents, Ca^{2+} currents, electrogenic Na-K ATPase, the Na-Ca exchanger, and the so-called funny, or pacemaker, current (I_f); however, the relative importance of those currents remain under scrutiny.[58]

Triggered automaticity and afterdepolarizations

Impulse initiation that is hooked into afterdepolarizations is known as triggered automaticity or activity. Membrane voltage oscillations that occur during (early afterdepolarizations) or after (delayed afterdepolarizations, DADs) a nerve impulse are known as afterdepolarizations. The cellular feature common to the induction of DADs is the presence of an increased Ca^{2+} load within the cytosol and sarcoplasmic reticulum.[59]

Digitalis glycoside toxicity, catecholamines, and ischemia all can enhance calcium ion loading enough to supply DADs. Accumulation of lysophospholipids

TABLE 13.3 Mechanism of arrhythmia.

Electrophysiologic property	Mechanism	Molecular components	Prototypic arrhythmias
Cellular			
Impulse initiation			
Automaticity	Suppression/ acceleration of phase 4	I_f, $I_{Ca\text{-}L}$, $I_{Ca\text{-}T}$, $I_{K'}$, I_{K1}	Sinus bradycardia, sinus tachycardia
Triggered automaticity	DADs	Calcium overload, I_T	Digitalis toxicity, reperfusion VT
	EADs	$I_{Ca\text{-}L}$, $I_{K'}$, I_{Na}	Torsades de pointes, congenital and acquired
Excitation			
	Suppression of phase 0	I_{Na}	Ischemic VF
	AP shortening, inexcitability	$I_{K\text{-}ATP}$	
Repolarization			
	Suppression	$I_{Ca\text{-}L}$	AV block
	AP prolongation, EADs, DADs	$I_{Na'}$, $I_{Ca\text{-}L}$, $I_{K'}$, $I_{K1'}$, Ca^{2+} homeostasis	Polymorphic VT (HF, LVH)
	AP shortening	$I_{Ca\text{-}L}$, K channels, Ca^{2+} homeostasis	Atrial fibrillation
Multicellular			
Cellular coupling	Decreased coupling	Connexins (Cx43), I_{Na}, $I_{K\text{-}ATP}$	Ischemic VT/VF
Tissue structure	Excitable gap and functional reentry	Extracellular matrix, collagen	Monomorphic VT, atrial fibrillation

in ischemic myocardium with subsequent Na^+ and Ca^{2+} overload might be a mechanism for DADs and triggered automaticity. Cells that go through a MI may display spontaneous release of calcium from the sarcoplasmic reticulum, and this might generate "waves" of intracellular calcium increase and arrhythmias (Fig. 13.3).[60]

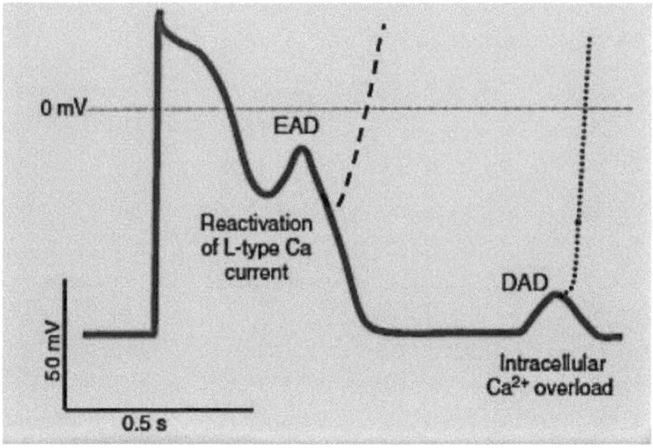

FIGURE 13.3 Schematic action potentials with EADs and DADs: afterdepolarizations are spontaneous depolarizations in cardiac myocytes. EADs occur before the top of the nerve impulse (phases 2 and 3), interrupting repolarization. DADs occur during phase 4 of the nerve impulse after completion of repolarization. The cellular mechanisms of EADs and DADs differ (see text).

Abnormal impulse conduction: reentry

The most common arrhythmia mechanism is known as reentry, which results from abnormal electrical impulse conduction and works by creating a circulation of an activation wave around an inexcitable obstacle. The reason for reentry is a couple of electrophysiologically dissimilar pathways for impulse propagation around an inexcitable region.[61] Reentry can occur around a fixed anatomical structure (e.g., myocardial lesion), with a stable pattern of cardiac depolarization occupation series over the antero-grade and retrograde limbs of the circuit. This type of reentry, known as anatomic reentry or excitable gap reentry, is initiated when a depolarizing wavefront confronts a neighborhood of unidirectional conduction block within the retrograde limb of the circuit. Conduction across the antero-grade limb occurs with a delay that, if of sufficient duration, allows for recovery of conduction within the retrograde limb with reentry of the depolarization wave into the retrograde limb of the circuit. Sustained reentry requires that the functional dimension of depolarized tissue or the tachycardia wavelength (λ = conduction velocity $\times$ refractory period) fits within the entire anatomic length of the circuit, mentioned because of the path length. When the trail length of the circuit exceeds the λ of the tachycardia, the region between the top of the activation wave and the refractory tail is called the excitable gap. Anatomically determined, excitable gap reentry can explain several clinically important tachycardias, like AV reentry, atrial flutter, bundle branch reentry VT, and VT in scarred myocardium (Fig. 13.4).[62]

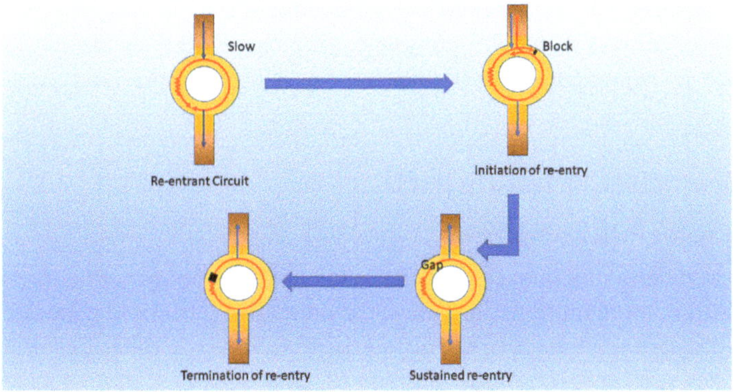

FIGURE 13.4 Diagram of reentry: (A) The circuit contains two limbs, one with slow conduction. (B) A premature impulse blocks within the fast pathway and conducts over the slow pathway, allowing the fast pathway to recover so that the activation wave can reenter the fast pathway from the retrograde direction. (C) During sustained reentry utilizing such a circuit, a niche (excitable gap) exists between the activating head of the wave and therefore the recovering tail. (D) One mechanism of termination of reentry occurs when the conduction and recovery characteristics of the circuit change and therefore the activating head of the wave collides with the tail, extinguishing the tachycardia.

Types of cardiac arrhythmias

Bradycardia

Sinoatrial node dysfunction

SND and AV conduction blocks are the foremost common causes of pathological bradycardia. SND may result from either extrinsic factors (e.g., drugs, hypothyroidism, sleep apnea) or intrinsic causes [e.g., SSS, arteria coronaria disease (CAD), inflammation].[63]

Atrioventricular conduction block

AV conduction block is defined as an impediment or intervention within the transmission of an impulse, either transient or permanent, from the atria to the ventricles thanks to an anatomic or functional impairment within the conduction system. The conductions are often delayed, intermittent, or absent. Conduction block from the atrium to the ventricle can occur for various reasons, including hypothyroidism, drugs, infections, inflammation, heritable/congenital diseases, and CAD.[64] The AV conduction blocks are often classified based on the severity of block into first-, second-, and third-degree block.

1. First-degree AV block: PR interval >0.21 s with all atrial impulses conducted. In other words, first-degree block is slowed conduction without missed beats.

2. Second-degree AV block: missed beats, often during a regular pattern, for instance, 2:1, 3:2, or higher degrees of block.
3. Third-degree AV block: complete Adams–Stokes syndrome, during which no supraventricular impulses are conducted to the ventricles.

Supraventricular tachyarrhythmia

Atrial premature complexes

Atrial premature complexes (APCs), also referred to as atrial premature beats, APDs, premature atrial beats, or premature atrial complexes, result from premature activation of the atria arising from a site other than the sinus node. They are observed on the surface ECG as a P wave that happens relatively early within the cycle (i.e., prematurely before subsequent sinus P wave should occur) and features a different morphology from the sinus P wave. APCs are the foremost common arrhythmia identified during extended ECG monitoring. APCs typically are asymptomatic although some patients experience palpitations or an irregularity of the pulse.[65]

Junctional premature complexes

Junctional premature complexes (JPCs), also referred to as junctional premature beats or junctional premature depolarizations, arise within the AV junction (e.g., AV node and His bundle). JPCs are very uncommon. They will cause no symptoms or cause symptoms, like palpitations.[66]

Sinus tachycardia

Sinus tachycardia is defined as a rise in sinus rate to >100 beats/min. Sinus tachycardia is assessed into physiological sinus tachycardia and inappropriate sinus tachycardia (IST). Physiological sinus tachycardia occurs in keeping with the extent of physical, emotional, pathological, or pharmacological stress. These include exercise, fever, and hyperthyroidism. IST, also called chronic nonparoxysmal sinus tachycardia, is an unusual condition that happens in individuals without apparent heart condition or other causes for sinus tachycardia, like hyperthyroidism or fever. Affected patients have an elevated resting pulse and/or an exaggerated pulse response to exercise; many patients have both.[67]

The underlying pathological basis for IST is probably going to be multifactorial, but two main mechanisms are proposed: (1) enhanced automaticity of the sinus node and (2) abnormal autonomic regulation of the sinus node with excess sympathetic and reduced parasympathetic tone. Sinus tachycardia is usually asymptomatic, although the patient may complain of a rapid heartbeat.[68]

Atrial fibrillation

AF is the commonest chronic arrhythmia, which is characterized by disorganized, rapid, and irregular atrial activation. The ventricular response to the rapid atrial activation is additionally irregular, and therefore the ventricular rate in untreated patients also tends to be rapid. Many patients with AF are asymptomatic. In some patients, it causes adverse consequences associated with a discount in flow (e.g., palpitation, exercise intolerance, and hypotension) and to atrial and atrial appendage thrombus formation (e.g., ischemic stroke and peripheral embolization).[69]

Atrial flutter

Macro-reentrant atrial tachycardias involving the atrial myocardium are collectively mentioned as atrial flutter (AFL). AFL and macro-reentrant atrial tachycardia are frequently used interchangeably, with both denoting a nonfocal source of an atrial arrhythmia. There are two sorts of AFL: typical and atypical. Typical (also referred to as counterclockwise) right AFL represents approximately 80% of all AFL. Typical right AFL has an atrial rate of 260–300 beats/min with a ventricular response that tends to be 2:1 or typically 130–150 beats/min. Typical AFL is caused by a macro-reentrant right atrial circuit around the tricuspid annulus, and intrinsically, it is also referred to as cavotricuspid isthmus dependent flutter.[70] AFL is a smaller amount common than AF. AFL occurs most frequently in patients with chronic obstructive pulmonary disease (COPD) but could also be seen in those with rheumatic or CAD, congestive coronary failure, atrial septal defect, or surgically repaired congenital heart condition. AFL is usually related to palpitation (acute) and fatigue (chronic). Almost like AF, AFL also predisposes the individual to thromboembolism.[71]

Atrial tachycardias

Multifocal atrial tachycardia

Multifocal atrial tachycardia (MAT), also called chaotic atrial tachycardia, is characterized by a minimum of three distinct P wave morphologies and sometimes a minimum of three different PR intervals, and therefore the associated atrial and ventricular rates are typically between 100 and 150 beats/min. MAT is the signature tachycardia of patients with severe pulmonary diseases, like COPD. It also can occur within the presence of coronary, valvular, hypertensive, and other sorts of heart diseases, particularly when associated with coronary failure and/or underlying lung disease. In most cases, the clinical manifestations of MAT differ from those of other tachyarrhythmias therein symptoms predominantly relate to the underlying precipitating illness instead of the arrhythmia. Patients rarely present with symptoms, such as palpitations.[72]

Focal atrial tachycardias

Focal atrial tachycardias (FATs) are caused by regular atrial activation from atrial areas with centrifugal spread. FATs are usually manifest by atrial rates between 150 and 250 beats/min, with a P wave contour different from that of the sinus P wave. Neither the sinus nor the AV node plays a task within the initiation or perpetuation of the tachycardia. FATs do not occur randomly throughout the atria, but rather cluster at predefined anatomic locations. Most patients with FAT report palpitations associated with their episodes of tachycardia. Rarely, patients may present with syncope or exacerbation of an underlying cardiac condition (e.g., angina).[73]

Atrioventricular nodal tachycardias

Atrioventricular nodal reentrant tachycardia

AVNRT is the commonest sort of paroxysmal supraventricular tachycardias (PSVTs) and is more prevalent in females. AVNRT is related to palpitations, dizziness, and neck pulsations. It is not usually related to structural heart condition. Rates of tachycardia are often between 140 and 250 beats/min. Although the reentrant circuit was initially thought to be confined to the compact AV node, a more contemporary view recognizes the standard participation of perinodal atrial tissue as the most common component of the reentrant circuit.[74]

Atrioventricular junctional tachycardias

Junctional tachycardias are further classified into different forms, including focal junctional tachycardia and nonparoxysmal junctional tachycardia. Focal junctional tachycardia, also known as automatic or paroxysmal junctional tachycardia, may be a very uncommon arrhythmia. It always presents in young adulthood. Nonparoxysmal junctional tachycardia may be a benign arrhythmia that is characterized by a narrow complex tachycardia with rates of 70–120 beats/min.[75] The arrhythmogenic mechanism is assumed to be related to an enhanced automaticity arising from a high junctional focus or in response to a triggered mechanism. It shows a typical "warm-up" and "cool-down" pattern and cannot be terminated by pacing maneuvers. The most important feature about this tachycardia is that it is going to be a marker for a significant underlying condition, like digitalis toxicity, postcardiac surgery, hypokalemia, or myocardial ischemia.[76]

Tachycardias associated with accessory atrioventricular pathways

They are reentrant tachycardias with an anatomically defined circuit that consists of two distinct pathways, the traditional AV conduction system and an AV accessory pathway, linked by common proximal (the atria) and distal (the ventricles) tissues. If sufficient differences in conduction time and refractoriness exist between the traditional conduction system and the accessory pathway, a properly timed premature impulse of atrial, junctional, or ventricular origin can initiate reentry.[77]

Two terms, distinguished by the presence or absence of arrhythmias, are wont to describe individuals with accessory pathways: (1) the WPW pattern is applied to the patient with preexcitation manifest on an ECG within the absence of symptomatic arrhythmias, and (2) the WPW syndrome is applied to the patient with both preexcitation manifest on an ECG and symptomatic arrhythmias [e.g., AV reentrant (or reciprocating) tachycardia (AVRT) and AF] involving the accessory pathway.[78]

The two major sorts of arrhythmias in persons with an AV accessory pathway are orthodromic AVRT (including permanent junctional reciprocating tachycardia) and antidromic AVRT. Orthodromic AVRT comprises 90%–95% of the reentrant tachycardias related to the WPW syndrome. The diagnosis of WPW syndrome is reserved for patients who have both preexcitation and tachyarrhythmias.[79]

Ventricular tachyarrhythmia

Premature ventricular complexes

Premature ventricular complexes (PVCs), also referred to as ventricular premature beats, ventricular premature complexes, premature ventricular beats, or ventricular extrasystoles, are triggered from the ventricular myocardium during a sort of situation. PVCs are common and occur during a broad spectrum of the population. This includes patients without structural heart condition and people with any sort of cardiac disease, independent of severity. PVCs produce few or no symptoms within the overwhelming majority of patients. Some patients may experience palpitations or dizziness.[3]

Ventricular tachycardia

VT is defined as an arrhythmia of three or more consecutive ventricular beats in duration at a rate of >100 beats/min (cycle length < 600 ms). VT is further classified into nonsustained VT and sustained VT. As described below, TdP is additionally a sort of VT.

Nonsustained ventricular tachycardia

Nonsustained VT is defined as a VT terminating spontaneously in <30 s. It is often monomorphic (with one QRS morphology) or polymorphic (with a changing QRS morphology at cycle length between 600 and 180 ms). Nonsustained VT is usually asymptomatic, but some patients experience palpitations, light-headedness, presyncope, or dyspnea.[80]

Sustained ventricular tachycardia

Sustained VT is defined as a VT >30 s in duration and/or requiring termination thanks to hemodynamic compromise in <30 s. It is often monomorphic or polymorphic. Sustained VT is potentially life threatening thanks to hemodynamic instability.[81]

Torsades de pointes

TdP may be a sort of polymorphic VT that happens within the setting of acquired or congenital QT interval prolongation[82] within the specific case of TdP, these variations take the form of a progressive, sinusoidal, cyclic alteration of the QRS axis. The peaks of the QRS complexes appear to "twist" around the isoelectric line of the recording, hence the name torsades de pointes or "twisting of the points."[83] Typical features of TdP include an antecedent prolonged QT interval, particularly within the last sinus beat preceding the onset of the arrhythmia; a ventricular rate of 160–250 beats/min; irregular RR intervals; and a cycling of the QRS axis through 180 degrees every 5–20 beats. TdP is typically short-lived and terminates spontaneously. However, most patients experience multiple episodes of the arrhythmia, and episodes can recur in rapid succession, potentially degenerating to fibrillation (VF) and SCD.[84]

Ventricular flutter

Ventricular flutter may be a regular (cycle length variability 30 ms or less) monomorphic VT that happens at a really rapid rate of 150–300 beats/min (usually around 200beats/min). Often, no distinctive T waves are discernible. There is no isoelectric interval between QRS complexes. P waves or evidence of atrial activity is absent since the ventricular rate is rapid (VF Rapid, usually >300 beats/min), and this grossly irregular ventricular rhythm is present with marked variability in QRS cycle length, morphology, and amplitude. Both ventricular flutter and VF represent severe derangements of the heartbeat that usually terminate fatally within 3–5 min unless corrective measures are undertaken promptly.[85]

Long-QT syndrome

The LQTS could also be a disorder of myocardial repolarization characterized by a protracted QT interval on the ECG.[86] As noted earlier, this syndrome is said to be an increased risk of TdP, a characteristic life-threatening cardiac arrhythmia. The LQTS could even be either congenital or acquired. Congenital LQTS consists of defects in cardiac ion channels that are responsible for cardiac depolarization.[87] Defects that enhance sodium or calcium inward currents or inhibit outward potassium currents during the plateau phase of the impulse prolong impulse duration and hence the QT interval. Acquired LQTS usually results from drug therapy, hypokalemia, or hypomagnesemia. The primary symptoms in patients with LQTS include palpitations, syncope, seizures, and SCD.[88]

Antiarrhythmic drugs

Classification of antiarrhythmic drugs

Antiarrhythmic drugs act primarily by suppressing or preventing abnormal formation or conduction of cardiac nerve impulse.[89] Because sodium channels are involved within the spontaneous depolarization of phase 4 of nerve impulse in nodal cells and within the phase 0 depolarization of nonpacemaker cells, drugs that block sodium channels can reduce abnormal automaticity and slow conduction of the cardiac impulse.[90] The automaticity is decided by the speed of phase 4 spontaneous depolarization in pacemaker cells, whereas the conduction velocity of nerve impulse in nonpacemaker cells is decided by the speed of phase 0 depolarization.[91]

Similarly, since calcium channels are involved within the phase 0 depolarization of pacemaker cells, calcium channel blockers (CCBs) inhibit the conduction of nerve impulse through the nodal cells or tissues.[92] Likewise, drugs that block repolarizing potassium channels can prolong repolarization and the nerve impulse duration (APD) and thereby increasing the biological time of cardiac tissue and hindering reentry.[93]

Drugs that block β-adrenergic receptors attenuate the sympathetic stimulation of cardiac automaticity and conduction velocity and thereby prevent the overstimulation of sympathetic tone that contributes to some sorts of cardiac arrhythmias.[94]

On the idea of the abovementioned mechanisms, E.M. Vaughan–Williams has divided the antiarrhythmic drugs into four main classes, with class I consisting of sodium channel blockers, class II consisting of β-blockers, class III consisting of potassium-channel blockers and other drugs that prolong the APD, and sophistication IV consisting of CCBs. The Vaughan–Williams classification has proven useful in helping understand the clinical effects of the antiarrhythmic agents. However, it represents an oversimplification of the electrophysiological events that occur with each of the drug classes. In addition, a couple of drugs (e.g., adenosine) do not fit into any of those categories, and a few drugs (e.g., amiodarone) might be included in additional than one category (Table 13.4).[95]

Class I antiarrhythmic drugs

General aspects of class I drugs

Sodium channel binding and dissociation properties

Class I drugs act by blocking the sodium channels, thereby inhibiting phase 0 depolarization in nonpacemaker cells and phase 4 spontaneous depolarization in pacemaker cells. These drugs are charged and may interact with

TABLE 13.4 Classification of antiarrhythmic drugs.

Class	Effect	Repolarization time	Example
IA	Sodium channel inhibition ↓↓	Prolongs	Quinidine, disopyramide, procainamide
IB	Sodium channel inhibition ↓	Shortens	Lidocaine, phenytoin, mexiletine, tocainide
IC	Sodium Channel Inhibition ↓↓↓	Unchanged	Flecainide, propafenone
II	I_f, a pacemaker and depolarizing current; indirect Ca^{2+} channel block	Unchanged	β--blockers (excluding sotalol, which has class III effects as well)
III	Repolarizing K^+ currents	Markedly prolongs	Amiodarone, sotalol, ibutilide, dofetilide
IV	AV nodal Ca^{2+} block	Unchanged	Verapamil, diltiazem
IV like	K^+ channel opener, hyperpolarization	Unchanged	Adenosine

specific aminoalkanoic acid residues within the internal pore of the sodium channels to cause inhibition.

Class I drugs are further divided into three subgroups. This subclassification is based on their different effects on sodium channels, which, in turn, result from the various binding and dissociation properties.[96]

Use-dependent blockage

Antiarrhythmic drugs preferentially bind to sodium channels when the channels are at active (open) and/or inactive states, and consequently, dissociation occurs when the channels are at rest. During faster heart rates, less time exists for the drugs to dissociate from the channels thanks to less time for the channels to be at rest, thereby leading to an increased number of blocked channels and enhanced blockade. These pharmacological effects may cause a progressive decrease in conduction velocity of action potential and a widening of the QRS complex in ECG. This property is understood as use-dependent blockage. This explains why antiarrhythmic drugs are simpler on tissue that's firing rapidly, that is, tachyarrhythmias (Table 13.5).[97]

TABLE 13.5 Sodium channel binding and dissociation properties for subclasses of class I drugs.

Subclass	Sodium channel blockage	Binding and dissociation from sodium channels	Affinity for sodium channels at open or inactivated state
IA	Moderate	Intermediate	High affinity for open state
IB	Weak	Rapid	High affinity for both open and inactive state
IC	Strong	Slow	High affinity for open state

Specific class IA drugs

- Disopyramide (Norpace)
- Procainamide (Pronestyl)
- Quinidine

Molecular mechanisms and pharmacological effects

- Quinidine

  Quinidine depresses the rapid inward depolarizing sodium current, thereby slowing phase 0 depolarization and reducing the amplitude of the nerve impulse without affecting the electric potential. In pacemaker cells and Purkinje fibers, it reduces the slope of phase 4 depolarization and shifts the edge voltage upward toward zero. The result is slowed conduction and reduced automaticity altogether parts of the heart, with an increase of the Effective Refractory Period (ERP) relative to the duration of the nerve impulse within the atria, ventricles, and Purkinje tissues. Quinidine also directly prolongs the biological time by blocking potassium channels.[98]

  Quinidine increases the fibrillation thresholds of the atria and ventricles, and it raises the ventricular defibrillation threshold also. By slowing conduction and prolonging the ERP, quinidine can interrupt or prevent reentrant arrhythmias and arrhythmias thanks to increased automaticity, including atrial flutter (AFL), fibrillation (AF), and PSVT. In patients with the SSS, quinidine can cause marked sinus node depression and bradycardia. In most patients, however, the use of quinidine is related to a rise within the sinus rate.[99]

  Quinidine prolongs the QT interval during a dose-related fashion. This might cause increased ventricular automaticity and polymorphic VT, including TdP. In addition, quinidine has anticholinergic activity and negative inotropic activity, and it acts peripherally as an α-adrenergic antagonist, causing vasodilation.[100]

Recently, the utilization of quinidine in treating cardiac arrhythmias has received renewed attention. Quinidine could also be particularly effective for the management of ventricular arrhythmias in BrS, a genetic disease caused by abnormalities in sodium channels.[101] However, quinidine is inaccessible in many countries thanks to its limited use in CV medicine and, consequently, a scarcity of incentives for drug manufacturing.[102]

- Disopyramide and procainamide

Disopyramide and procainamide are almost like quinidine with reference to electrophysiological effects. The anticholinergic activity of disopyramide is stronger than that of quinidine. Among the IA drugs, procainamide has the weakest anticholinergic activity.[103]

Specific class IB drugs

- Lidocaine (Xylocaine)
- Mexiletine (Mexitil)

Molecular mechanisms and pharmacological effects

Lidocaine and mexiletine inhibit the inward sodium current, thus reducing the speed of rise of the action potential (phase 0). They decrease the ERP in Purkinje fibers. The decrease in ERP is of lesser magnitude than the decrease in APD, with a resulting increase within the ERP/APD ratio. This increased ratio appears to be liable for the inhibition of reentry and thereby raise the fibrillation threshold.[104]

Because lidocaine and mexiletine have greater affinity for both open and inactivated states of sodium channels, they are particularly effective in blocking rapidly firing tissues, like ischemic tissue, where there's a higher likelihood of sodium channels being within the open or inactivated state. This explains their efficacy in suppressing ventricular arrhythmias resulting from myocardial ischemia (e.g., myocardial infarction) (Fig. 13.5).[105]

Specific class IC drugs

- Flecainide (Tambocor)
- Propafenone (Rythmol)

Molecular mechanisms and pharmacological effects

Among class I antiarrhythmic drugs, class IC drugs are the foremost potent sodium channel blockers. Both flecainide and propafenone dramatically reduce the speed of phase 0 of action potential, thereby slowing conduction velocity and inhibiting reentry altogether parts of the guts with the best effect on the His-Purkinje system. Blockage of sodium channels also slows down

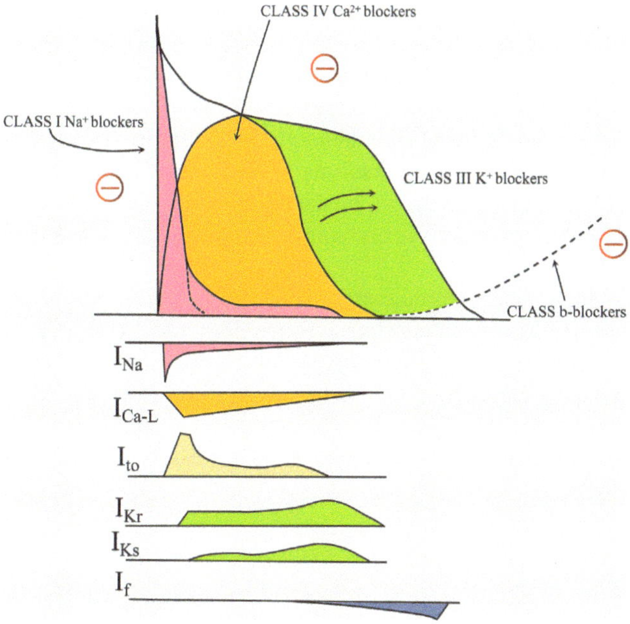

FIGURE 13.5 Types and actions of antiarrhythmic drugs: Class I agents decrease phase zero of the rapid depolarization of the nerve impulse (rapid sodium channel). Class II agents, b-blocking drugs, have complex actions including inhibition of spontaneous depolarization (phase 4) and indirect closure of calcium channels, which are less likely to be within the "open" state when not phosphorylated by cyclic AMP. Class III agents block the outward potassium channels to prolong the nerve impulse duration and hence refractoriness. Class IV agents, verapamil and diltiazem, and therefore the indirect calcium antagonist, adenosine, all inhibit the inward calcium channel, which is most prominent in nodal tissue, particularly the cardiac muscle. Most antiarrhythmic drugs have quite one action. Within the lower panel are shown the main currents on which antiarrhythmics act, consistent with the Sicilian gambit. *Ca-L*, long-lasting calcium; *I*, current; *If*, inward funny current; *Kr*, rapid component of repolarizing potassium current; *Ks*, slow component; *Na*, sodium; *to*, transient outward.

phase 4 depolarization in pacemaker cells, leading to decreased spontaneous automaticity.[106]

Class IC drugs depress triggered activity likely thanks to inhibition of inward sodium ion current mediated by partially recovered sodium ion channels during depolarization phase (phase 3). Class IB drugs, especially propafenone, exert cardiac depressing effects likely thanks to β-blocking activity.[106]

Class II antiarrhythmic drugs

General aspects

Class II antiarrhythmic drugs are β-blockers. These drugs block the proarrhythmic effects of β1-adrenergic receptor activation resulting from sympathetic stimulation. Sympathetic activation of β1-adrenergic receptors in SA nodal cells accelerates phase 4 depolarization, thereby increasing automaticity. Activation of β1-adrenergic receptors in AV nodal cells augments phase 0 Ca^{2+} currents, leading to increased conduction velocity and elevated risk of reentry. Activation of β1-adrenergic receptors in AV nodal cells also increases phase 3K + currents, resulting in shortened biological time.[106]

These β1-adrenergic receptor–mediated effects collectively contribute to the event of cardiac arrhythmias associated with sympathetic hyperactivation.

By blocking the aforementioned β1-adrenergic receptor–mediated actions, class II antiarrhythmic drugs reduce heart rate, slow AV conduction velocity, and prolong AV refractory period. Slowing AV nodal conduction velocity and prolongation of AV nodal biological time end in decreased reentry.[107]

AV nodal reentry may be a fundamental mechanism of supraventricular tachyarrhythmias.

β-Blockers commonly used for treating arrhythmias

Although many β-blockers are approved to be used in the United States, metoprolol, carvedilol, atenolol, propranolol, and esmolol are most generally wont to treat cardiac arrhythmias. It is generally considered that β-blockers possess class effects which if titrated to the right dose, all can be used effectively to treat cardiac arrhythmias also as other CV diseases. However, differences in pharmacokinetic or pharmacodynamic properties influence the choice of the actual β-blockers.

Class III antiarrhythmic drugs

Listed below are the US Food and Drug Administration (FDA)-approved class III antiarrhythmic drugs. Among them, dronedarone is the newest member of this drug class.[108]

Sotalol may be a β-blocker that also blocks potassium channels to prolong ERP, and intrinsically, it's usually classified as a class III drug.[109] It is sometimes also classified as a category II drug, some other examples are:

- Amiodarone (Cordarone)
- Dronedarone (Multaq)
- Dofetilide (Tikosyn)
- Ibutilide (Corvert)
- Sotalol (Betapace)

General aspects

Class III drugs block the repolarizing potassium channels, thereby prolonging repolarization and ERP. Prolongation of ERP reduces reentry. On the opposite hand, blockage of ventricular potassium currents leads to prolongation of the QT interval on ECG. Prolongation of QT interval may predispose to TdP, a polymorphic VT.[110]

In addition to the blockage of potassium channels, amiodarone and dronedarone also inhibit sodium channels in depolarized tissues, a characteristic effect of sophistication IB drugs.[111]

Amiodarone and dronedarone also block calcium channels as well as β-adrenergic receptors.[112]

Specific class III drugs

Amiodarone and dronedarone

Molecular mechanisms and pharmacological effects Amiodarone is usually considered a category III antiarrhythmic drug, but it possesses electrophysiological characteristics of all four classes of antiarrhythmics, including blockage of sodium channels, β-adrenergic receptors (as well as α-adrenergic receptors), potassium channels, and calcium channels.[113]

Like class I drugs, amiodarone blocks sodium channels at rapid pacing frequencies, and like class II drugs, it exerts a noncompetitive antisympathetic action (blockage of both β- and α-adrenergic receptors). One of its main effects is to lengthen the cardiac nerve impulse, a category III effect. This results in prolongation of ERP. The negative chronotropic effect of amiodarone in nodal tissues is analogous to the effect of class IV drugs. The antisympathetic action and therefore the block of calcium and potassium channels are liable for the negative dromotropic effects on the sinus node and the slowing of conduction and prolongation of ERP within the AV node. Its vasodilatory action can decrease cardiac workload and consequently myocardial oxygen consumption.[114]

As an amiodarone derivative, dronedarone is believed to possess similar mechanisms of actions of amiodarone, that is, dronedarone has antiarrhythmic properties belonging to all four Vaughan–Williams classes. However, the contribution of each of those activities to the clinical effect is not clear.

Ibutilide and dofetilide

Molecular mechanisms and pharmacological effects Ibutilide and dofetilide, like other class III drugs, are traditionally thought to dam outward potassium currents, thereby leading to prolongation of nerve impulse and ERP. While dofetilide at clinically relevant concentrations is known to dam the cardiac ion channel carrying the rapid component of the delayed rectifier potassium current and have no effects on sodium channels, ibutilide may primarily affect sodium channels. During this regard, voltage-clamp studies indicate that ibutilide, at nanomolar concentrations, delays repolarization mainly by activation of a slow, inward current (predominantly sodium), instead of by blocking outward potassium currents. This also results in prolongation of atrial and ventricular APD and refractoriness.[115]

Ibutilide produces mild slowing of the sinus rate and AV conduction. In contrast, dofetilide does not influence cardiac conduction velocity and sinus node function. Like other class III drugs, ibutilide and dofetilide cause prolongation of the QT interval, which can be related to TdP.[116]

Sotalol

Molecular mechanisms and pharmacological effects Sotalol blocks both β-androgenic receptors and repolarizing potassium channels and thus has both class II and III antiarrhythmic properties. The category II (β-blockade) electrophysiological effects of sotalol are manifested by increased sinus cycle length (slowed heart rate), decreased AV nodal conduction, and increased AV nodal refractoriness. The category III electrophysiological effects include prolongation of the atrial and ventricular monophasic action potentials and ERP prolongation of atrial muscle, ventricular muscle, and AV accessory pathways (where present) in both the anterograde and retrograde directions.[117]

Class IV antiarrhythmic drugs

- Diltiazem (Cardizem)
- Verapamil (Calan, Isoptin)

General aspects

Class IV drugs are nondihydropyridine CCBs and include diltiazem and verapamil. By blocking L-type calcium channels, class IV drugs can slow the sinus rate, increase the refractoriness of and prolong conduction through the AV node, and depress left ventricular contractility. Verapamil features a more pronounced effect on SA and AV nodes than diltiazem.[95]

Molecular mechanisms and pharmacological effects

Diltiazem and verapamil inhibit the influx of calcium ions during membrane depolarization of cardiac and vascular smooth muscle. The therapeutic efficacy of the drugs in supraventricular tachycardias is said to their ability to slow AV nodal conduction time and prolong AV nodal refractoriness.[118]

Diltiazem and verapamil exhibit frequency (use)-dependent effects on AV nodal conduction such that they may selectively reduce the guts rate during tachycardias involving the AV node with little or no effect on normal AV nodal conduction at normal heart rates. These drugs slow the ventricular rate in patients with a rapid ventricular response during AF or AFL. They convert PSVT to normal sinus rhythm by interrupting the reentry circuit in AV nodal reentrant tachycardias.[119]

Like other CCBs, due to their effect on vascular smooth muscle, diltiazem and verapamil reduce peripheral resistance, thereby decreasing vital sign. These drugs relax arteria coronaria and stop arteria coronaria spasm and reduce myocardial oxygen demand. As such, they are used to treat angina.[120]

Other antiarrhythmic drugs

- Adenosine (Adenocard)
- Digoxin (Digox)
- Magnesium
- Vernakalant (Brinavess)

Adenosine

Molecular mechanisms and pharmacological effects

The antiarrhythmic effects of adenosine are mediated by specific G protein–coupled receptor signaling. Adenosine activates acetylcholine (Ach)-sensitive potassium channels within the atrium and SA and AV nodes, leading to membrane hyperpolarization and therefore the subsequent inhibition of voltage-dependent calcium channels. Adenosine slows AV conduction time and inhibits reentry pathways through the AV node. The drug can restore normal sinus rhythm in patients with PSVT, including PSVT associated with WPW syndrome.[121]

Magnesium

Magnesium ion is the fourth most abundant cation within the human body. It is involved in multiple essential physiological, biochemical, and cellular processes regulating CV function. Magnesium plays a critical role in modulating vascular smooth muscular tone, endothelial cell function, and myocardial excitability, and intrinsically, dysregulation of magnesium may play a crucial part within the pathogenesis of CV disorders including hypertension, atherosclerosis, coronary artery disease, congestive coronary failure, and cardiac arrhythmias.[122] Probably the foremost widely accepted and practiced use of magnesium in CV medicine is for the prevention and/or treatment of cardiac arrhythmias. Multiple randomized clinical trials and/or metaanalyses of the randomized trials suggest a role for magnesium supplementation within the management of postoperative arrhythmias, AF, and ventricular arrhythmias (including TdP).[123] However, the precise efficacy of magnesium within the prevention and treatment of cardiac arrhythmias remain to be established in large-scale, randomized controlled trials. Likewise, basic research is warranted to further elucidate the underlying molecular mechanisms of magnesium-mediated antiarrhythmic activity.

Vernakalant

Vernakalant may be a novel and comparatively atrium-selective drug, which inhibits atrium-selective potassium ion currents with only a little inhibitory effect on the rapidly activating delayed rectifier potassium ion current within the ventricle. This results in prolongation of atrial refractoriness and slowing of atrial impulse conduction. The drug has been recently approved in Europe as an iv therapy for rapid conversion of recent-onset AF to sinus rhythm in adults.[124] Vernakalant is currently not a US FDA–approved drug for clinical use.[124–127]

New developments in antiarrhythmic therapy

1. The persistent imperfections of current antiarrhythmic drugs and rapidly expanding technologies have led to a continued explosion in the use of devices and ablative techniques for both supraventricular and ventricular arrhythmias.[128–130]
2. AF has become a very active focus of research, with the popularity that with our aging population it's now a serious hazard, yet with persisting problems in management like the continuing controversy regarding rate versus rhythm control with an ever-increasing trend toward intervention by ablation.[131–133]
3. There has been increasing interest in the use of so-called upstream therapy in arrhythmia management, particularly AF. Upstream therapy involves the targeting of processes resulting in the development of the arrhythmia substrate, with the hope of preventing initial arrhythmia occurrence (primary prevention) or reducing the likelihood of arrhythmia recurrence after initial presentation (secondary prevention).[134,135]
4. Stroke is recognized because the principal clinically significant complication of AF and therefore the introduction of latest antithrombotic agents, so that stroke prevention has become one among the first considerations within the science of AF management.[136–139]
5. Important gender differences in cardiac electrophysiology exist. Compared with men, women have higher resting heart rates and longer QT intervals with greater risk of drug-induced TdP. Women with AF are at a higher risk of stroke, and they are less likely to receive anticoagulation and ablation procedures. Women have a far better response to cardiac resynchronization therapy in terms of reduced numbers of hospitalizations and more robust reverse ventricular remodeling. Further studies are required to elucidate the underlying pathophysiologic characteristics of these sex differences in cardiac arrhythmias.[140–146]

Conclusion

Treatment is not required simply because an arrhythmia has been detected. In an otherwise normal heart, asymptomatic arrhythmias and those that do not compromise hemodynamics, such as most atrial extrasystoles (AES) and occasional ventricular extrasystoles (VES), first-degree A-V block, bundle branch block, and so on, do not require antiarrhythmic medication; reassurance is sufficient. Propranolol is the best solution if a patient is particularly bothered by AES. Except in a few chosen patients, chronic preventive therapy with class I and class IV antiarrhythmics does not appear to provide a survival benefit. Vigorous therapy, on the other side, is recommended in case life-threatening arrhythmias include sustained VT, TdP, and VF, Hypotension, dyspnea, activity limitation, or heart failure, palpitation noticeable in PSVT, persistent VT, AF, and TdP, when a minor arrhythmia can develop to a more serious one, such as after a heart attack (warning arrhythmias). Antiarrhythmics are usually only needed for a short time in the conditions described above. The majority of antiarrhythmic medications have a tight safety margin. The goal is to improve CV function by restoring sinus rhythm, regulating ventricular rate, or changing the electrical and mechanical activity pattern to a more desired pattern.

Despite substantial research, antiarrhythmic drug selection is still mostly empirical.

References

1. Hiss RG, Lamb LE. Electrocardiographic findings in 122,043 individuals. *Circulation*. 1962;25:947–961.
2. Weber BE, Kapoor WN. Evaluation and outcomes of patients with palpitations. *Am J Med*. 1996;100:138–148.
3. Baman TS, Lange DC, Ilg KJ, et al. Relationship between burden of premature ventricular complexes and left ventricular function. *Heart Rhythm*. 2010;7:865–869.
4. Kennedy HL, Whitlock JA, Sprague MK, Kennedy LJ, Buckingham TA, Goldberg RJ. Long-term follow-up of asymptomatic healthy subjects with frequent and complex ventricular ectopy. *N Engl J Med*. 1985;312:193–197.
5. Willich SN, Maclure M, Mittleman M, Arntz HR, Muller JE. Sudden cardiac death: support for a role of triggering in causation. *Circulation*. 1993;87:1442–1450.
6. Bayes de Luna A, Coumel P, Leclercq JF. Ambulatory sudden cardiac death: mechanisms of production of fatal arrhythmia on the basis of data from 157 cases. *Am Heart J*. 1989;117:151–159.
7. de Vreede-Swagemakers JJ, Gorgels AP, Dubois-Arbouw WI, et al. Circumstances and causes of out-of-hospital cardiac arrest in sudden death survivors. *Heart*. 1998;79:356–361.
8. Huikuri HV, Castellanos A, Myerburg RJ. Sudden death due to cardiac arrhythmias. *N Engl J Med*. 2001;345:1473–1482.
9. Gale CP, Camm AJ. Assessment of palpitations. *BMJ*. 2016;352.
10. Lopshire JC, Douglas PZ. Sudden cardiac death: better understanding of risks, mechanisms, and treatment. *Circulation*. 2006;114(11):1134–1136.
11. Moya A, et al. Mechanism of syncope in patients with isolated syncope and in patients with tilt-positive syncope. *Circulation*. 2001;104(11):1261–1267.
12. Puppala VK, Mehmet A, Oana D, David GB. Risk stratification of patients presenting with transient loss of consciousness. *Cardiol Clin*. 2015;33(3):387–396.

13. Ferris Jr EB, Capps RB, Weiss S. Carotid sinus syncope and its bearing on the mechanism of the unconscious state and convulsions: a study of 32 additional cases. *Medicine.* 1935;14(4):377.
14. Ungar A, et al. Fall prevention in the elderly. *Clin Cases Miner Bone Metab.* 2013;10 (2):91.
15. Alboni P, et al. An abnormal neural reflex plays a role in causing syncope in sinus bradycardia. *J Am Coll Cardiol.* 1993;22(4):1130–1134.
16. Myerburg RJ, Junttila MJ. Sudden cardiac death caused by coronary heart disease. *Circulation.* 2012;125(8):1043–1052.
17. Roberts WC. Sudden cardiac death: definitions and causes. *Am J Cardiol.* 1986;57 (15):1410–1413.
18. Singh M, Morin DP, Link MS. Sudden cardiac death in long QT syndrome (LQTS), Brugada syndrome, and catecholaminergic polymorphic ventricular tachycardia (CPVT). *Prog Cardiovasc Dis.* 2019;62(3):227–234.
19. Grossman P, Wilhelm FH, Spoerle M. Respiratory sinus arrhythmia, cardiac vagal control, and daily activity. *American Journal of Physiology-Heart and Circulatory Physiology.* 2004;287(2):H728–H734. Senguttuvan, NB, Patil, NC. Cannon waves in atrioventricular nodal re-entry tachycardia. *CMAJ.* 2013;185(2):E129.
20. Tester DJ, Ackerman MJ. Genetics of cardiac arrhythmias. In: Mann DL, Zipes DP, Libby P, Bonow RO, eds. *Braunwald's heart disease: a textbook of cardiovascular medicine.* 10th ed. St Louis, MO: Elsevier; 2015:617–628.
21. Fernández-Falgueras A, et al. Cardiac channelopathies and sudden death: recent clinical and genetic advances. *Biology.* 2017;6(1):7.
22. Schwartz PJ, Stramba-Badiale M, Crotti L, et al. Prevalence of the congenital long QT syndrome. *Circulation.* 2009;120(18):1761.
23. Schwartz PJ, et al. Genotype-phenotype correlation in the long-QT syndrome: gene-specific triggers for life-threatening arrhythmias. *Circulation.* 2001;103(1):89–95.
24. Patel SI, et al. QT prolongation and sudden cardiac death risk in hypertrophic cardiomyopathy. *Acta Cardiol.* 2019;74(1):53–58.
25. Sakaguchi T, et al. Age- and genotype-specific triggers for life-threatening arrhythmia in the genotyped long QT syndrome. *J Cardiovasc Electrophysiol.* 2008;19(8):794–799.
26. Jons C, et al. Risk of fatal arrhythmic events in long QT syndrome patients after syncope. *J Am Coll Cardiol.* 2010;55(8):783–788.
27. Kim JA, Lopes CM, Moss AJ, et al. Trigger-specific risk factors and response to therapy in long QT syndrome type 2. *Heart Rhythm.* 2010;7(12):1797–1805.
28. Larsen LA, et al. Recessive Romano-Ward syndrome associated with compound heterozygosity for two mutations in the KVLQT1 gene. *Eur J Hum Genet.* 1999;7(6):724–728.
29. Tranebjærg L, et al. Jervell and Lange-Nielsen syndrome: a Norwegian perspective. *Am J Med Genet.* 1999;89(3):137–146.
30. Wilders R, Verkerk AO. Long QT syndrome and sinus bradycardia–a mini review. *Front Cardiovasc Med.* 2018;5:106.
31. Yazawa M, et al. Using induced pluripotent stem cells to investigate cardiac phenotypes in Timothy syndrome. *Nature.* 2011;471(7337):230–234.
32. Tristani-Firouzi M, Etheridge SP. Kir 2.1 channelopathies: the Andersen–Tawil syndrome. *Pflügers Archiv—Eur J Physiol.* 2010;460(2):289–294.
33. Goldenberg I, Thottathil P, Lopes CM, et al. Trigger-specific ion-channel mechanisms, risk factors, and response to therapy in type 1 long QT syndrome. *Heart Rhythm.* 2012;9 (1):49–56.

34. Zareba W, Cygankiewicz I. Long QT syndrome and short QT syndrome. *Prog Cardiovasc Dis*. 2008;51(3):264–278.
35. Roden DM. Long QT syndrome: reduced repolarization reserve and the genetic link. *J Intern Med*. 2006;259(1):59–69.
36. O-Uchi J, Rice JJ, Ruwald MH, et al. Impaired IKs channel activation by Ca(2 +)-dependent PKC shows correlation with emotion/arousal-triggered events in LQT1. *J Mol Cell Cardiol*. 2015;4(7):10.
37. Bjerregaard P, Gussak I. Short QT syndrome: mechanisms, diagnosis and treatment. *Nat Clin Pract Cardiovasc Med*. 2005;2(2):84–87.
38. Schimpf R, et al. Short QT syndrome. *Cardiovasc Res*. 2005;67(3):357–366.
39. Borggrefe M, et al. Short QT syndrome: genotype-phenotype correlations. *J Electrocardiol*. 2005;38(4):75–80.
40. Fitzgerald PT, Ackerman MJ. Drug-induced torsades de pointes: the evolving role of pharmacogenetics. *Heart Rhythm*. 2005;2(11):S30–S37.
41. Itoh H, Sakaguchi T, Ding W-G, et al. Latent genetic backgrounds and molecular pathogenesis in drug-induced long-QT syndrome. *Circ Arrhythm Electrophysiol*. 2009;2(5):511–523.
42. Lee K, et al. IKr channel blockers: novel antiarrhythmic agents. *Curr Med Chem-Cardiovasc Hematol Agents*. 2003;1(3):203–223.
43. Brown AM. Drugs, hERG and sudden death. *Cell Calcium*. 2004;35(6):543–547.
44. Silva J, Rudy Y. Subunit interaction determines I Ks participation in cardiac repolarization and repolarization reserve. *Circulation*. 2005;112(10):1384–1391.
45. Napolitano C, et al. Evidence for a cardiac ion channel mutation underlying drug-induced QT prolongation and life-threatening arrhythmias. *J Cardiovasc Electrophysiol*. 2000;11(6):691–696.
46. Tester DJ, Kopplin LJ, Will ML, Ackerman MJ. Spectrum and prevalence of cardiac ryanodine receptor (RyR2) mutations in a cohort of unrelated patients referred explicitly for long QT syndrome genetic testing. *Heart Rhythm*. 2005;2(10):1099–1105.
47. Sumitomo N, et al. Catecholaminergic polymorphic ventricular tachycardia: electrocardiographic characteristics and optimal therapeutic strategies to prevent sudden death. *Heart*. 2003;89(1):66–70.
48. Schimpf R, et al. Channelopathies: Brugada syndrome, long QT syndrome, short QT syndrome, and CPVT. *Herz Kardiovaskuläre Erkrankungen*. 2009;34(4):281–288.
49. Richter S, et al. Variability of the diagnostic ECG pattern in an ICD patient population with Brugada syndrome. *J Cardiovasc Electrophysiol*. 2009;20(1):69–75.
50. Kapplinger JD, et al. An international compendium of mutations in the SCN5A-encoded cardiac sodium channel in patients referred for Brugada syndrome genetic testing. *Heart Rhythm*. 2010;7(1):33–46.
51. Letsas KP, et al. Meta-analysis on risk stratification of asymptomatic individuals with the Brugada phenotype. *Am J Cardiol*. 2015;116(1):98–103.
52. Strauss HC, et al. Electrophysiologic evaluation of sinus node function in patients with sinus node dysfunction. *Circulation*. 1976;53(5):763–776.
53. Nof E, Glikson M, Antzelevitch C. Genetics and sinus node dysfunction. *J Atr Fibrillation*. 2009;1(6):151.
54. Lei M, Huang CL-H, Zhang Y. Genetic Na + channelopathies and sinus node dysfunction. *Prog Biophys Mol Biol*. 2008;98(2-3):171–178.
55. Goldberger AL, Goldberger ZD, Shvilkin A. *Clinical electrocardiography: a simplified approach e-book. Goldberger's Clinical Electrocardiography – A Simplified Approach*. Elsevier Health Sciences; 2017.

56. Bartos DC, Grandi E, Ripplinger CM. Ion channels in the heart. *Compr Physiol.* 2011;5 (3):1423–1464.
57. Catterall WA. Structure and function of voltage-gated ion channels. *Annu Rev Biochem.* 1995;64(1):493–531.
58. Mangoni ME, Nargeot J. Genesis and regulation of the heart automaticity. *Physiol Rev.* 2008;88(3):919–982.
59. Fozzard HA. Afterdepolarizations and triggered activity. *Basic Res Cardiol.* 1992;87(Suppl 2):105–113.
60. Corr PB, Saffitz JE, Sobel BE. Lysophospholipids, long chain acylcarnitines and membrane dysfunction in the ischaemic heart. *Basic Res Cardiol.* 1987;82(Suppl 1):199–208.
61. Akhtar M, et al. Atrioventricular nodal reentry. Clinical, electrophysiological, and therapeutic considerations. *Circulation.* 1993;88(1):282–295.
62. Robert E, et al. Dispersion-based reentry: mechanism of initiation of ventricular tachycardia in isolated rabbit hearts. *American Journal of Physiology-Heart and Circulatory Physiology.* 1999;276(2):H413–H423.
63. Jabbour F, Kanmanthareddy A. *Sinus Node Dysfunction.* StatPearls; 2019.
64. Keener JP. On cardiac arrythmias: AV conduction block. *J Math Biol.* 1981;12 (2):215–225.
65. Schmitt C, et al. Biatrial multisite mapping of atrial premature complexes triggering onset of atrial fibrillation. *Am J Cardiol.* 2002;89(12):1381–1387.
66. Scheinman MM, et al. Clinical and electrophysiologic features and role of catheter ablation techniques in adult patients with automatic atrioventricular junctional tachycardia. *Am J Cardiol.* 1994;74(6):565–572.
67. Yusuf S, Camm AJ. Deciphering the sinus tachycardias. *Clin Cardiol.* 2005;28 (6):267–276.
68. Olshansky B, Sullivan RM. Inappropriate sinus tachycardia. *J Am Coll Cardiol.* 2013;61 (8):793–801. Davies, MJ, Pomerance, A. Pathology of atrial fibrillation in man. *Br Heart J.* 1972;34(5):520.
69. Davies MJ, Pomerance A. Pathology of atrial fibrillation in man. *Br Heart J.* 1972;34 (5):520.
70. Pérez FJ, et al. Long-term outcomes after catheter ablation of cavo-tricuspid isthmus dependent atrial flutter: a meta-analysis. *Circ Arrhythm Electrophysiol.* 2009;2 (4):393–401.
71. Granada J, et al. Incidence and predictors of atrial flutter in the general population. *J Am Coll Cardiol.* 2000;36(7):2242–2246.
72. Kastor JA. Multifocal atrial tachycardia. *N Engl J Med.* 1990;322(24):1713–1717.
73. Rosso R, Kistler PM. Focal atrial tachycardia. *Heart.* 2010;96(3):181–185.
74. Katritsis DG, Camm AJ. Classification and differential diagnosis of atrioventricular nodal re-entrant tachycardia. *Europace.* 2006;8(1):29–36.
75. Fishenfeld J, Desser KB, Benchimol A. Non-paroxysmal AV junctional tachycardia associated with acute myocardial infarction. *Am Heart J.* 1973;86(6):754–758.
76. Esberger D, Jones S, Morris F. Junctional tachycardias. *BMJ.* 2002;324(7338):662–665.
77. Watanabe Y, Dreifus LS. Inhomogeneous conduction in the AV node: a model for re-entry. *Am Heart J.* 1965;70(4):505–514.
78. Nihei K, et al. Wolff-Parkinson-White (WPW) syndrome in isolated noncompaction of the ventricular myocardium (INVM) three cases. *Circ J.* 2004;68(1):82–84.
79. Nair K, et al. Antidromic His capture during entrainment of orthodromic AVRT. *Pacing Clin Electrophysiol.* 2010;33(9):1153–1156.

80. Bogun F, et al. QT dispersion in nonsustained ventricular tachycardia and coronary artery disease. *Am J Cardiol*. 1996;77(4):256–259.
81. Newby KH, et al. Sustained ventricular arrhythmias in patients receiving thrombolytic therapy: incidence and outcomes. *Circulation*. 1998;98(23):2567–2573.
82. Yan G-X, et al. Phase 2 early afterdepolarization as a trigger of polymorphic ventricular tachycardia in acquired long-QT syndrome: direct evidence from intracellular recordings in the intact left ventricular wall. *Circulation*. 2001;103(23):2851–2856.
83. Cranefield PF, Aronson RS. Torsades de pointes and early afterdepolarizations. *Cardiovasc Drugs Ther*. 1991;5(2):531–537.
84. Hondeghem LM. QT and TdP QT: an unreliable predictor of proarrhythmia. *Acta Cardiol*. 2008;63(1):1–7.
85. Hayashi M, et al. Sudden nocturnal death in young males from ventricular flutter. *Jpn Heart J*. 1985;26(4):585–591.
86. Arking DE, et al. Genetic association study of QT interval highlights role for calcium signaling pathways in myocardial repolarization. *Nat Genet*. 2014;46(8):826–836.
87. Viskin S, et al. Mode of onset of torsade de pointes in congenital long QT syndrome. *J Am Coll Cardiol*. 1996;28(5):1262–1268.
88. El-Sherif N, Turitto G, Boutjdir M. Acquired long QT syndrome and torsade de pointes. *Pacing Clin Electrophysiol*. 2018;41(4):414–421.
89. Nattel S, Singh BN. Evolution, mechanisms, and classification of antiarrhythmic drugs: focus on class III actions. *Am J Cardiol*. 1999;84(9):11–19.
90. Echt DS, et al. Evaluation of antiarrhythmic drugs on defibrillation energy requirements in dogs. Sodium channel block and action potential prolongation. *Circulation*. 1989;79(5):1106–1117.
91. Buchanan Jr JW, Saito T, Gettes LS. The effects of antiarrhythmic drugs, stimulation frequency, and potassium-induced resting membrane potential changes on conduction velocity and dV/dtmax in guinea pig myocardium. *Circ Res*. 1985;56(5):696–703.
92. Hondeghem LM, Katzung BG. Antiarrhythmic agents: the modulated receptor mechanism of action of sodium and calcium channel-blocking drugs. *Annu Rev Pharmacol Toxicol*. 1984;24(1):387–423.
93. Fei H, Hanna MS, Frame LH. Assessing the excitable gap in reentry by resetting: implications for tachycardia termination by premature stimuli and antiarrhythmic drugs. *Circulation*. 1996;94(9):2268–2277.
94. Roden DM, Darbar D, Kannankeril PJ. *Antiarrhythmic drugs. Cardiovascular medicine*. London: Springer; 2007:2085–2102.
95. Frumin H, Kerin NZ, Rubenfire M. Classification of antiarrhythmic drugs. *J Clin Pharmacol*. 1989;29(5):387–394.
96. Sunami A, Dudley SC, Fozzard HA. Sodium channel selectivity filter regulates antiarrhythmic drug binding. *Proc Natl Acad Sci USA*. 1997;94(25):14126–14131.
97. Weirich J, Antoni H. Rate-dependence of antiarrhythmic and proarrhythmic properties of class I and class III antiarrhythmic drugs. *Basic Res Cardiol*. 1998;93(1):s125–s132.
98. Yang F, et al. Quinidine revisited. *Am J Med*. 2009;122(4):317–321.
99. Noujaim SF, et al. Structural bases for the different anti-fibrillatory effects of chloroquine and quinidine. *Cardiovasc Res*. 2011;89(4):862–869.
100. Bauman JL, et al. Torsade de pointes due to quinidine: observations in 31 patients. *Am Heart J*. 1984;107(3):425–430.
101. Belhassen B, Glick A, Viskin S. Efficacy of quinidine in high-risk patients with Brugada syndrome. *Circulation*. 2004;110(13):1731–1737.

102. Viskin S, et al. Quinidine, a life-saving medication for Brugada syndrome, is inaccessible in many countries. *J Am Coll Cardiol*. 2013;61(23):2383–2387.
103. Nakajima T, et al. Anti-cholinergic effects of quinidine, disopyramide, and procainamide in isolated atrial myocytes: mediation by different molecular mechanisms. *Circ Res*. 1989;64(2):297–303.
104. Sheets MF, et al. Sodium channel molecular conformations and antiarrhythmic drug affinity. *Trends Cardiovasc Med*. 2010;20(1):16–21.
105. Manolis AS, et al. Mexiletine: pharmacology and therapeutic use. *Clin Cardiol*. 1990;13 (5):349–359.
106. Hanley CM, Robinson VM, Kowey PR. Status of antiarrhythmic drug development for atrial fibrillation: new drugs and new molecular mechanisms. *Circ Arrhythm Electrophysiol*. 2016;9(3):e002479.
107. Brubaker S, Long B, Koyfman A. Alternative treatment options for atrioventricular-nodal-reentry tachycardia: an emergency medicine review. *J Emerg Med*. 2018;54(2):198–206.
108. Zareba KM. Dronedarone: a new antiarrhythmic agent. *Drugs Today (Barc)*. 2006;42 (2):75–86.
109. Anderson JL, Prystowsky EN. Sotalol: an important new antiarrhythmic. *Am Heart J*. 1999;137(3):388–409.
110. Roden DM. Current status of class III antiarrhythmic drug therapy. *Am J Cardiol*. 1993;72(6):B44–B49.
111. Gautier P, et al. Electrophysiologic characterization of dronedarone in guinea pig ventricular cells. *J Cardiovasc Pharmacol*. 2003;41(2):191–202.
112. Dorian P. Clinical pharmacology of dronedarone: implications for the therapy of atrial fibrillation. *J Cardiovasc Pharmacol Ther*. 2010;15(4_suppl):15S–18S.
113. Zipes DP, Troup PJ. New antiarrhythmic agents: amiodarone, aprindine, disopyramide, ethmozin, mexiletine, tocainide, verapamil. *Am J Cardiol*. 1978;41(6):1005–1024.
114. Rosenbaum MB, et al. Clinical efficacy of amiodarone as an antiarrhythmic agent. *Am J Cardiol*. 1976;38(7):934–944.
115. Naccarelli GV, et al. Electrophysiology and pharmacology of ibutilide. *Am J Cardiol*. 1996;78(8):12–16.
116. Murray KT. Ibutilide. *Circulation*. 1998;97(5):493–497.
117. Manoach M, Tribulova N. Sotalol: the mechanism of its antiarrhythmic-defibrillating effect. *Cardiovasc Drug Rev*. 2001;19(2):172–182.
118. Lee KS, Tsien RW. Mechanism of calcium channel blockade by verapamil, D600, diltiazem and nitrendipine in single dialysed heart cells. *Nature*. 1983;302(5911):790–794.
119. Mitchell LB, Schroeder JS, Mason JW. Comparative clinical electrophysiologic effects of diltiazem, verapamil and nifedipine: a review. *Am J Cardiol*. 1982;49(3):629–635.
120. Chaffman M, Brogden RN. Diltiazem. *Drugs*. 1985;29(5):387–454.
121. Wilbur SL, Marchlinski FE. Adenosine as an antiarrhythmic agent. *Am J Cardiol*. 1997;79(12):30–37.
122. Iseri LT. Magnesium and cardiac arrhythmias. *Magnesium*. 1986;5(3–4):111–126.
123. Tzivoni D, et al. Magnesium therapy for torsades de pointes. *Am J Cardiol*. 1984;53 (4):528–530.
124. Dobrev D, Hamad B, Kirkpatrick P. Vernakalant. *Nat Rev Drug Discov*. 2010;9(12):915–916.
125. Roy D, et al. Vernakalant hydrochloride for rapid conversion of atrial fibrillation. *Circulation*. 2008;117(12):1518–1525.
126. Fedida D. Vernakalant (RSD1235): a novel, atrial-selective antifibrillatory agent. *Expert Opin Investig Drugs*. 2007;16(4):519–532.

127. Stiell IG, et al. A multicenter, open-label study of vernakalant for the conversion of atrial fibrillation to sinus rhythm. *Am Heart J*. 2010;159(6):1095–1101.
128. Viola N, et al. The technology in use for the surgical ablation of atrial fibrillation. *Semin Thorac Cardiovasc Surg*. 2002;14(3).
129. Melby SJ, Schuessler RB, Damiano Jr. RJ. Ablation technology for the surgical treatment of atrial fibrillation. *ASAIO J (American Society for Artificial Internal Organs: 1992)*. 2013;59(5):461.
130. Lall SC, Damiano RJ. Surgical ablation devices for atrial fibrillation. *J Interv Cardiac Electrophysiol*. 2007;20(3):73–82.
131. Heijman J, et al. Translational challenges in atrial fibrillation. *Circ Res*. 2018;122(5):752–773.
132. Philip I, Berroëta C, Leblanc I. Perioperative challenges of atrial fibrillation. *Curr Opin Anesthesiol*. 2014;27(3):344–352.
133. Wood KA, et al. Symptom challenges after atrial fibrillation ablation. *Heart Lung*. 2017;46(6):425–431.
134. Savelieva I, et al. Upstream therapies for management of atrial fibrillation: review of clinical evidence and implications for European Society of Cardiology guidelines. Part I: primary prevention. *Europace*. 2011;13(3):308–328.
135. Smit MD, Van Gelder IC. Upstream therapy of atrial fibrillation. *Expert Rev Cardiovasc Ther*. 2009;7(7):763–778.
136. Tse H-F, et al. Stroke prevention in atrial fibrillation—an Asian stroke perspective. *Heart Rhythm*. 2013;10(7):1082–1088.
137. Lip GYH, et al. Stroke prevention in atrial fibrillation: past, present and future. *Thromb Haemost*. 2017;117(07):1230–1239.
138. Lip GYH, Lane DA. Stroke prevention in atrial fibrillation: a systematic review. *JAMA*. 2015;313(19):1950–1962.
139. Freedman B, Potpara TS, Lip GYH. Stroke prevention in atrial fibrillation. *Lancet*. 2016;388(10046):806–817.
140. Wolbrette D, et al. Gender differences in arrhythmias. *Clin Cardiol*. 2002;25(2):49–56.
141. Yarnoz MJ, Curtis AB. More reasons why men and women are not the same (gender differences in electrophysiology and arrhythmias). *Am J Cardiol*. 2008;101(9):1291–1296.
142. Larsen JA, Kadish AH. Effects of gender on cardiac arrhythmias. *J Cardiovasc Electrophysiol*. 1998;9(6):655–664.
143. Peters RW, Gold MR. The influence of gender on arrhythmias. *Cardiol Rev*. 2004;12(2):97–105.
144. Lampert R, et al. Gender differences in ventricular arrhythmia recurrence in patients with coronary artery disease and implantable cardioverter-defibrillators. *J Am Coll Cardiol*. 2004;43(12):2293–2299.
145. Milman A, et al. Gender differences in patients with Brugada syndrome and arrhythmic events: data from a survey on arrhythmic events in 678 patients. *Heart Rhythm*. 2018;15(10):1457–1465.
146. Curtis AB, Narasimha D. Arrhythmias in women. *Clin Cardiol*. 2012;35(3):166–171.
147. Karmakar Sanmoy, et al. Hypokalemia: a potent risk for QTc prolongation in clarithromycin treated rats. *Eur J Pharmacol*. 2013;709(1–3):80–84.
148. Karmakar Sanmoy, et al. QT prolongation by ranitidine in hypokalemia and arrhythmogen provoked rat heart. *Vasc Dis Ther*. 2017;2(4):1–5.

Chapter 14

Insights into the mode of action of antianginal and vasodilating agents

Susmita Patra[1], Pratibha Gupta[1], Reshma Kumari[2], Sandipan Jana[2], Pallab Kanti Haldar[2], Rudranil Bhowmik[2], Avishek Mandal[2], Md. Adil Shaharyar[2], Hindol Mazumdar[2], Kumar Anand[2] and Sanmoy Karmakar[2]

[1]*Department of Pharmaceutical Technology, Adamas University, Barasat, Kolkata, West Bengal, India,* [2]*Bioeuivalence Study Centre, Department of Pharmaceutical Technology, Jadavpur University, Kolkata, West Bengal, India*

Pathophysiology associated with angina pectoris

Angina pectoris is a clinical condition of ischemic heart disease outcome of transient myocardial ischemia. Generally, angina pectoris develops due to atherosclerosis occurring in the coronary arteries which is followed by imbalance between myocardial demand and coronary blood supply. It is characterized by paroxysmal pain in the substernal or precordial region of the chest, which is provoked by an increase in the demand of the heart. Angina is a preindicator symptomatic state for a variety of major cardiovascular events that propagate in a cyclic manner. Coronary arteries are lined by the endothelial cells, and these cells regulate the muscle tone and prevent thrombosis, and if any of the abovementioned function is affected, it results into coronary heart disease.[1–4] Any injury in the lining will trigger the immune system, which results into the development of fibrous tissue and consequently leads to stenosis. Coronary artery stenosis is one of the important factors for the development of myocardial ischemia. Angina pectoris is a clinical manifestation that develops from a dynamic myocardial ischemia. During angina, paroxysmal pain in the substernal or precordial region of the chest can be seen when the oxygen demand is not sufficient as per the need of myocardial cells, or when the coronary blood flow is obstructed due to various underlying comorbid conditions such as chronic stenosing coronary atherosclerosis, sudden vasospasm of coronary trunk induced by coronary atherosclerosis, complicated coronary plaques, platelet thrombi over atherosclerotic plaques, and vasospasm of the coronary artery.[5–7] Dilation of left ventricle during ischemia increases the myocardial oxygen demand; also, increase in the left

How Synthetic Drugs Work. DOI: https://doi.org/10.1016/B978-0-323-99855-0.00014-2

ventricular filling pressure decreases the coronary perfusion pressure, which ultimately results in the imbalance between the myocardial oxygen demand and supply.[8–12] Along with the increase in myocardial oxygen demand, there is an increase in heart rate, blood pressure, filling pressure in left ventricle, and catecholamine, which propagate the vicious cycle. Angina shows majorly three different types of clinical patterns with divergent pathogenesis, among which stable or atypical angina is the most common one. Stable angina is characterized by attacks of pain following physical exertion or emotional excitement, which is further relieved by rest. Epicardial vessels and intra-myocardial arteries and arterioles together perform the function of delivering oxygen to the heart. The main factors for determining the myocardial oxygen demand are heart rate, intra-myocardial wall tension, and contractility of the heart muscles. Increase in the end-diastolic volume will subsequently increase the left ventricular preload; also, increase in the systolic pressure will raise the left ventricular preload. Thus, after increase in the preload or afterload, the heart will demand more oxygen. Heart of a healthy person experiences very little resistance during the blood flow in the epicardial vessels. In the presence of atherosclerotic plaques, the blood flow is obstructed, which is again compensated with the autoregulation mechanism of the body. During autoregulation, the myocardial vessels dilate in response to the increased oxygen demand.[13–15] Various mediators that act as a vasodilator are involved in the myocardial perfusion. The most common symptoms in the stable angina are chest pain, which may extend to the left arm, shoulder, or jaw. Symptoms are exacerbated by stress, which can be subdued with sublingual nitroglycerine. The deficient oxygen supply to the heart can also occur because of various functional macrovascular and microvascular diseases, which reflects the heterogenicity of the disease. Aortic stenosis and anemia can also contribute to the disease.[16–20] The functional microvascular abnormalities occur in the microvessels and the epicardial arteries due to either enhanced vasoconstriction or impaired vasodilation. Concentration of some vasoactive substances like endothelin-1 also gets elevated. The vascular tone and the myocardial blood flow are maintained by the coronary endothelium via nitric oxide–dependent mechanism, and the abnormal vasodilation may occur due to resistance to NO, adenosine, and prostacyclin.[21–23] Variation in the neurogenic vascular tone, hormonal changes, and various environmental factors such as low temperature, stress, and exertion are also associated with the progression of pathology. The patient will feel heaviness in the precordium, retro sternum, or the epigastric region, which can be felt as crushing, tightening of the chest, or gripping of the chest. Patients having comorbid condition like diabetes may report symptoms other than precordial origin like dyspnea, diaphoresis, and emesis. Chest pain that usually lasts for more than 15 min and subsequently radiates to both the arms with an additional third heart sound or hypotension may suggest myocardial infarction. Generally, most of the people do not seek medical care at the beginning, which is a major cause for worsening of the symptoms. Around 17% ischemia is asymptomatic in the diabetic patients, and 75% of the patient's episodes occur without any symptom. Many noncoronary causes of chest pain exist such as peptic ulcer, GERD, pancreatic diseases, esophagitis, arthritis, myositis, pulmonary embolism, pneumonia, pericarditis, generalized anxiety disorder, panic disorder, and thyrotoxicosis. The other subtype of angina is unstable angina, which occurs due to the increase in the severity of the angina pectoris. Intracoronary grayish–white platelet-rich thrombus or yellow plaque is formed on the ruptured atherosclerotic artery with complex lesion. Inflammation causes rupturing of the fibrous plaque cups with secretion of matrix metalloproteinases. There is a higher chance for myocardial infraction in unstable angina patient. In classic angina, the attacks are more frequent during exercise, whereas in variant angina, attacks are unpredictable and are more common during sleep (Figs. 14.1 and 14.2).[24–26]

1. *Pathology of classic angina:* This is the most common form of angina. Coronary arteries are responsible for blood supply in epicardium, and its perforating branches supply blood in deeper tissue. In a healthy heart, there is little resistance to blood flow in coronary artery. In presence of atherosclerotic plaques (accumulation of cholesterol and other lipids), blood flow is impeded. Autoregulation system helps to compensate during this situation by dilation of myocardial vessels in response to decreased oxygen supply. Due to autoregulation, blood flow changes in heart rapidly as a result of higher oxygen stipulation. Due to coronary

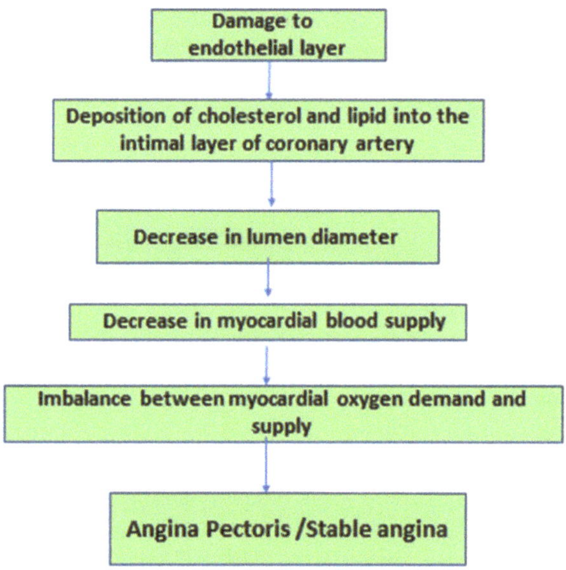

FIGURE 14.1 Pathophysiology of development of angina pectoris.

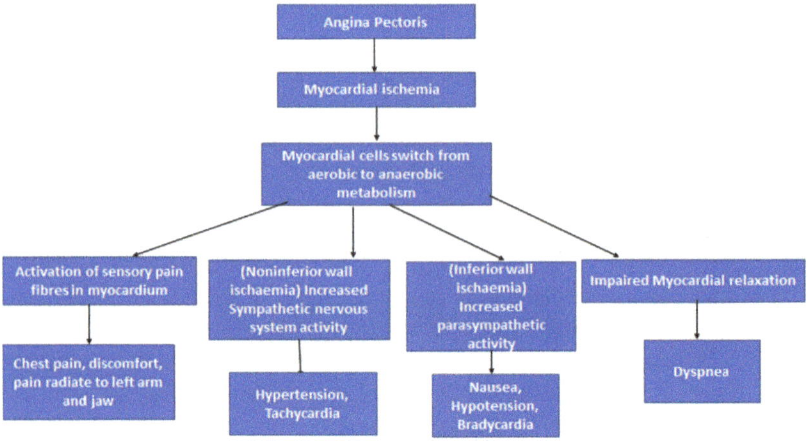

FIGURE 14.2 Consequences of angina pectoris.

blockage, blood flow fails to meet the increased oxygen demand, which causes ischemic pain. Endothelium damages, catecholamine surges cause vasoconstriction and variation in arterial tone. Pathological changes involved ischemic myocardium, coronary sinus blood pH falls, decrease cellular potassium level, accumulation of lactate in myocardium, ECG abnormalities, and deterioration of systolic and diastolic function.[27–32]

2. *Pathology of variant angina:* Variant angina, also known as vasospastic angina or prinzmetal angina, is unpredictable and attacks may occur during rest or sleep. Variant angina develops due to abnormal coronary artery spasm. Several factors are responsible for coronary artery spasm. Balance between sympathetic and parasympathetic tone is important for smooth blood flow through coronary vessels. Any injury in endothelial layer and primary smooth muscle cells of coronary artery may causes impaired regulation between vasoconstriction and vasodilation. This imbalance can predispose vasospasm during certain circumstances like cold weather, exercise, and exposure of certain drugs like alpha-agonists and cocaine. Some risk factors including cigarette smoking, inflammatory states (high hs-CRP level), and insulin resistance may precipitate variant angina.[33–36]

USFDA classification of antianginal drugs

Class of drugs	Name
Nitrates	*Short acting:* Glyceryl trinitrate (GTN, nitroglycerine) *Long acting*: Isosorbide dinitrate (short acting by sublingual route), isosorbide mononitrate, erythrityl tetranitrate, pentaerythritol tetranitrate

(*Continued*)

(Continued)

Class of drugs	Name
Beta-blockers	Propranolol, metoprolol, atenolol, and others
Calcium channel blockers	*Phenyl alkylamine*: Verapamil *Benzothiazepine:* Diltiazem *Dihydropyridines:* Nifedipine, felodipine, amlodipine, nitrendipine, nimodipine, lacidipine, lercanidipine, benidipine
Potassium channel opener	Nicorandil, cromakalim, pinacidil
Newer drugs	
Ranolazine	
3-Ketoacyl CoA thiolase blocker	Trimetazidine
Calcium channel blocker/ inhibition of the Rho-kinase signaling pathway	Fasudil
Inhibitor of the cardiac pacemaker current (If)	Ivabradine

Mechanism of action of nitrates

Organic nitrates are the most commonly used nitrates for the management of acute angina pectoris. These potent coronary vasodilators are obtained exogenously from nitric oxide. Nitrates almost act through same mechanism only time course can differ according to time course it can be short acting and long acting. They are available in a variety of preparations such as short acting as intravenous preparations, sublingual tablets, and sprays and long-acting transdermal ointments and patches, pills. Short-acting preparations are of use in acute ischemic events, whereas long-acting nitrates are frequently used in patients with stable angina. Nitrates mostly cause preload reduction with dilation of veins, which results into decreased preload venous return to the heart. The end-diastolic size and pressure of the heart are reduced which restore the pressure gradient across the walls of the ventricles. Nitrates also dilate some of the arteries, which reduce the total peripheral resistance and thus afterload on heart. Nitrates, if given in a large dose, may lead to subsequent events such as fall in blood pressure, sympathetic stimulation, tachycardia, increased cardiac contractility, and increased cardiac work, and thus angina may be precipitated.

Nitrates mainly target the coronary arteries and not the arterioles or resistance vessels due to which blood is redistributed and the blood flow is also increased in the ischemic area in angina patients. On the other hand, resistance vessels maintain their tone in the nonischemic zone in which the flow does not increase.[37–39]

Organic nitrates are first dinitrated with the help of an enzyme in the smooth muscles to release nitric oxide as a free radical. The expression and distribution of the mitochondrial aldehyde dehydrogenase enzyme, which help in the denitration of organic nitrates to nitric oxide, generally differ, and the concentration is found to be more in the veins and epicardial conducting arteries as compared to arteries and autoregulatory arterioles. Therefore, preferential dilation occurs in veins and epicardial conducting arteries due to differential distribution of the enzyme in such vessels. Nitric oxide further activates guanylyl cyclase, which results into increase in cyclic guanine monophosphate (cGMP) causing dephosphorylation of myosin light chain kinase (MLCK). Due to less amount of active MLCK, there is interference with the activation of myosin. Due to less myosin, there is no further contraction which subsequently causes relaxation. Another theory states that increase in the intracellular cGMP may also reduce Ca^{2+} entry which may also causes relaxation. The nitric oxides produced from organic nitrates can also activate cGMP synthesis in the platelets which gives antiaggregatory effect. The antiaggregatory effect is important and useful in unstable angina.[40]

The short-acting glyceryl trinitrate (GTN) is a direct acting vasodilator and also reduces pulmonary vascular resistance. In small doses, it causes decrease in the ventricular filling pressure which is also indicated as preload, and in high dose, it causes decrease in systemic vascular resistance which is indicated as afterload. This combined decrease in the preload and afterload causes increase in the cardiac output. GTN acts in a dose-dependent manner; it dilates the arteries and veins. It causes dilation of the large veins which can promote peripheral pooling of the blood and subsequently decreases venous return. Decrease in the venous return to the heart causes reduction in the left ventricular and end-diastolic pressure. Arteriolar relaxation due to GTN causes reduction in the systemic vascular resistance. With the action of GTN on the preload and afterload the myocardial oxygen consumption is also decreased. GTN provides relief within 3 min to most of the patients.

The long-acting isosorbide dinitrate causes relaxation of the vascular smooth muscle also in addition to dilation of the peripheral arteries and veins; dilation of the veins causes reduction in the left ventricular-end-diastolic pressure and preload. Dilation of the arteries causes decrease in the systolic arterial pressure, mean arterial pressure, vascular resistance, etc. Other long-acting organic nitrates like isosorbide mononitrate, erythrityl tetranitrate, and pentaerythritol tetranitrate work in a similar fashion.

Organic nitrates are effective in classical as well as variant angina. The sublingual formulation of GTN tablet or spray or isosorbide dinitrate can be taken to terminate the angina attack. Longer acting formulation of GTN can be included in the regular schedule for chronic prophylaxis. In the case of acute coronary syndromes also GTN is given initially through sublingual route, but if the pain persists, intravenous infusion of GTN is initiated.

The primary pharmacologic action of nitrodilators, arterial and venous dilation, makes these compounds useful in the treatment of hypertension, heart failure, angina, and myocardial infarction. Another beneficial action of nitrodilators is their ability to inhibit platelet aggregation.

Nitrates can be used to treat different pathologic conditions such as chronic primary or secondary hypertension emerging from pheochromocytoma, stenosis, acute and chronic heart failure ischemic heart disease, and angina pectoris. The drug can decrease preload, which may further decrease myocardial oxygen demand, decrease vascular resistance and thus reduce the pain.

The side effects associated with nitrates are headache, flushing, postural hypotension, and reflex tachycardia. Chronic use of sodium nitroprusside may cause thiocyanate toxicity because it forms cyanide and NO. Nitrates increase the production of cGMP, and drugs like sildenafil inhibit cGMP degradation. Combination of these two may cause hypotension and impaired coronary perfusion (Fig. 14.3).[41–43]

Mechanism of action of beta-blockers

The endogenous catecholamines such as epinephrine and norepinephrine bind to the β_1-adrenergic receptors and increase the automaticity as well as the conductivity of the heart. Through renin-angiotensin system also β_1-receptors cause increase in the blood pressure. On the other hand, binding of these catecholamines to the β_2-receptors causes relaxation of the smooth muscles along with some metabolic effects. Beta-blockers bind to their specific beta-adrenoceptors and block the binding of catecholamines from binding to their specific receptors, thus blocking the sympathetic responses. The type of action of beta-blockers shows that they are dependent upon the type of receptor and the type of organ system. Beta-blockers or sympatholytic

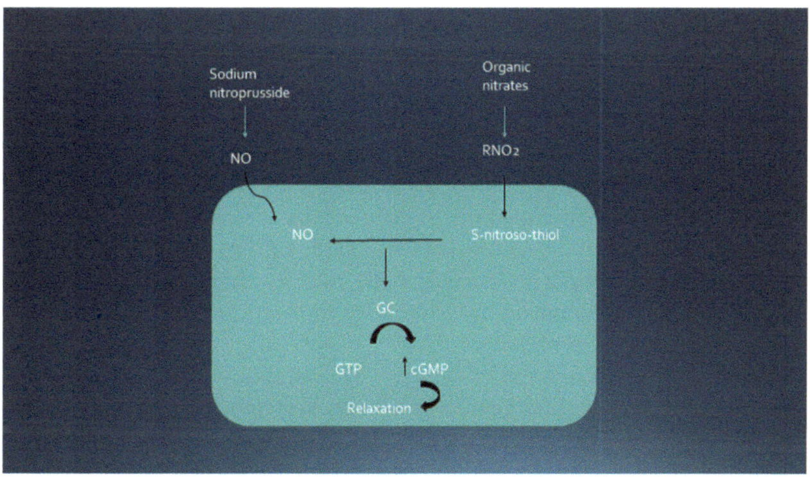

FIGURE 14.3 Mechanism of action of nitrates.

drugs are classified as beta-1 selective like atenolol, bisoprolol, metoprolol and esmolol and nonselective beta-blockers like propranolol, carvedilol, sotalol, and labetalol. Some of the beta-blockers when bind to its specific receptors act as a partial agonist as they can activate the adrenoceptors to some extent at the same time, they can inhibit the binding of norepinephrine to its receptor. These kinds of beta-blockers thus prevent very prominent sympathetic activity but evoke some sort of sympathetic action. These partial blockers are known to having intrinsic sympathomimetic activity. Beta-blockers also possess membrane stabilizing activity like sodium channel blockers. The nonselective beta-blockers are the first-generation drugs, while the selective beta-1 blockers are the second-generation drugs. The third-generation beta-blockers are also there, and they can block the alpha-adrenoceptors and possess vasodilating action. Beta-blockers inhibit the automaticity and conductivity of the heart and thus slow down the heart rate, which ultimately decreases the oxygen demand. They help decrease the blood pressure via renin-angiotensin pathway. All these activities of the beta-blockers help in the improvement of angina pectoris. Beta-blockers also prolong the arterial refractory periods, thus showing a potent antiarrhythmic effect. When beta-blockers bind to beta-adrenoceptors, which are present in the cardiac tissue, conducting tissue and contracting myocytes give the negative chronotropic and ionotropic effect. In the heart, both β1 and β2 adrenoceptors are there, but the former is the more prominent one. Beta-adrenoceptors belong to the G-protein coupled receptor family and through Gs-proteins, they have the potential to activate the adenylyl cyclase, which can generate cAMP from adenosine triphosphate (ATP). Increase in the cAMP activity can further activate cAMP-dependent protein kinase pathway, which can phosphorylate L-type calcium channels, which allow more calcium to enter into the cell during action potential. Due to more calcium entry into the cell, there is more release of calcium through the sarcoplasmic reticulum.[44–46] All these pathways lead to the increase inotropy and chronotropic effect in the heart. The protein kinase-A can also help in the phosphorylation at the site of sarcoplasmic reticulum which increases release of calcium through ryanodine receptors. As calcium is abundantly present this may help in the binding of more troponin C to increase the inotropy. Protein kinase-A can also phosphorylate myosin chains, which gives a positive ionotropic effect. Thus, beta-blockers decrease the heart rate, contractility, conductivity, in the heart. Vascular smooth muscles having β_2-adrenoceptors are activated by norepinephrine, the receptors are coupled to Gs-protein, which helps in the formation of cAMP, which can cause smooth muscle relaxation with the inhibition of MLCK. The inhibitory effect of cAMP is responsible for the phosphorylation of smooth muscle myosin. Beta-blockers show different cardiac as well as vascular effects among which the most common cardiac effect that can be observed by beta-blockers are decrease in contractility, relaxation rate, heart rate, and conduction velocity and the

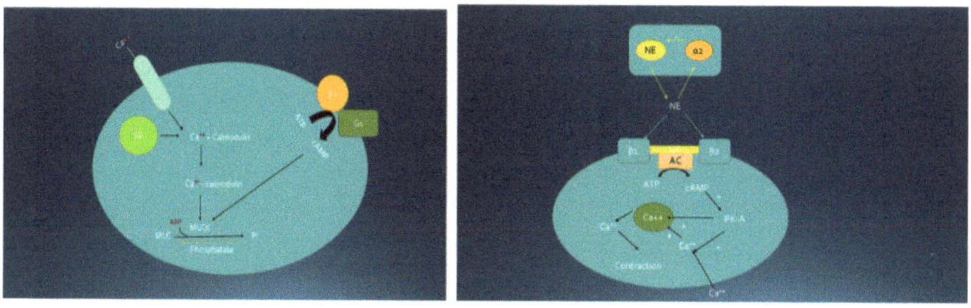

FIGURE 14.4 Mechanism of action of beta-blockers.

most common vascular effects is vasoconstriction due to smooth muscle contraction.[47–50]

The most common side effects associated with the use of beta-blockers due to blockage in the sympathetic tone of the heart are bradycardia, bronchoconstriction, reduced exercise capacity, heart failure, hypotension, and conduction block in the nodal tissue. Beta-blockers can cover the tachycardia like symptom in diabetic patients (Fig. 14.4).[51–54]

Mechanism of action of calcium channel blocker

Calcium channel blockers regulate the entry of calcium through binding with the L-type calcium channels which are present over the cardiac cells, nodal tissues and vascular smooth muscles. This class of drugs causes vasodilation, negative inotropy, negative chronotropy, decrease in conductivity, and negative dromotropy particularly in the nodal tissue. They are used in the treatment of hypertension, angina, and arrhythmias. Calcium channel blockers are classified chemically into dihydropyridines (nifedipine, amlodipine, lacidipine, benidipine, nimodipine, felodipine, nitrendipine, lercanidipine, cilnidipine, nicardipine), phenyl alkylamine (verapamil), and benzothiazepine (diltiazem) among which dihydropyridines are lipophilic in nature with greater potency, while the other two class of drugs are hydrophilic in nature with less potency. Three different types of calcium channels exist in the smooth muscles, which are voltage-sensitive channels (activated due to fluctuation in the voltage), receptor-operated channel (activated by adrenergic neurotransmitters), and leak channel (mechanical stretch causes the movement of calcium ions). The voltage-sensitive channel is made up of glycoproteins with major α_1 subunit enclosing the ion channel and associated subunits like α_2, β, δ, and γ. The voltage-sensitive calcium channels are further subdivided into L-type channel, T-type channel, and N-type channel. L-type channel causes excitation of the myocytes and contraction of the smooth muscles in the heart. It also regulates the conductivity in the heart. T-type channel regulate the activity of SA node and the N-type channel is mainly present in the central nervous system; it also regulates the neurotransmitter release in the sympathetic nervous system.[55–57] The L-type channels are found in different organs with specific isoform. Through calcium channel blocker only the L-type channel can be blocked. Depolarization occurs in the smooth muscle of the heart with the influx of calcium ion through drop down in the potential up to −40 mV, and the entered calcium triggers the release of more calcium from the calcium store in the cell. The increase in the intracellular calcium causes both excitation and contraction by phosphorylating the myosin light chain. The calcium channel blockers thus relax the vascular smooth muscles, and relaxation of artery is more prominent as compared to veins. It also relaxes the extravascular smooth muscles such as bronchial, biliary, intestinal smooth muscle, etc. Calcium plays a very important role in the ionotropic action of heart as it helps in the release of more calcium from the sarcoplasmic reticulum. Contraction occur due to surge in calcium concentration, it binds to the troponin protein which further allows the interaction of myosin and actin. Depolarization in the SA and AV node during the zero phase is calcium dependent. The refractory period, which is of longer duration in the L-type calcium channel, decides the conductivity and automaticity of the heart. Calcium channel blockers mainly targets the recovery period and prolongs that period so that the depolarization process can be delayed. The phenyl alkylamine (verapamil) and benzothiazepines (diltiazem) have negative chronotropic action while dihydropyridines does not have. Verapamil can decrease the conductivity in SA and AV nodes, but nifedipine does not show decrease in the conductivity. Diltiazem causes less decrease in the contractility as compared to the verapamil.[58–59]

The most common therapeutic use of calcium channel blocker is for hypertension, angina pectoris, and arrhythmia. With the chronic use of calcium channel blockers, side effects like cutaneous flushing, headache, hypotension, accumulation of fluid and reflex increase in the heart rate, bradycardia, defective conduction, systole heart failure etc. may occur. For stable angina, diltiazem and verapamil are most commonly used, because drugs like nifedipine lacks direct negative cardiac effect. Drugs like nifedipine and amlodipine, which act for a longer duration, can be used safely for hypertension, also because of reduced reflex responses they are the drug of choice for angina. Calcium channel blockers which belongs to the class non-dihydropyridines, should not be co-administered along with beta-blocker as they can together cause depression in the cardiac activity (Fig. 14.5).[60]

Mechanism of action of potassium channel opener

This class of drugs found helpful as an antianginal agent. These drugs have both vasodilatory and cardioprotective property. Potassium channel openers act on ATP-sensitive K + -channels present in vascular smooth muscle. Due to increased potassium efflux in smooth muscle cell, cells hold out hyperpolarized state. Hyperpolarized state reduces the chance of depolarization and

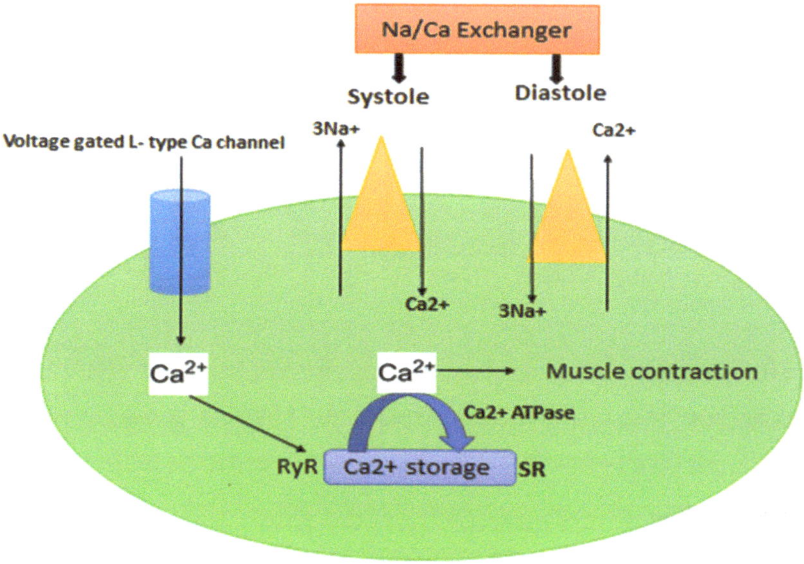

FIGURE 14.5 Mechanism of action of calcium channel blocker.

sensitivity toward any kind of stimuli. The other actions include reduced intracellular free Ca^{2+}. Both effects together relax vascular smooth muscle, which found to be helpful for angina patient as it dilates peripheral and coronary artery. Nicorandil also shows nitrate-like activity on vascular smooth muscle cells, responsible for relaxation of blood vessels by increasing cGMP. Thus, coronary blood flow is increased. It is beneficial for both stable as well as vasospastic angina, compare to calcium channel blocker and nitrates.[61–67]

Other drugs

Dipyridamole

It is an adenosine transport blocker that causes elevation of tissue adenosine levels. Adenosine stimulates angiogenesis due to reduced oxygen supply. Angiogenesis is formation of new blood vessels results of proliferation and migration of endothelial cells. Adenosine is released from vascular wall and platelets. Adenosine receptor (A1 and A2) present in endothelial cell surface stimulated during hypoxic condition and increase the proliferation of endothelial cells and reuptake by red blood cells. In addition, it acts on adenosine receptor of platelets and stimulates adenylyl cyclase cause increased level of cAMP, which is a potent inhibitor of platelet activation and thus inhibits platelet aggregation. Dipyridamole also inhibits cGMP PDE and stimulates the production of PGI2 and act as a coronary dilator and increase coronary blood flow. It also dilates resistance vessels and minimize anginal attack (Fig. 14.6).[68–74]

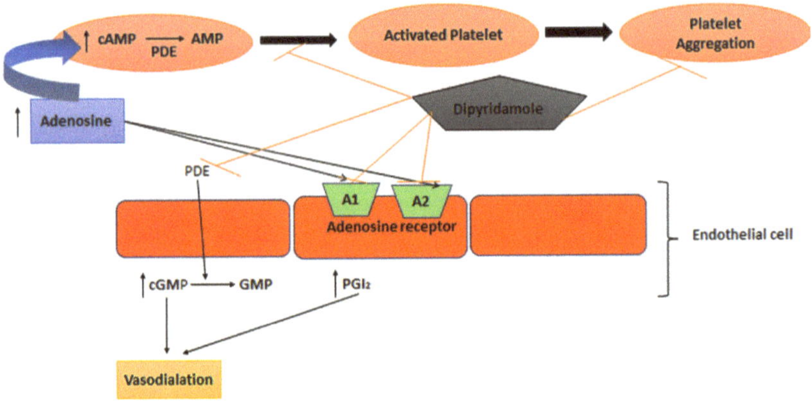

FIGURE 14.6 Mechanism of action of Dipyridamole. ↑ indicates increase, ⊥ indicates inhibition.

Trimetazidine

It is a cytoprotective drugs responsible for inhibition of enzyme long-chain 3-ketoacyl coenzyme A thiolase (LC 3-KAT), which is a final enzyme in free fatty acid (FFA) β-oxidation pathway. By inhibiting this enzyme, it reduces FFA metabolism in myocardium and increases glucose metabolism. During ischemia myocardium shifts to utilize fatty acid as a substrate for ATP generation and fatty acid oxidation requires more oxygen to generate the same amount of ATP. Thus, it worsens the situation. Trimetazidine inhibits this pathway and improves the ischemic condition. In addition, trimetazidine also increases pyruvate dehydrogenase activity, thus it restores the homeostasis between glucose oxidation and glycolysis. Combinedly trimetazidine decreased oxygen consumption required for ATP production, hydrogen ion production, reduced calcium ion accumulation, decreased reactive oxygen species generation, and reduced neutrophil infiltration (Fig. 14.7).[75–79]

Ranolazine

Ranolazine, a newer antianginal drug, acts as a specific inhibitor of late sodium current and reduces sodium overload intracellularly. Myocardial ischemia is accompanied with reduced ATP fluxes and thus energy supply decreased causes disturbances in homeostasis in cardiac myocytes. During ischemia, increased late sodium ion current causes intracellular increase of sodium ion and calcium responsible for disturbances ion homeostasis intracellularly. Ranolazine recorrects this ion disturbances by inhibiting late sodium current and causes symptomatic relief in angina patient. Ranolazine also inhibits reversible exchange of sodium–calcium and thus improves

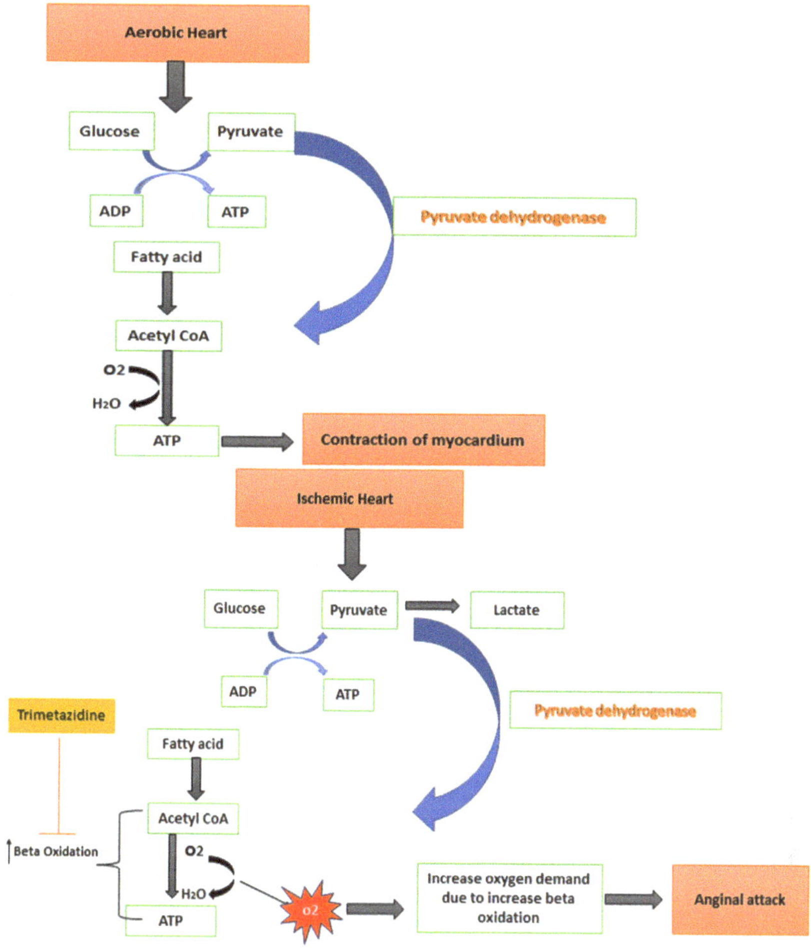

FIGURE 14.7 Mechanism of action of trimetazidine.

diastolic tone by accumulation of calcium and coronary blood flow enhanced (Fig. 14.8).[80–83]

Fasudil

Atherosclerosis is one of the reasons for developing stable angina, which is associated with progressive inflammation, lipid accumulation, and fibrosis occurred in coronary arterial wall. Rho kinase (ROCK) plays an important role for development of atherosclerotic arterial lesion. Fasudil acts as a ROCK inhibitor and upregulated eNOS and minimalizes endothelial dysfunction, ameliorates vascular cell contraction, proliferation and migration.

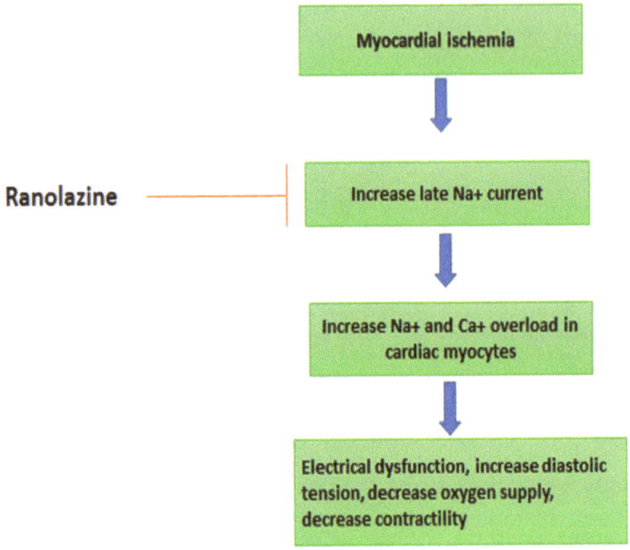

FIGURE 14.8 Mechanism of action of ranolazine.

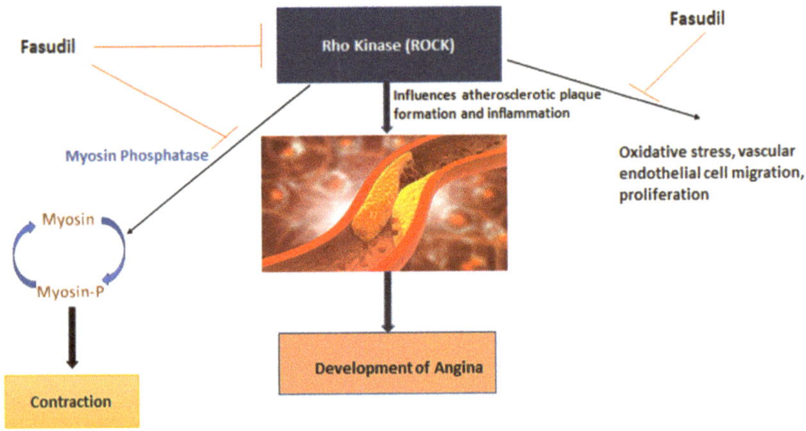

FIGURE 14.9 Mechanism of action of fasudil.

It also helps to reduce oxidative stress, vascular inflammation, macrophage infiltration, atherosclerosis plaque formation (Fig. 14.9).[84–87]

Ivabradine

This drug controls the heart rate by blocking the channel responsible for cardiac pacemaker current, which controls heart rate. Ivabradine prolongs

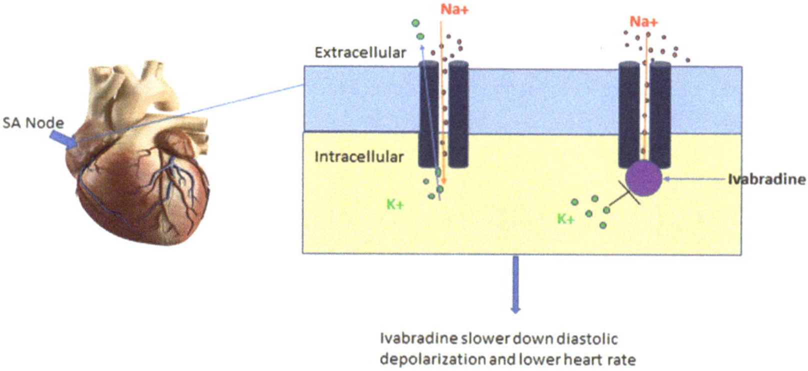

FIGURE 14.10 Mechanism of action of ivabradine.

diastolic time and reduced heart rate. Sinoatrial node has unique features in terms of alteration in their resting membrane potential, which is needed for spontaneous depolarization. Depolarization causes spontaneous repetitive action potential which is needed for automatic functioning. Depolarization is initiated by opening of mixed sodium–potassium current. Ivabradine selectively blocks hyperpolarization-activated cyclic nucleotide–gated transmembrane channel present in SA node and reduces the slope of diastolic depolarization of pacemaker action potential and thus reduces the heart rate. Ivabradine shows its effect in a dose-dependent manner (Fig. 14.10).[88–92]

Conclusion

Angina pectoris remains a serious health issue and large number populations, around 14.4% of women and 15.1% of men across the world, are diagnosed with angina pectoris.[93] Beta-blockers, nitrates, and calcium blockers remain first line drugs to treat angina pectoris, and these classes of drugs are the most extensively used. All these drugs give symptomatic relief, but they do not give any robust outcomes. The second line drugs, such as dipyridamole, fasudil, ranolazine developed to treat angina, have been extensively studied for their mechanism of action. Numerous clinical trials have been performed to study the effect of newer drugs. Still all antianginal drugs have similar efficacy and with no such survival benefit, it is hard to decide the first choice of drugs over other.

Several drugs are in pipeline to treat angina pectoris and its related comorbidities. The present study gives an idea about the mechanism of action of newer agents along with old drugs for angina pectoris. Recently, one diamond approach has been suggested to treat angina along with antihypertensive agents.[94,95] This therapeutic approach toward angina may solve the anginal complications more effectively.

References

1. Epstein SE, Redwood DR, Goldstein RE, Beiser GD, Rosing DR, Glancy DL, et al. Angina pectoris: pathophysiology, evaluation, and treatment. *Ann Intern Med.* 1971;75 (2):263–296.
2. Hinton TC, Chaitman BR. The prognosis in stable and unstable angina. *Cardiol Clin.* 1991;9:27–38.
3. da Costa JT. The physiopathology of angina pectoris. *Acta Med Port.* 1997;10 (4):233–241.
4. Procacci P, Zoppi M, Maresca M. Physiopathology of the cardiac pain. Critical review. *Recenti Prog Med.* 1974;56(6):520–546.
5. Tousoulis D, Androulakis E, Kontogeorgou A, Papageorgiou N, Charakida M, Siama K, et al. Insight to the pathophysiology of stable angina pectoris. *Curr Pharm Des.* 2013;19 (9):1593–1600.
6. Bourassa MG, Pasternac A. Douleurs angineuses avec coronaires normales ou peu lésées [Editorial: Anginal pain with normal or largely unaffected coronary vessels]. *Schweiz Med Wochenschr.* 1974;104(45):1605–1608.
7. James TN. Diseases of the large and small coronary arteries. *Arch Intern Med.* 1974;134 (1):163–176.
8. Weisman HF, Bulkley BH. Pathophysiology of atherosclerotic heart disease. *Cardiol Clin.* 1984;2(4):555–569.
9. Velican D, Iacob M. Anatomoclinical correlations in coronary heart disease: recent advances and unanswered questions. *Med Interne.* 1989;27(1):3–14.
10. Baroldi G, Giuliano G. Ischemic heart disease: clinical and pathological mismatch. *Can J Cardiol.* 1986;Suppl A:248–254.
11. Bashe Jr WJ, Baba N, Keller MD, Geer JC, Anthony JR. Pathology of atherosclerotic heart disease in sudden death. II. The significance of myocardial infarction. *Circulation.* 1975;52 (6):63–77.
12. Julius BK, Spillmann M, Vassalli G, Villari B, Eberli FR, Hess OM. Angina pectoris in patients with aortic stenosis and normal coronary arteries: mechanisms and pathophysiological concepts. *Circulation.* 1997;95(4):892–898.
13. Perper JA, Kuller LH, Cooper M. Arteriosclerosis of coronary arteries in sudden, unexpected deaths. *Circulation.* 1975;52(6):27–33.
14. Sontag TJ, Carnemolla R, Vaisar T, Reardon CA, Getz GS. Naturally occurring variant of mouse apolipoprotein A-I alters the lipid and HDL association properties of the protein. *J Lipid Res.* 2012;53(5):951–963.
15. Lambert CR. Pathophysiology of stable angina pectoris. *Cardiol Clin.* 1991;9(1):1–10.
16. Chierchia S, Smith G, Morgan M, Gallino A, Deanfield J, Croom M, et al. Role of heart rate in pathophysiology of chronic stable angina. *Lancet.* 1984;324(8416): 1353–1357.
17. Wilke A, Noll B, Maisch B. Angina pectoris bei extrakoronaren Erkrankungen [Angina pectoris in extracoronary diseases]. *Herz.* 1999;24(2):132–139.
18. Sylvén C. Mechanisms of pain in angina pectoris—a critical review of the adenosine hypothesis. *Cardiovasc Drugs Ther.* 1993;7(5):745–759.
19. Crea F, Gaspardone A. New look to an old symptom: angina pectoris. *Circulation.* 1997;96 (10):3766–3773.
20. Droste C. Pathophysiologie schmerzhafter und stummer Myokardischämie [Pathophysiology of painful and silent myocardial ischemia]. *Herz.* 1987;12(6):369–386.

21. Tenaglia AN, Peters KG, Sketch Jr MH, Annex BH. Neovascularization in atherectomy specimens from patients with unstable angina: implications for pathogenesis of unstable angina. *Am Heart J.* 1998;135(1):10–14.
22. Sadigh-Lindell B, Sylvén C, Berglund M, Eriksson BE. Role of adenosine and opioid-receptor mechanisms for pain in patients with silent myocardial ischemia or angina pectoris: a double-blind, placebo-controlled study. *J Cardiovasc Pharmacol.* 2003;42(6): 757–763.
23. Meller ST, Gebhart GF. A critical review of the afferent pathways and the potential chemical mediators involved in cardiac pain. *Neuroscience.* 1992;48(3):501–524.
24. Warren J. Remarks on angina pectoris. *N Engl J Med.* 1812;1812(1):1–11.
25. Himbert J. The angina pectoris state. *Ann Med Interne (Paris).* 1969;120(10):619–631.
26. Baba N, Bashe Jr WJ, Keller MD, Geer JC, Anthony JR. Pathology of atherosclerotic heart disease in sudden death. I. Organizing thrombosis and acute coronary vessel lesions. *Circulation.* 1975;52(6):53–59.
27. Balla C, Pavasini R, Ferrari R. Treatment of angina: where are we? *Cardiology.* 2018;140 (1):52–67.
28. Thadani U. Management of stable angina – current guidelines: a critical appraisal. *Cardiovasc Drugs Ther.* 2016;30(4):419–426.
29. Gayet JL, Paganelli F, Cohen-Solal A. Update on the medical treatment of stable angina. *Arch Cardiovasc Dis.* 2011;104(10):536–544.
30. Santucci A, Riccini C, Cavallini C. Treatment of stable ischaemic heart disease: the old and the new. *Eur Heart J Suppl.* 2020;22:54–59.
31. Kaski J, Arrebola-Moreno A, Dungu J. Treatment strategies for chronic stable angina. *Expert Opin Pharmacother.* 2011;12:2833–2844.
32. Wee Y, Burns K, Bett N. Medical management of chronic stable angina. *Aust Prescr.* 2015;38(4):131–136.
33. Picard F, Sayah N, Spagnoli V, Adjedj J, Varenne O. Vasospastic angina: a literature review of current evidence. *Arch Cardiovasc Dis.* 2019;112(1):44–55.
34. Tripathi KD. *Essentials of Medical Pharmacology.* 7th ed. Jaypee Brothers Medical Publishers; 2013:539–540.
35. Harris JR, Hale GM, Dasari TW, Schwier NC. Pharmacotherapy of vasospastic angina. *J Cardiovasc Pharmacol Ther.* 2016;21(5):439–451.
36. McMahon MT, McPherson MA, Talbert RL, Greenberg B, Sheaffer SL. Diagnosis and treatment of Prinzmetal's variant angina. *Clin Pharm.* 1982;1(1):34–42.
37. Torfgård KE, Ahlner J. Mechanisms of action of nitrates. *Cardiovasc Drugs Ther.* 1994;8 (5):701–717.
38. Tarkin JM, Kaski JC. Vasodilator therapy: nitrates and nicorandil. *Cardiovasc Drugs Ther.* 2016;30(4):367–378.
39. Horowitz JD. Role of nitrates in unstable angina pectoris. *Am J Cardiol.* 1992;70 (8):64–71.
40. Smith ER, Smiseth OA, Kingma I, Manyari D, Belenkie I, Tyberg JV. Mechanism of action of nitrates: role of changes in venous capacitance and in the left ventricular diastolic pressure-volume relation. *Am J Med.* 1984;76(6):14–21.
41. Winbury MM, Howe BB, Hefner MA. Effect of nitrates and other coronary dilators on large and small coronary vessels: an hypothesis for the mechanism of action of nitrates. *J Pharmacol Exp Ther.* 1969;168(1):70–95.
42. Thadani U, Opie LH. Nitrates for unstable angina. *Cardiovasc Drugs Ther.* 1994;8 (5):719–726.

43. Thadani U. Oral nitrates: more than symptomatic therapy in coronary artery disease? *Cardiovasc Drugs Ther*. 1997;11(1):213–218.
44. Liu X, Engelman RM, Agrawal HR, Das DK. Preservation of membrane phospholipids by propranolol, pindolol, and metoprolol: a novel mechanism of action of beta-blockers. *J Mol Cell Cardiol*. 1991;23(10):1091–1100.
45. Pedersen ME, Cockcroft JR. The vasodilatory beta-blockers. *Curr Hypertens Rep*. 2007;9 (4):269–277.
46. Robinson BF. Mechanism of action of beta-blocking drugs in angina pectoris: a review. *Postgrad Med J*. 1976;52(Suppl 4):43–45.
47. Elgendy IY, Mahmoud A, Conti CR. Beta-blockers in the management of coronary artery disease: are we on the verge of a new paradigm shift? *Recent Pat Cardiovasc Drug Discov*. 2014;9(1):11–21.
48. Wilson AG, Brooke OG, Lloyd HJ, Robinson BF. Mechanism of action of beta-adrenergic receptor blocking agents in angina pectoris: comparison of action of propranolol with dexpropranolol and practolol. *Br Med J*. 1969;4(5680):399–401.
49. Hadzi Pesić LJ. Beta blokatori u terapiji angine pektoris [Beta blockers in the treatment of angina pectoris]. *Srp Arh Celok Lek*. 1992;120(4):35–38.
50. Radović VV. [Studies of the outcome of the treatment with beta-blockers in secondary prevention of the ischemic heart disease]. *Med Pregl*. 2009;62(9–10):450–455.
51. Radović VV. [Use of beta blockers in various clinical states]. *Med Pregl*. 2011;64 (1–2):55–60.
52. Chierchia S, Gerosa S, Glazier JJ. Beta-blockers for the treatment of angina pectoris: indications in relation to pathophysiological mechanisms. *J Cardiovasc Pharmacol*. 1987;10 (2):29–33.
53. Chierchia S, Muiesan L, Davies A, Balasubramian V, Gerosa S, Raftery EB. Role of the sympathetic nervous system in the pathogenesis of chronic stable angina. Implications for the mechanism of action of beta-blockers. *Circulation*. 1990;82(3):71–81.
54. Di Somma S, de Divitiis M, Bertocchi F, Carotenuto A, Cudemo G, Petitto M, et al. Treatment of hypertension associated with stable angina pectoris: favourable interaction between new metoprolol formulation (OROS) and nifedipine. *Cardiologia*. 1996;41(7): 635–643.
55. Sueta D, Tabata N, Hokimoto S. Clinical roles of calcium channel blockers in ischemic heart diseases. *Hypertens Res*. 2017;40(5):423–428.
56. Opie LH, Yusuf S, Kübler W. Current status of safety and efficacy of calcium channel blockers in cardiovascular diseases: a critical analysis based on 100 studies. *Prog Cardiovasc Dis*. 2000;43(2):171–196.
57. Lopez LM, Santiago TM. Isradipine – another calcium-channel blocker for the treatment of hypertension and angina. *Ann Pharmacother*. 1992;26(6):789–799.
58. Beller GA. Calcium antagonists in the treatment of Prinzmetal's angina and unstable angina pectoris. *Circulation*. 1989;80(6):78–87.
59. Braunwald E. Mechanism of action of calcium-channel-blocking agents. *N Engl J Med*. 1982;307(26):1618–1627.
60. Katz AM. Pharmacology and mechanisms of action of calcium-channel blockers. *J Clin Hypertens*. 1986;2(3):28–37.
61. Ogawa N. Pharmacological properties of KRN2391, a novel vasodilator of the nitrate-potassium channel opener hybrid type. *Gen Pharmacol*. 1994;25(4):609–616.
62. Why HJ, Richardson PJ. A potassium channel opener as monotherapy in chronic stable angina pectoris: comparison with placebo. *Eur Heart J*. 1993;14:25–29.

63. Gvishiani M, Gabunia L, Makharadze T, Gongadze N. Nicorandil efficacy in the treatment of ischemic heart disease (review). *Georgian Med News*. 2018;280–281:152–155.
64. Ligtenberg JJ, van Haeften TW, Links TP, Smit AJ, Reitsma WD. Clinical relevance of ATP-dependent potassium channels. *Neth J Med*. 1995;47(5):241–251.
65. Miura T, Miki T. ATP-sensitive K+ channel openers: old drugs with new clinical benefits for the heart. *Curr Vasc Pharmacol*. 2003;1(3):251–258.
66. Andersson KE. Clinical pharmacology of potassium channel openers. *Pharmacol Toxicol*. 1992;70(4):244–254.
67. Chiariello M, Duilio C, Ambrosio G. Anti-angina activity of potassium-channel activators. *Cardiologia*. 1993;38(12):459–463.
68. Gresele P, Arnout J, Deckmyn H, Vermylen J. Mechanism of the antiplatelet action of dipyridamole in whole blood: modulation of adenosine concentration and activity. *Thromb Haemost*. 1986;55(1):12–18.
69. Bullough DA, Zhang C, Montag A, Mullane KM, Young MA. Adenosine-mediated inhibition of platelet aggregation by acadesine. A novel antithrombotic mechanism in vitro and in vivo. *J Clin Invest*. 1994;94(4):1524–1532.
70. Stafford NP, Pink AE, White AE, Glenn JR, Heptinstall S. Mechanisms involved in adenosine triphosphate–induced platelet aggregation in whole blood. *Arterioscler Thromb Vasc Biol*. 2003;23(10):1928–1933.
71. Gresele P, Zoja C, Deckmyn H, Arnout J, Vermylen J, Verstraete M. Dipyridamole inhibits platelet aggregation in whole blood. *Thromb Haemost*. 1983;50(4):852–856.
72. Harker LA, Kadatz RA. Mechanism of action of dipyridamole. *Thromb Res Suppl*. 1983;4:39–46.
73. Kim H-H, Liao JK. Translational therapeutics of dipyridamole. *Arterioscler Thromb Vasc Biol*. 2008;28:39–42.
74. Mills DC, Smith JB. The influence on platelet aggregation of drugs that affect the accumulation of adenosine 3:5-cyclic monophosphate in platelets. *Biochem J*. 1971;121: 185–196.
75. Chrusciel P, Rysz J, Banach M. Defining the role of trimetazidine in the treatment of cardiovascular disorders: some insights on its role in heart failure and peripheral artery disease. *Drugs*. 2014;74(9):971–980.
76. Marzilli M, Vinereanu D, Lopaschuk G, Chen Y, Dalal JJ, Danchin N, et al. Trimetazidine in cardiovascular medicine. *Int J Cardiol*. 2019;293:39–44.
77. Marzilli M. Cardioprotective effects of trimetazidine: a review. *Curr Med Res Opin*. 2003;19(7):661–672.
78. Lopaschuk GD. Optimizing cardiac energy metabolism: how can fatty acid and carbohydrate metabolism be manipulated? *Coron Artery Dis*. 2001;12(1):8–11.
79. Kantor PF, Lucien A, Kozak R, Lopaschuk GD. The antianginal drug trimetazidine shifts cardiac energy metabolism from fatty acid oxidation to glucose oxidation by inhibiting mitochondrial long-chain 3-ketoacyl coenzyme A thiolase. *Circ Res*. 2000;86(5):580–588.
80. Hasenfuss G, Maier LS. Mechanism of action of the new anti-ischemia drug ranolazine. *Clin Res Cardiol*. 2008;97(4):222–226.
81. Salazar CA, Basilio Flores JE, Veramendi Espinoza LE, Mejia Dolores JW, Rey Rodriguez DE, Loza Munárriz C. Ranolazine for stable angina pectoris. *Cochrane Database Syst Rev*. 2017;2(2):CD011747.
82. Stone PH, Chaitman BR, Stocke K, Sano J, DeVault A, Koch GG. The anti-ischemic mechanism of action of ranolazine in stable ischemic heart disease. *J Am Coll Cardiol*. 2010;56(12):934–942.

83. Antzelevitch C, Belardinelli L, Zygmunt AC, et al. Electrophysiological effects of ranolazine, a novel antianginal agent with antiarrhythmic properties. *Circulation.* 2004;110:904–910.
84. Shi J, Wei L. Rho kinases in cardiovascular physiology and pathophysiology: the effect of fasudil. *J Cardiovasc Pharmacol.* 2013;62(4):341–354.
85. Sato S, Ikegaki I, Asano T, Shimokawa H. Antiischemic properties of fasudil in experimental models of vasospastic angina. *Jpn J Pharmacol.* 2001;87(1):34–40.
86. Masumoto A, Mohri M, Shimokawa H, Urakami L, Usui M, Takeshita A. Suppression of coronary artery spasm by the Rho-kinase inhibitor fasudil in patients with vasospastic angina. *Circulation.* 2002;105(13):1545–1547.
87. Tsuno A, Nasu K, Kawano Y, Yuge A, Li H, Abe W, et al. Fasudil inhibits the proliferation and contractility and induces cell cycle arrest and apoptosis of human endometriotic stromal cells: a promising agent for the treatment of endometriosis. *J Clin Endocrinol Metab.* 2011;96(12):1944–1952.
88. Koruth JS, Lala A, Pinney S, Reddy VY, Dukkipati SR. The clinical use of ivabradine. *J Am Coll Cardiol.* 2017;70(14):1777–1784.
89. Giavarini A, de Silva R. The role of ivabradine in the management of angina pectoris. *Cardiovasc Drugs Ther.* 2016;30(4):407–417.
90. Mengesha HG, Weldearegawi B, Petrucka P, Bekele T, Otieno MG, Hailu A. Effect of ivabradine on cardiovascular outcomes in patients with stable angina: *meta*-analysis of randomized clinical trials. *BMC Cardiovasc Disord.* 2017;17(1):105.
91. Ide T, Ohtani K, Higo T, Tanaka M, Kawasaki Y, Tsutsui H. Ivabradine for the treatment of cardiovascular diseases. *Circ J.* 2019;83(2):252–260.
92. Pavasini R, Camici PG, Crea F, Danchin N, Fox K, Manolis AJ, et al. Anti-anginal drugs: systematic review and clinical implications. *Int J Cardiol.* 2019;283:55–63.
93. Pakhomov SS, Hemingway H, Weston SA, Jacobsen SJ, Rodeheffer R, Roger VL. Epidemiology of angina pectoris: role of natural language processing of the medical record. *Am Heart J.* 2007;153(4):666–673.
94. Ferrari R, Camici GP, Crea F, Danchin N, Fox K, et al. A 'diamond' approach to personalized treatment of angina. *Nat Rev Cardiol.* 2018;15:120–132.
95. Banerjee A, Roy D, Mazumdar H, et al. MicroRNA 155:145 ratio as a marker of atherogenic tilt manifested across different age groups and risk factor profiles. *Eur. Heart J.* 2022;43(1). Available from: https://doi.org/10.1093/eurheartj/ehab849.063.

Chapter 15

Mechanism of action of drugs used in hypertension

Rudranil Bhowmik[1], Md. Adil Shaharyar[1], Kumar Anand[1], Hindol Mazumdar[1], Avishek Mandal[1], Pallab Mandal[1], Suparno Chakraborty[2], Parag Panday[3] and Sanmoy Karmakar[1]

[1]Bioeuivalence Study Centre, Department of Pharmaceutical Technology, Jadavpur University, Kolkata, West Bengal, India, [2]TCG Life Sciences Pvt Ltd (formerly "Chembiotek Research International"), R&D Centre, Chemistry, Kolkata, West Bengal, India, [3]Infoclin Consultency, Kolkata, West Bengal, India

The most common cardiovascular disease is considered to be hypertension. Prevalence rate of hypertension increased with aging and aggravates further without proper intervention. Hypertension can be defined as pressure exerted by blood on inner wall of blood vessel. Elevated arterial hypertension for a prolong period damages blood vessels in different organs, with incidences like renal failure in kidney,[1] stroke, heart failure, coronary disease in heart,[2] and dementia in brain.[3]

Blood pressure levels of 120 mm Hg systolic and 80 mm Hg diastolic, or less, are regarded to be the lowest risk.[4] Hypertension is defined conventionally as elevated BP more than 140 mmHg as systolic and 90 mmHg as diastolic pressure. Such condition refers that a certain individual is prone to cardiovascular condition and could have needed medical attention. During very high BP, e.g, more than 210 and 120 mmHg systolic and diastolic, respectively, patients could develop fulminant arteriopathy characteristics, including injury of endothelium lining, leads to a marked inflammation in the intima, ultimately leading to arteriolar occlusion.[5,6]

Risk of cardiovascular disease augments with every 20/10 mmHg elevation of BP throughout range.[7] Hypertension is risky and cannot be ignored, because overtime it causes end-organ damage and both systolic, even isolated one and diastolic hypertension associated with it. Accurate detection of hypertension can prevent organ damage, though family history of cardiovascular disease and metabolic disorder like diabetes and other inflammatory factors also increases the chance of it along with other agonistic factors like obesity and smoking.[8] Hypertension does not show any early symptom,

How Synthetic Drugs Work. DOI: https://doi.org/10.1016/B978-0-323-99855-0.00015-4

usually asymptomatic unless end-organ damage surfaced, thus referred to as silent killer.[9,10]

Consideration of hypertension		
Blood pressure (mmHg)		
Classification	Systolic	Diastolic
Normal	Less than 120 mmHg	Less than 80 mmHg
Prehypertension or borderline	120–139 mmHg	80–89 mmHg
Hypertension with risk (stage 1)	140–159 mmHg	90–99 mmHg
Hypertension with high risk (stage 2)	Greater than 160 mmHg	Greater than 100 mmHg

BP is quantitative trait, so arbitrarily the dichotomy between hypertension and normotension is involved in positive relation with cardiovascular risk.[11] Dilatory sodium also plays an important role in hypertension. It is also reported that individuals prone to hypertension have kidneys unable to excrete excess sodium unless renal perfusion rate is increased over normal limit. Individual with genetically susceptible with hypertensive traits while exposed to high level of dietary sodium would develop salt and water retention, increased cardiac output (CO), peripheral vascular resistance (PVR) would increase, and hypertension would develop.[12,13]

Etiology of hypertension

In most cases, elevation of BP is associated with increased resistance to flow of blood through arterioles, often without any change in CO. There are many factors associated with integrally in PVR and essential hypertension, such as baroreceptor reflex, autonomic nervous system function, rennin angiotensin aldosterone system, and renal perfusion rate but none of them are responsible for it. Investigations suggest that hypertension is a cause of several abnormalities or a combination of those factors. Population with habit of daily low salt (sodium) intake does not show manifestation of hypertension with aging, whereas individuals with labile hypertension are prone to cardiac arrest after salt-enriched diet elevates BP. Other epidemiological factors are psychological stresses, genetic factors, reduced potassium and calcium in diet which develop the hypertension.[14]

Mutations in several genes play intricate and rare causes of hypertension. Functional variations of the genes for angiotensinogen (AGT), angiotensin-converting enzyme (ACE),[15] the β_2 adrenorecetor,[16,17] and α adducin[18,19] (a cytoskeletal protein) appear to contribute to some cases of essential hypertension.

Normal regulation of blood pressure

As per the hydraulic equation, arterial BP is directly proportionate to the product of CO and the PVR:[20]

$$BP = CO \times PVR$$

BP is maintained by three anatomic sites arterioles, postcapillary venules (capacitance vessels), and heart. Kidney is another important site to maintain BP by regulating volume of intravascular fluid. Autonomic nerves interact through baroreceptors known as baroreflex along with humoral controls. Renin–angiotensin–aldosterone system (RAAS) controls all the abovementioned sites for pressure homeostasis. Vasoactive substance like EDRF, released from vascular endothelium, may also involve local vascular resistance.

1. Postural baroreflex

   Baroreflex is related directly with posture of human body through baroreceptors. Baroreceptors are pressure receptors in simple terms. Sympathetic neurons centrally arise from vasomotor center of medulla and activated tonically by blood vessel. This tonic change reflects in adjustment of BP during postural changes. Baroreceptor in carotid artery is stimulated due to stretching of the vessel wall and prevents central sympathetic discharge. Similarly reduction of stretch reduces

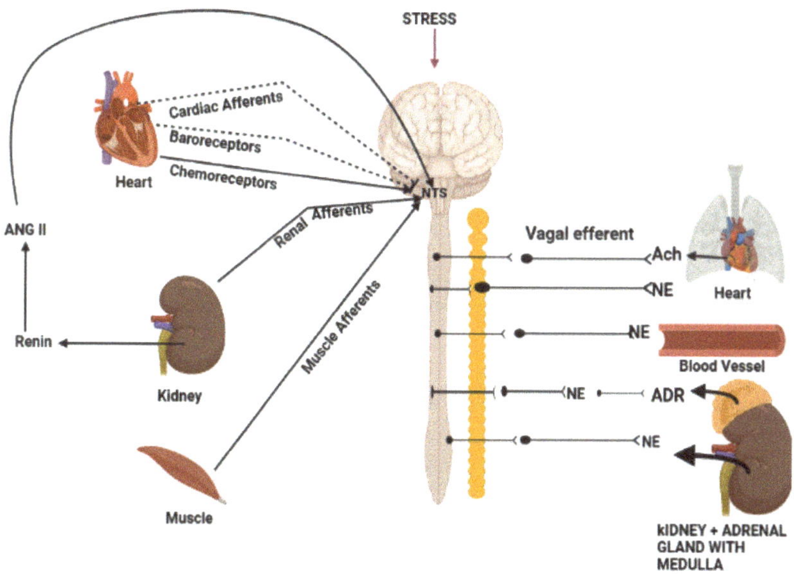

FIGURE 15.1 Different pathways of controlling blood pressure: NTS, Ach, NE, ADR. Different pathways contribute different aspects on hypertension. Activation of reflex baroreceptor reduces blood pressure by inhibiting catecholamine discharges. Reduced adrenergic discharge reduces heart rate, contraction of blood vessel, reduction of adrenalin liberation. Reduced blood pressure affects on salt reabsorption and activates RAAS. Renin activates AngII production and resulting increased blood pressure. Adrenalin also elevates heart rate and blood pressure. The dotted lines indicate reducing effect, and straight lines indicate inducing effects. *Ach*, Acetylcholine; *ADR*, adrenalin; *AngII*, angiotensin-II; *NE*, Norepinephrine; *NTS*, nucleus tractus solitarius; *RAAS*, renin–angiotensin–aldosterone system.

baroreceptor activity. To clarify, in an upright position, baroreceptors detect reduced pressure in ascending blood arteries as blood pools near the lower extremities of the body due to gravity. Thus reduced stress or tone withdraws inhibition of sympathetic discharge. As a result, sympathetic output increases through nerve endings and also increases PVR by artery constriction and increased CO through stimulation of heart and narrowing of capacitance vessels which lead to increased venous return, final restoration of BP.[21–24]

2. Renal response BP

Kidney controls blood volume and is primarily responsible for controlling long-term BP. When renal perfusion rate decreases, pressure change in Bowman's capsule causes internal redistribution of blood flow and reabsorption of salt and water will be increased in nephron. Simultaneously, reduced pressure in afferent blood vessels or arterioles in glomerulus stimulates production of renin (through sympathetic outlets via β-adrenoceptors) in juxtaglomerular apparatus through macula dense pathway. Renin increases production of angiotensin-II (AngII) that is responsible for direct vasoconstriction in resistance vessels and induces aldosterone synthesis. Angiotensin-II is product of angiotensin I (AngI) by ACE and AngI is product of AGT, a circulating protein produced in liver. The function of aldosterone is to increase absorption of salt (sodium) and water, thus increasing circulating blood volume. To maintain pressure homeostasis, vasopressin is released from posterior pituitary gland and regulates water balance through kidney (Fig. 15.1).[25–28]

Control of renin secretion

The renin secretion from juxtaglomerular cells is controlled by the following pathways: the macula densa pathway, intrarenal baroreceptor pathway, and β_1 adrenergic receptor pathway.

The juxtaglomerular apparatus is a specialized structure formed by the ascending distal convoluted tubule and the glomerular arterioles. The macula densa is a collection of specialized epithelial cells which lies adjacent to the juxtaglomerular cell in the distal convoluted tubule that detects sodium concentration of the fluid in the tubule. Change in salt reabsorption modifies renin release. In the case of increased NaCl (specially sodium) reabsorption, cells of macula densa contract afferent arterioles, reduce blood flow in glomerulus and glomerular filtration rate, and simultaneously prevent renin release resulting reduced BP in arterioles whereas reduction in NaCl flux stimulates renin release (Fig. 15.2).[29–32]

ATP, adenosine, and prostaglandins (PGs) modulate the macula densa pathway. During NaCl, reabsorption adenosine diphosphate (ADP) is utilized to fuel sodium–potassium antiport in renal tubule. Adenosine is produced by renal tissue and has potent effects on renal blood flow. More NaCl reabsorption causes depletion of ADP, as a result adenosine level increases. Adenosine acts as metabolic

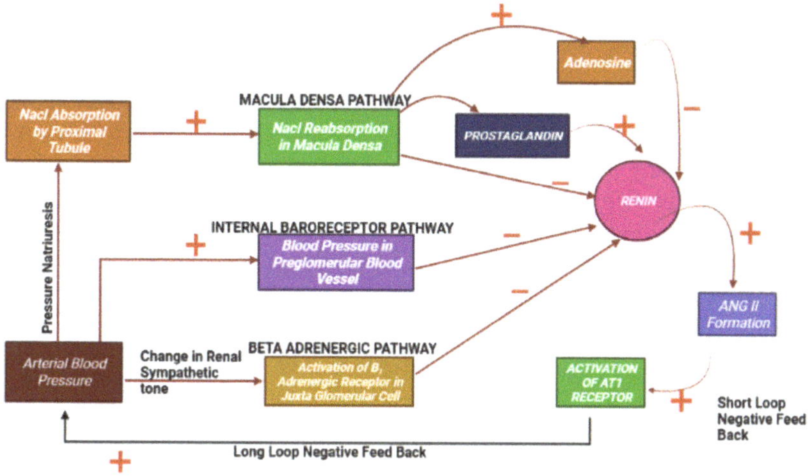

FIGURE 15.2 Different pathways that interfere renin release. " + " refers to increasing activity and "–" refers to decreasing activity.

regulator to maintain renal hemodynamics. By acting on A_1 adenosine receptor that is an inhibitory, G protein–coupled receptor (G_i) prevents activation of adenylyl cyclase (AC), hence cAMP concentration is diminished and renin release prevented.[33–35] Decreased renin concentration in blood reduces concentration of AngII, thus BP decreases which leads to reduction of glomerular filtration rate and decreases NaCl transportation. Reduced Na^+ concentration in macula densa induces cyclooxygenase-2 (COX-2) and neuronal nitric oxide synthase. Upregulation of nNOS also helps in induction of COX-2. PGs mainly PGE_2, PGI_2 are released when NaCl reabsorption decreases as a result of COX-2. These PGs act on a stimulatory G-protein receptor (Gs) and increase renin release followed by cAMP formation by AC activation.[36–38] ATP is also released when NaCl transport increases and inhibits renin release by working on P2Y receptors.

Renin release is also controlled by *internal baroreceptor pathway*. Increased BP or increased renal perfusion rate inhibits renin release and decreases in BP in preglomerular vessels stimulates it. The *β-adrenergic receptor pathway* is controlled by the release of norepinephrine (NE) from postganglionic sympathetic nerves; activation of β_1 receptors on juxtaglomerular cells enhances renin secretion.[39–41]

Renin and prorenin receptor

Renin is secreted as prorenin. Prorenin is inactive due to accessibility of AGT which is blocked by a propeptide chain. Prorenin can be activated by binding with catalytic site of prorenin receptor (PPR), where propertied chain is cleaved. Angiotensinogen is the substrate for renin, an abundant globular glycoprotein. It contains 452 amino acids and is synthesized secreted primarily from the liver. AngI is produced by cleaved amino terminus of angiotensinogen.[42–44]

ACE (kininase II, dipeptidyl carboxypeptidase) is a glycoprotein and an ectoenzyme. ACE is identical to kininase II, which acts and inactivates bradykinin and many prominent vasodilator peptides. ACE helps in the conversion of AngI to AngII, process occurs in plasma. Another carboxypeptidase is reported to work in angiotensin, which is termed ACE2.[45,46] ACE2 has a stronger affinity for AngII than AngI. A group of researchers says ACE2 also serves as SARS coronavirus receptor.[47]

Most recognized biological effects are observed by AngII on angiotensin I (AT_1) receptor. Upon acting on AT_1 receptor, AngII is responsible for vasoconstriction of coronary artery, hypertrophic cardiomyopathy and directly is associated with hypertension. AT_1 receptors involved in variety of signal transduction system result primary and secondary response depending upon cell types. AT_1 receptors are coupled with different G proteins, including excitatory (G_q), inhibitory (G_1), and $G_{12/13}$. Largely AT_1 receptors are coupled with G_q in most of the cell types by activating the IP_3, through Ca^{2+} pathway, via PLCβ.[48,49] As a result, activation of phosphokinase C, phospholipase A_2, phospholipase D, and other eicosanoids production leads to activation of calcium-dependent MAP kinases (primary response) and the Ca^{2+}–calmodulin-dependent activation of NOS may occur through secondary response. Reactive oxygen species (ROS) is also generated from the activity of membrane-bound nicotinamide adenine dinucleotide/nicotinamide adenine dinucleotide phosphate (NADH/NADPH) oxidase stimulated by AT_1 receptors.[50] Various biochemical activities are associated with ROS like activation of MAP kinase, tyrosine kinase, and phosphatases and inactivation of NO. These biochemical changes lead to physiological change in acute renal function variation, chronic effect on BP, and vascular hypertrophy and inflammation in cellular level.[51,52]

Classification of antihypertensive drugs

1. Diuretics
   - a Thiazides: hydrochlorothiazide, chlorothiazide, methyclothiazide, chlorthalidone, metolazone, bendroflumethiazide, indapamide, chlortalidone, cyclopenthiazide, indapamide, xipamide.
   - b Loop diuretics: furosemide, bumetanide, torasemide, ethacrynic acid.
   - c Potassium sparing diuretics: spironolactone, eplerenone, triamterene, amiloride.
2. Sympatholytic agents
   - a β-Receptor antagonist: metoprolol, atenolol, betaxolol, bisoprolol, esmolol, nadolol, carteolol, nebivolol, penbutolol, pindolol, timolol, propranolol.

b α-Receptor antagonist: prazosin, terazosin, doxazosin, phentolamine, phenoxybenzamine.
c Mixed α–β-receptor antagonist: labetalol, carvedilol, nebivolol.
d Centrally acting adrenergic agents: methyldopa, clonidine, guanabenz, guanfacine.
e Adrenergic neuron blocking agents: reserpine, guanadrel.

3. Ca^{2+} channel blocking agents
a Verapamil, diltiazem, amlodipine, nisoldipine, felodipine, nicardipine, isradipine, clevidipine, nifedipine, nitrendipine, nimodipine.

4. ACE inhibitors
a Enalapril, captopril, lisinopril, quinapril, ramipril, benazepril, fosinopril, moexipril, perindopril, trandolapril.

5. AngII receptor antagonist
a Losartan, candesartan, irbesartan, valsartan, telmisartan, eprosartan, olmesartan, eprosartan, azilsartan.

6. Direct renin inhibitor
a Aliskiren.

7. Vasodilators
a Arterial: hydralazine, minoxidil, diazoxide, fenoldopam.
b Arterial and venous: nitroprusside.

8. D1 receptor agonist: fenoldopam.

Diuretics

The strategy to use diuretics is to control sodium ion balance pharmacologically, although early management of hypertension is to restrict Na^{+} in diet.

Thiazides decrease extracellular volume initially in the distal convoluted tubule in the nephrons by interacting with a thiazide-sensitive NaCl cotransporter expressed, influencing Na^{+} excretion in the urine, and leading to a fall in CO. Although the exact mechanism is not certain, study refers that reduction of arterial BP by thiazides may open Ca^{2+}-activated K^{+} channels. According to abovementioned hypothesis, vascular smooth muscle cells get hyperpolarized. Hyperpolarization results closing of L-type Ca^{2+} channels, hence Ca^{2+} permeability becomes low, resulting vasodilation due to lack of calcium.[53] The major action of these drugs is NaCl cotransporter (genetic code: SLC12A3) found predominantly in the distal convoluted tubule (DCT) but not in the heart or vascular smooth muscle. By acting on NaCl cotransporter, thiazides reduce BP by decreasing peripheral resistance through reduced sodium concentration.[54]

In the thick ascending limb of the loop of Henle, loop diuretics inhibit activity of the $Na^{+}-K^{+}-2Cl^{-}$ symporter.[55] Loop diuretics are known to produce rapid and profound natriureses make them most efficient in diuretic class. Acute diuresis produced by loop diuretics may lead to other side effects in patients rather than other mild- or slow-acting diuretics. It is more useful in patient with edema or congestive heart failure, where reduction of body fluid is a fundamental. Still, by reducing body fluid, they reduce blood volume and manage hypertension.[56,57]

Late distal tubule and collecting duct contain epithelial cells where cytosolic mineralocorticoid receptor is expressed with affinity toward aldosterone. Aldosterone enters the epithelial cell and binds to aldosterone receptor that regulates the expression of multiple gene products called aldosterone-induced proteins (AIPs). AIPs are associated with sodium channel expression, and consequently, trans-epithelial NaCl transport is enhanced. This physiology greatly enhances the driving force for K^+ and H^+ secretions into the tubular lumen.[58] Potassium-sparring diuretics like spironolactone and eplerenone prevent binding of aldosterone to aldosterone receptor, thus preventing NaCl reabsorption and increase luminal fluid, thus decreasing blood volume and BP.[59,60]

Sympatholytic agents

Antagonism of β-adrenergic receptors affects reduction of myocardial contractility, heart rate, and CO. Another important consequence is blockade of the β-receptors of the juxtaglomerular complex which causes reducing renin secretion and thereby diminishing production of circulating AngII. This action likely contributes to the antihypertensive action of this class of drugs, in concert with the cardiac effects.

Metoprolol has rapid distribution in blood and extravascular fluids and is eliminated as metoprolol and metabolites also. Two of the metabolites have mild β_1-antagonistic activity. Metoprolol is also used in angina pectoris though it is reported that metoprolol is less effective than any other β-blockers.[61,62] Atenolol is well-tolerated and an effective drug having β-adrenoceptor antagonistic activity. Atenolol is selective β_1-receptor antagonist it significantly reduces systolic and diastolic BP and increases the consumption of oxygen in myocardial infraction. Due to its low lipid solubility, it likely has limited penetration in brain and effect on central nervous system (CNS), compared to propranolol.[63] Propranolol has potency to reduce hypertension both through renin-dependent and renin-independent pathways.[64] Although propranolol is a nonselective β-adrenergic blocker, betaxolol is more cardio-selective drug as it does not have partial agonistic activity toward β-adrenergic receptors. It significantly reduces systolic and diastolic BP as is myocardial oxygen demand and heart rate. It has a long duration of action and about four times more potent than propranolol.[65] Bisoprolol is a long-acting highly selective β_1 antagonist having no partial agonistic- or membrane-stabilizing activity. It is less potent than propranolol and betaxolol but more potency than atenolol or metoprolol.[66,67] Esmolol is a very short-acting relatively cardio-selective β-adrenoceptor antagonist, while used in infusion it prevents myocardial infraction, ischemia, and postoperative hypertension.[68,69] Nadolol was introduced and approved after propranolol by FDA for treatment of hypertension, angina, and arrhythmia induced by adrenalin.[70] Nebivolol is highly selective β_1-adrenergic receptor antagonist, also having vasodilatory activity through nitric oxide pathway. With BP lowering and NO-mediated effects, nebivolol not only improves systolic and diastolic function but also reduces peripheral resistance.[71,72] Penbutolol and pindolol are nonspecific adrenal receptor antagonist and having serotonin antagonistic activity, which are also used in behavioral syndromes.[73,74] Carteolol and timolol both are ocular nonselective β-adrenergic antagonist which are used to improve nasolacrimal occlusion.[75]

Sympathomimetic agents are used to activation of α-adrenergic receptors in vascular smooth muscle. As a result, PVR is increased and BP is maintained or elevated. α_1-Adrenergic receptor antagonists reduce arteriolar resistance and increase venous capacitance.[76] α_1-Adrenergic blockers also cause a variable amount of postural hypotension due to persisted vasodilation, but CO, heart rate, and plasma renin activity return to normal.

Prazosin exerts antihypertensive action by reducing vascular resistance and is a potent α1-adrenoceptor antagonist acting on postsynaptic neurones with competitive inhibition.[77,78] Terazosin has similar activity like prazosin and is used in mild-to-moderate hypertension having mild affinity toward nonselective α_2-adrenoceptors. Difference of terazosin from prazosin is that it has longer plasma half-life, effectively reduces urethral pressure and bladder outlet resistance, and also improves symptoms associated with benign prostate hyperplasia.[79–81] Doxazosin produces reduction of left ventricular hypertrophy and reduces risk of coronary heart disease.[82,83] Phentolamine causes vasodilation followed by reduction of afterload during systolic contraction, although it also produces inotropic effect in heart to increase blood ejection.[84] Phenoxybenzamine is a nonselective irreversible α-receptor antagonist used in benign prostate hyperplasia.[85]

Labetalol is an equimolar mixture stereoisomer. One isomer is an α_1-antagonist, another is a nonselective β-antagonist with partial agonist activity, and the other two isomers are inactive.[86] Carvedilol is a β-receptor antagonist with α_1-receptor antagonist activity. The drug has been approved for the treatment of hypertension and symptomatic heart failure. Carvedilol reduces risk of heart failure associated with systolic dysfunction.[87] Nebivolol is a β_1-selective adrenergic antagonist that also promotes vasodilatation rather than blocking α_1 receptors, nebivolol augments arterial smooth muscle relaxation via nitric oxide pathway.[88]

Methyldopa is converted to α-methyldopamine, again converted to α-methylnoradrenaline followed by metabolism in adrenergic neurons by the L-aromatic amino acid decarboxylase. After conversion to α-methylnoradrenaline, it is stored in the secretory vesicles of adrenergic neurons, instead of NE, substituting it. When the adrenergic neuron stimulates to discharges its neurotransmitter, α-methylnoradrenaline is released instead of NE. α-Methylnoradrenaline acts in the CNS to inhibit adrenergic neuronal outflow from the brainstem and probably acts as an agonist at presynaptic α_2-adrenergic receptors in the brainstem, attenuating NE release and thereby reducing the output of vasoconstrictor adrenergic signals to the peripheral sympathetic nervous system.[89]

Clonidine, guanabenz, and guanfacine, these drugs stimulate the α_{2A} subtype of α_2-adrenergic receptors in the brainstem, resulting in a reduction in sympathetic outflow from the CNS.[90]

Clonidine is an α-adrenergic receptor agonist that preferably stimulates postsynaptic adrenergic receptors (α_{2A} subtype), although it can also stimulate preganglionic neuron in the depressor site of the vasomotor center of the medulla oblongata in the region of the nucleus tractus solitarius (NTS). Activation of postsynaptic adrenergic receptors in NTS declines the efferent sympathetic neuronal vasoconstrictor tone to the heart, kidneys, and peripheral vasculature causing vasodilatation and lowering BP.[91]

The α_2-adrenergic agonists lower arterial pressure by an effect on both CO and peripheral resistance.

Guanadrel is an exogenous false neurotransmitter. Guanadrel is absorbed, stored, and released like NE but does not interact with monoamine oxidase. It specifically inhibits the function of peripheral postganglionic adrenergic neurons. Because of sympathetic blockade, adrenergic activity is reduced in both the vasculature of blood vessels and on CO and heart rate.[92,93]

Rauwolfia serpentina produces reserpine, an alkaloid obtained from the root of it. Reserpine tends to binds at the storage vesicles in central and peripheral adrenergic neurons. This intracellular interaction is strong enough to reduce adrenergic flow due to its prolong binding time. This interaction prevents the vesicular catecholamine transporter (VMAT2) thus inhibiting reuptake of catecholamine, so that nerve endings lose their physiological capacity to concentrate and store NE and dopamine. Catecholamines are metabolized followed by spontaneous liberation due to leakage into the cytoplasm. As a result active neurotransmitter no longer exists to release from nerve endings. Depletion of amine leads to antihypertensive activity both centrally and peripherally.[94,95]

Ca^{2+} channel blockers

Ca^{2+} channel blockers are one of the most important groups of antihypertensive agents. The general perception of hypertension is increased PVR in several types of blood vessels. Vascular smooth muscle contracts because of free calcium-ion concentration in intracellular fluid. Ca^{2+} activate myosin lite chain kinase through calcium–calmodolin complex, thus, initiates muscle contraction. Movements of calcium ions are controlled by various voltage-sensitive channels and inhibition of such channels decreases total amount of intracellular calcium ions. Calcium channel blocking agents reduces BP by relaxing vascular smooth muscle of arteries and lowering PVR.[96]

Decreased PVR induces a sympathetic discharge through baroreceptors. Cases of tachycardia may occur during adrenalin stimulation of SA node during use of dihydropyridines, which is almost absent with verapamil and diltiazem due to negative chronotropic effect.

Long-lasting calcium channels (L-type calcium channels) are responsible for the slow inward current of calcium in normal cardiac tissues, also responsible for prolonged action potential in cardiac cells. Verapamil blocks L-type channels in SA node and AV node, reduces myocardial contractility, and produces negative inotropic effect electrophysiologically. Verapamil is effective for essential hypertension as it produces systemic vasodilation and reduces systemic vascular resistance.[97,98] Diltiazem reduces stimulation of SA node and produces negative chronotropic effect and also improves vernacular function. Diltiazem is a potent vasodilator greatly which reduces vascular and coronary resistance.[99]

Amlodipine like other dihydropyridine antagonizes L-type calcium channels and is more vasoselective unlike verapamil and diltiazem. As it is a vasoselective agent, it does not have cardio-depressant effect and as it has a relatively long plasma presence, it prevents reflex tachycardia and subsequently manages catecholamine and renin activity.[100] Nifedipine also acts like amlodipine, along with treatment of different kinds of angina.[101] Nisoldipine produces coronary and peripheral vasodilation.[102] Felodipine relaxes vascular smooth muscle by acting on peripheral arterioles and it lowers peripheral resistance.[103] Nicardipine lowers mean BP by decreasing systemic and PVR.[104] Isradipine inhibits slow voltage–gated calcium channels in cardiac and vascular tissues, although it prefers vascular tissue. Like other dihydropyridine, it also increases coronary, skeletal muscle, and cerebral blood flow but has unchanged to reduced renal blood flow.[105] Clevidipine is newer generation drug used in both pre and postoperative cases where necessary. It shows high degree of vasoselectivity and has great effect on lowering arterial pressure.[106] Cilnidipine is a newer generation calcium channel blocker that acts both on L- and N-type calcium channels.[107]

Angiotensin-converting enzyme inhibitors

Angiotensin-II inhibitors lower BP principally by decreasing PVR. CO and heart rate are not significantly changed. Unlike direct vasodilators, these agents do not result in reflex sympathetic activation and can be used safely in persons with ischemic heart disease. The absence of reflex tachycardia may be due to downward resetting of the baroreceptors or to enhanced parasympathetic activity. This class of drug inhibits the converting enzyme peptidyl-dipeptidase that hydrolyzes AngI to AngII. This class of drug also inactivates bradykinin, a potent vasodilator, which works partly by stimulating release of nitric oxide and prostacyclin. Icatibant is an example of bradykinin receptor antagonist.

Enalapril is an oral prodrug that is converted by hydrolysis to a converting enzyme inhibitor, enalaprilat. Enalaprilat itself is available only for intravenous use, primarily for hypertensive emergencies. All Benazepril, fosinopril, moexipril, perindopril, quinapril, ramipril, and trandolapril are other long-acting members of the class, are prodrugs like enalapril, and are converted to the active agents by hydrolysis, primarily in the liver.[108,109] Benazepril exerts hemodynamic effects that benefited through decreasing vascular resistance by prevision of angiotensin-II formation.[110] Captopril reported to decrease kallikrein level and that elevates level of bradykinin.[111,112] Along with ACE inhibition, fosinopril was reported to reduce mass of left ventricle and thinning of cardiac wall.[113] Lisinopril is well tolerated and gives symptomatic relief in congestive heart failure.[114] Quinapril lowers BP both through renin-dependant and nondependant pathways. It reduces systemic vascular resistance and heart rate but increases CO, although pressure changes are not observed in normotensive subjects.[115,116] Moexipril and ramipril are comparative less effective, less effective but enough hypotensive effect.[117,118] Perindopril is prodrug, converted into perindoprilat which exerts ACE inhibiting activity. Perindopril significantly reduces arterial and hemodynamic abnormalities.[119] Trandolapril is converted into trandolapril and the metabolite is more potent than other metabolites like enalaprilat, ramiprilat, pendolaprilat.[120]

AngII receptor antagonist

The AngII receptor blockers (ARBs) bind to the AT_1 receptor with high affinity and are more than 10,000-fold selective for the AT_1 receptor over the AT_2 receptor. The mechanism of insurmountable antagonism by ARBs may be due to slow dissociation kinetics of the compounds from the AT_1 receptor; however, a number of other factors may contribute, such as ARB-induced receptor internalization and alternative binding sites for ARBs on the AT_1 receptor.[121]

ARBs potently and selectively inhibit most of the biological effects of AngII,[122,123] including AngII-induced contraction of vascular smooth muscle, rapid and slow pressor responses, thirst, vasopressin release, aldosterone secretion, release of adrenal catecholamines, enhancement of noradrenergic neurotransmission, increases in sympathetic tone, changes in renal function, and cellular hypertrophy and hyperplasia.

Valsartan is oral angiotensin-II receptor antagonist used in hypertension management with rapid activity.[124] Losartan is a potent AT_1 receptor antagonist. A metabolite of losartan E_{3174} is 15–20 times more potent over AT_1 receptor. Losartan improves left ventricular mass index, vascular resistance, heart rate while reduces renal function.[125] Candesartan often gives in a salt form to prevent primary metabolism. It binds with AT_1 receptor competitively and nonselectively and is used in every kind of hypertension.[126] Irbesartan selectively binds with AT1 receptor and inhibits AngII activity longer and greater than valsartan and losartan.[127] Telmisartan is a nonpeptide, competitive, highly selective AT1 receptor antagonist.[128] Eprosartan is another drug that has high affinity for AT1 receptor (1000 times more than AT2 receptor) effecting on RAAS in management of high BP. It does not have selectivity for serotonin, adrenalin, or any other receptors.[129,130] Olmesartan is newer generation with high affinity toward angiotensin-II receptor, often used as active metabolite of a salt prodrug form.[131] Azilsartan is new generation of the same group used in essential hypertension.[132]

Direct renin inhibitor

Aliskiren is an oral active, low-molecular-weight nonpeptide that is a potent competitive inhibitor of renin and only molecule to be used clinically. Enalkiren, zankiren, CGP38560A, and remikiren are other drugs of this class but do not prove satisfactory in clinical trial, due to either poor bioavailability, low potency, or very short half-life. It binds the active site of renin and prevents binding of angiotensinogen to block conversion of it to AngI and, consequently decreases the production of AngII. Aliskiren also has negative impact on aldosterone levels and enhances natriuresis.[133–135]

Vasodilators

Action of hydralazine is on arteriolar smooth muscle directly. Mechanism of it is unclear but somehow involves in reduction of intracellular calcium concentration. Variety of cellular pathway would be interfered due to calcium-ion concentration and sting probability suggests inhibition of Ca^{2+} through IP_3-induced pathway that leads to diminished contraction.[136] Another evidence is opening of calcium-mediated potassium channel which promotes arterial dilation.[137]

Minoxidil is reported to be not active but when metabolized by hepatic sulfotransferase and it becomes active compound minoxidil *N-O* sulfate. Minoxidil sulfate causes hyperpolarization by activation of K^+ channel mediated by ATP in smooth muscle, hence permitting potassium ion efflux. Hyperpolarization effecting relaxation of smooth muscle causes vasodilation and fall of BP.[138] This agent is also used in the treatment of alopecia.

Nitroprusside, like a nitrovasodilator, releases NO that activates the guanylyl cyclase. Guanylyl cyclase acts on GTP and converts it into cGMP through PKG pathway, leading to vasodilation,[139] simulating the generation of NO by vascular endothelium, which is impaired in many hypertensive individuals.[140]

D1 receptor agonist

Fenoldopam is a D1 receptor selective agonist that causes peripheral vasodilation. It reduces BP in a dose-dependent manner in patients with severe hypertension. Along with vasodilatory activity, it also has diuretic activity.[141–143]

Conclusion

Strategies in the management of hypertension are continuously evolving. Broad-spectrum pharmacological strategies are being employed. Additionally, drugs targeting cardiovascular and renal diseases are promising and their exploration at the Genetic and molecular level could start an era of targeted and personalized drug therapies in the management of hypertension. These technologies will be a source of decoration for the future antihypertensive therapies, but currently, available medications should be pharmacologically optimized in such a way so as to improve patient compliance, dose and appropriate access to the health-care system in the management of hypertension and associated complications.

References

1. Hall JE. The kidney, hypertension, and obesity. *Hypertension*. 2003;41(3):625–633.
2. Diamond EL. The role of anger and hostility in essential hypertension and coronary heart disease. *Psychol Bull*. 1982;92(2):410.
3. Meissner A. Hypertension and the brain: a risk factor for more than heart disease. *Cerebrovasc Dis*. 2016;42(3–4):255–262.
4. Guyton AC. Blood pressure control—special role of the kidneys and body fluids. *Science*. 1991;252(5014):1813–1816.
5. Wagenvoort CA. Plexogenic arteriopathy. *Thorax*. 1994;49(Suppl):S39.
6. Hsu CY, McCulloch CE, Darbinian J, Go AS, Iribarren C. Elevated blood pressure and risk of end-stage renal disease in subjects without baseline kidney disease. *Arch Intern Med*. 2005;165(8):923–928.
7. Chobanian AV, Bakris GL, Black HR, Cushman WC, Green LA, Izzo Jr JL, et al. Seventh report of the joint national committee on prevention, detection, evaluation, and treatment of high blood pressure. *Hypertension*. 2003;42(6):1206–1252.
8. Schmieder RE. End organ damage in hypertension. *Dtsch Ärzteblatt Int*. 2010;107(49):866.
9. Sawicka K, Szczyrek M, Jastrzebska I, Prasal M, Zwolak A, Daniluk J. Hypertension – the silent killer. *J Pre-Clin Clinical Res*. 2011;5(2).
10. Kalehoff JP, Oparil S. The story of the silent killer. *Curr Hypertension Rep*. 2020;22 (9):1–4.
11. Clarke R, Collins R, Lewington S, Donald A, Alfthan G, Tuomilehto J, et al. Homocysteine and risk of ischemic heart disease and stroke: a *meta*-analysis. *J Am Med Assoc*. 2002;288(16):2015–2022.
12. Guyton AC, Coleman TG, Cowley Jr AW, Manning Jr RD, Norman Jr RA, Ferguson JD. Brief reviews: a systems analysis approach to understanding long-range arterial blood pressure control and hypertension. *Circ Res*. 1974;35(2):159–176.

13. Sullivan JM, Prewitt RL, Josephs JA. Attenuation of the microcirculation in young patients with high-output borderline hypertension. *Hypertension.* 1983;5(6):844–851.
14. Dahlöf B. Cardiovascular disease risk factors: epidemiology and risk assessment. *Am J Cardiol.* 2010;105(1):3A–9A.
15. Te Riet L, van Esch JH, Roks AJ, van den Meiracker AH, Danser AJ. Hypertension: renin–angiotensin–aldosterone system alterations. *Circ Res.* 2015;116(6):960–975.
16. Timmermann B, Mo R, Luft FC, Gerdts E, Busjahn A, Omvik P, et al. β-2 adrenoceptor genetic variation is associated with genetic predisposition to essential hypertension: the Bergen Blood Pressure Study. *Kidney Int.* 1998;53(6):1455–1460.
17. Luft FC. Molecular genetics of human hypertension. *J Hypertens.* 1998;16 (12):1871–1878.
18. Cusi D, Barlassina C, Azzani T, Casari G, Citterio L, Devoto M, et al. Polymorphisms of α-adducin and salt sensitivity in patients with essential hypertension. *Lancet.* 1997;349 (9062):1353–1357.
19. Casari G, Barlassina C, Cusi D, Zagato L, Muirhead R, Righetti M, et al. Association of the α-adducin locus with essential hypertension. *Hypertension.* 1995;25(3):320–326.
20. Milnor WR, Bergel DH, Bargainer JD. Hydraulic power associated with pulmonary blood flow and its relation to heart rate. *Circ Res.* 1966;19(3):467–480.
21. Kirchheim HR. Systemic arterial baroreceptor reflexes. *Physiol Rev.* 1976;56(1):100–177.
22. Robbe HW, Mulder LJ, Rüddel HE, Langewitz WA, Veldman JB, Mulder G. Assessment of baroreceptor reflex sensitivity by means of spectral analysis. *Hypertension.* 1987;10 (5):538–543.
23. Bristow JD, Honour AJ, Pickering GW, Sleight P, Smyth HS. Diminished baroreflex sensitivity in high blood pressure. *Circulation.* 1969;39(1):48–54.
24. Bertinieri G, Di Rienzo M, Cavallazzi A, Ferrari AU, Pedotti A, Mancia G. A new approach to analysis of the arterial baroreflex. *J Hypertens Suppl.* 1985;3(3):S79–S81.
25. Guilluy C, Brégeon J, Toumaniantz G, Rolli-Derkinderen M, Retailleau K, Loufrani L, et al. The Rho exchange factor Arhgef1 mediates the effects of angiotensin II on vascular tone and blood pressure. *Nat Med.* 2010;16(2):183–190.
26. Lindeman RD, Tobin JD, Shock NW. Association between blood pressure and the rate of decline in renal function with age. *Kidney Int.* 1984;26(6):861–868.
27. Page IH, Heuer GJ. The effect of renal denervation on the level of arterial blood pressure and renal function in essential hypertension. *J Clin Invest.* 1935;14(1):27–30.
28. Carey RM, Wang ZQ, Siragy HM. Role of the angiotensin type 2 receptor in the regulation of blood pressure and renal function. *Hypertension.* 2000;35(1):155–163.
29. Vander AJ. Control of renin release. *Physiol Rev.* 1967;47(3):359–382.
30. Morgan TR. A microperfusion study of influence of macula densa on glomerular filtration rate. *Am J Physiol-Legacy Content.* 1971;220(1):186–190.
31. Briggs JP, Schnermann J. Macula densa control of renin secretion and glomerular vascular tone: evidence for common cellular mechanisms. *Kidney Blood Press Res.* 1986;9 (4):193–203.
32. Velazquez HE, Good DW, Wright FS. Mutual dependence of sodium and chloride absorption by renal distal tubule. *Am J Physiol-Renal Physiol.* 1984;247(6):F904–F911.
33. Spielman WS, Thompson CI. A proposed role for adenosine in the regulation of renal hemodynamics and renin release. *Am J Physiol-Renal Physiol.* 1982;242(5):F423–F435.
34. Churchill PC. Second messengers in renin secretion. *Am J Physiol-Renal Physiol.* 1985;249 (2):F175–F184.

35. Osswald H. The role of adenosine in the regulation of glomerular filtration rate and renin secretion. *Trends Pharmacol Sci*. 1984;5:94–97.
36. Francisco LL, Osborn JL, DiBona GF. Prostaglandin in renin release during sodium deprivation. *Am J Physiol-Renal Physiol*. 1982;243(6):F537–F542.
37. Freeman RH, Davis JO, Villarreal D. Role of renal prostaglandins in the control of renin release. *Circ Res*. 1984;54(1):1–9.
38. Wang JL, Cheng HF, Harris RC. Cyclooxygenase-2 inhibition decreases renin content and lowers blood pressure in a model of renovascular hypertension. *Hypertension*. 1999;34(1):96–101.
39. Berl TO, Henrich WL, Erickson AL, Schrier RW. Prostaglandins in the beta-adrenergic and baroreceptor-mediated secretion of renin. *Am J Physiol-Renal Physiol*. 1979;236(5):F472–F477.
40. Pilowsky PM, Goodchild AK. Baroreceptor reflex pathways and neurotransmitters: 10 years on. *J Hypertens*. 2002;20(9):1675–1688.
41. Winer N, Chokshi DS, Yoon MS, Freedman AD. Adrenergic receptor mediation of renin secretion. *J Clin Endocrinol Metab*. 1969;29(9):1168–1175.
42. Nguyen G, Delarue F, Burcklé C, Bouzhir L, Giller T, Sraer JD. Pivotal role of the renin/prorenin receptor in angiotensin II production and cellular responses to renin. *J Clin Invest*. 2002;109(11):1417–1427.
43. Danser AJ, Deinum J. Renin, prorenin and the putative (pro) renin receptor. *Hypertension*. 2005;46(5):1069–1076.
44. Batenburg W, Danser AJ. Prorenin and the (pro)renin receptor: binding kinetics, signalling and interaction with aliskiren. *J Renin Angiotensin Aldosterone Syst*. 2008;9:181–184.
45. Donoghue M, Hsieh F, Baronas E, et al. A novel angiotensin-converting enzyme–related carboxypeptidase (ACE2) converts angiotensin I to angiotensin (1–9). *Circ Res*. 2000;87:E1–E9.
46. Tipnis SR, Hooper NM, Hyde R, et al. A human homolog of angiotensin-converting enzyme: Cloning and functional expression as a captopril-insensitive carboxypeptidase. *J Biol Chem*. 2000;275:33238–33243.
47. Li W, Moore MJ, Vasilieva N, et al. Angiotensin-converting enzyme 2 is a functional receptor for the SARS coronavirus. *Nature*. 2003;426:450–454.
48. Smrcka AV, Brown KO, Sternweis PC. Regulation of polyphosphoinositide-specific phospholipase C activity by purified Gq. *Science*. 1991;251(4995):804–807.
49. Siehler S. Regulation of RhoGEF proteins by G12/13-coupled receptors. *Br J Pharmacol*. 2009;158(1):41–49.
50. Zafari AM, Ushio-Fukai M, Akers M, Yin Q, Shah A, Harrison DG, et al. Role of NADH/NADPH oxidase–derived H_2O_2 in angiotensin II–induced vascular hypertrophy. *Hypertension*. 1998;32(3):488–495.
51. Mehta PK, Griendling KK. Angiotensin II cell signaling: physiological and pathological effects in the cardiovascular system. *Am J Physiol Cell Physiol*. 2007;292:C82–C97.
52. Higuchi S, Ohtsu H, Suzuki H, et al. Angiotensin II signal transduction through the AT1 receptor: Novel insights into mechanisms and pathophysiology. *Clin Sci*. 2007;112:417–428.
53. Pickkers P, Garcha RS, Schachter M, et al. Inhibition of carbonic anhydrase accounts for the direct vascular effects of hydrochlorothiazide. *Hypertension*. 1999;33:1043–1048.
54. Mastroianni N, De Fusco M, Zollo M, Arrigo G, Zuffardi O, Bettinelli A, et al. Molecular cloning, expression pattern, and chromosomal localization of the human Na–Cl thiazide-sensitive cotransporter (SLC12A3). *Genomics*. 1996;35(3):486–493.

55. Saier MH, Boyden DA. Mechanism, regulation and physiological significance of the loop diuretic-sensitive NaCl/KCl symport system in animal cells. *Mol Cell Biochem.* 1984;59 (1):11–32.
56. Musini VM, Rezapour P, Wright JM, Bassett K, Jauca CD. Blood pressure-lowering efficacy of loop diuretics for primary hypertension. *Cochrane Database Syst Rev.* 2015;(5).
57. Malha L, Mann SJ. Loop diuretics in the treatment of hypertension. *Curr Hypertens Rep.* 2016;18(4):27.
58. Freel EM, Connell JM. Mechanisms of hypertension: the expanding role of aldosterone. *J Am Soc Nephrol.* 2004;15(8):1993–2001.
59. Tanaka H, Watanabe K, Harima M, Thanikachalam PV, Yamaguchi KI, Tachikawa H, et al. Effects of various diuretics on cardiac function in rats with heart failure. *Yakugaku zasshi: J Pharm Soc Jpn.* 2009;129(7):871–879.
60. Ferreira JP, Eschalier R, Duarte K, Damman K, Gustafsson F, Schou M, et al. Reduced diuretic dose in patients treated with eplerenone: data from the EPHESUS trial. *Circulation: Heart Fail.* 2020;13(5):e006597.
61. Regårdh CG, Johnsson G. Clinical pharmacokinetics of metoprolol. *Clin Pharmacokinet.* 1980;5(6):557–569.
62. Benfield P, Clissold SP, Brogden RN. Metoprolol. *Drugs.* 1986;31(5):376–429.
63. Wadworth AN, Murdoch D, Brogden RN. Atenolol. *Drugs.* 1991;42(3):468–510.
64. Hollifield JW, Sherman K, Vander Zwagg R, Shand DG. Proposed mechanisms of propranolol's antihypertensive effect in essential hypertension. *N Engl J Med.* 1976;295 (2):68–73.
65. Beresford R, Heel RC. Betaxolol. *Drugs.* 1986;31(1):6–28.
66. Lancaster SG, Sorkin EM. Bisoprolol. *Drugs.* 1988;36(3):256–285.
67. McGavin JK, Keating GM. Bisoprolol. *Drugs.* 2002;62(18):2677–2696.
68. Benfield P, Sorkin EM. Esmolol. *Drugs.* 1987;33(4):392–412.
69. Garnock-Jones KP. Esmolol. *Drugs.* 2012;72(1):109–132.
70. Frishman WH. Nadolol: a new β-adrenoceptor antagonist. *N Engl J Med.* 1981;305 (12):678–682.
71. Kamp O, Metra M, Bugatti S, Bettari L, Dei Cas A, Petrini N, et al. Nebivolol. *Drugs.* 2010;70(1):41–56.
72. Moen MD, Wagstaff AJ. Nebivolol. *Drugs.* 2006;66(10):1389–1409.
73. Castro ME, Harrison PJ, Pazos A, Sharp T. Affinity of (±)-pindolol,(-)-penbutolol, and (-)-tertatolol for pre-and postsynaptic serotonin 5-HT1A receptors in human and rat brain. *J Neurochem.* 2000;75(2):755–762.
74. Artigas F, Celada P, Laruelle M, Adell A. How does pindolol improve antidepressant action? *Trends Pharmacol Sci.* 2001;22(5):224–228.
75. Freedman SF, Freedman NJ, Shields MB, Lobaugh B, Samsa GP, Keates EU, et al. Effects of ocular carteolol and timolol on plasma high-density lipoprotein cholesterol level. *Am J Ophthalmol.* 1993;116(5):600–611.
76. Grimm Jr RH. Alpha 1-antagonists in the treatment of hypertension. *Hypertension.* 1989;13 (5_supplement):I131.
77. Graham RM, Pettinger WAPrazosin. *N Engl J Med.* 1979;300(5):232–236.
78. Stanaszek WF, Kellerman D, Brogden RN, Romankiewicz JA. Prazosin update. *Drugs.* 1983;25(4):339–384.
79. Titmarsh S, Monk JP. Terazosin. *Drugs.* 1987;33(5):461–477.
80. Wilde MI, Fitton A, Sorkin EM. Terazosin. *Drugs Aging.* 1993;3(3):258–277.
81. Kyncl JJ. Pharmacology of terazosin. *Am J Med.* 1986;80(5):12–19.

82. Fulton B, Wagstaff AJ, Sorkin EM. Doxazosin. *Drugs*. 1995;49(2):295–320.
83. Young RA, Brogden RN. Doxazosin. *Drugs*. 1988;35(5):525–541.
84. Gould L. Phentolamine. *Am Heart J*. 1969;78(2):276–278.
85. Yoham AL, Casadesus D. *Phenoxybenzamine*. StatPearls; 2020.
86. Goa KL, Benfield P, Sorkin EM. Labetalol. *Drugs*. 1989;37(5):583–627.
87. McTavish D, Campoli-Richards D, Sorkin EM. Carvedilol. *Drugs*. 1993;45(2):232–258.
88. Mangrella M, Rossi F, Fici F, Rossi F. Pharmacology of nebivolol. *Pharmacol Res*. 1998;38(6):419–431.
89. Day MD, Roach AG, Whiting RL. The mechanism of the antihypertensive action of α-methyldopa in hypertensive rats. *Eur J Pharmacol*. 1973;21(3):271–280.
90. MacMillan LB, Hein L, Smith MS, et al. Central hypotensive effects of the α2A-adrenergic receptor sub-type. *Science*. 1996;273:801–803.
91. Houston MC. Clonidine hydrochloride: review of pharmacologic and clinical aspects. *Prog Cardiovasc Dis*. 1981;23(5):337–350.
92. Finnerty FA, Brogden RN. Guanadrel. *Drugs*. 1985;30(1):22–31.
93. Dunn MI, Dunlap JL. Guanadrel: a new antihypertensive drug. *JAMA*. 1981;245(16):1639–1642.
94. Shamon SD, Perez MI. Blood pressure-lowering efficacy of reserpine for primary hypertension. *Cochrane Database Syst Rev*. 2016;(12).
95. Freis ED. Mental depression in hypertensive patients treated for long periods with large doses of reserpine. *N Engl J Med*. 1954;251(25):1006–1008.
96. Weber MA. Calcium channel antagonists in the treatment of hypertension. *Am J Cardiovasc Drugs*. 2002;2:415–431.
97. McTavish D, Sorkin EM. Verapamil. *Drugs*. 1989;38(1):19–76.
98. Brogden RN, Benfield P. Verapamil. *Drugs*. 1996;51(5):792–819.
99. Buckley MM, Grant SM, Goa KL, McTavish D, Sorkin EM. Diltiazem. *Drugs*. 1990;39(5):757–806.
100. Nayler WG. Amlodipine. *Clin drug investigation*. 1997;13(1):1.
101. Sorkin EM, Clissold SP, Brogden RN. Nifedipine. *Drugs*. 1985;30(3):182–274.
102. Friedel HA, Sorkin EM. Nisoldipine. *Drugs*. 1988;36(6):682–731.
103. Saltiel E, Ellrodt AG, Monk JP, Langley MS. Felodipine. *Drugs*. 1988;36(4):387–428.
104. Frampton JE, Faulds D. Nicardipine. *Drugs Aging*. 1993;3(2):165–187.
105. Fitton A, Benfield P. Isradipine. *Drugs*. 1990;40(1):31–74.
106. Deeks ED, Keating GM, Keam SJ. Clevidipine. *Am J Cardiovasc Drugs*. 2009;9(2):117–134.
107. Ozawa Y, Hayashi K, Kobori H. New generation calcium channel blockers in hypertensive treatment. *Curr Hypertens Rev*. 2006;2(2):103–111.
108. Salvetti A. Newer ACE inhibitors. *Drugs*. 1990;40(6):800–828.
109. Todd PA, Heel RC. Enalapril. *Drugs*. 1986;31(3):198–248.
110. Balfour JA, Goa KL. Benazepril. *Drugs*. 1991;42(3):511–539.
111. Brogden RN, Todd PA, Sorkin EM. Captopril. *Drugs*. 1988;36(5):540–600.
112. Vidt DG, Bravo EL, Fouad FM. Captopril. *N Engl J Med*. 1982;306(4):214–219.
113. Davis R, Coukell A, McTavish D. Fosinopril. *Drugs*. 1997;54(1):103–116.
114. Simpson K, Jarvis B. Lisinopril. *Drugs*. 2000;59(5):1149–1167.
115. Wadworth AN, Brogden RN. Quinapril. *Drugs*. 1991;41(3):378–399.
116. Culy CR, Jarvis B. Quinapril. *Drugs*. 2002;62(2):339–385.
117. Todd PA, Benfield P. Ramipril. *Drugs*. 1990;39(1):110–135.
118. Brogden RN, Wiseman LR. Moexipril. *Drugs*. 1998;55(6):845–860.

119. Hurst M, Jarvis B. Perindopril. *Drugs*. 2001;61(6):867–896.
120. Peters DC, Noble S, Plosker GL. Trandolapril. *Drugs*. 1998;56(5):871–893.
121. McConnaughey MM, McConnaughey JS, Ingenito AJ. Practical considerations of the pharmacology of angiotensin receptor blockers. *J Clin Pharmacol*. 1999;39(547–559):122.
122. Timmermans PBMWM, Wong PC, Chiu AT, et al. Angiotensin II receptors and angiotensin II receptor antagonists. *Pharmacol Rev*. 1993;45:205–251.
123. Csajka C, Buclin T, Brunner HR, Biollaz J. Pharmacokinetic–pharmacodynamic profile of angiotensin II receptor antagonists. *Clin Pharmacokinet*. 1997;32:1–29.
124. Croom KF, Keating GM. Valsartan. *Am J Cardiovasc Drugs*. 2004;4(6):395–404.
125. Simpson KL, McClellan KJ. Losartan. *Drugs Aging*. 2000;16(3):227–250.
126. Gleiter CH, Jägle C, Gresser U, Mörike KCandesartan. *Cardiovasc Drug Rev*. 2004;22 (4):263–284.
127. Croom KF, Curran MP, Goa KL, Perry CM. Irbesartan. *Drugs*. 2004;64(9):999–1028.
128 Nandi U, Karmakar S, Das AK, et al. Pharmacokinetics, pharmacodynamics and toxicity of a combination of metoprolol succinate and telmisartan in Wistar albino rats: safety profiling. *Regul Toxicol Pharmacol*. 2013;65(1):68–78. Available from: https://doi.org/10.1016/j.yrtph.2012.11.001. Epub 2012 Nov 27, PMID: 23201407.
129. Robins GW, Scott LJ. Eprosartan. *Drugs*. 2005;65(16):2355–2377.
130. Plosker GL. Eprosartan. *Drugs*. 2009;69(17):2477–2499.
131 Gorain B, Choudhury H, Kundu A, et al. Nanoemulsion strategy for olmesartan medoxomil improves oral absorption and extended antihypertensive activity in hypertensive rats. *Colloids Surf B Biointerfaces*. 2014;115:286–294. Available from: https://doi.org/10.1016/j.colsurfb.2013.12.016. Epub 2013 Dec 16, PMID: 24388859.
132. Perry CM. Azilsartan medoxomil. *Clin Drug Invest*. 2012;32(9):621–639.
133. Nussberger J, Wuerzner G, Jensen C, et al. Angiotensin II suppression in humans by the orally active renin inhibitor Aliskiren (SPP100): comparison with enalapril. *Hypertension*. 2002;39:E1–E8.
134. Brown MJ. Aliskiren. *Circulation*. 2008;118(7):773–784.
135. Frampton JE, Curran MP. Aliskiren. *Drugs*. 2007;67(12):1767–1792.
136. Ellershaw DC, Gurney AM. Mechanisms of hyralazine induced vasodilation in rabbit aorta and pulmonary artery. *Br J Pharmacol*. 2001;134:621–631.
137. Bang L, Nielsen-Kudsk JE, Gruhn N, et al. Hydralazine-induced vasodilation involves opening of high conductance Ca2 + -activated K + channels. *Eur J Pharmacol*. 1998;361:43–49.
138. Leblanc N, Wilde DW, Keef KD, Hume JR. Electrophysio-logical mechanisms of minoxidil sulfate-induced vasodilation of rabbit portal vein. *Circ Res*. 1989;65:1102–1111.
139. Linder A, McCluskey L, Cole K, et al. Dynamic association of nitric oxide downstream signaling molecules with endothelial caveolin-1 in rat aorta. *J Pharmacol Exp Ther*. 2005;. Epub ahead of print.
140. Ramchandra R, Barrett C, Malpas S. Nitric oxide and sympathetic nerve activity in the control of blood pressure. *Clin Exp Pharmacol Physiol*. 2005;32:440–446.
141. Brogden RN, Markham A. Fenoldopam. *Drugs*. 1997;54(4):634–650.
142. Tumlin JA, Dunbar LM, Oparil S, Buckalew V, Ram CV, Mathur V, et al. Fenoldopam Study Group Fenoldopam, a dopamine agonist, for hypertensive emergency: a multicenter randomized trial. *Acad Emerg Med*. 2000;7(6):653–662.
143. Murphy MB, Murray C, Shorten GD. Fenoldopam—a selective peripheral dopamine-receptor agonist for the treatment of severe hypertension. *N Engl J Med*. 2001;345 (21):1548–1557.

Chapter 16

Mechanism of action of diuretic and anti-diuretic drugs

Raja Chakraverty[1], Kalyan Samanta[2], Pallab Mandal[3] and Samit Karmakar[4]

[1]ICMR Research Scholar, Department of Pharmacology, IPGMER-SSKM Hospital, Kolkata, West Bengal, India, [2]MD-PGT, Department of Pharmacology, IPGMER-SSKM Hospital, Kolkata, West Bengal, India, [3]Bioeuivalence Study Centre, Department of Pharmaceutical Technology, Jadavpur University, Kolkata, West Bengal, India, [4]Medical College Kolkata, Kolkata, West Bengal, India

Introduction

Diuretics are drugs those increase the rate of flow of urine.[1−9] These drugs increase the rate of $Na+$ and $Cl-$ excretion and reduce extracellular fluid (ECF) volume by decreasing total body NaCl. Diuretics exert their action by acting on different parts of nephron that is the structural and functional unit of kidney.

To know the mechanisms of action of various diuretics, we have to know the renal physiology regarding the formation of urine and concentration mechanisms.

We shall discuss briefly the anatomy and physiology of nephron regarding flow of urine in different parts starting from glomerulus to collecting duct (CD).

Brief anatomy and physiology of the nephron

Each nephron (Fig. 16.1) consists of two parts, renal corpuscle (also known as Malpighian corpuscle) and renal tubule.[10−14] Renal corpuscle is formed by Glomerulus and Bowman's capsule. Renal tubule is the continuation of Bowman capsule and its different parts are proximal convoluted tubule (PCT), Henle's loop and distal convoluted tubule (DCT), and CD.

Urine formation is the blood purifying function of the kidneys. Normally, about 1200−1300 mL of blood, which is around 24%−26% of total cardiac output, enter the kidneys. Kidneys excrete unwanted and toxic substances

How Synthetic Drugs Work. DOI: https://doi.org/10.1016/B978-0-323-99855-0.00016-6

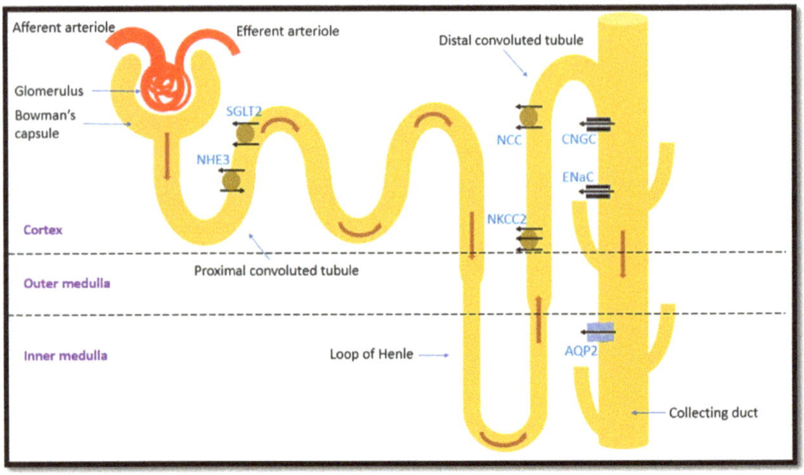

FIGURE 16.1 Structure of nephron and location of various channels in apical membrane. *AQP2*, Aquaporin-2; *ENaC*, epithelial Na channel; *NHE3*, Na^+/H^+ exchanger; *NKCC2*, $Na^+/K^+/2Cl^-$ cotransporter; *NCC*, Na^+/Cl^- cotransporter; SGLT2, sodium-glucose cotransporter, isoform 2.

along with water from blood as urine. Normal urinary output is around 1000–1500 mL per day.

In short, as blood passes through glomerular capillaries, the plasma gets filtered into Bowman capsule (this is called glomerular filtration). This filtrate from the Bowman capsule passes through tubular portion and undergoes many changes. Some wanted substances (e.g., glucose, amino acids, water, and electrolytes) are reabsorbed from the tubules and this process is called tubular reabsorption, while unwanted substances are secreted into tubule from peritubular blood vessels (this is called tubular secretion or excretion). So, urine formation consists of three mechanisms: (1) glomerular filtration, (2) tubular reabsorption, and (3) tubular secretion.

Classification of diuretics (according to site of their action)

1. *Drugs acting on glomerulus*[14–17]
   a. Adenosine receptor antagonist: caffeine, theophylline, theobromine.
2. *Drugs acting on PCT*
   a. Carbonic anhydrase (CA) inhibitors: acetazolamide, dorzolamide, ethoxzolamide, methazolamide, etc.
3. *Drugs acting on loop of Henle*
   a. Loop diuretics: furosemide, torsemide, bumetanide, ethacrynic acid.
4. *Drugs acting on DCT*
   a. Thiazide diuretics: chlorothiazide, hydrochlorothiazide, chlorthalidone, indapamide, metolazone.

5. *Drugs acting on DCT and CD*
   a. Potassium sparing diuretics: aldosterone antagonists: spironolactone and eplerenone.
   b. Inhibitors of renal epithelial Na^+ channel (ENaC): triamterene and amiloride.
6. *Others*
   a. Osmotic diuretics: mannitol, glycerol, urea, and isosorbide, etc.

Normal physiology of different parts of nephron and related diuretics

Glomerulus and Bowman's capsule

As blood passes through glomerular capillaries, plasma is filtered into Bowman capsule.[15–27] All the substances of plasma are filtered (such as Na^+, K^+, Ca^{2+}, Cl^-, HCO_3^-, amino acids, and some organic solutes) except few plasma proteins having relatively high molecular weight. The filtrate then reaches tubular portion and moves toward CDs.

Adenosine plays very important role in regulating the glomerular filtration rate (GFR). Adenosine is released from macula densa and acts on adenosine receptor (A1 receptor) which is present in afferent arteriole and causes constriction of the afferent arteriole which leads to decreased GFR. A1 receptors are also present in PCT and stimulate the reabsorption of Na^+.

Diuretic acting on glomerulus

Adenosine receptor antagonist: caffeine, theophylline, theobromine

Mechanism of action

They inhibit the A1 receptors. Dilatation of afferent arterioles occurs in glomerulus. Also, Na^+ reabsorption from the PCT in inhibited. This results in diuresis and natriuresis.

Proximal convoluted tubule

PCT is the coiled segment arising from the Bowman's capsule and is situated in cortex.[28–57] The wall of PCT is made up of a single-layer cuboidal epithelial cells with hair like projections toward lumen and called brush bordered epithelial cells.

About 80%–85% of filtrate is reabsorbed in PCT. The brush borders of epithelial cells increase the surface area and facilitate the reabsorption. CA enzyme plays an important role in reabsorption in this portion. Type IV CA enzyme is found in brush border of the luminal membrane and basolateral membranes and type II in the cytoplasm. Substances reabsorbed from PCT are sodium (almost 85% of filtered sodium bicarbonate and 40% of sodium chloride), glucose, phosphate, amino acids, lactate, chloride, potassium, calcium, bicarbonates, urea, and uric acid via specific transport systems. There is passive reabsorption of water for maintaining constant osmolality.

In the middle third of PCT, there are organic acid secretory systems that secrete few organic acids such as uric acid, penicillin antibiotics, diuretics like loop, and thiazide diuretics. There are organic base secretory systems in the proximal and middle third of PCT which secretes bases like creatinine, choline, etc.

There are various transporters in the epithelial cells. Na + /H + exchanger is present in luminal membrane and involved in Na + uptake and H + extrusion. In the basolateral side, there is Na + K + ATPase transporter that pumps K + into the cell in exchange of Na + ion. In the basolateral membrane, there is another cotransporter Na + /HCO3 − which moves Na + along with HCO3 − in the interstitium.

$NaHCO_3$ reabsorption in PCT is started by the action of the Na + /H + exchanger (Fig. 16.2). Na + enters into the cell from tubular lumen in exchange for an intracellular H + . Na + /K + −ATPase transporters are situated in the basolateral membrane pumps and these reabsorbed Na + ions into the interstitium for maintaining a low-intracellular Na + ion concentration.

The secreted H + combines with bicarbonate HCO3 − to form carbonic acid into the lumen. Carbonic acid is rapidly dissociated into CO_2 and H_2O by the CA (CA-type IV) enzyme. CO_2 being lipid soluble enters the

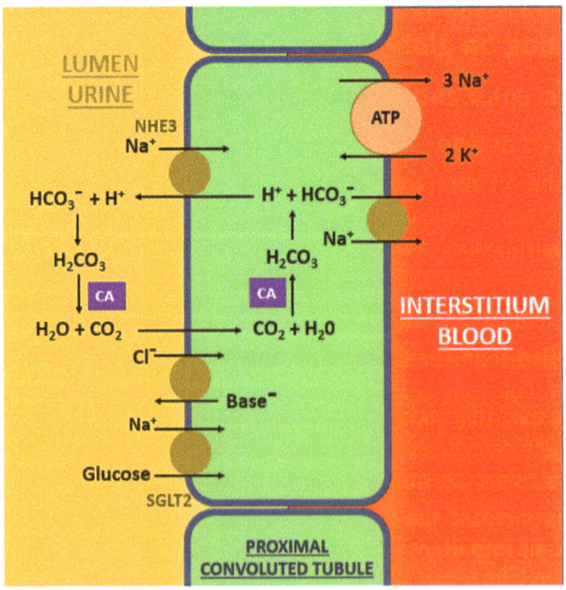

FIGURE 16.2 Na + reabsorption in PCT. *CA*, Carbonic anhydrase; *NHE3*, Na + /H + exchanger; *PCT*, proximal convoluted tubule; *SGLT2*, sodium-glucose cotransporter, isoform 2.

proximal tubule (PT) cells by simple diffusion. Then it is rehydrated back to H_2CO_3 by intracellular CA (CA-type II) enzyme.

This H_2CO_3 ionizes spontaneously to form $H+$ ion and $HCO3-$ ion and an electrochemical gradient for $HCO3-$ is created across basolateral membrane. This electrochemical gradient for $HCO3-$ is used by the $Na+/HCO3-$ symporter in the basolateral membrane to transport $Na+$ and $HCO3-$ into the interstitial space.

Thus bicarbonate reabsorption in the PCT is dependent on CA activity. Net effect is transport of $NaHCO_3$ from tubular lumen to interstitial space followed by movement of water by isotonic reabsorption.

PCT reabsorbs almost all of the glucose filtered by the glomeruli in normal individuals. Around 90% of the glucose reabsorption occurs through sodium-glucose cotransporter 2 which reabsorbs glucose along with $Na+$.

Drugs acting on proximal convoluted tubule

Carbonic anhydrase inhibitors: acetazolamide, dorzolamide, ethoxzolamide, methazolamide, etc

Mechanism of action

CA inhibitors, by acting on proximal tubular epithelial cells, inhibit CA enzyme (Flow diagram 16.1) and thus block the abovementioned pathway. H_2CO_3 is not dissociated into H_2O and CO_2 which enter the epithelial cell to form H_2CO_3 again in cytoplasm to supply free $HCO3-$ ions to be transported along with $Na+$ to interstitium by cotransporter in basolateral membrane. As a result, transport of $NaHCO_3$ from tubular lumen to interstitial space is inhibited. This is associated with inhibition of water reabsorption. CA inhibitor thus causes increased excretion of $HCO3-$ along with $Na+$, $K+$, and water.

However, CA inhibitors also act on distal part of distal tubule. Due to inhibition of CA enzyme here, the physiological mechanism of acidification of urine also fails.

Net excretion of alkaline urine contains $NaHCO_3$, $KHCO_3$, and water with mild metabolic acidosis. Body tries to conserve $Na+$ by increasing its reabsorption from the remaining tubule in the nephron. As a result, over couple of days, action of CA inhibitor becomes self-limiting.

Sodium-glucose cotransporter 2 inhibitors: dapagliflozin, canagliflozin, empagliflozin, etc

Mechanism of action

They inhibit this sodium-glucose cotransporter (Flow diagram 16.2) and hence $Na+$ reabsorption also stops along with glucose.[58–60] This leads to $Na+$ excretion and exerts their diuretic effect. Further, due to the presence

Na+ enters PT cell via Na^+/H^+ exchanger (LM), H^+ moves into lumen

↓

Na^+/K^+-ATPase transporter (BM) pumps Na^+ into the interstitium to maintain a low intracellular Na+ concentration.

↓

Secreted H^+ combines with $HCO3^-$ to form H2CO3 (L)

↓

H2CO3 dissociates to CO2 and H2O

By CA IV ↓**X blocked by CA inhibitor**

CO2 being lipid soluble enters the PT cells by simple diffusion

↓**X**

CO2 rehydrated back to H2CO3 by intracellular CA II

By CA IV ↓**X blocked by CA inhibitor**

H2CO3 ionizes spontaneously to form H^+ and $HCO3^-$

↓**X**

Electrochemical gradient for $HCO3^-$ is created across BM

↓**X**

$Na^+/HCO3^-$ symporter (BM) transport Na^+ & $HCO3^-$ into the interstitial space

↓**X**

Movement of water by isotonic reabsorption.

FLOW DIAGRAM 16.1 Mechanism of action of CA inhibitor. *CA*, Carbonic anhydrase.

SGLT2 in proximal convoluted tubule (LM)

X ↓ **blocked by SGLT2 inhibitor**

Na+ enters PT cell along with glucose

X ↓

Na^+/K^+-ATPase transporter (BM) pumps Na^+ into the interstitium

to maintain a low intracellular Na^+ concentration

X ↓

Movement of water by isotonic reabsorption

FLOW DIAGRAM 16.2 Mechanism of action of SGLT2 inhibitor. *SGLT2*, Sodium glucose co transporter-2 inhibitor.

of unabsorbed glucose hypertonicity of the luminal fluid increases, this inhibits the water reabsorption from the tubule and urine volume increases.

Loop of Henle

The PCT straightens and the next portion of each nephron is the loop of Henle. Loop of Henle consists of (1) descending limb, (2) hairpin bend, and

(3) ascending limb. Descending limb has two segments, continuation of PCT is thick (6 mm) followed by thin segment up to hairpin bend. Ascending limb also consists of two segments, continuation of hairpin bends as thin segment followed by thick segment (9 mm). Thin segment consists of thin permeable cells with flattened epithelium while thick portion of the ascending limb is made up of thick cells containing many mitochondria.

Thin descending limb does not participate in salt reabsorption but is permeable to water and site of water reabsorption. So, tubular fluid is concentrated here.

Thick ascending limb (TAL) is impermeable to water but is site of NaCl reabsorption and so regarded as diluting segment. In the luminal membrane, there are Na + K + 2Cl − cotransporter, Na + /H + exchanger, and K + channels. The Na + K + ATPase pumps are located in the basolateral membrane.

From this region, active reabsorption of sodium ion is mediated by Na + K + 2Cl − cotransporter system. There are actually two isoforms of Na + K + 2Cl − cotransporter: absorptive and secretory isoform. The absorptive isoform is expressed at the luminal membrane and secretory isoform is expressed on the basolateral membrane.

Sodium, potassium, and chloride ions are reabsorbed by these Na + K + 2Cl − cotransporter (Fig. 16.3). One Na +, one K +, and two

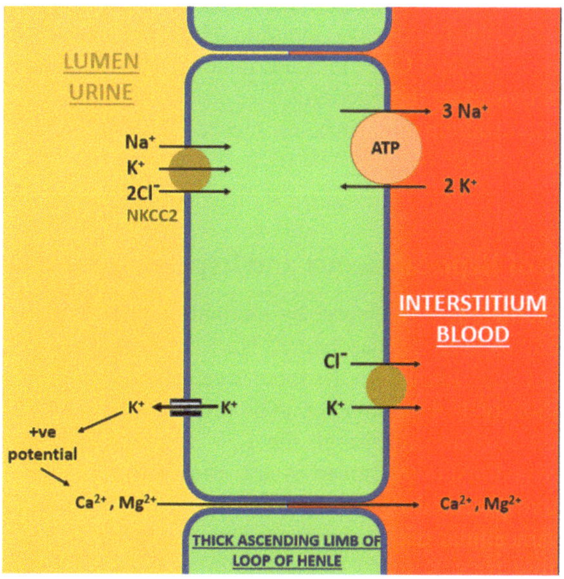

FIGURE 16.3 Na + ion reabsorption in thick ascending limb of Henle's loop. *NKCC2*, Na + / K + /2Cl − cotransporter.

Cl^- ions are transported together to the epithelial cells via this cotransporter. These $Na^+K^+2Cl^-$ cotransporters are electrically neutral because two cations are transported along with two anions.

Na^+/K^+-ATPase transporter in the basolateral membrane extrudes the reabsorbed Na^+ ion into the interstitium to maintain a low-intracellular Na^+ concentration and pumps K^+ into the cell. Thus Na^+ is reabsorbed in TAL.

Due to K^+ transport by luminal $Na^+K^+2Cl^-$ cotransporters and basolateral Na^+/K^+-ATPase pump, there is accumulation of K^+ within the tubular cell.

Accumulation of K^+ within the cells promotes its back diffusion from the tubular cell into the lumen through K^+ channels. Now a positive potential is created inside the lumen by this back diffusion of K^+.

This positive potential drives divalent cations Ca^{2+} and Mg^{2+} reabsorption via paracellular pathway into the interstitium.

Diuretics acting on thick ascending limb

Loop diuretics: furosemide, torsemide, bumetanide and ethacrynic acid, etc

Mechanism of action

Loop diuretics primarily act on TAL of loop of Henle.[61–63] Loop diuretics bind to the chloride binding site of $Na^+K^+2Cl^-$ cotransport proteins and inhibit them (Fig. 16.3 and Flow diagram 16.3) the reabsorption of Na^+ and Cl^- ions. Na^+ and Cl^- ions are retained in the lumen and excreted. Loop diuretics thus exert their action.

The increased sodium concentration reaches the DCT and promotes loss of H^+ and K^+ ions.

Mechanism of hypocalcaemia and hypomagnesemia

As discussed earlier, K^+ transport by luminal $Na^+K^+2Cl^-$ cotransporters (Fig. 16.3) as well as basolateral Na^+/K^+-ATPase pump leads to accumulation of K^+ ion within the tubular cell.

Accumulation of K^+ within the cells promotes its back diffusion from the tubular cell into lumen through the K^+ ion channels. Now a positive potential is created inside the lumen by this back diffusion of K^+.

This positive potential drives divalent cations Ca^{2+} and Mg^{2+} reabsorption via paracellular pathway into the interstitium.

By inhibiting $Na^+K^+2Cl^-$ cotransporter (Flow diagram 16.3), loop diuretics inhibit these reabsorptions of Ca^{2+} and Mg^{2+} leading to hypocalcemia and hypomagnesemia.

NKCC2 in thick ascending limb of loop of Henle (LM)
X ↓ **Loop diuretics bind to Cl^- biding site of NKCC2 and inhibits it**
NKCC2 transports 1 Na^+, 1 K^+ & 2 Cl^- ions
X ↓
Na^+/K^+-ATPase transporter (BM) extrudes reabsorbed Na+ into interstitium to maintain a low intracellular Na^+ concentration and pumps K^+ into the cell
X ↓
Na^+ is reabsorbed in TAL
X ↓
Accumulation of K^+ within the tubular cell
X ↓
Back diffusion of K^+ from tubular cell into the lumen through K^+ channels (LM)
X ↓
Positive potential created by back diffusion of K^+
X ↓
This potential drives Ca^{2+} & Mg^{2+} into the interstitium via paracellular pathway
X ↓
Ca^{2+}, Mg^{2+} reabsorption

FLOW DIAGRAM 16.3 Mechanism of action of Loop diuretics.

Mechanism of hypokalemia and metabolic alkalosis

Loop diuretics bind to chloride binding sites of Na + K + 2Cl − cotransport (Flow diagram 16.3) proteins and inhibit the reabsorption of Na +, K +, and Cl − ions. Na +, K +, and Cl − ions are retained in the lumen and excreted. The increased sodium concentration that reaches the distal tubule promotes loss or hydrogen and potassium iron (discussed later). Loop diuretics in high dose, particularly, may produce metabolic alkalosis as there is loss of hydrogen and potassium and also increased excretion of calcium and magnesium as already stated.

Distal convoluted tubule

DCT is the continuation of TAL starting at medulla and occupies the cortex of nephron and is continued as CD.[64–66] DCT is lined by single-layer cuboidal epithelial cells without any brush border and these cells are called intercalated cells (I cell). Na +, Ca2 +, bicarbonate, and water are reabsorbed from DCT.

There are Na + Cl − cotransporters, Ca2 + ion channels in the luminal membrane and Na + K + ATPase pump, Ca2 + H + ATPase pump, and Na + /Ca2 + exchanger in the basolateral membrane.

From this region, active reabsorption of sodium ion is mediated by Na^+Cl^- cotransporter system. This part is also impermeable to water and 8%–10% of filtered sodium chloride is reabsorbed in this segment.

This Na^+Cl^- cotransporters are electrically neutral because one cation is transported along with one anion.

Na^+K^+ATPase pump, located in the basolateral membrane, pumps K^+ into the cell in exchange of Na^+ ion for maintaining a low-intracellular Na^+ ion concentration. Na^+ is transported the interstitium.

Unlike TAL segment, in DCT there is no excess accumulation of K^+ within the tubular cell. There is no back diffusion of K^+ ions from the tubular cell into the lumen and hence inside the lumen no positive potential is created. So, there is no drive of divalent cations Ca^{2+} and Mg^{2+} ion reabsorption via paracellular pathway into the interstitium like in case of TAL of loop of Henle.

Instead calcium is actively reabsorbed from this segment via calcium channels located in the luminal membrane. Both parathyroid hormone and calcitriol promote calcium ion reabsorption.

Diuretics acting on distal convoluted tubule

Thiazide diuretics: chlorothiazide, chlorthalidone, hydrochlorothiazide, indapamide, metolazone

They have moderately powerful diuretic action not to that extent of loop diuretics.[59,67]

Mechanism of action

Thiazide diuretics are secreted in PCT by the organic acid secretory systems and reach early DCT via tubular fluid. In the early part of DCT, they inhibit electro neutral Na^+Cl^- cotransporter system. Na^+ and Cl^- ion reabsorption stops (Flow diagram 16.4). The Na^+ and Cl^- ions are excreted along with water.

Loop diuretic action of thiazide is also partially mediated by renal PGE2 and PGI2 synthesis. They also inhibit CA enzyme in PCT.

Mechanism of no hypocalcemia

Thiazide diuretics inhibit electro neutral Na^+Cl^- cotransporter system. So, there is no excess accumulation of intracellular K^+ and no back diffusion of K^+ in the lumen and no Ca^{2+} reabsorption due to lumen positive potential created by K^+ ions.

Instead calcium is actively reabsorbed from this segment via calcium channels (Fig. 16.4 and Flow diagram 16.4) located in the luminal membrane by the help of parathyroid hormone and calcitriol. Thiazide causes low-intracellular sodium that promotes enhanced Na^+/Ca^{2+} exchange in the

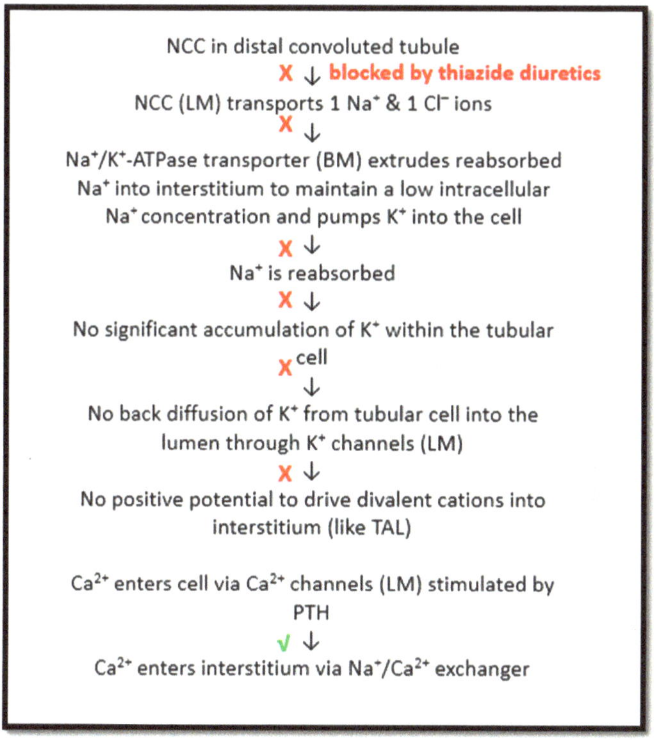

FLOW DIAGRAM 16.4 Mechanism of action of thiazide diuretics.

basolateral membrane and overall absorption of Ca2 + is increased. Unlike the situation in the TAL of Henle's loop where loop diuretics directly inhibit the calcium reabsorption as discussed earlier, thiazide diuretics rather enhance parathyroid hormone-regulated calcium reabsorption from the DCT.

When more sodium reaches the CD from the DCT, the high flow rate of the filtrate produced by thiazides also increases K + excretion by continuously flashing it away increasing the gradient from the principal cells to the lumen. Potassium loss is significant.

Thiazide diuretics decrease the calcium concentration of urine promoting calcium reabsorption in the DCT. During diuresis by thiazides, urine is reach in sodium and chloride but almost free of bicarbonate. Increased bicarbonate and decreased ECF volume lead to increased concentration of bicarbonate per unit volume of ECF.

Aldosterone stimulation in collecting tubule promotes hypokalemia and hydrogen ion secretion which stimulates bicarbonate reabsorption from the proximal tubule.

All these events lead to development of hypochloremic metabolic alkalosis.

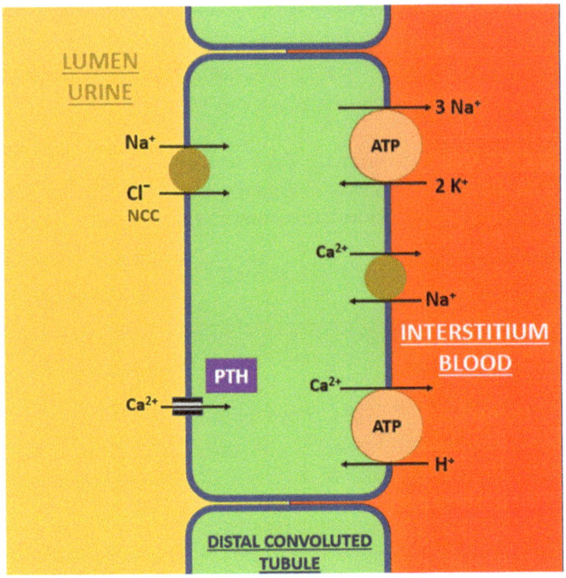

FIGURE 16.4 Na + reabsorption in distal convoluted tubule. *NCC*, Na + /Cl − cotransporter; *PTH*, Parathyroid hormone.

Collecting tubule system

Several distal tubules open into each collecting tubules and the collecting tubules join to form the CDs.[68,69] Lower part of the CD is located in medulla. 7−10 initial CD s join to form the straight CD passing through medulla. CD is formed by two types of epithelial cells; principal cell (P cell) and intercalated cell (I cell).

There are no apical cotransport systems for sodium and other ions in principal cells. Instead, in the apical membrane, they have different ion channels for Na + absorption and K + excretion, but no channel for anions. In the basolateral side, there are Na + K + ATPase pumps.

In the intercalated cells, there is H + /ATPase pump in luminal membrane and HCO3 − /Cl − exchanger in the basolateral membrane.

These cells are normally impermeable to water in absence of antidiuretic hormone (ADH) and to sodium in absence of aldosterone. Aldosterone enters the epithelial cell (Fig. 16.5) from interstitial side and combines with mineralocorticoid receptor (Mr) in cytosol to form drug−receptor complex. The Mr aldosterone complex translocates to the nucleus. This promotes gene-mediated mRNA synthesis that regulates the expression aldosterone-induced proteins (AIPs). AIPs activate Na + ion channels and translocate them from cytosolic site to luminal membrane and Na + K + ATPase pumps to basolateral membrane. They also increase production of ATP by mitochondria. All these changes increase Na + ion reabsorption.

By the epithelial Na + channels (ENaC), Na + ions enter the principal cell (Fig. 16.6) from tubular fluid and via basolateral Na + /K + -ATPase, transported

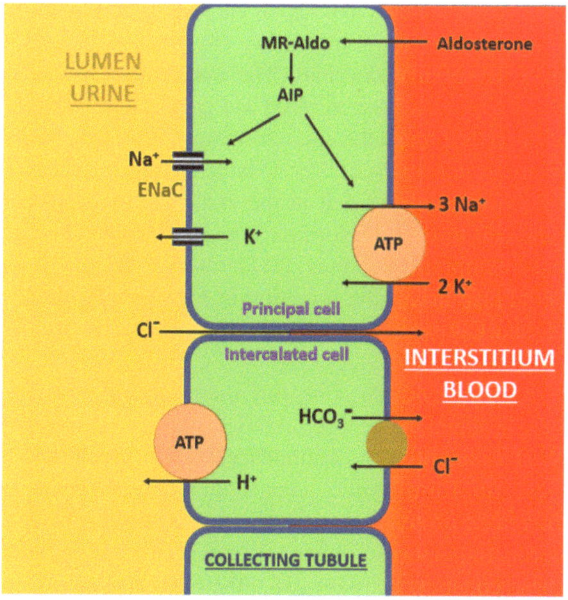

FIGURE 16.5 Mineralocorticoid receptor–mediated Na + reabsorption. *Mr–Aldo*, mineralocorticoid receptor–aldosterone complex; *AIP*, aldosterone-induced protein; *ENaC*, epithelial sodium channel.

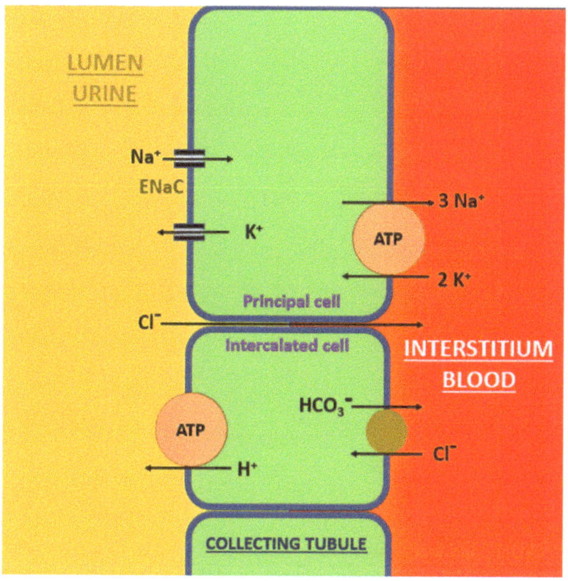

FIGURE 16.6 Na + reabsorption via epithelial sodium channels. *ENaC*, Epithelial sodium channel.

to the blood. K + ion is secreted into lumen via K + channels. Na + entry inside cell predominates over K + ion secretion into the lumen and lumen-negative electrical potential of 10–50 mV develops. The lumen-negative electrical potential drives transport of Cl − ion back to blood via paracellular pathway and secretes K + ion out of the cells through the apical membrane K + ion channel.

Via the HCO3 − /Cl − exchanger located in the basolateral membrane, chloride enters the intercalated cell in the exchange of bicarbonate which is driven out of the cell to the interstitium. The ATP-driven H + pump situated in the luminal membrane secretes the hydrogen to the lumen. Lumen-negative potential also drives the secretion of hydrogen by these pumps.

From DCT and CD water is reabsorbed in facultative way by the action of ADH.

Normally, the DCT and the collecting duct are impermeable to H_2O but become permeable when ADH acts. ADH combines with vasopressin (V2) receptors in the basolateral side of tubular epithelial membrane and activates adenylyl cyclase, to form cyclic adenosine monophosphate (AMP). This cyclic AMP increases protein kinase A (PKA) activity which leads to activation of aquaporins (aquaporin-2) channels and their transportation to luminal membrane. These channels increase make these segments permeable to water and increase water reabsorption (Fig. 16.7).

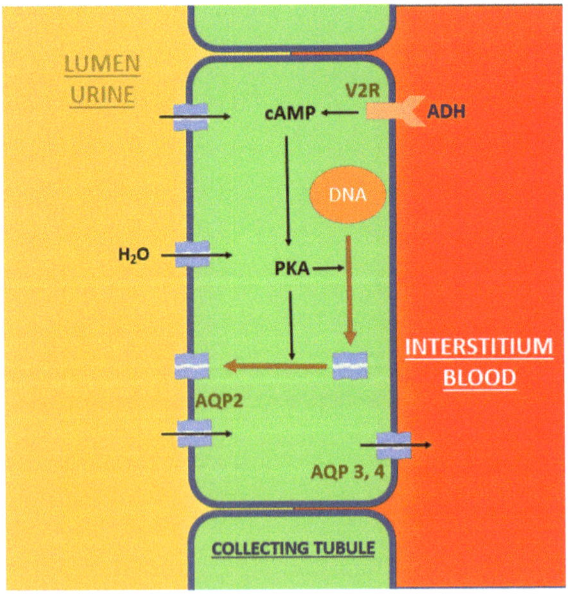

FIGURE 16.7 ADH induced aquaporin channel-mediated water reabsorption. *ADH*, Antidiuretic hormone; *AQP2*, aquaporin channel 2; *AQP3,4*, aquaporin channel 3,4; *cAMP*, cyclic adenosine monophosphate; *DNA*, deoxyribonucleic acid; *PKA*, protein kinase A; *V2R*, vasopressin receptor.

Diuretics acting on tubule system

Aldosterone receptor antagonist or mineralocorticoid receptor antagonist (K + sparing diuretics): spironolactone, eplerenone

Mechanism of action

Aldosterone receptor antagonist acts on distal part of distal tubule and collecting tubules.[53,69] They bind to Mrs (Flow diagram 16.5) and prevent mRNA synthesis followed by AIPs expressions. Thus activation of sodium channel is inhibited. So, Na + reabsorption decreases. As a result, potassium secretion is also decreased. H + secretion is decreased. Uric acid secretion is decreased.

Inhibitors of renal epithelial Na + channel (K + sparing diuretics): triamterene, amiloride

Mechanism of action

Epithelial sodium channel inhibitors (like amiloride and triamterene) are secreted through organic base secretory system at the PCT and act at the distal part of DCT and collecting tubule. They inhibit this epithelial Na + ion channel (Flow diagram 16.6) and thus inhibit the entry of Na + in the cell. This promotes the excretion of Na + as lumen-negative potential does not

Aldosterone enters epithelial cell (BM)
↓
Combines with the cytosolic MR to form drug receptor complex
X ↓ **blocked by MRA**
MR aldosterone complex translocate to the nucleus
↓
Gene mediated mRNA synthesis which regulates
X ↓
Expression of AIPs
X ↓
AIPs activate Na^+ channels
and
translocate them from cytosolic site to LM
and
translocate Na^+/K^+ATPase pumps to BM
and
increase ATP production by mitochondria.
X ↓
All these changes increase Na^+ reabsorption

FLOW DIAGRAM 16.5 Mechanism of action of aldosterone receptor antagonist.

ENaC in collecting tubule (BM)
X ↓ **blocked by ENaC inhibitors**
By ENaC, Na^+ enters P cell from the tubular fluid
X ↓
Na^+/K^+-ATPase transporter extrudes reabsorbed Na^+ into interstitium to maintain a low intracellular Na^+ concentration and pumps K^+ into P cell
X ↓
K^+ is secreted into lumen via K^+ channels.
X ↓
Na+ entry inside cell predominates over K+ secretion into the lumen
X ↓
Lumen negative potential of 10 – 50 mV develops
X ↓
Drives transport of Cl^- to the blood via the paracellular pathway
and
secretes K^+ out of cells through K^+ channel (LM)

FLOW DIAGRAM 16.6 Mechanism of action of epithelial sodium channel inhibitor.

develop, and Cl − ion is also not transported back to blood via paracellular pathways. So, this facilitates Na + and Cl − excretion and exerts their diuretic effects.

So, by blocking up this channel, they inhibit Na + reabsorption. Thus the lumen-negative potential decreases. Lumen-negative potential is the driving force of potassium secretion. So, potassium secretion is also inhibited.

Net loss of sodium is minor; potassium excretion is prevented in significant level.

The lumen-negative potential is also the driving force of H + ion secretion. So, these drugs by reducing the lumen-negative potential also inhibit the secretion of hydrogen ions as well. This leads to metabolic acidosis.

Since their mode of action is independent of aldosterone, so, they have diuretic activity even in patients of Addison's disease. Amiloride is not metabolized in the liver and therefore is 10 times more potent and longer-acting compared to triamterene. Both are mild uricosurics.

Antidiuretic hormone receptor (vasopressin) antagonist: tolvaptan, conivaptan

Mechanism of action

As discussed earlier, Anti diuretic hormone (ADH) combines with V2 receptors which activates cAMP which increases the activity of PKA and aquaporin channels are formed leading to water reabsorption.[63–66] ADH receptor

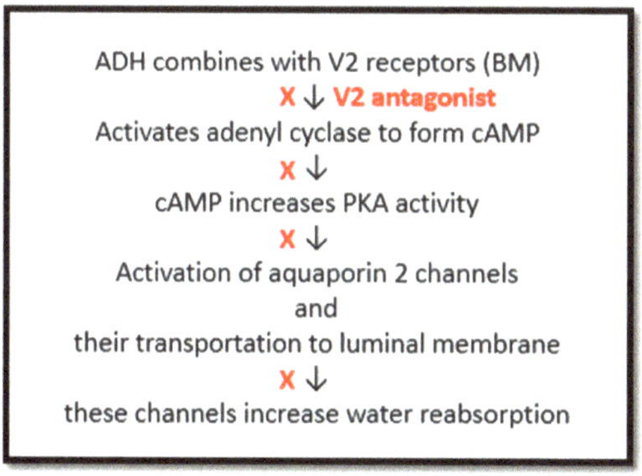

FLOW DIAGRAM 16.7 Mechanism of action of ADH receptor (V2) antagonist. *ADH*, antidiuretic hormone.

antagonists inhibits (Flow diagram 16.7) the receptors and thereby inhibit aquaporin channel activation. This leads to inhibition of water reabsorption and thus exerts diuretic effect.

Nonspecific cation channel inhibitor: natriuretic peptides: (1) atria natriuretic peptide, (2) brain natriuretic peptide, (3) C-type natriuretic peptide and urodilatin

Mechanism of action

They inhibit sodium absorption by acting on the nonspecific cationic channels in the inner medullary CDs (Fig. 16.8).[64–67] Natriuretic peptides (NPs) bind to cell surface receptors that are isoforms of particulate guanylyl cyclase. Guanylyl cyclase synthesizes cGMP which directly inhibit those cation channels (cyclic nucleotide gated cation channel or CNGC). They also inhibit the cation channels indirectly by activating protein kinase G (PKG). PKG also inhibits the Na + K + ATPase pump on the basolateral membrane. As a result, Na + absorption is inhibited.

Others

Osmotic diuretics: mannitol, urea, isosorbide, glycerol

Mechanism of action

They act indirectly in water-permeable segments of nephron: PCT and descending limb of Henle's loop, and collecting tubules.[68,69]

They are minimally metabolized in human body and freely filter edat the glomerulus and undergo minimal reabsorption. Due to the presence of nonreabsorbable solutes along with other electrolytes, the hypertonicity of the luminal fluid increases. This limits osmosis of water into interstitium and

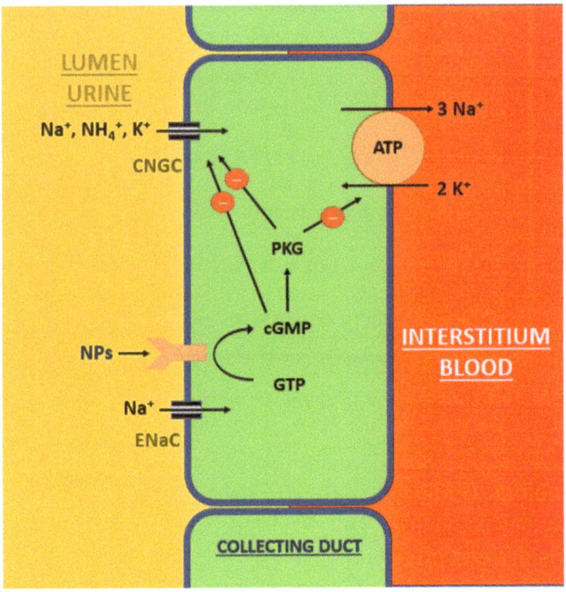

FIGURE 16.8 Mechanism of action of natriuretic peptides.

thereby reduces the Na + ion concentration in the lumen till Na + reabsorption stops. This inhibits the water reabsorption from the tubule and urine volume increases.

They extract water from intracellular compartments and expand ECF volume and thus decrease viscosity of blood and inhibit renin release. These effects increase renal blood flow. The increase in renal medullary blood flow helps in removal of NaCl and urea from the renal medulla and reduces medullary tonicity. This reduction in medullary tonicity promotes a decrease in the excretion of water from the descending thin limb, which in turn limits the concentration of NaCl in tubular fluid which enters ascending thin limb. This latter effect inhibits the passive reabsorption of NaCl in the ascending thin limb.

Mannitol when given intravenously first increases the osmolarity of the ECF. To equalize the osmolarity, water shifts from the intracellular space to the extracellular space which increases filtration load at Glomerulus.

Conclusion

Therefore the main effect of osmotic diuresis is to increase the amount of water, with a relatively small increase in sodium excretion. They increase urinary excretion of almost all electrolytes (e.g., Na + , K + , Cl − , HCO − , Ca2 + , Mg2 + , and phosphate). This chapter sheds light on the various sites and pharmacological actions of drugs affecting these. The chapter mainly focuses on loop diuretics, which are the primary line of treatment in case of patients with chronic kidney disease (CKD). The chapter deals not only with thiazides and mineralocorticoid antagonists but also with other class of diuretics dealing with subsets of CKD patients.

References

1. Bauersachs J, et al. Mineralocorticoid receptor activation and mineralocorticoid receptor antagonist treatment in cardiac and renal diseases. *Hypertension*. 2015;65:257–263.
2. Benarroch EE. Oxytocin and vasopressin: social neuropeptides with complex neuromodulatory functions. *Neurology*. 2013;80:1521–1528.
3. Berl T, et al. Oral tolvaptan is safe and effective in chronic hyponatremia. *J Am Soc Nephrol*. 2010;21:705.
4. Berl T. Vasopressin antagonists. *N Engl J Med*. 2015;372(23):2207–2216.
5. Bernstein PL, Ellison DH. Diuretics and salt transport along the nephron. *Semin Nephrol*. 2011;31(6):475–482.
6. Brater DC. Diuretic therapy. *N Engl J Med*. 1998;339:387–395.
7. Brater DC. *Mechanism of Action of Diuretics*. UpToDate; 2013. <http://www.uptodate.com>.
8. Brenner BM, ed. *Brenner & Rector's the Kidney*. 8th ed. Saunders; 2008.
9. Brown J, et al. Spironolactone vs placebo or in combination with steroids for hirsutism and/or acne. *Cochrane Database Syst Rev*. 2009;(2)CD000194.
10. Cooper BE. Diuresis in renal failure: treat the patient, not the urine output. *Crit Care Med*. 2009;37:761.
11. Costello-Boerrigter LC, Boerrigter G, Burnett Jr. JC. Revisiting salt and water retention: new diuretics, aquaretics, and natriuretics. *Med Clin North Am*. 2003;87:475.
12. D'Elia E, Krum H. Mineralcorticoid antagonists in heart failure. *Heart Fail Clin*. 2014;10:559–564.
13. Edelmann F, et al. Effect of spironolactone on diastolic function and exercise capacity in patients with heart failure with preserved ejection fraction: the Aldo-DHF randomized controlled trial. *JAMA*. 2013;309:781–791.
14. Ernst ME, Moser M. Use of diuretics in patients with hypertension. *N Engl J Med*. 2009;361:2153.
15. Faris R, et al. Current evidence supporting the role of diuretics in heart failure: a meta analysis of randomised controlled trials. *Int J Cardiol*. 2002;82:149–158.
16. Forssmann WG, Meyer M, Forsmann K. The renal urodilatin system. Clinical implications. *Cardiovasc Res*. 2001;51(3):450.
17. Garcia ML, Kaczorowski GJ. Targeting the inward-rectifier potassium channel ROMK in cardiovascular disease. *Curr Opin Pharmacol*. 2014;15:1–6.
18. Ginès P, Schrier RW. Renal failure in cirrhosis. *N Engl J Med*. 2009;361:1279.
19. Hao C-M, Breyer MD. Physiological regulation of prostaglandins in the kidney. *Annu Rev Physiol*. 2008;70:357.
20. Hays RM. Vasopressin antagonists: progress and promise. *N Engl J Med*. 2006;355:146.
21. Hill JA, Yancy CW, Abraham WT. Beyond diuretics: management of volume overload in acute heart failure syndromes. *Am J Med*. 2006;119:S37.
22. Hocher B. Adenosine A1 receptor antagonists in clinical research and development. *Kidney Int*. 2010;78(5):438.

23. Iovino M, et al. Molecular mechanisms involved in the control of neurohypophyseal hormones secretion. *Curr Pharm Des*. 2014;20:6702–6713.
24. Jackson EK. Drugs affecting renal excretory function. In: Brunton LL, Dandan RH, Knollmann BC, eds. *Goodman & Gilman's the Pharmacological Basis of Therapeutics*. 13th ed. New York: McGraw Hill Education; 2018:445–470.
25. Kaplan NM. The place of diuretics in preventing cardiovascular events. *J Hum Hypertens*. 2004;18:S29.
26. Kellenberger S, Schild L. International Union of Basic and Clinical Pharmacology. XCI. Structure, function, and pharmacology of acid-sensing ion channels and the epithelial Na^+ channel. *Pharmacol Rev*. 2015;67:1–35.
27. Kim GH, et al. Antidiuretic effect of hydrochlorothiazide in lithium-induced nephrogenic diabetes insipidus is associated with upregulation of aquaporin-2, Na-Cl cotransporter, and epithelial sodium channel. *J Am Soc Nephrol*. 2004;15:2836.
28. Kishore BK, Ecelbarger CM. Lithium. A versatile tool for understanding renal physiology. *Am J Physiol Ren Physiol*. 2013;304:F1139–F1149.
29. Kortenoeven MLA, et al. Amiloride blocks lithium entry through the sodium channel thereby attenuating the resultant nephrogenic diabetes insipidus. *Kidney Int*. 2009;76:44–53.
30. Kortenoeven MLA, et al. Demeclocycline attenuates hyponatremia by reducing aquaporin-2 expression in the renal inner medulla. *Am J Physiol Ren Physiol*. 2013;305: F1705–F1718.
31. Layek A, et al. Efficacy of vasopressin during cardio-pulmonary resuscitation in adult patients: a meta-analysis. *Resuscitation*. 2014;85:855–863.
32. Lee C, Burnett J. Natriuretic peptides and therapeutic applications. *Heart Fail Rev*. 2007;12:131.
33. Lüss H, et al. Renal effects of ularitide in patients with decompensated heart failure. *Am Heart J*. 2008;155:1012.
34. Mitrovic V, et al. Cardio-renal effects of the A1 adenosine receptor antagonist SLV320 in patients with heart failure. *Circ Heart Fail*. 2009;2:523.
35. Na KY, et al. Upregulation of Na^+ transporter abundance in response to chronic thiazide or loop diuretic treatment in rats. *Am J Physiol*. 2003;284:F133.
36. Nejsum LN. The renal plumbing system: aquaporin water channels. *Cell Mol Life Sci*. 2005;62:1692–1706.
37. Nigwekar SU, Waikar SS. Diuretics in acute kidney injury. *Semin Nephrol*. 2011;31: 523–534.
38. Nijenhuis T, et al. Enhanced passive Ca^{2+} reabsorption and reduced Mg^{2+} channel abundance explains thiazide-induced hypocalciuria and hypomagnesemia. *J Clin Invest*. 2005;115:1651.
39. Nirdé P, et al. Antimineralocorticoid 11β-substituted spirolactones exhibit androgen receptor agonistic activity: a structure function study. *Mol Pharmacol*. 2001;59:1307–1313.
40. O'Connor CM, et al. Effect of nesiritide in patients with acute decompensated heart failure. *N Engl J Med*. 2011;365:32–43.
41. Olde Engberink RHG, et al. Effects of thiazide-type and thiazide-like diuretics on cardiovascular events and mortality: systematic review and meta-analysis. *Hypertension*. 2015;65:1033–1040.
42. Palmer BF. Metabolic complications associated with use of diuretics. *Semin Nephrol*. 2011;31:542–552.

43. Pitt B, et al. Spironolactone for heart failure with preserved ejection fraction. *N Engl J Med.* 2014;370:1383–1392.
44. Potter LR. Natriuretic peptide metabolism, clearance and degradation. *FEBS J.* 2011;278: 1808–1817.
45. Ritchie ND, et al. Acetazolamide for the prevention of acute mountain sickness—a systematic review and meta-analysis. *J Travel Med.* 2012;19:298–307.
46. Rodenburg EM, et al. Thiazide-associated hyponatremia: a population based study. *Am J Kidney Dis.* 2013;62:67–72.
47. Ronchetti S, et al. GILZ as a mediator of the anti-inflammatory effects of glucocorticoids. *Front Endocrinol (Lausanne).* 2015;6. Available from: https://doi.org/10.3389/fendo.2015.00170. Accessed 10.04.17.
48. Ronzaud C, Staub O. Ubiquitylation and control of renal Na^+ balance and blood pressure. *Physiology.* 2014;29:16–26.
49. Roush GC, et al. Diuretics: a review and update. *J Cardiovasc Pharmacol Ther.* 2014;19: 5–13.
50. Roush GC, et al. Head-to-head comparisons of hydrochlorothiazide with indapamide and chlorthalidone: antihypertensive and metabolic effects. *Hypertension.* 2015;65:1041–1046.
51. Sam R, Ives HE, David Pearce D. Diuretic agents. In: Katzung BG, ed. *Basic & Clinical Pharmacology.* 14th ed. New York: McGraw Hill Education; 2018:254–275.
52. Schnermann J, Huang Y, Mizel D. Fluid reabsorption in proximal convoluted tubules of mice with gene deletions of claudin-2 and/or aquaporin1. *Am J Physiol Ren Physiol.* 2013;305:F1352.
53. Scozzafava A, Supuran CT. Glaucoma and the applications of carbonic anhydrase inhibitors. *Subcell Biochem.* 2014;75:349–359.
54. Serpa Neto A, et al. Vasopressin and terlipressin in adult vasodilatory shock: a systematic review and meta-analysis of nine randomized controlled trials. *Crit Care.* 2012;16:R154.
55. Shargorodsky M, et al. Treatment of hypertension with thiazides: benefit or damage—effect of low- and high-dose thiazide diuretics on arterial elasticity and metabolic parameters in hypertensive patients with and without glucose intolerance. *J Cardiometab Syndr.* 2007;2:16.
56. Sharma HL, Sharma KK. Diuretics. In: Sharma HL, Sharma KK, eds. *Principles of Pharmacology.* 3rd ed. New Delhi: Paras Medical Publisher; 2017:227–240.
57. Shlipak MG, Massie BM. The clinical challenge of cardiorenal syndrome. *Circulation.* 2004;110:1514.
58. Sica DA, Gehr TWB. Diuretic use in stage 5 chronic kidney disease and end-stage renal disease. *Curr Opin Nephrol Hypertens.* 2003;12:483.
59. Sundar S, Dickinson PD. Spironolactone, a possible selective androgen receptor modulator, should be used with caution in patients with metastatic carcinoma of the prostate. *BMJ Case Rep.* 2012;25:2012.
60. Tamargo J, et al. Diuretics in the treatment of hypertension. Part 1: Thiazide and thiazide-like diuretics. *Expert Opin Pharmacother.* 2014;15:527–547.
61. Tavares M, et al. New pharmacologic therapies in acute heart failure. *Crit Care Med.* 2008;36:S112.
62. Tovar-Palacio C, et al. Ion and diuretic specificity of chimeric proteins between apical Na^+-K^+-$2Cl^-$ and Na^+-Cl^- cotransporters. *Am J Physiol.* 2004;287:F570.
63. Tripathi KD. Diuretics. In: Tripathi KD, ed. *Essentials of Medical Pharmacology.* 8th ed. New Delhi: Jaypee Brothers Medical Publishers; 2019:625–638.

64. Vasilakou D, et al. Sodium-glucose cotransporter 2 inhibitors for type 2 diabetes: a systematic review and meta-analysis. *Ann Intern Med.* 2013;159:262.
65. Wakai A, et al. Mannitol for acute traumatic brain injury. *Cochrane Database Syst Rev.* 2013;(8):CD001049.
66. Wakai R, Roberts IG, Schierhout G. Mannitol for acute traumatic brain injury. *Cochrane Database Syst Rev.* 2008; (online publication) Issue 4.
67. Welling PA. Regulation of renal potassium secretion: molecular mechanisms. *Semin Nephrol.* 2013;33:215–228.
68. Wilcox C. New insights into diuretic use in patients with chronic renal disease. *J Am Soc Nephrol.* 2002;13:798.
69. Wile D. Diuretics: a review. *Ann Clin Biochem.* 2012;49:419–431.

Further reading

Bruderer S, et al. Use of diuretics and risk of incident gout: a population based case-control study. *Arthritis Rheumatol.* 2014;66:185–196.

Buggey J, et al. A reappraisal of loop diuretic choice in heart failure patients. *Am Heart J.* 2015;169:323–333.

Chapter 17

Mechanism of action of drugs used in gastrointestinal diseases

Himani Nautiyal[1], Imran Kazmi[2], Mohammed Kaleem[2], Muhammad Afzal[3], Muhammad Masood Ahmad[4], Ameeduzzafar Zafar[4] and Rupinder Kaur[5]

[1]Siddhartha Institute of Pharmacy, Dehradun, Uttarakhand, India, [2]Department of Biochemistry, Faculty of Science, King Abdulaziz University, Jeddah, Saudi Arabia, [3]Department of Pharmacology, College of Pharmacy, Jouf University, Sakaka, Aljouf, Saudi Arabia, [4]Department of Pharmaceutics, College of Pharmacy, Jouf University, Sakaka, Aljouf, Saudi Arabia, [5]Chandigarh College of Pharmacy, Landran, Mohali, Punjab, India

Overview

Oxygen and food provide energy and are the building blocks for the survival of the human body.[1] Direct respiration is responsible for oxygen intake; this oxygen is further utilized for metabolic processes inside the body, while food undergoes a long process called digestion and absorption to provide nutrition values for metabolic reactions. Digestion is basic function of the gastrointestinal tract (GIT); along with this function,[2] it also servers as important part of endocrine system. As specific enteric nervous system, integrative neuronal networks are present in GIT, where almost similar number of neurons is present in the spinal cord. This organ system is the site for different diseases ranging from short modalities (dyspepsia) to complicated diseases like Crohn's disease. In this chapter, we will discuss about physiological functions of GIT and pharmacological activities of synthetic drugs used for the treatment of different illnesses associated with GIT.[3]

Introduction

The gastrointestinal tract (GIT) comprises almost 9-m long tube starting in the mouth and ending into anus, and different accessory organs, liver, gall bladder, and pancreases, are also associated with GIT. The food enters in mouth, where it is chewed by teeth and then swallowed through esophagus to reach stomach, and it stays there for several hours depending on stomach

How Synthetic Drugs Work. DOI: https://doi.org/10.1016/B978-0-323-99855-0.00017-8

motility and nature of food, food further processed in intestine for absorption and finally for elimination thought rectum. Two muscular rings (lower esophagus sphincter and pyloric sphincter) are responsible for food strict storage in the stomach for digestion and to avoid its unwanted availability in esophagus and duodenum. Lower esophagus sphincter helps to avoid damage of esophagus resulting due to acidic backup; pyloric sphincter precedes the semidigested food in duodenum only when it is not occupied and intestine gets enough time to absorb nutritional substances from this semidigested food.[4]

Neuronal and hormonal control over gastrointestinal tract

Various pathways are responsible for mutual communication between central nervous system and GIT.[5] Intestinal metabolic compounds and bacterial contents indirectly stimulate the vagus nerve and amalgamate details to central nervous system to produce balance between nervous system and intestinal tract.[6] Afferent fibers of vagus nerve express toll receptors and neurotransmitter receptors at fibers end, on which different subtracts bind directly such as bacterial metabolites, short-chain polysaccharides, and lipopolysaccharides. The stimuli-receptor binding generated signals transmit information to the brain, which is responsible for intestinal motility and immunity.[7] Intestinal hormones such as serotonins [5-hydroxytryptamine (5-HT)] and cholecystokinin (CCK) are produced in the small intestine, in response to activation of endocrine cells by food components (carbohydrates, proteins, and lipids) present in GIT, and these hormones also bind to afferent nerve receptors and regulate intestinal movement.[8]

Gastrointestinal acid regulation

When acid secretion was discovered in the stomach earlier last century, scientists were convinced regarding the role of acid in pathogenesis of different diseases associated with stomach and other neighboring organs (esophagus and duodenum).[9] Gastric acid regulation is initiated by different pathways (hormonal, paracrine, and neuronal). When we ingest the food, these pathways get activated by stimuli either in brain or in the stomach such as proteins (chemical stimuli), stomach distension (mechanical stimuli). Acetylcholine (neurotransmitter), histamine (paracrine), gastrin (hormone), and also somatostatin (paracrine inhibitory hormone) are important secretory agents responsible for regulation of acids in the GIT.[10]

Peripheral regulation of acid

About 2.5-L gastric juice is secreted in a day. Prorenins and pepsinogens are exocrine secretions produced in peptic cells, along with these hydrochloric acids, and some intrinsic factors are also produced and secreted from oxyntic cells.[11] Gastric mucosa is surrounded by mucus-producing cells, which works as protective layer (trapped bicarbonate ions produce gel-like protective structure and maintain pH 6–7) in the acidic environment of GIT. Disturbance among secretion and protection mechanism is responsible for the development of gastric ulcers which also are the target sites for treatment drugs.[12]

Gastric partial cells contain G-cells, which are responsible for the initiation of acid secretion in terms of release of gastrin, which further activates CCK B receptor present in enterochromaffin-like cells resulting in the series cascade of calcium ions. Histamine release from exocytotic cells results in activation of Cl current. Histamine released during the process also activates partial cell H_2 receptor–mediated H^+/K^+/ATPase. This is the final pathway for gastric acid secretion.[13]

Initially, isotonic hydrochloric acid (15 mmol) with pH <1 is produced in the parietal cells, which has hydrogen concentration more than million than in the plasma. Active chloride ions transport occurs into canaliculi in the cells that communicate with gastric gland lumen and then with stomach.[14] Chloride ion secretion is accompanied by potassium ion secretion that is exchanged for hydrogen ion within the cell (K^+H^+/ATPase) and bicarbonate ions. The bicarbonate ion also exchanges for chloride ions in the parietal cells. Parietal cells activated by different stimuli include gastrin (stimulatory hormone), acetylcholine (stimulatory neurotransmitter), histamine (stimulatory autacoid), prostaglandin (inhibitory autacoid).[15]

Gastrin

A gastric antrum and duodenum mucosa contain endocrine cell that produces gastrin, which is further transported to portal vein; the gastrin stimulates acid production in parietal cells and mucosa production in acid-secreting part of stomach. During and after meal, production of acid is also regulated by circulating gastrin.[16]

Acetylcholine

Neurotransmitters released from vagus nerve (acetylcholine) activate muscarinic receptors of parietal cells and on the histamine-containing cell surfaces.[17]

Histamine

Within the stomach, mast cells (or histamine-containing cells similar to mast cells) lying close to the parietal cell release a steady basal release of histamine, which is further increased by gastrin and acetylcholine. The hormone acts on parietal cell H_2 receptors, which are responsive to histamine concentrations that are below the threshold required for vascular H_2 receptor activation[18] (Table 17.1 and Fig. 17.1).

TABLE 17.1 Summary of factors involved in regulation of acid secretion.

S. no.	Acid regulation
1	The proton pump ($K^{+}H^{+}$ATPase) in gastric parietal cells is responsible for secretion of acid.
2	Acetylcholine, gastrin, and histamine act like endogenous secretory agents for acid in gastrointestinal tract.
3	Prostaglandins ($I_2$and E_2) are responsible for mucus and bicarbonate secretion, and blood vessels dilation also inhibits acid production.

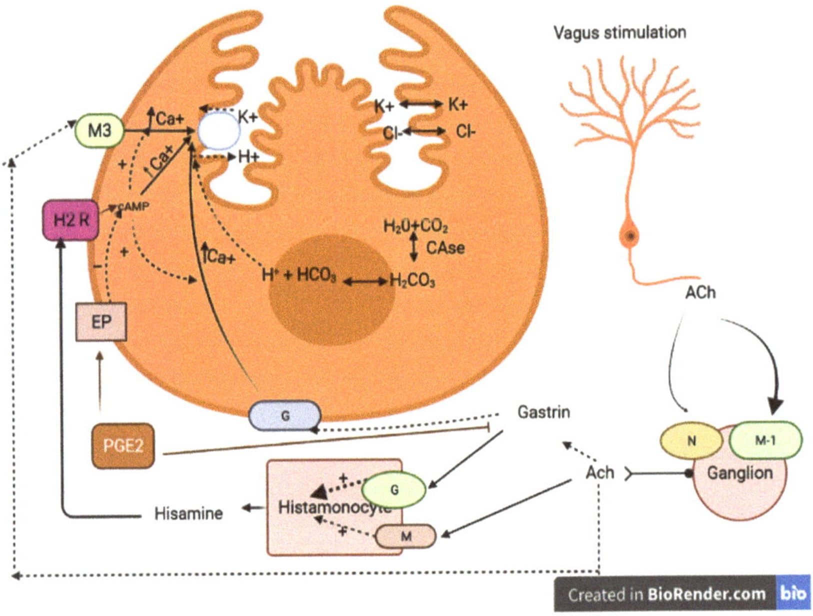

FIGURE 17.1 Physiology of acid secretion, M3/M1, Ach, G, H2, PGE2, HCO3. *Ach*, Acetylcholine; *G*, gastrin receptors protein; *H2*, histaminergic receptor type-2; *M3/M1*, muscarinic receptor types 3 and 1; *PGE2*, prostaglandin E2; *HCO3*, bicarbonate ions.

Peptic ulcer

One of the common diseases related to acid disturbance is peptic ulcer, which requires gastric acid for its formation. Peptic ulcer is divided into three main categories, including *Helicobacter pylori* (HP) associated, nonsteroidal antiinflammatory drugs (NSAIDs) induced, and ulcers induced by stress.[19] Almost every gastric ulcer results due to an imbalance between defensive and aggressive factors (pepsin and gastric acid) in the presence of HP, NSAIDs, and other causative agents (Table 17.2) associated with it.

TABLE 17.2 Comparison of common forms of peptic ulcer.

Characteristic	*H. pylori* induced	NSAID induced	SRMD
Condition	Chronic	Chronic	Acute
Site of damage	Duodenum > stomach	Stomach > duodenum	Stomach > duodenum
Intragastric pH	More dependent	Less dependent	Less dependent
Symptoms	Usually epigastric pain	Often asymptomatic	Asymptomatic
Ulcer depth	Superficial	Deep	Most superficial
GI bleeding	Less severe, single vessel	More severe, single vessel	More severe, superficial mucosal capillaries

H. pylori, Helicobacter pylori; NSAID, nonsteroidal antiinflammatory drug; *SRMD*, Stress related mucosal disease

Histamine released by muscarinic stimulation of gastrin may integrate and interact with the local secretory and circulatory in responses to hormones such as histamine, acetylcholine, and gastrin regulate H^+ secretion by the parietal cell (Table 17.2).

Potential causes of peptic ulcer

Common causes
Helicobacter pylori infection
Nonsteroidal antiinflammatory drugs
Critical illness (stress-related mucosal damage)
Uncommon causes
Hypersecretion of gastric acid (e.g., Zollinger–Ellison syndrome)
Viral infections (e.g., cytomegalovirus)
Vascular insufficiency (crack cocaine associated)
Radiation
Chemotherapy (e.g., hepatic artery infusions)
Rare genetic subtypes

The bacterium HP is a Gram-negative microaerophilic microorganism, which is involved in broad spectrum infections associated with digestive tract. It was first isolated by Warren and marshal in 1982.[20] The vaca gene and urease molecular complex are universally present as essential virulence factor in any HP strain. Gastric mucosa is damaged directly or indirectly by ammonia and bicarbonate, either produced by urease enzyme or by compounds produced in ammonia processing. Local inflammatory reactions result due to excessive production of urease enzymes.[21] NSAIDs are most commonly prescribed medicines that are dispensed over the counter in many countries also in India. Chronic administration of nonselective NSAIDs is widely linked with gastrointestinal injuries.[22–24] It has been found that two mechanisms are involved in progression of GIT mucus damage, that is, inhibition of systemic prostaglandin synthesis and direct damage to gastric epithelium. Acidic nature of different NSAIDs results in direct damage to gastric mucosa. Inhibition of cyclooxygenase enzyme (COX) is predominantly responsible for mucosal damage, as COX is key enzyme for the synthesis of protective endogenous molecule called prostaglandin[25] (Fig. 17.2).

Drugs used for neutralizing and inhibiting acid release

Antacids

These are alkaline compounds used to neutralize acid content in stomach. These drugs are being used for such conditions for more than 100 years.[26] Aluminum, magnesium, and calcium hydroxide, and also sodium bicarbonate, counteract acid in the stomach due to their alkaline nature, increase pH to neutral, reduce pepsin activity, and increase prostaglandin and bicarbonate secretion.

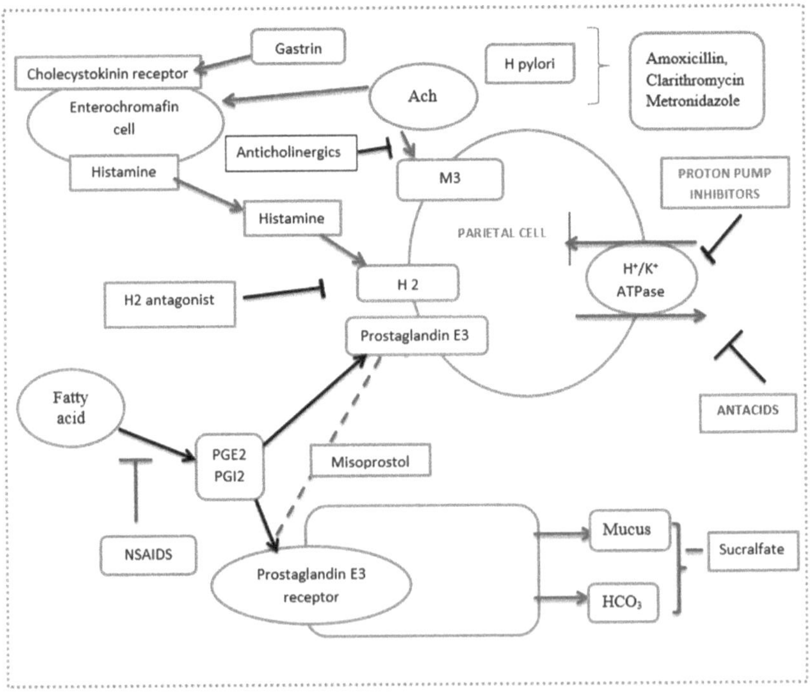

FIGURE 17.2 Sites of action of antisecretory drugs and other antiulcer agents. *H. pylori*, *Helicobacter pylori*; *H2*, histaminergic receptor type-2; *HCO3*, bicarbonate ions; *M3*, muscarinic receptor type 3; *PGE2*, prostaglandin E2, *NSAIDs*, nonsteroidal antiinflammatory drugs.

Classification

On the basis of digestive absorbance nature, it can be classified into the following:

- Absorbable
  - sodium carbonate
  - magnesium oxide
  - magnesium carbonate
  - calcium carbonate
- Nonabsorbable
  - aluminum phosphate
  - aluminum hydroxide
  - magnesium silicate
  - magnesium hydroxide
  - aluminum–magnesium combination

Due to various systemic side effects, absorbable antacids are rarely used for clinical practices. These are quick acting but have short duration of action (15–20 min), also these antacids may provoke rebound syndrome (secondary acid secretion).[26,27]

Nonabsorbable antacids have lesser side effects compared to absorbable antacids and these drugs have longer duration of action 2–3 h. The therapeutic mechanism of action is associated with hydrochloric acid absorption. Acid-neutralizing capacity is effective until pH reaches 3–4. Other beneficial effects include absorption of pepsin (reducing proteolytic activity), connecting lysolecithin and bile acid to protect gastric mucosa, stimulate prostaglandin synthesis that further stimulates mucin and bicarbonate secretion to improve microcirculation. Antacids are also capable to bind epithelial growth factor in ulcerous region and stimulate cell proliferation and angiogenesis.

Acid-neutralizing capacity expressed in mEq of hydrochloric acid, neutralized by standard dose of antacids to increase pH to 3.5 in approximately 15 min (predetermined).[28] Acid-neutralizing capacity is evaluation of antacid efficiency. Types of cation present in antacid determine pharmacodynamics of antacids.

Aluminum-containing antacids have more beneficial effects than other antacids[29,30] that include neutralizing, cytoprotective, and absorbing effects. But due to these effects, gastric motility also gets affected, and constipation results. Magnesium-containing antacids have laxative effect on gastric motility. A combination of aluminum and magnesium antacids has better therapeutics as aluminum hydroxide provides longer duration of action and magnesium hydroxide shows quick onset of action (Table 17.3).

Antacid side effects

1. On short-term administration, absorbable antacids produce (rebound syndrome) secondary hypersecretion.

TABLE 17.3 Comparison of antiulcer effects of different ion salts.

Action	Calcium	Magnesium	Aluminum
Neutralizing effect	+	++	+++
Cytoprotective effect	–	–	++
Absorbing effect	+	–	++

2. On long-term application, antacids produce milk acidity syndrome and hyperacidity.
3. Water salt metabolism is adversely affected by sodium bicarbonate.
4. Magnesium and sodium antacids produce urinary alkalization, which leads to settling of phosphate molecules in the form of phosphate stones.
5. Calcium-containing antacids produce hypercalcemia, which leads to kidney stone formation.
6. A combination milk and calcium antacid is not administered together as it promotes milk-alkali syndrome (vomiting, polyuria, and mental disordcr).
7. Nonabsorbable antacids have lesser side effects as compared to absorbable ones. These drugs show side effects only in long duration of uses. Aluminum antacids cause constipation and magnesium salts are responsible for laxative effects.

Contraindication

Aluminum antacids are not used in pregnancy; other contraindications are severe kidney failure and Alzheimer's disease.

Histamine receptor antagonist

Gastric parietal cells embedded in stomach epithelium are responsible for the release of hydrochloric acid, and histamine is important stimuli for this process that is secreted from neighboring enterochromaffin cells.[31] H_2-type histamine receptor is present on parietal cells. Pharmacological antagonist of H_2 receptor on GIT is used for different GIT diseases from acidity to peptic ulcers, erosions to gastroesophageal reflex disease (GERD).

These drugs are responsible for inhibition of acid production due to histamine, gastrin, and acetylcholine; also pepsin secretion is reduced. Nocturnal and basal acid secretion is affected mostly, which helps in peptic ulcer healing by these drugs.[32]

H_2 blocker drugs are well tolerated, used widely by prescription, and over the counter. The Binding site for H_2 blocker drugs is basolateral membrane of gastric parietal cells. Selectivity of histamine receptor is key importance, as selective H_2 blocker drugs do not bind to H_1 receptor which is blocked by antiallergic drugs.

S. no.	Antiulcer drug
1	Cimetidine
2	Ranitidine
3	Famotidine
4	Nizatidine

These drugs are safe for use; only some minor side effects are produced, including diarrhea, constipation, fatigue, and headache. These drugs are metabolized in liver by cytochrome P450 enzyme[33] (Table 17.1). **Therapeutic uses:** Treatment of conditions associated with excessive acid production including: 1. Dyspepsia or heart burn à using low dose formulation given 30 mins before meals (high acidic condition inactivates pepsin).2. Treatment of gastric & duodenal ulcer à Decrease acid secretion which ultimately decrease pain and allow complete healing of the ulcer; this require 6-8 weeks treatment with.3. Prophylaxis against stress induced peptic ulcer (1 tablet at bed time).4. Treatment of gastroesophageal reflux disease (GERD) & esophageal ulcer.5. Second choice drugs in treatment of hypersecretory conditions as Zollinger Ellison syndrome (gastrinoma) , as it requires high doses to control excess acid secretion. **Adverse effects:** Dizziness, headache, confusion, diarrhea & skin rashes. **2. Cimetidine binds to androgen receptors and cause antiandrogen effects** Male: gynecomastia, decreased sperm count, low testicular weight & reversible impotence in patients receiving high doses.Female: galactorrhea. Rantidine, famotidine & nizatidine à don't bind to androgen receptors **3. Liver toxicity:** cimetidine causes reversible cholestatic effects while ranitidine causes reversible hepatitis with or without jaundice. **4. CNS dysfunction** à delirium and confusion (most common in elderly patients receiving cimetidine). **5. Cimetidine can inhibit cytochrome P450** (mixed function oxidase) à inhibits the metabolism of co-administered drugs as phenytoin, warfarin & hypoglycemic drugs (drug-drug interaction). Ranitidine is weak inhibitor of cytochrome P450.

H^+/K^+ ATPase inhibitor/ Proton pump inhibitor (PPIs): Omeprazole, Lansoprazole, Rabeprazole, Pantoprazole, Esomeprazole Mechanism of Action

They are acid labile pro-drugs administered orally as enteric coated preparations, after absorption from the gut, the prodrug then distributed to the canaleculi of parietal cells where converted to the active metabolite (sulfoxide derivative) that binds to H^+,K^+ ATPase enzyme (proton pump) located at the luminal membrane of gastric parietal cells and inhibits the excretion of H^+. They are very potent anti-secretory agents at a single dose of 20 mg omeprazole can produce 95% inhibition of gastric acid secretion for 2 days (40mg can cause 100%

inhibition). **Therapeutic Uses:** 1. Drugs of first choice for Zollinger Ellison syndrome (gastrinoma). 2. Peptic ulcer disease (together with antibiotic to eliminate H. pylori which is the main cause of peptic ulcer). 3. Most effective in treating Gastroesophageal reflux disease. **Adverse effects:** 1. PPIs generally are well tolerated. Adverse drug reactions are rare: Headache, confusion & rarely skin rashes or affect liver causing liver damage. 2. Gastric tumors (gastrinoma) in rats not human, so not used for more than 1 month, as it reduces acid secretion which can contribute to Hypergastrinemia & gastric tumours. They can increase Bacterial growth in stomach which secrete nitroso compounds which are known for carcinogenicity. 3. Reduces secretion of intrinsic factor which contributes to decrease absorption of B_{12} that serve major reason to cause pernicious anemia.

Antimuscarinic drugs: Pirenzipene & Telenzepine. **Mechanism of Action:** These are selective M_1 antagonist which block M_1 receptors on enterochromaffin-like (ECL) cells and decrease histamine release ultimately stimulation of parietal H2 receptors does not take place and reduction of HCl secretion results finally. Less potent than H_2 inhibitors & has many side effects. These drugs are not in use now, because of the availability of safer and more efficacious drugs. **Adverse effects:** Blurred vision, photophobia, enhances Intraocular pressure (IOP), cycloplegia, declines sweating, urinary retention, constipation, dry mouth & difficulty in swallowing. Contraindicated in glaucoma or elder patients (urinary retention).

PG analogue: Misoprostol, Enprostil, Rioprostil Mechanism of Action: PGE2 and PGI2 are produced by gastric mucosal cells and considered to be cytoprotective by decreasing gastric acid secretion and enhancing the mucus and HCO_3^- secretion. Further Prostaglandins also inhibit Gastrin secretion and improve mucosal blood flow. PGE_1 analogue found to increase thickness of mucous layer, HCO_3 secretion and to decrease gastric HCl production (through stimulating PGs receptors in parietal cells which inhibit cAMP generation inracellularly and finally inhibit the proton pump, hence serve as the cytoprotective & antisecretory (dual mechanism). **Therapeutic Uses:** It is used for prophylaxis (prevention) against NSAIDs induced ulcers when used for long term as in rheumatoid arthritis. **Adverse effects:** 1. Nausea, vomiting, diarrhea, intestinal colic & may cause fever. 2. Have oxytocic effect can cause contraction of the uterus which lead to induction of abortion for pregnant female (abortifacient), so contraindicated in pregnancy (can be used safely for men),proton pump inhibitors are preferred over these. Antibiotics for *Helicobacter pylori* infection.

Antibiotics for Helicobacter pylori infection: Helicobacter pylorus is pathogenic bacteria present in acidic condition of GIT. HP infection produces different gastrointestinal disorders that include heartburn, gastritis, GERD, and duodenal ulcer and gastric cancers. More than 90% duodenal ulcer occurs due to HP infection.[34,35]

Most widely used method for bacterial eradication is antibiotic combination such as amoxicillin + clarithromycin or proton pump inhibitor and metronidazole.[36]

Antibiotic resistance is major cause of treatment failure. Low drug concentration, short gastric residence time, and poor drug penetration are the causes for antibiotic resistance.[37]

Standard treatment regimen for this infection is clarithromycin + proton pump inhibitor + amoxicillin and metronidazole for 7, 10, and 14 days. Different studies showed drug regimen that provides 80%–90% eradication rate always consists of PPIs, amoxicillin, and clarithromycin[38] (Tables 17.4 and 17.5).

Antiemetics and emetics

Vomiting

Unpleasant urge of vomit is called nausea and forceful expulsion of gastrointestinal content is called emesis (vomiting), when gastrointestinal content is forced into esophagus, without expulsion is termed retching[40,41]

Mechanism of evacuation

Bidirectional interaction (due to different stimuli), between gut and brain, leads to nausea and vomiting. Systemic emetic stimuli circulating in blood and cerebrospinal fluid act directly on central receptor sites in area postrema that lacks blood–brain barrier. A systemically administered drug activates receptors present on vagal afferents projecting sensory signals to solitary tract nucleus.[42,43] When toxic drugs and various microorganisms (virus, bacteria, fungi) enter, the gastrointestinal lumen leads to release of emetic modulators and local neurotransmitters that act on vagal afferent receptors and via circulating in blood the sesecretions stimulate brainstem area postrema.[44,45] Diseases associated with visceral organs (kidney, heart) produce sensation that reaches nucleus of solitary tract, through splanchnic nerve. Motion sickness and opioid analgesic-related signals reach vestibular apparatus or cerebellum, and these signals are further collected by brainstem vestibular nuclei. Emotional and cognitive stimuli are collected and processed by cerebral cortex and limbic system.[46–48] The dorsal motor nucleus is output pathway of nucleus solitary tract, which projects to upper GIT for emetic reflexes. For the nausea perceptions the mid and forebrain works as projections for solitary tract nucleus[49–52] (Fig. 17.3).

5-HT (serotonin) and substance P (SP) are fundamentals of gastric motility, nausea, and vomiting and these components are synthesized largely in gastric enterochromaffin cells (> 90% total body content).[53,54] Emetogenic stimuli (chemical, mechanical, and neurological) stimulate release of 5-HT and SP in calcium-dependent manner from gastrointestinal enterochromaffin cells.[55–58] These released constituents further activate their corresponding receptors to produce nausea and vomiting (Fig. 17.4).

TABLE 17.4 Current treatment regimen of *Helicobacter pylori* infection.[39]

S. no.	Standard regimen (7–14 d)	Sequent regimen (5 d)	Quadruple bismuth regimen (7, 10, 14 d)	Concomitant regimen (7–10 d)	Levofloxacin regimen (5–7 d)
1	PPI (standard dose bid) + amoxicillin (1 g bid) + clarithromycin (500 mg)	PPI (standard dose bid) + amoxicillin (1 g)		PPI (standard dose, bid) + clarithromycin (500 mg) + amoxicillin (1 g) + metronidazole (500 mg) + tinidazole (500 mg bid)	PPI (standard dose, bid) + levofloxacin (500 mg, bid) + either amoxicillin (1000 mg or tinidazole 500 mg, bid)
2	PPI (standard dose bid) + metronidazole (400 mg, bid) + clarithromycin (500 mg)	PPI (standard dose bid) + amoxicillin (1 g) followed by PPI + clarithromycin (500 mg) + metronidazole (500 mg)	PPI	PPI (standard dose, bid) + amoxicillin (750 mg, bid) + sitafloxacin (100 mg)	Esomeprazole (40 mg, bid) + amoxicillin (1000 mg, bid) + Levofloxacin (500 mg, bid)
3	PPI (standard dose bid) + amoxicillin (1 g bid) + metronidazole (400 mg)	PPI (standard dose bid) + amoxicillin (1 g) followed by PPI + clarithromycin (500 mg) + tinidazole (500 mg)			Esomeprazole (20 mg, bid) + amoxicillin (1 g, bid) + levofloxacin (250 mg, bid)

TABLE 17.5 Different classes of antiulcer drugs, mechanism of action, and adverse effects currently in use.

Pharmacological agents	Mechanism of action	Adverse effect
Antacids	Proteolytic inhibition of pepsin and increase in gastric pH	Nausea, vomiting, constipation
Histamine receptor blocker	Inhibition of H_2 receptor in parietal cells	Headache, anxiety, cardiovascular effects
Proton Pump inhibitor	H^+/K^+ATPase inhibition	Nausea, vomiting, constipation, flatulence
Cytoprotective agents	Increases mucus production and blood circulation	Nausea, vomiting, diarrhea, abdominal pain

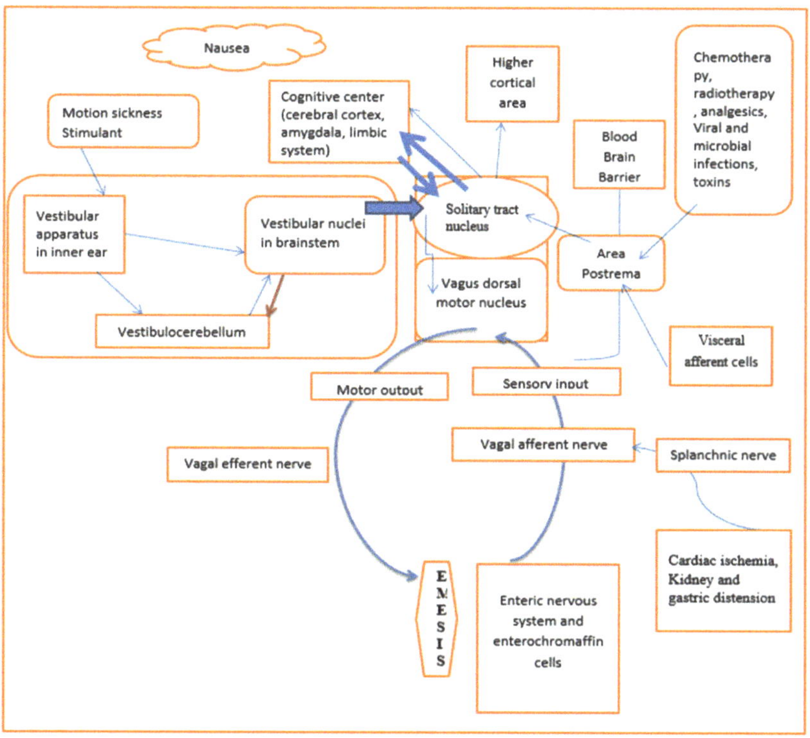

FIGURE 17.3 Pathways involved in nausea and vomiting.

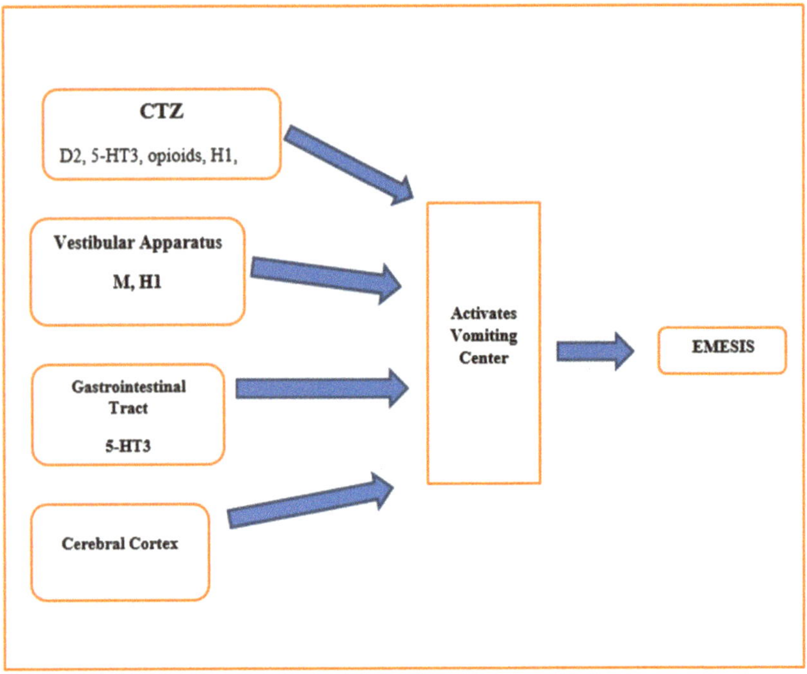

FIGURE 17.4 Pathways involved in nausea and vomiting.

Stimulants for vomiting

See Table 17.6.

Classification of antiemetics

See Table 17.7.

5-Hydroxytryptamine 3 receptor antagonist

Area postrema, vagal afferents, solitary tract nucleus are different sites where 5-HT3 receptors are found. 5-HT3 receptors are ligand-gated ion channels that cause fast depolarization via modulating the influx and outflux of Na^+/K^+ ions.[59] The others biological actions involving 5-HT3 receptors are gut peristalsis, decreased heart rate, decreased blood pressure (transient), apnea, pain, and itch.

Drugs that block 5-HT3 receptors include ondansetron, granisetron, palonosetron, dolasetron, and alosetron (Table 17.7).

Adverse effects: relatively safe antiemetic, the most common include headache, mild constipation and abdominal discomfort, rashes and mild allergies observed when injected IV

TABLE 17.6 Potential stimulants of nausea and vomiting.

S. no.	Stimulants for vomiting	Mechanism of stimulation
1	Drugs, bacteria, toxins, viruses	These agents enter the gastric lumen and indirectly activate emetic centers located in dorsal vagal complex (as local emetogenic neurotransmitters are released in upper gastrointestinal tract and further stimulation of vagus nerves receptors).
2	Infectious organism and drugs (which enters directly systemically)	Act directly on dorsal vagal complex emetic area in brainstem.
3	Pathological abnormalities in gastrointestinal tract	Stimulation of vagal afferents directly or via visceral organs (heart).
4	Emotional and cognitive	Stimuli within CNS.
5	Motion sickness	Disturbance in vestibular nuclei and cerebellum.

Uses: ondansetron blocks emetogenic impulses peripherally as well as at central relays. It has weak gastrokinetic activity because of 5-HT3 antagonism.

The first choice drugs for treatment of chemotherapy-induced vomiting, for other types of vomiting such as postoperative nausea and vomiting are now being treated with ondansetron.[60]

D_2 receptors antagonists/neuroleptics

- chlorpromazine
- prochlorperazine
- haloperidol
- domperidone

These drugs antagonize D_2 receptors in CTZ. These drugs show extended spectrum of antiemetic activity and found promising effects.[61]

1. drug induced and in the treatment nausea and vomiting after anesthesia
2. gastritis, migraine, liver diseases, and other disease-induced vomiting
3. chemotherapy and cancer-associated vomiting
4. treatment of radiation sickness
5. treatment of motion sickness: indicated only in hyperemesis gravidarum

Less effective in motion sickness because dopaminergic link is absent in vestibular pathway

Most of these drugs produce sedation and acute muscle dystonia especially in children and girls. Antiemetic dose is much lower than antipsychotic.

TABLE 17.7 Summarizing different classes of antiemetic drugs and their special uses.

S. no.	Class of drugs	Drugs	Uses
1	5-HT3 antagonist	Ondansetron Palonosetron	Chemotherapy-induced nausea, vomiting Postoperative nausea vomiting
2	D_2 antagonist	Phenothiazines Butyrophenone	Motion sickness, migraine, viral gastroenteritis, radiotherapy, chemotherapy, pregnancy-associated nausea and vomiting
3	H_1 antagonist	Promethazine Diphenhydramine	Increased Intracranial pressure, motion sickness, and pregnancy-induced nausea and vomiting
4	Anticholinergic	Hyoscine (scopolamine)	Used as prophylactic drug for motion sickness
5	Synthetic cannabinoids	Dronabinol Nabilone	Used in patients who failed to respond to other antiemetics in chemotherapy- and radiotherapy-induced nausea vomiting
6	corticosteroids	Dexamethasone	Hyperemesis associated with cancer chemotherapy and pregnancy
7	SP/NK1 antagonist	Aprepitant	Postoperative nausea vomiting and chemotherapy-induced nausea vomiting in combination with corticosteroids and serotonin antagonist

Prochlorperazine is a labyrinthine suppressant and has antivertigo and antivomiting effects. It is available for parenteral use in the treatment of vertigo associated with vomiting, primarily effective in vomiting rather than psychosis.

Adverse effects: sedation (chlorpromazine), extrapyramidal adverse effects because of D_2 receptors blockade (domperidone doesn't have these adverse effects because it does not cross blood–brain barrier).

Prokinetic drugs

- metoclopramide
- cisapride
- mosapride

Metoclopramide is the prototype drug of this class; it is highly effective against chemotherapy-induced emetogenic influences (especially cisplatin high dose–related emesis) and is found to prevent emesis in 30%–40% of patients and decrease emesis in majority.[62] The pharmacological actions are mediated through D_2 antagonism, 5HT-3 antagonism, and 5-HT4 agonism. Antagonism of D_2 and 5-HT3 receptors is responsible for antiemetic effects while 5-HT4 agonism causes prokinetic influences. Cisapride use is found to cause acute death because of severe cardiac adverse events.[63]

Metoclopramide is also used for the treatment of concurrent hiccups, GERD, and heartburn because of its prokinetic activities and its influences on lower esophagus sphincter tone.[64]

The adverse effects associated with metoclopramide use are extrapyramidal adverse events, sedation, and diarrhea which limit its use.

Antihistamines and anticholinergic

Antihistamines

- diphenhydramine
- dimenhydrinate
- cyclizine
- meclizine (with B_6)
- promethazine

Anticholinergics

- dicyclomine
- hyoscine

Mechanism of action

Antihistamines and anticholinergic are believed to be most efficacious in the treatment of motion sickness because of the involvement of histaminergic (H_1) and muscarinic (M_1) receptors between vestibular nerve and vomiting center.[65]

Uses: treatment of motion sickness and morning sickness. Treatment of vertigo, nausea and vomiting associated with Meniere's disease (distension of membrane of labyrinth of inner ear from excess fluids due to inflammation of the inner ear and dilated endolymph sac). Prophylactic against motion sickness (0.5-mg orally before traveling or 1.5-mg transdermal patches behind the pinna to give prolonged effect for 3 days).

Adverse effects: atropine-like side effects → blurred vision, urinary retention, constipation, sunstroke, and dryness of mouth; sedation (atropine causes central nervous system (CNS) stimulation).

Cannabinoids

tetrahydrocannabinol (THC)
dronabinol
nabilone

The exact mechanism of action is still under debate but the current proposed mechanisms suggested as cannabinoids interact with the central CB1 and 5-HT3 receptors in the dorsal vagal complex, which are well established mediator of emesis, in the area postrema. Researchers have studied and confirmed that the endogenous cannabinoid, THC, inhibits 5-HT3 receptors action. Preclinical research finding concludes that cannabinoids agonize CB1-mediated action and diminish serotonin release, and prevent nausea/emesis.[66] The mechanism for the 5-HT3 inhibition suggested that CBN-1 receptors activate 5-HT1A receptor that are inhibitory in nature and decline serotonin release, which is responsible for lower prospective to elicit emesis. Gastrointestinal CB1 receptors via activation of inhibitory G protein coupled to receptors decrease the motility also.[67]

Uses: treatment of cancer chemotherapy-induced emesis → by blocking 5-HT3 receptors in the vomiting center in medulla but less effective than ondansetron and metoclopramide.

Mild appetite stimulant → in AIDs or cancer patients to treat anorexia (by blocking 5-HT receptors in satiety centers leading to increase the appetite).

Adverse drug rections (ADRs): hallucination, confusion, and CNS depression.

Glucocorticoids

- dexamethasone
- prednisolone
- methylprednisolone

The glucocorticoids are now used as adjuvant to manage the chemotherapy-induced nausea and vomiting.[68]

The antiemetic mechanisms of glucocorticoids are suggested as:

1. They are potent antiinflammatory as they can block the generation of inflammatory mediators; cytotoxic drugs and radiation therapy are well established to cause inflammatory mediator generations that can contribute to the emesis.
2. Findings of the research demonstrated that glucocorticoids decline the serotonin expressions in rat brain.
3. Glucocorticoids are found to have antiadrenergic activities and the research studies conclude adrenergic involvement in the emesis.

Uses: insomnia and can worsen the situation of diabetes.

Vitamin B6

It acts as cofactor in the decarboxylation of glutamic acid to form gamma amino butyric acid (GABA) that is an inhibitory transmitter in the brain causing inhibition of vomiting center.[69]

Vitamin B6 is not used alone as it has weak effect.

Emetics

Emetics are used to treat toxicity within short period of intoxication.

Ipecacuanha

Ipecac sirup contains emetine and cephaline.

Mechanism of action

Ipecacuanha centrally activates chemoreceptor triggor zone (CTZ) and peripherally, causes irritation of gastric mucosa, stimulates afferent vagus nerve, and induces vomiting and treatment of poisoning.

(Child dose: 5–15 m—adult dose: 15–30 mL)→if no vomiting, repeat the dose→if no vomiting, make gastric lavage to remove ipecac as it is toxic.

Extract is 14 times more concentrated than sirup→so toxic.

Apomorphine

Mechanism of action

Apomorphine centrally stimulates D_2 receptors at CTZ and vomiting. It has weak depressant effect on respiratory centers→should be avoided in toxicity with morphine and opioids.[70]

Contraindications

- The emetics should be avoided in case ingestion of acid or alkali→corrosion of stomach or esophagus (use milk or egg white)
- In case of unconsciousness.
- In case of convulsions (such as toxicity due to colchicine and strychnine).
- In case of gas and petroleum distillate.
- In case of esophageal varices→bleeding

Laxatives, purgatives, and cathartics

Laxatives→ ↑motility→facilitate defecation→treat constipation.

Purgatives (cause diarrhea)→evacuation of bowel before surgery or X-ray examination and treatment of poisoning (Hg poisoning) and with some antiparasitic drugs (to expel the worms or larvae to prevent reinfection).[71]

Cathartic (large-dose purgative)→severe diarrhea→dehydration and shock.

Classification (laxatives, purgatives, and cathartics)

See Table 17.8.

Antidiarrheal agents

Diarrhea is a condition of frequent watery feces, which is commonly escorted by abdominal cramps and with nausea and vomiting sometimes. Mostly, it is a physiological response for rapid ridding the gut of poisonous or irritating substances. Many causes suggested infection, toxins, and even anxiety. Side effects of drug or radiation therapy have also been suggested as etiological factors for this disease. Manifestations include from mild discomfort to a medical emergency which require hospitalization and parenteral water and electrolyte replacement. Globally, acute diarrheal disease is one of the principal causes of death in malnourished infants, especially in developing countries where medical care is compromised.[72]

During diarrhea, increase gastrointestinal motility is accompanied by an increased secretion coupled with a decreased absorption of fluid, which leads to a loss of electrolytes (particularly Na +) and water. Cholera toxins and some other bacterial toxins produce a profound increase in electrolyte and fluid secretion by irreversibly activating the guanine nucleotide regulatory proteins that couple the surface receptors of the mucosal cells to adenylate cyclase.

There are three approaches generally employed for the treatment of severe/acute diarrhea:

- maintenance of fluid and electrolyte balance
- use of antiinfective agents
- use of spasmolytic or other antidiarrheal agents

Oral rehydration supplements

The maintenance of fluid and electrolyte balance by means of oral rehydration is the first priority, and wider application of this cheap and simple remedy could save the lives of many infants in the developing world. Many patients require no other treatment. In the ileum, as in parts of the nephron, there is cotransport of Na^+ and glucose across the epithelial cell. The presence of glucose (and some amino acids) therefore enhances Na^+ absorption and thus water uptake. Preparations of sodium chloride and glucose for oral rehydration are available in powder form, ready to be dissolved in water before use.[73]

Other types of antidiarrheal drug that mitigate the symptoms of the condition include:

- spasmolytic or antimotility agents,
- adsorbents, and
- agents that modify fluid and electrolyte transport (Table 17.9).

TABLE 17.8 Different classes of anticonstipating drugs their uses and adverse effects.

S. no.	Drug classes	Examples	Mechanism of actions	Uses	Adverse effects
1	**Bulk-forming agents**	Psyllium seeds, Nigella sativa, methylcellulose, carboxymethylcellulose, and agar-agar Dietary fibers → bran and other vegetable fibers	Nondigestible fibers → induce water retention in intestinal lumen → ↑mass or bulk of intestinal materials → distension of intestinal wall → stimulate peristaltic activity of GIT → facilitate defecation	laxative and protect against colon cancer	Gases in colon
2	**Osmotic laxatives or purgatives**				
2a.	**Saline osmotic laxative**	1. $MgSO_4$ (Epsom's salt) → 10–15 mg in 300-mL water 2. MgO (milk of magnesia) → 7%–10%	Only 1% absorbed and 99% remain in intestine → hypertonic solution → attract and retain water in the intestinal lumen by osmosis (*acting by physical mechanism*) → ↑ intraluminal pressure → ↑peristaltic motility → copious watery diarrhea → evacuation of GIT	Evacuate the bowel before surgery/radiology used after treatment of parasites, e.g., *Taenia solium*	Not suitable in renal failure

(*Continued*)

TABLE 17.8 (Continued)

S. no.	Drug classes	Examples	Mechanism of actions	Uses	Adverse effects
2b.	**Lactulose**	Nondigestible synthetic disaccharide→formed of fructose–galactose Taken in high dose 10 g	It is not digested and not absorbed→reach colon→bacteria cause hydrolysis of lactulose→lactic acid + acetic + other acids→retain water by osmosis→bulk→stimulate peristaltic movement→laxative effect	1. Laxative to treat constipation→effect appear after 2 days 2. In prophylaxis and treatment of **hepatic coma** (in case of liver cirrhosis or alcohol or bilhariziasis): a. Lactic and acetic acids formed react with NH_3 in colon and neutralize it to salt→prevent absorption of NH3 from colon. b. To treat constipation→prevent hydrolysis of protein in feces by bacteria. Used orally or by enema (usually with neomycin tablets to kill normal bacterial flora→↓ formation of ammonia)	
2c.	**Sorbitol 40%**	**Polyalcohol and used in high concentration**	Sweet taste→not absorbed→hyperosmosis→bulk→↑ motility→diarrhea	Used in the treatment of toxicity with activated charcoal→sweet taste make charcoal more acceptable and it is not adsorbed on charcoal &facilitates excretion of charcoal after absorbing the toxins.	Less toxic than saline cathartics

3	**Stimulant laxatives and purgatives**				
		Castor oil	Hydrolyzed by pancreatic lipase in the intestine→ricinoleic acid (irritant fatty acid)→irritation of intestinal mucosa and stimulate **myenteric plexus** in GI mucosa→release 5-HT and substance P→↑motility→severe diarrhea→complete evacuation of GIT Taken 15–30 mL orally late at evening→diarrhea after 4–5 h in the morning→action continues till complete evacuation of GIT	Before surgery or radiological examination of the abdomen as purgative.	1. Cramps, colic and dehydration and abortion in pregnant women (contraindication) 2. Not used in toxicity→as it may help in absorption of lipid-soluble toxic material.
		Anthraquinone glycosides: senna, cascara, rhubarb, and aloes	1. Glycosides (**sennosides A and B**) hydrolyzed at colon by bacterial flora→free aglicone rhein anthrone→stimulate **myenteric plexus**→↑motility→defecation 2. Also, ↑ PGE_2 synthesis in intestine→↑ contraction and motility In small dose→laxative/higher dose→purgative/toxic dose→cathartic		Allergic reactions→skin rashes. Cramps (colic). In large doses→excessive purgation→may cause dehydration &shock. Excreted in milk→diarrhea in breast-fed infants. Chronic use→damage myenteric plexus→colonic atony **(cathartic colon = laxative abuse)** Coloration of urine depending on the pH of the patient's urine (alkaline→reddish> acidic→yellow).
		Bisacodyl	Not absorbed orally →but cause irritant effect on intestinal mucosa Available as: Enteric-coated tablets (to prevent irritation of stomach→vomiting) (not with antacids→dissolve enteric coating) Suppositories	Used in the treatment of constipation and before radiological examination	
		Glycerol	Mild irritant	Used as rectal suppository	

(*Continued*)

TABLE 17.8 (Continued)

S. no.	Drug classes	Examples	Mechanism of actions	Uses	Adverse effects
4	**Surfactant laxatives: (stool softeners)**				
		Docusate (dioctyl sodium sulfosuccinate)	An anionic surfactant → stimulates the incorporation of water into fatty intestinal material → emulsification of fat → softens the feces	Used in the treatment of hemorrhoids and anal fissures	Hepatotoxicity, abdominal cramps, increased absorption of some drugs
5	**Tegaserod**		5-HT_4 agonist used orally before meals as its bioavailability is low enhanced motility	Used (2- to 6-mg tab) in the treatment of chronic constipation.	Headache, diarrhea in high dose.
6	**Lubricant laxatives**	**Paraffin oil**	It is an inert hydrocarbon, neither digested nor absorbed, used as lubricant	1. To avoid straining during defecation → in hemorrhoids &painful anal fissures. 2. As laxative during pregnancy (may also use bulk-forming agent—but not stimulant laxatives)	1. Dissolve fat-soluble vitamins (A,D,E,K) → inhibit their absorption → deficiency. 2. If aspirated to lungs → **lipid pneumonia**. 3. Leak from anal sphincter → staining of clothes 4. Slightly absorbed if given with docusate → deposited in myenteric lymph nodes → granulomas 5. **(Paraffinomas)** → inflammatory reaction resulting in tumor formation.

Bold means defining the new class and drugs.

TABLE 17.9 Different classes of antidiarrheal agents, mechanism of action, and uses.

S. no.	Drug class	Examples of the drugs	Mechanism of action	Adverse effect
1	Antimotility drugs	Diphenoxylate and loperamide	These drugs activate presynaptic opioid receptors in the enteric nervous system to inhibit acetylcholine release and decrease peristalsis.	Drowsiness, dizziness, abdominal cramps, because these drugs can contribute to toxic megacolon, should not be used in young children or in patients with severe colitis.
2	Adsorbents	Aluminum hydroxide and methylcellulose They are much less effective than antimotility agents	Act by adsorbing intestinal toxins or microorganisms and/or by coating or protecting the intestinal mucosa.	They can interfere with the absorption of other drugs.
3	Agents that modify fluid and electrolyte transport	Bismuth subsalicylate	Its action may be due to its salicylate component as well as its coating action. Used for travelers' diarrhea	Black tongue and black stools.

References

1. Bellstedt DU. The building blocks and origins of life. *HTS Theological Stud*. 2020;76 (1):1–7.
2. Li C, Yu W, Wu P, Chen XD. Current in vitro digestion systems for understanding food digestion in human upper gastrointestinal tract. *Trends Food Sci Technol*. 2020;96:114–126.
3. Dumic I, Nordin T, Jecmenica M, Lalosevic MS, Milosavljevic T, Milovanovic T. Gastrointestinal tract disorders in older age. *Can J Gastroenterol Hepatol*. 2019;2019.
4. Cogan T, Cogan M, Tamil L. MAPGI: accurate identification of anatomical landmarks and diseased tissue in gastrointestinal tract using deep learning. *Comput Biol Med*. 2019;111:103351.
5. Cussotto S, Sandhu KV, Dinan TG, Cryan JF. The neuroendocrinology of the microbiota-gut-brain axis: a behavioural perspective. *Front Neuroendocrinol*. 2018;51:80–101.

6. Davis KL, Montag C. Selected principles of pankseppian affective neuroscience. *Front Neurosci*. 2019;12:1025.
7. Bonaz B, Sinniger V, Pellissier S. The vagus nerve in the neuro-immune axis: implications in the pathology of the gastrointestinal tract. *Front Immunol*. 2017;8:1452.
8. Gunawardene AR, Corfe BM, Staton CA. Classification and functions of enteroendocrine cells of the lower gastrointestinal tract. *Int J Exp Pathol*. 2011;92(4):219–231.
9. Sachs G, Prinz C, Loo D, Bamberg K, Besancon M, Shin JM. Gastric acid secretion: activation and inhibition. *Yale J Biol Med*. 1994;67(3–4):81.
10. Schubert ML. Regulation of gastric secretion. *Curr Opin Gastroenterol*. 1997;13 (6):441–450.
11. Thomas A. Gastrointestinal secretions and vomiting. *Anaesth Intensive Care Med*. 2006;7 (2):54–56.
12. Repetto MG, Llesuy SF. Antioxidant properties of natural compounds used in popular medicine for gastric ulcers. *Braz J Med Biol Res*. 2002;35:523–534.
13. Engevik AC, Kaji I, Goldenring JR. The physiology of the gastric parietal cell. *Physiol Rev*. 2020;100(2):573–602.
14. Wilson RL, Stevenson CE. *Anatomy and physiology of the stomach. Shackelford's Surgery of the Alimentary Tract*. Elsevier; 2019:634–646. 2 Volume Set.
15. Arin RM, Gorostidi A, Navarro-Imaz H, Rueda Y, Fresnedo O, Ochoa B. Adenosine: direct and indirect actions on gastric acid secretion. *Front Physiol*. 2017;8:737.
16. Walsh JH. Role of gastrin as a trophic hormone. *Digestion*. 1990;47(suppl 1):11–16.
17. Singh R. *Digestive System*. 2008.
18. Haas HL, Sergeeva OA, Selbach O. Histamine in the nervous system. *Physiol Rev*. 2008;.
19. Iijima K, Kanno T, Koike T, Shimosegawa T. *Helicobacter pylori*-negative, non-steroidal anti-inflammatory drug: negative idiopathic ulcers in Asia. *World J Gastroenterol*. 2014;20 (3):706.
20. Marshall BJ, McGechie DB, Rogers PA, Clancy RJ. Pyloric campylobacter infection and gastroduodenal disease. *Med J Aust*. 1985;142(8):439–444.
21. Stingl K, Uhlemann E-M, Schmid R, Altendorf K, Bakker EP. Energetics of *Helicobacter pylori* and its implications for the mechanism of urease-dependent acid tolerance at pH 1. *J Bacteriol*. 2002;184(11):3053–3060.
22. Laine L. Approaches to nonsteroidal anti-inflammatory drug use in the high-risk patient. *Gastroenterology*. 2001;120(3):594–606.
23. Hawkey CJ. Nonsteroidal anti-inflammatory drug gastropathy. *Gastroenterology*. 2000;119 (2):521–535.
24. Wolfe MM, Lichtenstein DR, Singh G. Gastrointestinal toxicity of nonsteroidal antiinflammatory drugs. *N Engl J Med*. 1999;340(24):1888–1899.
25. Kumar A, Ashwlayan V, Verma M. Diagnostic approach & pharmacological treatment regimen of peptic ulcer disease. *Pharm Pharm Res Open Acc J*. 2019;1:1–12.
26. Belousov YB, Moiseev VS, Lepakhin VK. *Clinical Pharmacology and Pharmacotherapy*. Medical News Agency; 2010:884 p.
27. Uenishi K, Fujita T, Ishida H, et al. Fractional absorption of active absorbable algal calcium (AAACa) and calcium carbonate measured by a dual stable-isotope method. *Nutrients*. 2010;2(7):752–761.
28. Ayensu I, Bekoe SO, Adu JK, Brobbey AA, Appiah E. Evaluation of acid neutralizing and buffering capacities of selected antacids in Ghana. *Sci Afr*. 2020;8:e00347.
29. Kirpalani H, Huang LH. *Manual of Pediatric Intensive Care*. PMPH-USA; 2009.

30. Zhang Y-F, Dai X-J, Wang T, et al. Effects of an Al^{3+}-and Mg^{2+}-containing antacid, ferrous sulfate, and calcium carbonate on the absorption of nemonoxacin (TG-873870) in healthy Chinese volunteers. *Acta Pharmacol Sin*. 2014;35(12):1586–1592.
31. Hersey SJ, Sachs G. Gastric acid secretion. *Physiol Rev*. 1995;75(1):155–189.
32. Wolfe MM, Sachs G. Acid suppression: optimizing therapy for gastroduodenal ulcer healing, gastroesophageal reflux disease, and stress-related erosive syndrome. *Gastroenterology*. 2000;118(2):S9–S31.
33. LiverTox N. *Clinical and Research Information on Drug-Induced Liver Injury*. Bethesda, MD: National Institute of Diabetes and Digestive and Kidney Diseases; 2012.
34. Rana R, Wang SL, Li J, Wang YX, Rao QW, Yang CQ. *Helicobacter pylori* infection: a recent approach to diagnosis and management. *J Biomed*. 2017;2(1):45–56.
35. Zhao S, Lv Y, Zhang J-B, Wang B, Lv G-J, Ma X-J. Gastroretentive drug delivery systems for the treatment of *Helicobacter pylori*. *World J Gastroenterol*. 2014;20(28):9321.
36. Safavi M, Sabourian R, Foroumadi A. Treatment of *Helicobacter pylori* infection: current and future insights. *World J Clin Cases*. 2016;4(1):5.
37. Paul B, Adimoolam S, Quereshi MJ, Eva JJ. Current status of *H. pylori* infection treatment 2017. *J Appl Pharm Sci*. 2017;7(10):190–195.
38. Papastergiou V, Georgopoulos SD, Karatapanis S. Treatment of *Helicobacter pylori* infection: past, present and future. *World J Gastrointest Pathophysiol*. 2014;5(4):392.
39. Kuna L, Jakab J, Smolic R, Raguz-Lucic N, Vcev A, Smolic M. Peptic ulcer disease: a brief review of conventional therapy and herbal treatment options. *J Clin Med*. 2019;8(2):179.
40. Zhong W, Shahbaz O, Teskey G, et al. Mechanisms of nausea and vomiting: current knowledge and recent advances in intracellular emetic signaling systems. *Int J Mol Sci*. 2021;22(11):5797.
41. Singh P, Kuo B. Central aspects of nausea and vomiting in GI disorders. *Curr Treat Options Gastroenterol*. 2016;14(4):444–451.
42. Wickham RJ. Revisiting the physiology of nausea and vomiting—challenging the paradigm. *Supportive Care Cancer*. 2020;28(1):13–21.
43. Navari RM. Olanzapine for the prevention and treatment of chronic nausea and chemotherapy-induced nausea and vomiting. *Eur J Pharmacol*. 2014;722:180–186.
44. Bashashati M, McCallum RW. Neurochemical mechanisms and pharmacologic strategies in managing nausea and vomiting related to cyclic vomiting syndrome and other gastrointestinal disorders. *Eur J Pharmacol*. 2014;722:79–94.
45. McKenzie E, Chan D, Parsafar S, et al. Evolution of antiemetic studies for radiation-induced nausea and vomiting within an outpatient palliative radiotherapy clinic. *Supportive Care Cancer*. 2019;27(9):3245–3252.
46. Porreca F, Ossipov MH. Nausea and vomiting side effects with opioid analgesics during treatment of chronic pain: mechanisms, implications, and management options. *Pain Med*. 2009;10(4):654–662.
47. Smith HS, Laufer A. Opioid induced nausea and vomiting. *Eur J Pharmacol*. 2014;722:67–78.
48. Horn CC, Wallisch WJ, Homanics GE, Williams JP. Pathophysiological and neurochemical mechanisms of postoperative nausea and vomiting. *Eur J Pharmacol*. 2014;722:55–66.
49. Wood JD, Alpers DH, Andrews PLR. Fundamentals of neurogastroenterology. *Gut*. 1999;45(suppl 2):II6–II16.
50. Barmack NH. Central vestibular system: vestibular nuclei and posterior cerebellum. *Brain Res Bull*. 2003;60(5–6):511–541.

51. Gagliuso AH, Chapman EK, Martinelli GP, Holstein GR. Vestibular neurons with direct projections to the solitary nucleus in the rat. *J Neurophysiol*. 2019;122(2):512–524.
52. Cai Y-L, Ma W-L, Li M, et al. Glutamatergic vestibular neurons express Fos after vestibular stimulation and project to the NTS and the PBN in rats. *Neurosci Lett*. 2007;417(2):132–137.
53. Diwakarla S, Fothergill LJ, Fakhry J, Callaghan B, Furness JB. Heterogeneity of enterochromaffin cells within the gastrointestinal tract. *Neurogastroenterol Motil*. 2017;29(6):e13101.
54. Obara Y, Machida T, Takano Y, et al. Cisplatin increases the number of enterochromaffin cells containing substance P in rat intestine. *Naunyn Schmiedebergs Arch Pharmacol*. 2018;391(8):847–858.
55. Chappa AK, Audus KL, Lunte SM. Characteristics of substance P transport across the blood–brain barrier. *Pharm Res*. 2006;23(6):1201–1208.
56. Freed AL, Audus KL, Lunte SM. Investigation of substance P transport across the blood-brain barrier. *Peptides*. 2002;23(1):157–165.
57. Babic T, Browning KN. The role of vagal neurocircuits in the regulation of nausea and vomiting. *Eur J Pharmacol*. 2014;722:38–47.
58. Alcaino C, Knutson KR, Treichel AJ, et al. A population of gut epithelial enterochromaffin cells is mechanosensitive and requires Piezo2 to convert force into serotonin release. *Proc Natl Acad Sci USA*. 2018;115(32):E7632–E7641.
59. Mastitskaya S, Turovsky E, Marina N, et al. Astrocytes modulate baroreflex sensitivity at the level of the nucleus of the solitary tract. *J Neurosci*. 2020;40(15):3052–3062.
60. Gan TJ, Belani KG, Bergese S, et al. Fourth consensus guidelines for the management of postoperative nausea and vomiting. *Anesth Analg*. 2019;131(2):411–448.
61. Sanger GJ, Andrews PLR. A history of drug discovery for treatment of nausea and vomiting and the implications for future research. *Front Pharmacol*. 2018;9:913.
62. Levitt M. *Cannabinoids as antiemetics in cancer chemotherapy. Cannabinoids Therapeutic Agents*. Chapman and Hall/CRC; 2019:71–84.
63. Uribe AA, Bergese SD. What is the ideal combination antiemetic regimen? *Best Pract Res Clin Anaesthesiol*. 2020;.
64. Kuriakose TM, Raj RA. *A Review on Multiple Sclerosis and Persistent Hiccups Management*, n.d.
65. Greenlee H, Darwin L. Postoperative nausea and vomiting. *Anaesth Intensive Care Med*. 2021;.
66. Fakhfouri G, Rahimian R, Dyhrfjeld-Johnsen J, Zirak MR, Beaulieu J-M. 5-HT3 receptor antagonists in neurologic and neuropsychiatric disorders: the iceberg still lies beneath the surface. *Pharmacol Rev*. 2019;71(3):383–412.
67. Darmani NA, Belkacemi L, Zhong W. Δ9-THC and related cannabinoids suppress substance P-induced neurokinin NK1-receptor-mediated vomiting via activation of cannabinoid CB1 receptor. *Eur J Pharmacol*. 2019;865:172806.
68. Qiu T, Men P, Xu X, Zhai S, Cui X. Antiemetic regimen with aprepitant in the prevention of chemotherapy-induced nausea and vomiting: an updated systematic review and *meta*-analysis. *Medicine*. 2020;99(33).
69. Muñiz-Castrillo S, Vogrig A, Joubert B, et al. Transient neurological symptoms preceding cerebellar ataxia with glutamic acid decarboxylase antibodies. *Cerebellum*. 2020;19(5):715–721.
70. Auffret M, Drapier S, Vérin M. The many faces of apomorphine: lessons from the past and challenges for the future. *Drugs R&D*. 2018;18(2):91–107.

71. Malik AA, ul Bari S. *Human Abdominal Hydatidosis*. Springer; 2019.
72. Schiller LR. Evaluation of chronic diarrhea and irritable bowel syndrome with diarrhea in adults in the era of precision medicine. *J Am Coll Gastroenterol*. 2018;113(5):660–669.
73. Sollanek KJ, Kenefick RW, Cheuvront SN. Osmolality of commercially available oral rehydration solutions: impact of brand, storage time, and temperature. *Nutrients*. 2019;11 (7):1485.

Chapter 18

Mechanisms of action of antibacterial agents (AMA)

Raja Chakraverty[1], Kalyan Samanta[1], Pallab Mandal[2], Samit Karmakar[3] and Sanmoy Karmakar[2]
[1]ICMR Research Scholar, Department of Pharmacology, IPGME&R-SSKM Hospital, Kolkata, West Bengal, India, [2]Bioeuivalence Study Centre, Department of Pharmaceutical Technology, Jadavpur University, Kolkata, West Bengal, India, [3]Medical College Kolkata, Kolkata, West Bengal, India

Introduction

An important aspect for any antimicrobial drug is its inherent selectivity, owing to which the drugs inhibit the growth of the pathogenic microbe preferentially or selectively is used in the pharmacotherapy of a broad spectrum of infectious diseases.[1–6] Both in terms of the spectrum of activity, the antimicrobial drugs and its selectivity are important grading considerations in the therapeutic modality of antimicrobial therapy.

A list of classification of β-lactams is given next.

Classification of β-lactams

1. Acid-resistant penicillin: penicillin V (semisynthetic)
2. Penicillinase- or β-lactamase resistant (antistaphylococcal): methicillin, oxacillin, and cloxacillin
3. Extended spectrum
    a. aminopenicillins (also active against *Haemophilus influenzae* Pneumococci): ampicillin and amoxicillin
    b. carboxypenicillin (Pseudomonas and Proteus or antipseudomonal): carbenicillin and ticarcillin
    c. ureidopenicillin (Pseudomonas and Klebsiella): piperacillin and mezlocillin
4. β-lactamase inhibitors: clavulanic acid and sulbactam
5. Miscellaneous β-lactam antibiotics:

How Synthetic Drugs Work. DOI: https://doi.org/10.1016/B978-0-323-99855-0.00018-X

a. carbapenem drugs: imipenem
b. monobactam: aztreonam

Cell wall biosynthesis inhibitors[7–9]

These groups of drugs are also known as β-lactams or penicillins that have been synthesized as a by-product of *Penicillium chrysogenum* and as also from *Penicillium notatum*. Benzylpenicillin (PnG) was first discovered followed by phenoxymethylpenicillin (PnV).

After the drug gets attached to the various specific penicillin-binding proteins in the cell wall, they proceed to cleave the transpeptidase as well as carboxypeptidase enzymes, thereby inhibiting the formation transpeptidation process and cross-linking.

The diagrammatic representation of the mechanism of β-lactam antibiotics with their mechanism is discussed.

Carbapenems

The treatment modality of enterobacteria infection involves the use of carbapenems, because it is resistant to destruction by the β-lactamase produced by these organisms. Imipenem, an example of a carbapenem, acts in the same way as the other β-lactams. It has a very broad spectrum of antimicrobial activity, being active against many aerobic and anaerobic Gram-positive and Gram-negative organisms.

Unwanted effects are, in general, similar to those of other β-lactam antibiotics, but this agent does not necessarily cross-react immunologically with penicillin and its products, and so it does not usually cause allergic reactions in penicillin-sensitive individuals.

Cephalosporins

Cephalosporin C was originally extracted from the fungus *Cephalosporium acremonium* in the 1950s and has a similar spectrum of activity to that of penicillin against Gram-positive bacteria but is active against more Gram-negative bacteria than penicillin.[10–12] Another important structural difference is that cephalosporin C possesses two R groups, compared with just one R group for penicillin, and this provides for greater diversity in chemical alterations and the development of semisynthetic cephalosporins.

Protein synthesis inhibitors that bind the 30S subunit

Aminoglycosides are large, highly polar antibacterial drugs that bind to the 30S subunit of bacterial ribosomes, impairing the proofreading ability of the ribosomal complex.[13–19] This impairment causes mismatches between codons and anticodons, resulting in the production of proteins with incorrect amino acids and shortened proteins that insert into the cytoplasmic membrane. The disruption of the cytoplasmic membrane by the faulty proteins kills the bacterial cells.

Protein synthesis inhibitors that bind the 50S and 30S ribosomal subunits

There are several classes of antibacterial drugs that work through binding to the 50S subunit of bacterial ribosomes.[20–26] The macrolide antibacterial drugs have a large, complex ring structure and are part of a larger class of naturally produced secondary metabolites called polyketides (Fig. 18.1).

Complex compounds are produced in a stepwise fashion through the repeated addition of two-carbon units by a mechanism similar to that used for fatty acid synthesis. Macrolides are broad-spectrum, bacteriostatic drugs that block the elongation of proteins by inhibiting peptide-bond formation between specific combinations of amino acids. The first macrolide was erythromycin. The lincosamides include the naturally produced lincomycin and semisynthetic clindamycin. Although structurally distinct from

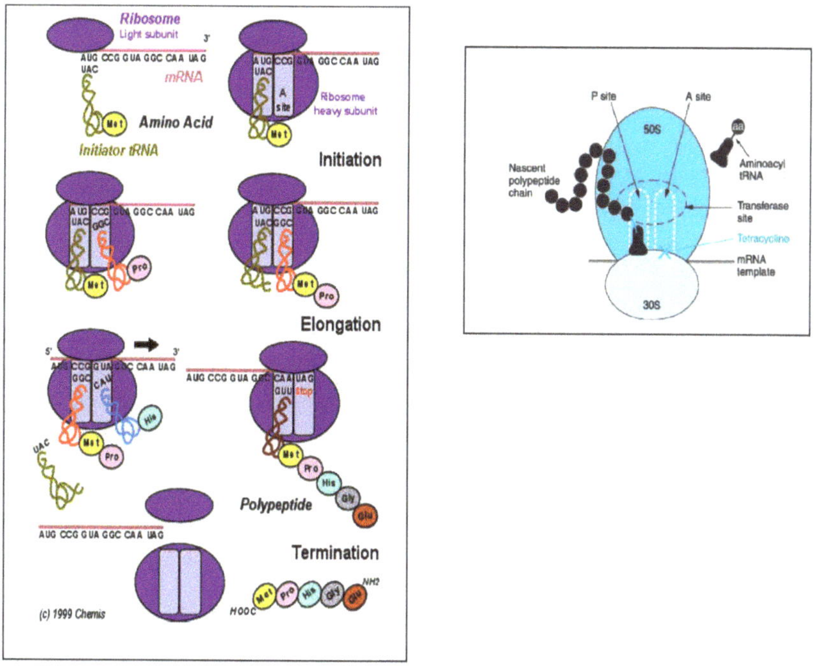

FIGURE 18.1 The mechanisms of action of protein synthesis inhibitor drugs acting at 50S and 30S ribosomal sites. *Adopted from Polikanov YS, Aleksashin NA, Beckert B and Wilson DN (2018).*

macrolides, lincosamides are similar in their mode of action to the macrolides through binding to the 50S ribosomal subunit and preventing peptide bond formation. Lincosamides are particularly active against streptococcal and staphylococcal infections.

Chloramphenicol also reportedly causes anemia in two different ways. One mechanism involves the targeting of mitochondrial ribosomes within hematopoietic stem cells, causing a reversible, dose-dependent suppression of blood cell production. Once chloramphenicol dosing is discontinued, blood cell production returns to normal. This mechanism highlights the similarity between 70s ribosomes of bacteria and the 70s ribosomes within our purview.

Membrane function inhibitors

A small group of antibacterials target the bacterial membrane as their mode of action. The polymyxins are natural polypeptide antibiotics that were first discovered in 1947 as products of *Bacillus polymyxa*; only polymyxin B and polymyxin E (colistin) have been used clinically.[27–35] They are lipophilic with detergent-like properties and interact with the lipopolysaccharide component of the outer membrane of Gram-negative bacteria, ultimately disrupting both their outer and inner membranes and killing the bacterial cells. Unfortunately, the membrane-targeting mechanism is not a selective toxicity, and these drugs also target and damage the membranes of cells in the kidney and nervous system when administered systemically.

Because of these serious side effects and their poor absorption from the digestive tract, polymyxin B is used in over-the-counter topical antibiotic ointments (e.g., Neosporin), and oral colistin was historically used only for bowel decontamination to prevent infections originating from bowel microbes in immunocompromised patients or for those undergoing certain abdominal surgeries. However, the emergence and spread of multidrug-resistant pathogens have led to increased use of intravenous colistin in hospitals, often as a drug of last resort to treat serious infections. The antibacterial daptomycin is a cyclic lipopeptide produced by *Streptomyces roseosporus* that seems to work like the polymyxins, inserting in the bacterial cell membrane and disrupting it. However, in contrast to polymyxin B and colistin, which target only Gram-negative bacteria, daptomycin specifically targets Gram-positive bacteria. It is typically administered intravenously and seems to be well tolerated, showing reversible toxicity in skeletal muscles.

Inhibitors of nucleic acid synthesis

Some antibacterial drugs work by inhibiting nucleic acid synthesis.[36–41] For example, metronidazole is a semisynthetic member of the nitroimidazole family that is also an antiprotozoan. It interferes with DNA replication in target cells. The drug rifampin is a semisynthetic member of the rifamycin family and functions by blocking RNA polymerase activity in bacteria.

ATP synthase inhibitors

Bedaquiline and delamanid represent the synthetic antibacterial class of compounds called the diarylquinolines; they use a novel mode of action that specifically inhibits mycobacterial growth.[42–52] Although the specific mechanism has yet to be elucidated, these compounds appear to interfere with the function of ATP synthases, perhaps by interfering with the use of the hydrogen ion gradient for ATP synthesis by oxidative phosphorylation, leading to reduced ATP production. Due to their side effects, including hepatotoxicity and potentially lethal heart arrhythmia, the use is reserved for serious, otherwise untreatable cases of tuberculosis.

Conclusion

Antibacterial drugs serve as the pillar of the pharmacotherapeutic treatment of infections and allied disorders. They serve as a major group of drugs in surgery in both pre and postsurgery stages but antimicrobial resistance has limited the effectiveness of antimicrobials that has to be counteracted.

References

1. Giske CG, Monnet DL, Cars O, Carmeli Y. Clinical and economic impact of common multidrug-resistant Gram-negative bacilli. *Antimicrob Agents Chemother.* 2008;52 (3):813–821 [PMC free article] [PubMed] [Google Scholar].
2. The Global Antibacterials Market: R&D Pipelines. *Market Analysis and Competitive Landscape.* 2007 August 28 [Google Scholar].
3. Boucher HW, Talbot GH, Bradley JS, et al. Bad bugs, no drugs: no ESKAPE! An update from the Infectious Diseases Society of America. *Clin Infect Dis.* 2009;48(1):1–12 [PubMed] [Google Scholar] • good article on restructuring infrastructure to develop new antimicrobial drugs.
4. Talbot GH, Bradley J, Edwards Jr JE, Gilbert D, Scheld M, Bartlett JG. Bad bugs need drugs: an update on the development pipeline from the Antimicrobial Availability Task Force of the Infectious Diseases Society of America. *Clin Infect Dis.* 2006;42(5):657–668 [PubMed] [Google Scholar].
5. Outterson K, Samora JB, Keller-Cuda K. Will longer antimicrobial patents improve global public health? *Lancet Infect Dis.* 2007;7(8):559–566 [PubMed] [Google Scholar] • Excellent article on incentives to uplift antibacterial drug discovery.
6. Colca JR, McDonald WG, Waldon DJ, et al. Cross-linking in the living cell locates the site of action of oxazolidinone antibiotics. *J Biol Chem.* 2003;278(24):21972–21979 [PubMed] [Google Scholar].
7. Lin AH, Murray RW, Vidmar TJ, Marotti KR. The oxazolidinone eperezolid binds to the 50S ribosomal subunit and competes with binding of chloramphenicol and lincomycin.

Antimicrob Agents Chemother. 1997;41(10):2127–2131 [PMC free article] [PubMed] [Google Scholar].
8. Qin Y, Polacek N, Vesper O, et al. The highly conserved LepA is a ribosomal elongation factor that back-translocates the ribosome. *Cell.* 2006;127(4):721–733 [PubMed] [Google Scholar].
9. Leach KL, Swaney SM, Colca JR, et al. The site of action of oxazolidinone antibiotics in living bacteria and in human mitochondria. *Mol Cell.* 2007;26(3):393–402 [PubMed] [Google Scholar] • in depth analysis of mechanism of action of oxazolidinones.
10. Wilson DN, Nierhaus KH. The oxazolidinone class of drugs find their orientation on the ribosome. *Mol Cell.* 2007;26(4):460–462 [PubMed] [Google Scholar].
11. French G. Safety and tolerability of linezolid. *J Antimicrob Chemother.* 2003;51(suppl 2): ii45–ii53 [PubMed] [Google Scholar].
12. Lee E, Burger S, Shah J, et al. Linezolid-associated toxic optic neuropathy: a report of 2 cases. *Clin Infect Dis.* 2003;37(10):1389–1391 [PubMed] [Google Scholar].
13. Brickner SJ, Hutchinson DK, Barbachyn MR, et al. Synthesis and antibacterial activity of U-100592 and U-100766, two oxazolidinone antibacterial agents for the potential treatment of multidrug-resistant Gram-positive bacterial infections. *J Med Chem.* 1996;39 (3):673–679 [PubMed] [Google Scholar].
14. Jorgensen JH, McElmeel ML, Trippy CW. In vitro activities of the oxazolidinone antibiotics U-100592 and U-100766 against *Staphylococcus aureus* and coagulase-negative *Staphylococcus* species. *Antimicrob Agents Chemother.* 1997;41(2):465–467 [PMC free article] [PubMed] [Google Scholar].
15. Mason Jr EO, Lamberth LB, Kaplan SL. In vitro activities of oxazolidinones U-100592 and U-100766 against penicillin-resistant and cephalosporin-resistant strains of *Streptococcus pneumoniae. Antimicrob Agents Chemother.* 1996;40(4):1039–1040 [PMC free article] [PubMed] [Google Scholar].
16. Molicotti P, Ortu S, Bua A, Cannas S, Sechi LA, Zanetti S. In vitro efficacy of linezolid on clinical strains of *Mycobacterium tuberculosis* and other mycobacteria. *N Microbiol.* 2006;29(4):275–280 [PubMed] [Google Scholar].
17. Brown-Elliott BA, Ward SC, Crist CJ, Mann LB, Wilson RW, Wallace Jr RJ. In vitro activities of linezolid against multiple Nocardia species. *Antimicrob Agents Chemother.* 2001;45(4):1295–1297 [PMC free article] [PubMed] [Google Scholar].
18. Moylett EH, Pacheco SE, Brown-Elliott BA, et al. Clinical experience with linezolid for the treatment of Nocardia infection. *Clin Infect Dis.* 2003;36(3):313–318 [PubMed] [Google Scholar].
19. Vara Prasad JV. New oxazolidinones. *Curr Opin Microbiol.* 2007;10(5):454–460 [PubMed] [Google Scholar].
20. File JRT, Bagheri F, Bush L, et al. A phase 2 study comparing two doses of radezolid to linezolid in adults with uncomplicated skin and skin structure infections (uSSSI) (L-1515c). In: *48th Annual Interscience Conference on Antimicrobial Agents and Chemotherapy (ICAAC) and the Infectious Disease Society of America (IDSA) 46th Annual Meeting*, October 25–28, Washington, DC; 2008 [Google Scholar].
21. Schaadt R, Sweeney D, Shinabarger D, Zurenko G. In vitro activity of TR-700, the active ingredient of the antibacterial prodrug TR-701, a novel oxazolidinone antibacterial agent. *Antimicrob Agents Chemother.* 2009;53(8):3236–3239 [PMC free article] [PubMed] [Google Scholar].

22. Foleno BD, Abbanat D, Goldschmidt RM, et al. In vitro antibacterial activity of the pyrrolopyrazolyl-substituted oxazolidinone RWJ-416457. *Antimicrob Agents Chemother.* 2007;51(1):361–365 [PMC free article] [PubMed] [Google Scholar].
23. Livermore DM, Warner M, Mushtaq S, North S, Woodford N. In vitro activity of the oxazolidinone RWJ-416457 against linezolid-resistant and -susceptible staphylococci and enterococci. *Antimicrob Agents Chemother.* 2007;51(3):1112–1114 [PMC free article] [PubMed] [Google Scholar].
24. Xiong L, Kloss P, Douthwaite S, et al. Oxazolidinone resistance mutations in 23S rRNA of *Escherichia coli* reveal the central region of domain V as the primary site of drug action. *J Bacteriol.* 2000;182(19):5325–5331 [PMC free article] [PubMed] [Google Scholar].
25. Shaw KJ, Poppe S, Schaadt R, et al. In vitro activity of TR-700, the antibacterial moiety of the prodrug TR-701, against linezolid-resistant strains. *Antimicrob Agents Chemother.* 2008;52(12):4442–4447 [PMC free article] [PubMed] [Google Scholar].
26. Feng J, Lupien A, Gingras H, et al. Genome sequencing of linezolid-resistant *Streptococcus pneumoniae* mutants reveals novel mechanisms of resistance. *Genome Res.* 2009;19(7):1214–1223 [PMC free article] [PubMed] [Google Scholar].
27. Chatterjee A, Mondal J, Bhowmik R, Bhattachayra A, Roy H, Kundu S. In-vitro anti-oxidant and antimicrobial study of *Ficus hispida. J Pharm Technol Res Manag.* 2015;3 (2):153–166.
28. Allen NE, Hobbs Jr JN, Nicas TI. Inhibition of peptidoglycan biosynthesis in vancomycin-susceptible and -resistant bacteria by a semisynthetic glycopeptide antibiotic. *Antimicrob Agents Chemother.* 1996;40(10):2356–2362 [PMC free article] [PubMed] [Google Scholar].
29. Kim SJ, Cegelski L, Stueber D, et al. Oritavancin exhibits dual mode of action to inhibit cell-wall biosynthesis in *Staphylococcus aureus. J Mol Biol.* 2008;377(1):281–293 [PMC free article] [PubMed] [Google Scholar].
30. Allen NE, LeTourneau DL, Hobbs Jr JN. Molecular interactions of a semisynthetic glycopeptide antibiotic with D-alanyl-D-alanine and D-alanyl-D-lactate residues. *Antimicrob Agents Chemother.* 1997;41(1):66–71 [PMC free article] [PubMed] [Google Scholar].
31. Allen NE, LeTourneau DL, Hobbs Jr JN. The role of hydrophobic side chains as determinants of antibacterial activity of semisynthetic glycopeptide antibiotics. *J Antibiot (Tokyo).* 1997;50(8):677–684 [PubMed] [Google Scholar].
32. Beauregard DA, Williams DH, Gwynn MN, Knowles DJ. Dimerization and membrane anchors in extracellular targeting of vancomycin group antibiotics. *Antimicrob Agents Chemother.* 1995;39(3):781–785 [PMC free article] [PubMed] [Google Scholar].
33. Buckwalter M, Dowell JA. Population pharmacokinetic analysis of dalbavancin, a novel lipoglycopeptide. *J Clin Pharmacol.* 2005;45(11):1279–1287 [PubMed] [Google Scholar].
34. Higgins DL, Chang R, Debabov DV, et al. Telavancin, a multifunctional lipoglycopeptide, disrupts both cell wall synthesis and cell membrane integrity in methicillin-resistant *Staphylococcus aureus. Antimicrob Agents Chemother.* 2005;49(3):1127–1134 [PMC free article] [PubMed] [Google Scholar].
35. Lunde CS, Hartouni SR, Janc JW, Mammen M, Humphrey PP, Benton BM. Telavancin disrupts the functional integrity of the bacterial membrane through targeted interaction with the cell wall precursor lipid II. *Antimicrob Agents Chemother.* 2009;53(8):3375–3383 [PMC free article] [PubMed] [Google Scholar] • good article on mechanism underlying telavancin effect on bacteria membrane integrity.

36. Candiani G, Abbondi M, Borgonovi M, Romano G, Parenti F. In-vitro and in-vivo antibacterial activity of BI 397, a new semi-synthetic glycopeptide antibiotic. *J Antimicrob Chemother.* 1999;44(2):179–192 [PubMed] [Google Scholar].
37. Lin G, Credito K, Ednie LM, Appelbaum PC. Antistaphylococcal activity of dalbavancin, an experimental glycopeptide. *Antimicrob Agents Chemother.* 2005;49(2):770–772 [PMC free article] [PubMed] [Google Scholar].
38. Streit JM, Sader HS, Fritsche TR, Jones RN. Dalbavancin activity against selected populations of antimicrobial-resistant Gram-positive pathogens. *Diagn Microbiol Infect Dis.* 2005;53(4):307–310 [PubMed] [Google Scholar].
39. King A, Phillips I, Kaniga K. Comparative in vitro activity of telavancin (TD-6424), a rapidly bactericidal, concentration-dependent anti-infective with multiple mechanisms of action against Gram-positive bacteria. *J Antimicrob Chemother.* 2004;53(5):797–803 [PubMed] [Google Scholar].
40. Krause KM, Renelli M, Difuntorum S, Wu TX, Debabov DV, Benton BM. In vitro activity of telavancin against resistant Gram-positive bacteria. *Antimicrob Agents Chemother.* 2008;52(7):2647–2652 [PMC free article] [PubMed] [Google Scholar].
41. Saravolatz LD, Pawlak JLJ. In vitro activity of oritavancin against CA-MRSA, VISA and daptomycin-non-susceptible *Staphylococcus aureus* (DNSSA) (C1–187). In: *48th Annual Interscience Conference on Antimicrobial Agents and Chemotherapy (ICAAC) and the Infectious Diseases Society of America (IDSA) 46th Annual Meeting*, October 25th–28th, Washington, DC; 2008 [Google Scholar].
42. Stryjewski ME, O'Riordan WD, Lau WK, et al. Telavancin vs standard therapy for treatment of complicated skin and soft-tissue infections due to Gram-positive bacteria. *Clin Infect Dis.* 2005;40(11):1601–1607 [PubMed] [Google Scholar].
43. Rubinstein E, Corey GR, Stryjewski ME, et al. Telavancin for treatment of hospital-acquired pneumonia (HAP) caused by MRSA and MSSA: the ATTAIN studies (K-530). In: *48th Annual Interscience Conference on Antimicrobial Agents and Chemotherapy (ICAAC) and the Infectious Disease Society of America (IDSA) 46th Annual Meeting*, October 25–28, Washington, DC; 2008 [Google Scholar].
44. Corey GR, Rubinstein E, Lalani T, et al. Telavancin for hospital-acquired pneumonia caused by *S. aureus*: efficacy analysis according to the in vitro susceptibility to vancomycin (K-528). In: *48th Annual Interscience Conference on Antimicrobial Agents and Chemotherapy (ICAAC) and the Infectious Disease Society of America (IDSA) 46th Annual Meeting*, October 25–28, Washington, DC; 2008 [Google Scholar].
45. Hartman CS, Wasilewski MM, Bates BM. Oritavancin in the treatment of complicated skin and skin structure infections (cSSSI): combined results of two phase 3 multinational trials (L-1514). In: *48th Annual Interscience Conference on Antimicrobial Agents and Chemotherapy (ICAAC) and the Infectious Diseases Society of America (IDSA) 46th Annual Meeting*, October 25–28, Washington, DC; 2008 [Google Scholar].
46. Fierce Biotech. *FDA: Targanta Must Conduct New Oritavancin Study.* Fierce Biotech; 2008. <http://www.fiercebiotech.com/story/fda-targanta-must-conduct-new-oritavancin-study/2008-12-09>; Last accessed 11.08.09.
47. Carrol J. *FDA Seeks More Telavancin Data.* Fierce Biotech; 2009. <http://www.fiercebiotech.com/story/fda-seeks-more-telavancin-data/2009-02-27>; Last accessed 11.08.09.
48. Arthur M, Courvalin P. Genetics and mechanisms of glycopeptide resistance in enterococci. *Antimicrob Agents Chemother.* 1993;37(8):1563–1571 [PMC free article] [PubMed] [Google Scholar].

49. Walsh CT, Fisher SL, Park IS, Prahalad M, Wu Z. Bacterial resistance to vancomycin: five genes and one missing hydrogen bond tell the story. *Chem Biol.* 1996;3(1):21–28 [PubMed] [Google Scholar].
50. Leuthner KD, Cheung CM, Rybak MJ. Comparative activity of the new lipoglycopeptide telavancin in the presence and absence of serum against 50 glycopeptide non-susceptible staphylococci and three vancomycin-resistant *Staphylococcus aureus*. *J Antimicrob Chemother.* 2006;58(2):338–343 [PubMed] [Google Scholar].
51. Goldstein BP, Draghi DC, Sheehan DJ, Hogan P, Sahm DF. Bactericidal activity and resistance development profiling of dalbavancin. *Antimicrob Agents Chemother.* 2007;51 (4):1150–1154 [PMC free article] [PubMed] [Google Scholar].
52. Seth M, Khan H, Bhowmik R, Karmakar S, Jana S. Facile fabrication of fluorine free zirconium zinc stearate based superhydrophobic and superoleophilic coating on cotton fabric with superior antibacterial property. *J Sol-Gel Sci Technol.* 2020;94:127–140.

Chapter 19

Mechanism of action of antifungal agents

Sandipan Jana[1], Srijon Gayen[1], Reshma Kumari[1], Susmita Patra[2], Pallab Kanti Haldar[1], Rudranil Bhowmik[1], Md. Adil Shaharyar[1], Avishek Mandal[1], Hindol Mazumdar[1] and Sanmoy Karmakar[1]

[1]*Bioeuivalence Study Centre, Department of Pharmaceutical Technology, Jadavpur University, Kolkata, West Bengal, India,* [2]*Department of Pharmaceutical Technology, Adamas University, Barasat, Kolkata, West Bengal, India*

Introduction

In the recent world scenario, human fungal diseases are a notable global health complication with inflated morbidity and mortality.[1,2] Fungi exist in nature and they are very common part of normal flora in humans and animals.[3] Especially in immunocompromised patients, there can be a wide range of fungal infection in human, including effect as a common, mild-to-superficial infection (SFI), as well as life-threatening invasive one. It is worth noticing that the fungal infection affects immunocompromised, cancer patients; premature infants are more affected compared to immunocompetent individuals.[3,4] Pathogenic fungi cause approximately 1.5 million death every year.[5,6]The pathogenicity of fungi, host immune response, and the site of infection ultimately determine the consequences. "In general, fungal infections are classified as superficial, cutaneous/mucosal, subcutaneous and Invasive."[7] Cutaneous infections in the skin and mucous membrane are sometimes caused by yeast pathogen, of which *Candida* species is an individual one.[6,8] "Subcutaneous infections (e.g., chromoblastomycosis) are associated with deeper layers of skin dermis and subcutaneous tissue."[3] On the other hand, lungs, heart, brain, kidneys, liver, and other internal organs of the body can be affected by to SFIs, invasive infection; observed mostly in immunocompromised patients.[3] These three species *Candida*, *Aspergillus*, and *Cryptococcus* cause more than 80% of the 1.5 million invasive fungal deaths occur every year globally.[5,6] This chapter provides a recent study on brief mechanism of action of antifungal agents on the recent development of fungal diseases.

How Synthetic Drugs Work. DOI: https://doi.org/10.1016/B978-0-323-99855-0.00019-1

Fungal infections that are also known as "mycoses" are sometimes chronic in nature.[9] Infections caused by fungi are superficial as well as systemic in nature. Fungi (singular:fungus) are generally nonmotile eukaryotic cells having a rigid cell wall composed of chitin and sterol.[9,10] Fungi are often mistaken for their plant-like appearances. Some are parasitic in nature, while others like mushrooms have economic importance due to their edible nature; they are also useful in the production of antibiotics and in the brewing industry.[9,11] Fungal diseases in humans are predominantly caused by pathogenic fungi. There are approximately 300 fungi pathogenic to humans but only a few are infective. Fungal infections are conventionally opportunistic in nature and attack the host when the immune system is weak or weakened due to some conditions like diabetes or due to the use of immunosuppressive agents and corticosteroids, etc. Fungal infections are aggravated due to the action of broad-spectrum antibiotics that kill the nonpathogenic bacteria originally competing with the fungi. Fungal infections are generally resistant to antibiotic therapy. A well-known fungal infection candidiasis affects a wounded human host or a pregnant woman.[11]

Fungi are classified into four types according to their morphological and some physical characteristics like the formation of hyphae.[9,11]

1. Yeast—*Cryptococcus neoformans* is the only pathogenic yeast that causes meningitis.[9]
2. Yeast-like fungi—which partly grows like yeast and hyphae also; *Candida albicans*, the pathogenic fungus in this group, causes systemic candidiasis and vaginal thrush.[9] *Pityrosporum orbiculare* is yeast-like fungus that causes superficial mycosis pityriasis versicolor.[9]
3. Molds—it is a true mycelium with filamentous fungi; *Aspergillus fumigatus* is to cause pulmonary aspergillosis.[9] Dermatophytes are the pathogenic molds that cause skin and nail infections.[9]
4. Dimorphic fungi which may grow as filaments or as yeast depending on their nutritional elements, for example, *Histoplasma capsulatum* causing histoplasmosis, *Coccidioides immitis* causing coccidioidomycosis, *Blastomyces dermatitidis* causing blastomycosis, etc.[9,11] *Pneumocystis carinii* is another opportunistic organism that has both protozoa- and fungi-like character and is resistant to antifungal drugs. It typically affects immunocompromised patients.[11]

Pathophysiology fungal diseases

Aspergillosis—Lung is the most commonly affected site of aspergillosis.[12] Respiratory tract is the common route of entry of aspergillosis spore and other entry site is gastrointestinal tract, including skin on rare side.[13] Inhaled aspergillosis spore makes cavity in lungs or it may found colonize mucus within the bronchi. Patient may deteriorate with moderately severe asthma with tenacious mucous and also produce a gradually progressive and destructive process in lungs containing centrilobular emphysema.[14] Infection may also involve asymmetric facial swelling, epistaxis, proptosis and cranial nerve abnormalities, bone erosion, and some nonspecific effects like cough, fever, and dyspnea that are frequent in pulmonary aspergillosis.[13] Pleuritic chest pain from pulmonary infection may occur with vascular invasion, which without adequate therapy may lead to mediastinal extension.[13] The involvement of central nervous system is a catastrophic consequence of disseminated aspergillosis and may manifest by seizures or focal neurologic effect.[15]

Blastomycosis—It is generally a systemic pyogranulomatous infection caused by spore of dermatitis.[16] Most infected patients are asymptomatic. Blastomycosis mainly involves the lungs and also has an effect on different organs like skin, oesteoarticular structure and genitourinary system, eye, peritoneum, and breast with pulmonary infection, which varies from subclinical pneumonia to ARDS (acute respiratory distress syndrome).[17] Symptoms and radiographic finding for pulmonary blastomycosis are nonspecific like fever, chills headache, malaise and chest pain, hemoptysis, anorexia, and weight loss.[18] Radiography can show nodules in the case of disseminated infection; cutaneous lesion often appears on neck, head, or extremities genitourinary, whereas prostates are more common involvement for men. Some symptoms include perineal discomfort, dysuria, and obstructive symptoms.[17,18]

Candidiasis—*C. albicans* and *Candida tropicalis* are most common causative organisms for candidiasis.[19] Generally, candidiasis are present as normal flora of the skin and mucocutaneous area and intestines.[20] Candidiasis in immunocompromised patients may occur due to the presence of diabetes mellitus or excessive use of contraceptive pills, antibiotic, and corticosteroid.[20] There are generally four types of candidiasis:

1. Oral thrush: Also known as mucocutaneous candidiasis. In this type of candidiasis the tongue, soft palate and buccal mucosa is covered with creamy white pseudomembrane composed of fungi.[21]
2. Candidal vaginitis: It is characterized by thick yellow curdy discharge from vagina; pseudomembrane lesions are also seen in vaginal mucosa.[20]
3. Cutaneous candidiasis: It involves changes in the shape of nail plate and colonized lesions seen in the intertriginous area of skin, axilla, groin, and intermammary area.[22]
4. Systemic candidiasis: It is rare in case and generally occurs in immunocompromised patients. Organism enters into body via mucous membrane, skin, or via intravenous infusion.[20] Most common type of disease like pyelonephritis and endocarditis occurs in this case.[20]

Coccidioidomycosis—Coccidioidomycosis infects through the inhalation of spores that travel through air. Farmers, construction workers, and people with outdoor activities are at high risk of this type of infection. Heavy rains followed by drought and winds accelerate the growth of mycelia. Traveling of the infectious person to other places and delayed onset of action also increase the spreadability of the mycelia.[23] The spherules grow in a size of 75 μm in diameter and divide internally by developing an internal septa and separating it into compartments consisting of endospores. The impregnated spherules rupture and release the endospores in the alveolar sac to start the infection. An airborne coccidioidomycosis *C. immitis* when enters the alveolar tissue, it has the ability to convert the spores into large tissue-invasive spherules. As spherules enlarge and rupture, each releases thousands of small endospores, which may form new spherules. In the alveolar sacs the macrophages pick up the endospores leading to acute inflammation. The remaining endospores either multiply within the tissues or are released in the environment again and further can lead to the regeneration of mycelia.[24]

The pulmonary diseases caused are characterized by acute, subacute, or chronic granulomatous reaction with varying degrees of fibrosis. In susceptible patients the spherules may also set up an extrapulmonary infection in the lungs. The infection generally branches with either or both widespread lung or systemic dissemination. Focal lesions may form in almost any tissue, most commonly in skin, subcutaneous tissues, bones (osteomyclitis), joints, and meningitis.[23]

Cryptococcosis—Cryptococcosis is also caused by the inhalation of the fungal propagules (either poorly encapsulated yeast cells or basidiospores) and affects the alveoli in lungs. The patients become asymptomatic with self-limited primary lung lesions.[25] After inhalation, *Cryptococcus* generally disseminates to the brain and meninges exhibiting microscopic multifocal intracerebral lesions with meningeal granulomas and larger focal brain lesions. In immunocompetent patients the pulmonary lesions can heal without antifungal therapy but cryptococcal meningitis is life-threatening and requires aggressive therapy.[25,26]

Focal sites of dissemination may occur in skin, bones, joints, liver, spleen, kidneys, prostate, and other tissues, but only the skin lesions have symptoms. Rarely, pyelonephritis occurs with renal papillary necrosis. The accumulated cryptococcal capsular polysaccharide causes cyst in the infected tissues with lesser inflammation.[25]

Histoplasmosis—Lungs are the most commonly affected organ for histoplasmosis, fungi phagocytized by pulmonary macrophages and neutrophils and spread via lymph nodes.[27] Pneumonitis occurs as a local infection. Disease generally does not occur in healthy individual due to histoplasma-mediated cellular immunity; if not controlled by cellular immunity, dissemination occurs in reticuloendothelial site.[27,28] Disease may depend on waving cellular immunity from primary to acute, granulomatous inflammation develops as cell-mediated immunity controls infection, and immunodeficient patient may develop acute or chronic progressive disseminated infection.[28]

Mucormycosis—it is a life-threatening fungal infection affecting immunocompromised host.[29–32] Burn, traumatic disruption of skin, and implantation causes cutaneous mucormycosis and ingestion cause's GI mucormycosis and inhalation of Mucorales may develop pulmonary mucormycosis.[33] Neutrophils help to destroying fungal hyphae. Monocyte and macrophages also help in host defense mechanism.[34] Acidosis, hyperglycemia, and corticosteroid treatment may increase the risk of mucormycosis. Iron plays an important role in the growth of fungi.[35] In the case of diabetes, iron-sequestering proteins in acidotic conditions decrease the iron-binding capacity, and fungi may damage endothelial cells that cause mucormycosis to lead to vascular invasion, dissemination, and tissue necrosis. In the case of diabetic ketoacidosis, increased concentration of glucose and iron in the body helps to increase grp78 protein and to increase the ability of Mucorales to penetrate endothelial cell.[36]

Mycetoma—it is generally subcutaneous infection manifested by *Madurella mycetomatis* and reported other causative organisms like *Madurella grisea*, *Leptosphaeria senegalensis*, and *Scedosporium apiospermum*.[37] It is a noncontagious chronic infectious disease that remains localized and involves cutaneous and subcutaneous tissues, fasciae, and bones.[38] Some characterizations are tumefaction, the presence of sclerotia, draining sinuses, etc. Materials discharged from the sinuses generally consist of colonies of fungi or bacteria.[20]

Sporotrichosis—sporotrichosis is caused by a fungus named Sporothrix.[39] Red nodular lesion that appears on skin also displays in central and peripheral area of granulomas.[40] Lymphocutaneous is the most common condition, indicating lymphatic area, and in the case of immunocompromised patients disseminated diseases occur like subcutaneous or lymphocutaneous forms that are left untreated.[41] There are some other types of condition generally include some specific organs or tissues.

1. Osteoarticular generally includes body joints and leads to tenosynovitis and arthritis.
2. In the case of tuberculosis, alcoholism, sarcoidosis causes pulmonary sporotrichosis, which may cause pleural effusion, lymphadenopathy, cavity, and pulmonary infiltrate.
3. In chronic and rare cases, meningitis occurs sometimes.[40]

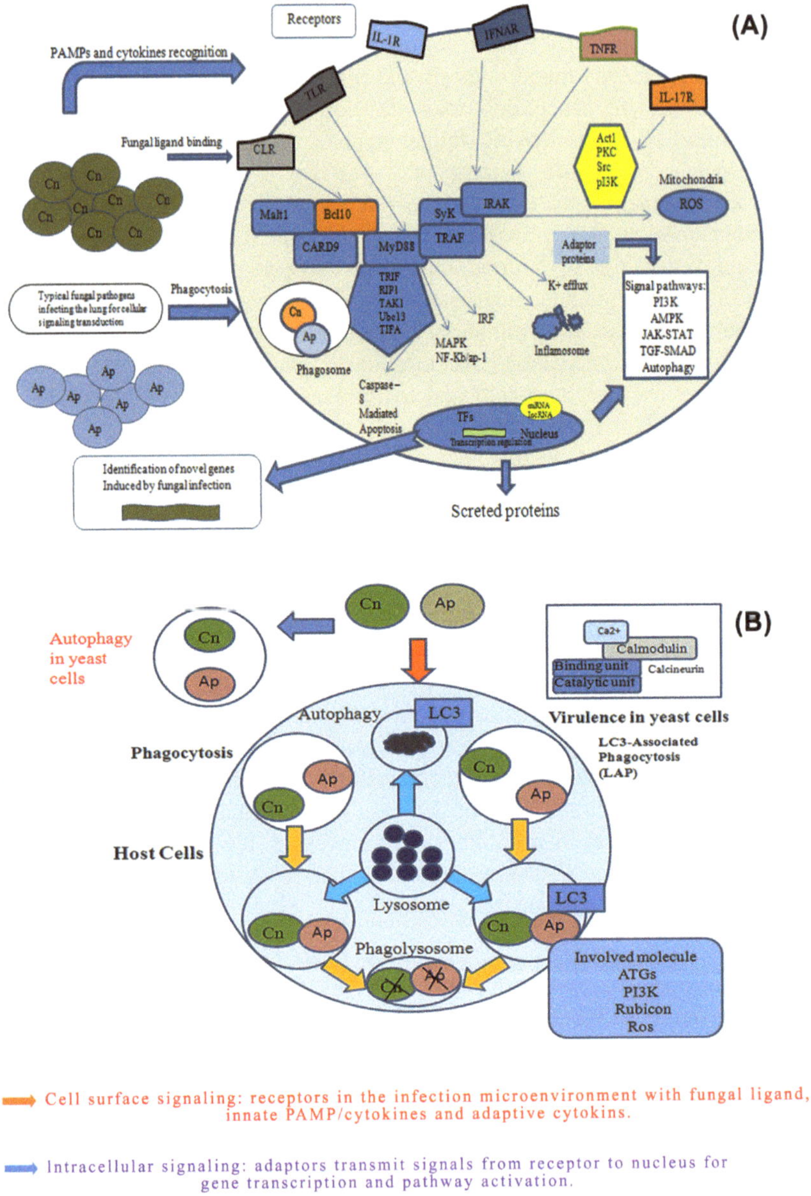

Classification of antifungal drugs

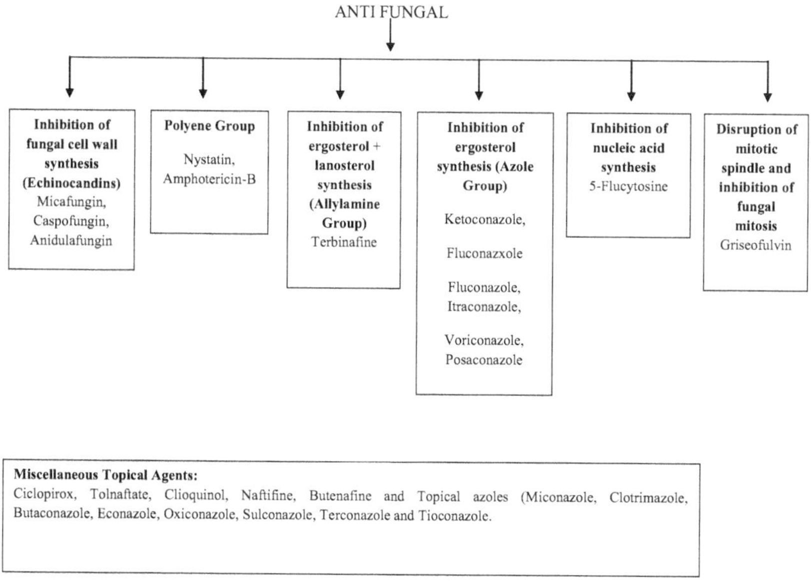

Mechanism of antifungal agents

Compared with bacteria, fungi often cause chronic infection and they have rigid cell walls and ergosterol-containing cell membrane and mostly resistant to antibiotic. Mycoses are fungal infection that can be superficial, systemic, or subcutaneous. Systemic mycoses are mostly life-threatening and usually difficult to treat when most patients are immunocompromised such as those who have HIV infection, those with cancer, or those who have a complicated surgery procedure or long-term use of antibiotics and have increased the risk of nosocomial fungal infection. Some opportunistic fungal pathogens are *C. albicans*, *Aspergillus*, *Cryptococcus*, etc.; and some antifungal agents like caspofungin, voriconazole, and amphotericin B and some imidazole and tetrazole derivatives are used to treat systemic fungal infection.[42]

Azole antifungal: Imidazole and triazole are the major groups that effect fungi by the inhibition of 1, 4-ά-demethylase enzyme on cytochrome P-450 of the gene ERG11,[9,43] causing demethylation of lanosterol to ergosterol and resulting the accumulation of the toxic product 14ά-methyl-3,6-diol that leads to growth arrest and also hinders the function of membrane-bound enzyme via diminishing the close packing of acyl chain of phospholipid.[43] Some other types of azole may effect on cytoplasmic membrane of fungi by increasing membrane permeability and also block respiratory chain electron transport.[9]

Terbinafine: Terbinafine inhibits the conversion of squalene to lanosterol by the inhibition of fungal enzyme squalene epoxidase.[9,43] It reduces ergosterol production by the inhibition of lanosterol production that effects fungal cell function ability.[9]

Flucytosine: Cytosine permease helps to transport of flucytosine into the fungal cell membrane and converts to 5-flurouracil with the help of cytosine deaminase enzyme and further metabolizes into 5-flurodeoxyuridine monophosphate.[9,43] It also inhibits the thymidylate synthases and diminishes the formation of thymidine monophosphate from deoxyuridine monophosphate that inhibits fungal DNA synthesis due to the lack of cytosine deaminase in mammalian cells; that is why it blocks the metabolism of fluorouracil and that helps to exhibit the selective action flucytosine.[9,43]

Griseofulvin: Griseofulvin causes the inhibition of microtubule function thereby blocking fungal mitosis and metaphase and also disrupts the assembly of mitotic spindle, which causes the blockage of fungal cell division.[9,43] Griseofulvin also blocks the fungal invasion via binding with newly synthesized keratin.[9]

Echinocandins: Echinocandins block the fungal cell wall synthesis and disrupt cellular integrity via the inhibition of 1, 3-β-D-glucan synthesis.[9]

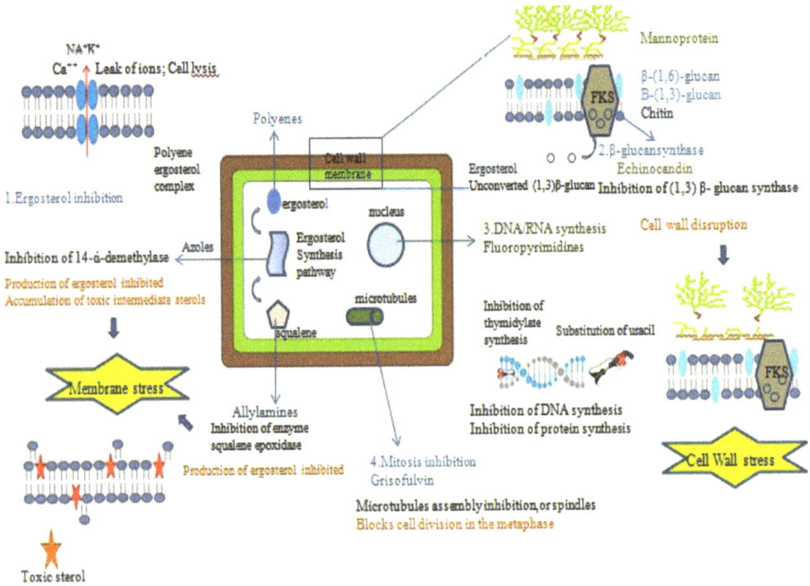

Polyene antibiotic—polyene antibiotic is an antifungal used systemically for many years. It is a typical antimicrobial molecule generally used in visceral infection.[44] It causes leakage of cellular contents, cytosolic molecules, and ions by binding with ergosterol that is the main component of sterol in fungal membrane and intercepts with fungal membrane, leading to the loss of membrane integrity.[44,45] The main fungicidal effect remains unclear.[44] However, current evidence shows that Amphotericin B aggregates the molecules of sequester ergosterol from bilayers of lipid and causes fungal cell death.[45] Amphotericin B has a greater affinity toward ergosterol over cholesterol because of its three-dimensional structure over cholesterol. Amphotericin B has a greater selectivity as an antifungal due to ergosterol: phospholipid ratio in fungi. Amphotericin B has a potential toxicity on mammalian cell.[44]

Class	Sl no	Drug	Drug, route and dosage, ADR, therapeutic uses Route and dosage	Adverse drug reaction	Therapeutic uses
Allylamines	1	Naftifine	Topical 1% cream or gel	Burning, stinging, irritation, redness, dry skin, or itching	Onychomycosis
	2	Terbinafine	Oral, topical 125-200-mg tab 1% cream	Rash, headache, diarrhea, stomach ache, indigestion, muscle or joint pain	• Ringworm • Onychomycosis
Antimetabolite	3	Flucytosine	Oral 50–150 mg/kg In 4 doses	Bone marrow depression, thrombocytopenia, rash, nausea, vomiting, diarrhea, and severe enterocolitis	Cryptococcosis (with amphotericin B)
Imidazole	4	Ketoconazole	Oral, topical 200-mg tab 0.5% cream	Eye dryness, irritation, prickling irritation, and discoloration of toenails	Athlete's foot, jock itch, ringworm, and seborrhea
	5	Clotrimazole	Oral, topical 100-mg vaginal tab 1% cream	Rash, hives, stomach pain, and foul-smelling vaginal discharge	Dermatophytosis (ringworm), candidiasis, tinea versicolor, piedra, tinea nigra, and fungal keratitis
	6	Econazole	Oral, topical 150-mg vaginal tab 1% cream/lotion	Burning, stinging, redness, tenderness, and irritation	Candidiasis, pityriasis
	7	Miconazole	Topical 100-mg vaginal ovules 2% cream/lotion	Headache, vaginal/urethral burning/itching/pain, or lower abdominal cramps	Candidiasis, pityriasis
	8	Oxiconazole	Topical 1% cream/lotion	Burning, stinging, swelling, redness, pimple-like bumps, tenderness, or flaking of the treated skin	Pityriasis
Triazole	9	Fluconazole	Oral, IV 100-mg/d mg caps 200 mg/100 mL IV infusion	Nausea, vomiting, diarrhea, stomach upset/pain, headache, dizziness, or hair loss	• Invasive candidiasis • Cryptococcosis • Coccidioidomycosis • Prophylaxis and empirical therapy in immunocompromised host
	10	Itraconazole	Oral, IV		• Invasive aspergillosis

(Continued)

(Continued)

Class	Sl no	Drug	Drug, route and dosage, ADR, therapeutic uses Route and dosage	Adverse drug reaction	Therapeutic uses
			200-mg IV/ bid 2 d Then 200 mg/d	Dry mouth, fever, increased thirst, irregular heartbeat, loss of appetite, mood changes, muscle pain, or cramps	• Blastomycosis • Coccidioidomycosis • Histoplasmosis • Pseudallescheriasis • Sporotrichosis • Ringworm • Onychomycosis
	11	Voriconazole	Oral, IV 400 mg/bid Then 200 mg/bid	Abnormal vision, diarrhea, headache, dry mouth, and dizziness	• Invasive aspergillosis • Invasive candidiasis • Pseudallescheriasis
	12	Posaconazole	Oral, IV 300 mg bid/ d 1d Then 300 mg/d Oral 200 mg/ tid	Skin rash, fluid retention in the legs, feet, arms or hands, muscle pain, and dizziness	• Oropharyngeal candidiasis • Prophylaxis in the immunocompromised host against aspergillosis and candidiasis
	13	Isavuconazole Isavuconazonium sulfate (prodrug)	Oral, IV 372-mg PO/ IV	Dyspnea, hypotension, chills, hypokalemia, and rash	• Invasive aspergillosis • Mucormycosis
Echinocandins	14	Caspofungin	IV70 mg/ dThen 50 mg/d	Swelling/redness/irritation At the injection site, nausea, vomiting, diarrhea, and headache	• Invasive candidiasis • Empirical therapy in the immunocompromised host
	15	Micafungin	IV100 mg/d	Black tarry stools, cough, decreased frequency or amount of urine, fast, pounding, or irregular heartbeat or pulse, fever, or chills	• Invasive candidiasis • Prophylaxis in the immunocompromised host
Polyene antibiotic	16	Amphotericin B	IV0.5–1 mg/ kg/d	Fever, shaking, chills, flushing, loss of appetite, upset stomach, headache, shortness of breath, and muscle or joint aches	• Invasive candidiasis • Invasive aspergillosis • Blastomycosis • Histoplasmosis • Coccidioidomycosis • Cryptococcosis • Mucormycosis • Sporotrichosis • Empirical therapy In immunocompromised host
Newer drug	17	Ibrexafungerp	Oral150-mg tab	Vaginal bleeding, rash/ hypersensitivity reaction, diarrhea, and nausea	Vaginal yeast infection

Black fungus and COVID-19

In the case of the immunocompromised patient, opportunism takes place for microorganism that surrounded by externally as well as inside our body.[45] Extend use of some steroid or some drugs quells the immune system; diseases like HIV, diabetes, and cancer make a person more susceptible to such infection.[45] The present worldwide pandemic Coronavirus disease 2019 is a new disease caused by SARS-CoV-2 with a variety of complication and manifestations that make patient's immune system feebler and make susceptible to secondary infection.[45,46] In some cases, in patients with post-COVID-19 stages, Mucormycosis or BLACK FUNGUS is the most commonly observed secondary infection as a case of highly use of steroid and uncontrolled diabetes.[46] Mucormycosis is fatal but rare opportunistic fungal infection caused by the inhalation of Mucorales.[46] Dark pigment–producing fungi are currently popular as BLACK FUNGUS after COVID-19, which blacken infected patient's tissue and overall give a black appearance in affected area.[45]

Source

The general sources of Mucorales are environmental plant, soil, dead materials, and discarded fruit and vegetable. In the case of a healthy person, the inhalation of spore from air does not cause any harm. On the other hand, for patients with SARS-CoV-2 and compromised immunity, mold or fungal spore generally came from humid environment and repeatedly using of one mask can become life-threatening. So it is needed to maintain proper ventilation of room, dispose mask after use, and avoid dust-polluted area.[45]

Reasons for sudden development

The reasons are as follows[45]:

- Some possible attributes behind the severity of mucormycosis.
- Improper and early use of steroid in COVID-19 treatment without any expert advice.
- Taking oral steroid with normal SpO_2 level under self-quarantine situation.
- COVID-19 patients after discharge from hospital need to maintain proper caution.
- A population with uncontrolled diabetes in SARS-CoV-2 infection is a significant cause of Mucormycosis.
- In pandemic situation, overcrowded hospitals with COVID-19 patients interrupt the maintenance of proper hygienic ventilators, humidifiers, oxygen mask, etc.

- Some studies show that there was a possibility in extensively use of zinc supplements for COVID-19 treatment and taking excessive stem inhalation.
- Clinically found that there were five types of mucormycosis infection happened with patients in COVID-19:[47,48]
  - rhinocerebral (44%–49%),
  - cutaneous (10%–16%),
  - pulmonary (10%–11%),
  - disseminated (6%–11.6%), and
  - gastrointestinal (2%–11%).

Symptoms

The symptoms are as follows[48]:

- swelling in the face
- pain and numbness, unusual (bloody or black-brown) discharge from the nose
- swollen eyes
- nasal or sinus congestion
- black lesions on nasal bridge or upper inside of the mouth
- loss of eyesight
- blurred vision

Treatments

In this situation of medical emergency, early diagnosis and treatment is the key to relief from this fatal disease. Some factors correlated with mucormycosis treatment are immunosuppressive drugs, proper antifungal therapy, hyperglycemia, metabolic acidosis, use of desferrioxamine, neutropenia, and proper surgical debridement of infected tissue.[32,49,50]

Depending on present difficulties and risk factors, as an antifungal therapy, Amphotericin B is the main drug of choice for initial treatment. Generally, liposomal amphotericin B was used 5 or 10 mg/kg/day continuously for several weeks till a sign of improvement, then oral posaconazole or isavuconazole was used for stand down the therapy. If patients can't tolerate Amphotericin B, IV posaconazole or isavuconazole was used for retrieve therapy.[49]

Conclusion

The final milestone of antifungal drug therapy in the 21st century was the identification and development of molecular mechanism of antifungal agents. However, the new antifungal therapy needs an increase in awareness due to the limitation in their spectrum of activity, pharmacokinetics, and drug interaction. Novel antifungal agents such as Ibrexafungerp are triterpenoids branched from enfumafungin with well-tolerated gastrointestinal adverse effect. The antifungal activity of orally induced Ibrexafungerp is exhibited by the inhibition of (1–3)-β-D-glucan synthase. Currently, the research is focused on the development of new molecular mechanism of antifungal drug with long-term memory response, particularly in immunocompromised and immunocompetent patients. Nevertheless, some of the drugs in clinical trials have given promising result; still there are many changes to overcome.

References

1. Zhang Y, Li R, Wang X. Monogenetic causes of fungal disease: recent developments. *Curr Opin Microbiol.* 2020;58:75–86. Available from: https://doi.org/10.1016/j.mib.2020.09.002.
2. Bongomin F, Gago S, Oladele R, Denning D. Global and multi-national prevalence of fungal diseases—estimate precision. *J Fungi.* 2017;3(4):57. Available from: https://doi.org/10.3390/jof3040057.
3. Pathakumari B, Liang G, Liu W. Immune defence to invasive fungal infections: a comprehensive review. *Biomed Pharmacother.* 2020;130:110550. Available from: https://doi.org/10.1016/j.biopha.2020.110550.
4. Spellberg B. Vaccines for invasive fungal infections. *F1000 Med Rep.* 2011;3.
5. Brown GD, Denning DW, Gow NA, Levitz SM, Netea MG, White TC. Hidden killers: human fungal infections. *Sci Transl Med.* 2012;4(165):165rv113.
6. Kaushik N, Pujalte GG, Reese ST. Superficial fungal infections. *Prim Care Clin Pract.* 2015;42(4):501–516.
7. Zhan P, Liu W. The changing face of dermatophytic infections worldwide. *Mycopathologia.* 2017;182(1–2):77–86.
8. Ameen M. Epidemiology of superficial fungal infections. *Clin Dermatol.* 2010;28:197–201.
9. Sharma HL, Sharma KK. *Principles of Pharmacology.* 3rd ed. Paras Medical Publisher; 2017.
10. Kee JL, Hayes ER, Mccuistion LE. *Pharmacology: A Patient-Centered Nursing Process Approach.* 8th ed. Elsevier; 2015.
11. Rang HP, Dale MM, Ritter JM, Flower RJ, Henderson G. *Rang and Dale's Pharmacology.* 7th ed. Elsevier Churchill Livingstone; 2012.
12. Chabi ML, Goracci A, Roche N, Paugam A, Lupo A, Revel MP. Pulmonary aspergillosis. *Diagn Interv Imaging.* 2015;96(5):435–442.
13. Segal BH. Aspergillosis. *N Engl J Med.* 2009;360(18):1870–1884.
14. Patel G, Greenberger PA. *Allergy Asthma Proc.* 2019;40(6):421–424.
15. Walsh TJ, Anaissie EJ, Denning DW, et al. Treatment of aspergillosis: clinical practice guidelines of the Infectious Diseases Society of America. *Clin Infect Dis.* 2008;46(3):327–360.
16. Storms TN, Clyde VL, Munson L, Ramsay EC. Blastomycosis in nondomestic felids. *J Zoo Wildl Med.* 2003;34(3):231–238.
17. Smith JA, Kauffman CA. Blastomycosis. Ann Arbor, MI: Division of Infectious Diseases, University of Michigan Medical School, Veterans Affairs Ann Arbor Healthcare System; 2010.

18. Castillo CG, Kauffman CA, Miceli MH. Blastomycosis. *Infect Dis Clin North Am.* 2016;30 (1):247–264.
19. Silva S, Negri M, Henriques M, Oliveira R, Williams DW, Azeredo J. Candida glabrata, Candida parapsilosis and Candida tropicalis: biology, epidemiology, pathogenicity and antifungal resistance. *FEMS Microbiol Rev.* 2012;36(2):288–305.
20. Mohon H. *Textbook of Pathology.* 7th ed. Jaypee Brothers Medical Publishers (P) Ltd; 2015.
21. Millsop JW, Fazel N. Oral candidiasis. *Clin Dermatol.* 2016;34(4):487–494.
22. McKay M, Gardner SS. Seborrhea, psoriasis and the papulosquamous dermatoses. *Primary Care.* 1989;16(3):739–763.
23. Revankar SG. Coccidioidomycosis (San Joaquin Fever; *Valley Fever*). Wayne State University School of Medicine; 2021. MSD Manual Professional Journal.
24. Akram SM, Koirala J. *Coccidioidomycosis. StatPearls.* Treasure Island, FL: StatPearls Publishing; 2021, PMID:. Available from: 28846274.
25. Revankar SG. Cryptococcosis (San Joaquin Fever; *Valley Fever*). Wayne State University School of Medicine; 2021. MSD Manual Professional Journal.
26. Maziarz EK, Perfect JR. Cryptococcosis. *Infect Dis Clin North Am.* 2016;30(1):179–206. Available from: https://doi.org/10.1016/j.idc.2015.10.006, PMID: 26897067; PMCID. Available from: PMC5808417.
27. McKinsey DS, McKinsey JP. Pulmonary histoplasmosis. *Semin Respir Crit Care Med.* 2011;32(6):735–744.
28. Azar M, Bahr N, Loyd J, Hage C, Wheat L. Histoplasmosis: up-to-date evidence-based approach to diagnosis and management. *Semin Respir Crit Care Med.* 2015;36 (05):729–745.
29. Boelaert JR, Fenves AZ, Coburn JW. Deferoxamine therapy and mucormycosis in dialysis patients: report of an international registry. *Am J Kidney Dis.* 1991;18(6):660–667, PMID. Available from: 1962650.
30. Boelaert JR, Fenves AZ, Coburn JW. Registry on mucormycosis in dialysis patients. *J Infect Dis.* 1989;160(5):914.
31. Ribes JA, Vanover-Sams CL, Baker DJ. Zygomycetes in human disease. *Clin Microbiol Rev.* 2000;13(2):236–301, PMC 100153. PMID. Available from: 10756000.
32. Spellberg B, Edwards Jr J, Ibrahim A. Novel perspectives on mucormycosis: pathophysiology, presentation, and management. *Clin Microbiol Rev.* 2005;18(3):556–569. Available from: https://doi.org/10.1128/CMR.18.3.556-569.2005, PMC 1195964. PMID. Available from: 16020690.
33. Castrejón-Pérez AD, Welsh EC, Miranda I, Ocampo-Candiani J, Welsh O. Cutaneous mucormycosis. *An Bras Dermatol.* 2017;92(3):304–311. Available from: https://doi.org/10.1590/abd1806-4841.20176614.
34. Waldorf AR. Pulmonary defense mechanisms against opportunistic fungal pathogens. *Immunol Ser.* 1989;47:243–271, PMID. Available from: 2490078.
35. Artis WM, Fountain JA, Delcher HK, Jones HE. A mechanism of susceptibility to mucormycosis in diabetic ketoacidosis: transferrin and iron availability. *Diabetes.* 1982;31 (12):1109–1114, PMID. Available from: 6816646.
36. Liu M, Spellberg B, Phan QT, et al. The endothelial cell receptor GRP78 is required for mucormycosis pathogenesis in diabetic mice. *J Clin Invest.* 2010;120(6):1914–1924. Available from: https://doi.org/10.1172/JCI42164, PMC 2877958. PMID. Available from: 20484814.
37. McGinnis MR. Mycetoma. *Dermatol Clin.* 1996;14(1):97–104.

38. Lichon V, Khachemoune A. Mycetoma. *Am J Clin Dermatol.* 2006;7(5):315–321. Available from: https://doi.org/10.2165/00128071-200607050-00005.
39. Barros MB, de Almeida Paes R, Schubach AO. Sporothrix schenckii and Sporotrichosis. *Clin Microbiol Rev.* 2011;24(4):633–654.
40. Dowd FJ. Sporotrichosisin. In: *xPharm: The Comprehensive Pharmacology Reference.* 2007.
41. Verma S, Verma G, Rattan R. *Indian Dermatol Online J.* 2019;10(3):303–306. Available from: https://doi.org/10.4103/idoj.IDOJ_272_18, PMID. Available from: 31149578.
42. Raffa RB, Rawls SM. *Netter's Illustrated Pharmacology.* Updated ed. PhD Temple University School of Pharmacy Philadelphia, Pennsylvania, Elena Portyansky Beyzarov, PharmD Director of Scientific Affairs.
43. Brunton LL, Dandan RH, Knollmann BC. *Goodman and Gilman's the Pharmacological Basis of Therapeutics.* 13th ed. McGraw-Hill Education; 2018.
44. Odds FC, Brown AJP, Gow NAR, Aberdeen Fungal Group. *Antifungal Agents: Mechanisms of Action.* Aberdeen: Department of Molecular and Cell Biology, Institute of Medical Sciences, University of Aberdeen.
45. Gokulshankar S, Mohanty BK. COVID-19 and black fungus. *Asian J Med Health Sci.* 2021;4(1):137.
46. Shevade S. Mucormycosis: black fungus, a deadly post-COVID infection. *MAR Microbiol.* 2021;2(5).
47. Chander J, Kaur M, Singla N, et al. Mucormycosis: battle with the deadly enemy over a five-year period in India. *J Fungi (Basel, Switzerland).* 2018;4(2):46. Available from: https://doi.org/10.3390/jof4020046.
48. Raghunath V, Rose KHP, Geetha KC, Deepthi RM. Mucormycosis – can the diagnosis be challenging at times? *SRM J Res Dental Sci.* 2018;9:191–196.
49. McCarthy M, Rosengart A, Schuetz AN, Kontoyiannis DP, Walsh TJ. *N Engl J Med.* 2014;371(2):150–160.
50. Garg D, Muthu V, Sehgal IS, et al. Coronavirus disease (Covid-19) associated mucormycosis (CAM): case report and systematic review of literature. *Mycopathologia.* 2021;186 (2):289–298.

Further reading

Global guideline for the diagnosis and management of mucormycosis: an initiative of the European Confederation of Medical Mycology in cooperation with the Mycoses Study Group Education and Research Consortium. Lancet Infect Dis. 2019 Dec;19(12):e405-e421. doi: 10.1016/S1473-3099(19)30312-3. *Management of Mucormycosis*2020;.

Chapter 20

Insights into the mechanism of action of antiviral drugs

Reshma Kumari[1], Sandipan Jana[1], Susmita Patra[2], Pallab Kanti Haldar[1], Rudranil Bhowmik[1], Avishek Mandal[1], Kumar Anand[1], Hindol Mazumdar[1], Md. Adil Shaharyar[1] and Sanmoy Karmakar[1]

[1]*Bioeuivalence Study Centre, Department of Pharmaceutical Technology, Jadavpur University, Kolkata, West Bengal, India,* [2]*Department of Pharmaceutical Technology, Adamas University, Barasat, Kolkata, West Bengal, India*

Introduction

Viruses are ultramicroscopic infectious parasites that have a genome (either RNA or DNA) or enzymes stored in a capsid (capsule made of protein). In some viruses, capsid is also covered with a lipid layer (envelope).[1]

Viruses are obligate parasites because they require host cells to reproduce and complete their life cycle. These host cells may include mammalian or insect or plant or bacterial cells. Virus not only depends on nutrition but also uses metabolic machinery of the host cell for their growth. Therefore it is considered difficult to find antiviral drug that would selectively target virus without harming the infected host cells.[2–4]

Virus life cycle and pathogenesis

Viruses propagate using a host cell to produce its clones, as a means of reproduction for further generation. Life cycles of all viruses share a general pattern:

- attachment to the host cell.
- penetration of genome into its host cell
- dominate and use the host cell machinery to replicate its viral component
- assembly of viral components into complete viral structure
- burst the host cell to release new viral clones to infect new host cells[5,6]

Depending upon the genomic material, virus can be classified as DNA viruses or RNA viruses. DNA virus replicates within the host cell nucleus where RNA polymerase transcripts DNA into viral mRNA, then viral m-RNA is

How Synthetic Drugs Work. DOI: https://doi.org/10.1016/B978-0-323-99855-0.00020-8

translated into viral proteins and enzymes by the host cell's ribosomes. DNA virus examples are poxviruses (causes smallpox), herpesviruses (causes chickenpox, shingles, oral, and genital herpes), papillomaviruses (causes warts), adenoviruses (causes pharyngoconjunctival), and hepadnaviruses (causes hepatitis B).[7,8]

Mostly, RNA virus replicates in host cell cytoplasm, whereas influenza (RNA) virus replicates in host cell nucleus. Viral RNA polymerase synthesizes mRNA from genomic viral RNA that gets translated to proteins which then directs the synthesis of more viral RNA. RNA virus examples are rubella virus, rhabdoviruses (causes rabies), picornaviruses (causes poliomyelitis, meningitis, colds, hepatitis A), flaviviruses (West Nile meningoencephalitis, yellow fever, hepatitis C, Zika virus); orthomyxoviruses (includes influenza); paramyxoviruses (causes measles, mumps), and coronaviruses [cause colds, severe acute respiratory syndrome (SARS)] (Fig. 20.1).[2,3]

The antiviral drugs based on their common mechanisms of action can be of two types, that is, drugs targeting virus and drugs targeting host.[9] Interference of viral transcription and replication or direct inactivation of viral structural proteins are the main aim of drugs targeting virus,[10–12] whereas drugs acting on host concentrate on binding host cell–specific receptor, inhibiting viral interaction and adsorption,[11,13] inhibition of important cellular factors that are under control of the virus during its replication cycle,[9] the use of interferons and other immunomodulators and gamma globulins.[14]

Some studies have reported that many RNA and DNA viruses and some retroviruses cause apoptosis by generating reactive species. Endogenous antioxidants are superoxide dismutase (SOD), catalase (CAT), and glutathione peroxidase (GPx).[15,16] The virus shares a common pathogenic pathway emphasizing respiratory syncytial production. During viral infection, there is antioxidant depletion, therefore the generation of oxidative stress and decrease in immune system. The nonenzymatic antioxidants are plant polyphenols, vitamins C and E (a-tocopherol), carotenoids, organosulfur compounds, minerals, and cofactors that are obtained from diet and it plays an important role in the maintenance of human health along with antivirals.[17,18]

Classification of drugs based on viral targets

1. Antiretro virus
   a. Nucleoside reverse transcriptase inhibitors (NRTIs): zidovudine, stavudine, lamivudine, abacavir, emtricitabine
   b. Nucleotide reverse transcriptase inhibitors: Tenofovir (TFV) disoproxil fumarate (TDF), tenofovir alafenamide (TAF)
   c. Non-NRTIs (NNRTIs): nevirapine (NVP), delavirdine, efavirenz, etravirine, rilpivirine (RPV), doravirine, elsulfavirine

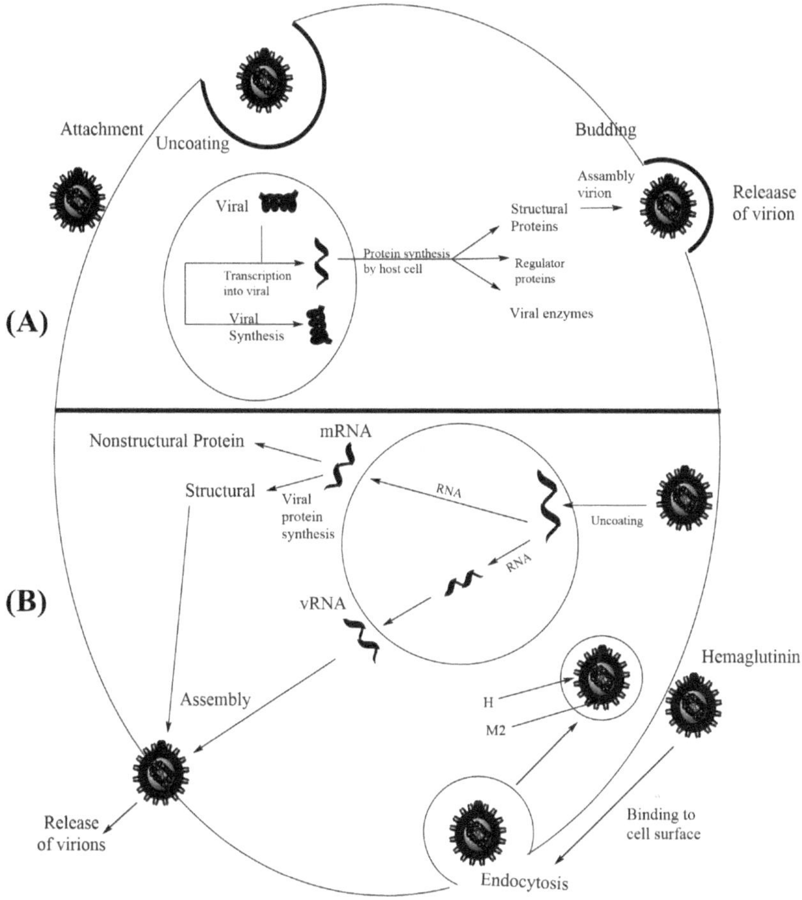

FIGURE 20.1 Replicative cycles of (A) DNA and (B) RNA viruses.

d. Protease inhibitors: saquinavir, amprenavir, ritonavir, indinavir, nelfinavir, lopinavir, atazanavir, fosamprenavir, tipranavir, darunavir
e. Integrase inhibitors (integrase strand transfer inhibitor): raltegravir, elvitegravir, dolutegravir, bictegravir
f. Fusion peptide inhibitor (GP41 inhibitor): enfuvirtide, albuvirtide
g. Adhesion inhibitor (GP120 inhibitor): fostemsavir
h. CCR5 receptor inhibitor: maraviroc

2. Antiherpesvirus:
   a. DNA polymerase UL30 inhibitors: Acyclovir, valaciclovir, idoxuridine, trifluridine, foscarnet, fomivirsen, famciclovir, and penciclovir.
   b. Envelope protein inhibitor: docosanol

3. Antiinfluenza virus:
   a. RNA polymerase inhibitors: Baloxavir marboxil, favipiravir
   b. Neuraminidase inhibitors: oseltamivir, zanamivir, peramivir, laninamivir
   c. Matrix protein 2 (M2): amantadine, rimantadine
4. Antihepatitis B virus:
   a. HBV DNA polymerase inhibitor: adefovir dipivoxil, besifovir, entecavir, telbivudine, TAF, TDF.
5. Antihepatitis C virus:
   a. HCV NS3/4A protease inhibitors: glecaprevir, grazoprevir, paritaprevir, simeprevir, vaniprevir, danoprevir
   b. HCV NS5A phosphoprotein inhibitors: ombitasvir, elbasvir, velpatasvir, daclatasvir, ledipasvir, pibrentasvir
   c. HCV NS5B polymerase inhibitors: sofosbuvir, dasabuvir
6. Antivaricella virus:
   a. VZV DNA polymerase inhibitor: acyclovir, brivudine, famciclovir, valaciclovir, vidarabine
7. Anticytomegalovirus:
   a. DNA polymerase inhibitors: cidofovir, ganciclovir, foscarnet, valganciclovir
8. Antirespiratory syncytial virus (RSV):
   a. Monoclonal antibody: palivizumab
9. Anti-SARS CoV-2 (coronavirus 2):
   a. SARS CoV-2 polymerase inhibitor: remdesivir, favipiravir

Elsulfavirine was approved in Russia; albuvirtide was approved in China; favipiravir and laninamivir were approved in Japan; danoprevir was approved in China and the Philippines; besifovir was approved in South Korea (Table 20.1).[19,20]

Pathophysiology of viruses

Human immunodeficiency virus

Human immunodeficiency virus (HIV) is a common retrovirus which belongs to a family lentivirus.[21] HIV impairs the body defense mechanism by targeting and depleting $CD4^+$ lymphocyte/T cells. The surface glycoprotein (gp120) of HIV has strong affinity for cells containing CD4 receptor on their surface which is predominantly present on $CD4^+$ T cells (T-helper cells); other cells like microphage, monocytes, microglial cells also possess CD4 receptor in less density. HIV enters the $CD4^+$ cells by attaching itself to the CD4 receptor and a coreceptor chemokine. Once it enters the CD4 cell cytoplasm, viral RNA gets converted to DNA with the help of viral enzyme reverse transcriptase (RT). This viral DNA is integrated with the nucleus of the CD4 + cell in the presence of the viral integrase enzyme. This process is

TABLE 20.1 List of viruses with their specific targets and novel inhibitors.

Sl. no.	Human viruses	Viral targets	Novel inhibitors
1.	HIV	Protease	TMB-607, TMC-310911, GRL-09510
		NRTIs	MK-8504, MK-8583, racivir, islatravir, rovafovir etalafenamide, stavudine, amdoxovir, elvucitabine
		NNRTIs	KM-023
		Integrase	Cabotegravir
		Gp41	GSK373239
2.	Hepatitis C virus	NS3/4A protease	Asunaprevir, faldaprevir, furaprevir, narlaprevir, seraprevir, vaniprevir, vedroprevir
		NS5A phosphoprotein	Ravidasvir, ruzasvir, odalasvir
		NS5B polymerase	sofosbuvir, deleobuvir, lomibuvir, mericitabine, radalbuvir
3.	Human influenza virus	RNA polymerase	Pimodivir
		Neuraminidase	Isocorilagin
4.	HSV	DNA polymerase UL30	Synguanol, filociclovir, MBX-2168, mitoxantrone dihydrochloride
		Envelope proteins	NGI-1, C19
5.	HCMV	DNA polymerase UL54	Filociclovir
6.	Hepatitis B virus	DNA polymerase	Tenofovir exalidex

HCMV, Human cytomegalovirus; *HIV*, human immunodeficiency virus; *HSV*, herpes simplex virus; *NRTIs*, nucleoside reverse transcriptase inhibitors; *NNRTIs*, nonnucleoside reverse transcriptase inhibitors.

called integration. Now, at this stage, $CD4^+$ cell (host cell) acts as a factory to produce more HIV. The new DNA formed then undergoes transcription and translation process, enabling the production of new viral proteins. All new viral particles replicated in $CD4^+$ T cells gather and bud out of the host cell and through circulation, it enters the lymphoid tissues where it multiplies and spread the infection. Under the influence of enzyme protease, the new virus becomes infectious virions.[22–24]

Pathophysiological changes in different organs & systems are briefly mentioned next[25–30]:

1. *Wasting syndrome:* The drastic fall in body's immune system is indicated as wasting syndrome, which refers to unintended decrease in body weight >10%; factors that are responsible are malnutrition, high BMR, malabsorption, problems of multiple opportunistic infections.
2. *Persistent generalized lymphadenopathy:* At initial stage, some patients may develop persistent generalized lymphadenopathy. It refers to massive enlargement of lymph nodes >1 cm at two or more extrainguinal sites. Proliferation of lymphocytic cells causes marked cortical follicular hyperplasia. At an advanced stage of AIDS, there are progressive destructions of lymphoid cells, or appearance of secondary tumors (e.g., Kaposi's sarcoma, lymphoma) or opportunistic infections.
3. *GI lesions manifestations:* GI manifestations include chronic dysentery, oral candidiasis, mucosal ulcers, and abdominal pain. In advanced cases, there is the development of secondary tumors in gastrointestinal tract (GIT).
4. *Pulmonary lesions and manifestations:* There are more chances of opportunistic infections causing pneumonia and tuberculosis, lung abscess, adult respiratory distress syndrome, and secondary tumors which may also develop.
5. *Mucocutaneous lesions and manifestations:* Erythematous rash and other allergic reactions occur. Secondary viral infections such as herpes, varicella zoster, and bacterial and fungal infections are more susceptible to occur.
6. *Hematologic lesions and manifestations:* Bone marrow suppression causes anemia, thrombocytopenia, and leucopenia.
7. Central nervous system *lesions and manifestation:* AIDS, neurological conditions are HIV encephalopathy or AIDS-associated dementia complex. Other pathological lesions are demyelinating and degenerative spinal cord and peripheral neuropathy and lymphoma of the brain.
8. *Renal lesions and manifestations:* HIV-associated nephropathy and genitourinary tract infections.
9. *Hepatobiliary lesions and manifestations:* Factors that are responsible are the development of coinfection with hepatitis B or C or other infectious and drug-induced hepatic toxicity. The hepatic lesions include steatoses and granulomatous hepatitis.
10. *Cardiovascular lesions and manifestations:* It includes dilated cardiomyopathy and pericardial effusion due to opportunistic infection and secondary neoplasm.
11. *Musculoskeletal lesions:* It includes osteoporosis, osteopenia, septic arthritis, polymyositis, and osteomyelitis.

12. *Endocrine lesions:* It is associated with a syndrome of lipodystrophy, which may be the result of dyslipidemia, hyperinsulinemia, and hyperglycemia. Thyroid function may alter, hypogonadism may occur, and ADH secretion may be inappropriate.

Antihuman immunodeficiency virus drugs

Nucleoside reverse transcriptase inhibitors

NRTIs are the first category of HIV drugs to be approved by food and drug administration (FDA). NRTIs are administered as prodrugs that undergo phosphorylation by cellular kinases[31,32] prior mounting its effect. 3′-hydroxyl group lacks at 2′-deoxyribosyl moiety of the NRTIs which obstruct 3′-5′-phosphodiester bond development between the NRTIs and incoming 5′-nucleoside triphosphates thus ending the formation of new viral DNA chain. Chain elongation can be stopped during DNA- or RNA-dependent DNA synthesis, inhibiting the formation of either the sense or antisense strands of the HIV-1 proviral DNA.[33,34]

Zidovudine

It is a thymidine analog (AZT) that is phosphorylated to triphosphate in host cell and selectively blocks viral RT and terminates proviral DNA synthesis. It is effective against HIV-1, HIV-2, and human T-cell lymphotropic virus.[35–38]

Stavudine

Stavudine is synthetic thymidine analog that function as AZT. It is used in multidrug regimen for the treatment of HIV infections. But it should not be combined with AZT as it antagonizes its action and also with didanosine because both cause peripheral neuropathy.[38–40]

Lamivudine (3TC) and emtricitabine (FTC)

Lamivudine and emtricitabine are analogs of deoxycytidine (ddC) where the 3′ carbon has been replaced by sulfur.

Cellular enzymes Phosphorylate emtricitabine to emtricitabine 5′-triphosphate.

These prodrugs are nucleoside analog inhibitors of HIV RT, which are needed to be converted in their active triphosphate forms by cellular kinases. The triphosphate forms compete with nucleotide substrates for internalization into new DNA chain. Usually, they function as chain terminators due to the absence of a 3′-OH.[38,41]

Abacavir

Abacavir is not a traditional NRTI. Along with the incorporation in the proviral DNA and termination of chain elongation, it selectively acts against HIV RT. Abacavir is converted to carbovir triphosphate (CBV-TP) which is an activated form of abacavir.[42]

Protein priming in viral RT delivers an additional site for nucleoside inhibitors. Since dGTP is the initiating nucleotide for HIV protein priming, guanosine analogs like abacavir are potential drugs interfering in this step of HIV replication.[41]

Nucleotide reverse transcriptase inhibitors

Tenofovir

TFV is an analog of adenosine 5′-monophosphate,[38] available in the form of prodrug, TDF, and TAF. The prodrugs are hydrolyzed to TFV in liver that later gets phosphorylated by cellular kinase to active diphosphate form. The activated TFV gets incorporated into viral DNA and terminates chain elongation by inhibiting HIV RT enzyme.[43,44]

NNRTIs are a very promising class of anti-HIV drugs which blocks the polymerization of HIV RT, an enzyme responsible for conversion of single-stranded viral RNA genome to double-stranded viral DNA genomes. The accurate mode of action of NNRTIs is yet to be elucidated; but it has been confirmed that by binding to the drug-binding site of HIV-1, RT leads to change in position of the attachment of the template primer, thereby inhibiting the binding of dNTP to form an RT–DNA–dNTP complex.

HIV RT, an asymmetric heterodimer contains two subunits: (1) p66 subunit (560 amino acids)—it has a role in performing the enzymatic functions of the RT; (2) p51 subunit (440 amino acids)—it works to provide the structural and conformational support. The noncompetitive NNRTIs are targeted allosterically to a hydrophobic domain. The NNRTIs act against HIV-1 strains only, because HIV-2 RT has been found to possess amino acids that render innate resistance to NNRTIs.

Efavirenz (EFV) is given in combination with two other NRTIs (e.g., EFV + TDF + FTC, EFV + TDF + 3TC) for initial treatment. It is a benzoxazinone compound having oral bioavailability of 40%–45%. It is observed that when administered once daily, it is highly effective in reducing HIV-1 viral loads, but it affects neuropsychiatric nervous system.

RPV was approved by the US FDA in 2011. RPV, a diarylpyrimidine compound, is used to overcome the resistance of NNRTI that was caused due to mutation. It is widely used due to its high efficacy, specificity, high oral bioavailability, easy synthesis, and minimum harmful effects. RPV is often suggested for treating patients having low RNA copies/mL, but not for those with high RNA copies/mL.

NVP is first NNRTI to be approved by US FDA in 1996. From studies, it is said that NVP has a poor resistance barrier, less efficacy, and serious life-threatening effects. The development of new-generation NNRTIs declined the use of NVP in initial therapy or the postexposure prophylaxis. NVP is a dipyridodiazepinone inhibitor and known for its low solubility and high intestinal permeability.

Elsulfavirine, a prodrug of VM-1500A, has been approved only in Russia (2017). The recommended dose is 20 mg/day, which is to be taken 15 min prior to a meal. Elsulfavirine has shown excellent antiviral properties in treatment-naive patients. It has shown to be well tolerated with some side effects, including headache, dizziness, and diarrhea.

Doravirine possesses excellent antiviral property, favorable safety, better tolerability, high barrier to drug resistance, and drug–drug interactions. The daily single dose of DOR + TDF + 3TC is offered as an initial regimen for treatment-naive patients. Its pharmacodynamic profiles are better compared to other drugs of this group. It is highly potent in suppressing viral replication. Furthermore, it possesses a broad-spectrum inhibitory activity against different subtypes of HIV-1 strains.

Etravirine belongs to second-generation NNRTI for HIV-1 treatment. It is recommended in patients who have undergone treatment experience due to its high genetic barrier and clinical effectiveness. It is a diarylpyrimidine compound with a low solubility and permeability, and also oral bioavailability is less. It shows little activity against HIV.[38,45]

Protease inhibitors

These group of drugs are potent inhibitors of viral protease enzyme. The enzyme protease is responsible for the cleavage of viral structural and replicative proteins such as gag-pol proteins, essential for the production of virions. Inhibition of this enzyme causes disruption in the production of infectious virions.

Ritonavir

Ritonavir is an inhibitor of HIV protease enzyme that also acts as potent CYP3A4 inhibitor. It has poor tolerability so mostly given in combination regimens. It is also employed in low doses to enhance the activity of other protease inhibitors because of its potency to inhibit CYP3A4 enzyme.[46–48]

Saquinavir

Saquinavir is a protein-like substrate that attaches to the active region of protease and inhibits its action. Saquinavir comes in two forms (soft gel and hard gel capsules) with different bioavailability. When saquinavir is combined with ritonavir, maximum bioavailability is achieved. The common side effects are vomiting, nausea, and diarrhea.[46,49,50]

Indinavir

Indinavir is a protein-like substrate and shares common features like other protease inhibitors. Its use has been decreased because of adverse effects like nephrolithiasis and other renal insufficiencies. Bioavailability is decreased when taken with meals.[51,52]

Nelfinavir

Nelfinavir is effective in treating both HIV-1 and -2. It is mostly used because of its relatively low toxicity profile. For treating HIV infection, nelfinavir is generally combined with other antiretroviral drugs. Nelfinavir is the only protease inhibitor not boosted by ritonavir because CYP3A4 has less effect on its metabolism.[53,54]

Lopinavir

Lopinavir is available in fixed-dose combination with ritonavir. The combination is effective against both HIV-1 and HIV-2 infections. Ritonavir increases the plasma concentration of lopinavir by reducing its metabolism. Side effects are abdominal pain, nausea, and diarrhea.[54,55]

Atazanavir

Atazanavir is azapeptide protease inhibitor effective against both HIV-1 and -2. It is absorbed well when taken with light meal while H2 blocker/proton pump inhibitors that supress acid secretion, decrease its absorption. The efficacy is enhanced by combining with ritonavir. Side effects are the same as described earlier.[56–58]

Fosamprenavir

It is a prodrug of amprenavir. It has better bioavailability and well tolerated compared to amprenavir. It is effective in the treatment of HIV-1 and -2. It is usually provided in combination for long efficacy.[59–61]

Tipranavir

Tipranavir is a new protease inhibitor effective against both HIV-1 and -2. It has been approved for treating-experienced patients. When combined with ritonavir its bioavailability is increased. Side effect is hepatotoxicity.[62,63]

Darunavir

Darunavir is also a new protease inhibitor effective against HIV-1 and -2. It has been approved for treating resistant mutants. It is used in combination form for improved efficacy.[64,65]

Integrase inhibitors

1. *Raltegravir:* It was the first integrase strand transfer inhibitor (INSTI), with antiviral activity against HIV-1. Raltegravir is a first-line drug to be approved. It inhibits the integrase of HIV-1 thereby preventing the DNA of the virus from getting inserted into the host genome leading to the reduced propagation of infection. Human phosphoryl transferases (e.g., DNA polymerases) are not inhibited by the drug.[66]
2. *Elvitegravir:* It is an INSTI. It was first approved in a merge with cobicistat (a CYP3A4 inhibitor) to be consumed once daily. The formulation is a recommended first-line treatment.[66]
3. *Dolutegravir:* Dolutegravir is an HIV-1 antiviral agent. It is a second-generation integrase strand transfer inhibitor (INSTI). It binds to the active site of HIV integrase and thereby blocks the strand transfer step (an essential step in replication) of viral DNA integration into the host cell.[67]
4. *Bictegravir:* Bictegravir is a potent integrase strand transfer inhibitor (INSTI). Its antiviral activity is same as dolutegravir. Bictegravir is manufactured in combination with TAF and emtricitabine (FTC) in one tablet BIKTARVY.

TAF is the prodrug of TFV and is the more targeted, potent, and safe form compared to TDF. TDF is an ester analog of the nucleotide reverse transcriptase inhibitor (NRTI) TFV. In vivo, TDF is first hydrolyzed to TFV and then phosphorylated by enzyme kinases to an active metabolite TFV diphosphate, which inhibits the activity of HIV RT due to competition with the nucleotide deoxyadenosine 5′-triphosphate for getting incorporated into viral DNA and finally terminating the DNA elongation.

Emtricitabine is a nucleoside RT inhibitor related to cytosine having activity against HIV-1 infection and can be used either alone or merge with other antiretroviral drugs. It is converted intracellularly to triphosphate. This triphosphate plays a significant role in halting the DNA synthesis of HIV strains by competitive inhibition of RT.[68–71]

Fusion peptide inhibitor

1. *Enfuvirtide:* Enfuvirtide is a synthetic peptide containing 36 amino acids that mimic the heptad region 2 and inhibit the formation of stable 6-helix configuration of gp41 which is vital for the entry of HIV-1 into the host

cells. Enfuvirtide binds to HR1 region and inhibits the hairpin formation and thereby the fusion. It is the first fusion inhibitor that was used clinically. The second-generation fusion inhibitors also mimic the HR2 sequence but overlap at other regions, represented by T-1249. It is active against enfuvirtide-resistant strains.[72–75]

2. *Albuvirtide:* Albuvirtide (ABT) is a synthetic peptide derivative of N-terminal sequence of HIV-1 gp41. Studies have shown that on IV Injection, ABT rapidly binds to serum albumin and increases half-life. A recent study demonstrated its potent activity against a broad spectrum of HIV-1 strains, including those strains observed in China and some variants resistant to T20.[76,77]

Adhesion inhibitor

Fostemsavir: It is a prodrug, the active metabolite being temsavir, is the first adhesion inhibitor drug. Temsavir binds to gp120 protein present on the surface of the HIV-1 and selectively interferes between the virus and CD4 receptor interaction with the host cell, thereby stopping the attachment and further configurational changes of gp41 on HIV-1. The drug was approved in the United States on 2 July 2020 to treat HIV-1 infection in adults who are heavily treated-experienced and experiencing multiple drug resistance (MDR) HIV-1 infection, thereby disrupting their current antiretroviral regimen due to resistance, intolerance, or safety considerations.[78]

CCR5 receptor inhibitor

Maraviroc: It is a noncompetitive, slowly reversible, specific antagonist of chemokine receptor 5 coreceptor that helps in the entry of CCR5-tropic HIV-1 into host cells by interacting with the HIV-1 envelope protein gp120 and CD4 receptors, resulting in a structural modification of the viral envelope protein gp41 thereby permitting fusion of the viral envelope with the host cell membrane. The drug shows its effectiveness when combined with other antiretroviral drugs in adults who have already undergone treatment. It has potent activity against MDR CCR5-tropic HIV-1 strains. It is the first CCR5 coreceptor antagonist to be approved by US FDA.[79]

Herpesvirus

Herpes simplex virus (HSV) is of two types—HSV1 and HSV2.

HSV1 is responsible for vascular lesions on skin, lips, and mucous membranes, whereas HSV2 causes primarily genital infection (Fig. 20.2).[80,81]

It transmits through close contact with an infected person or through their genital or oral secretions.[82]

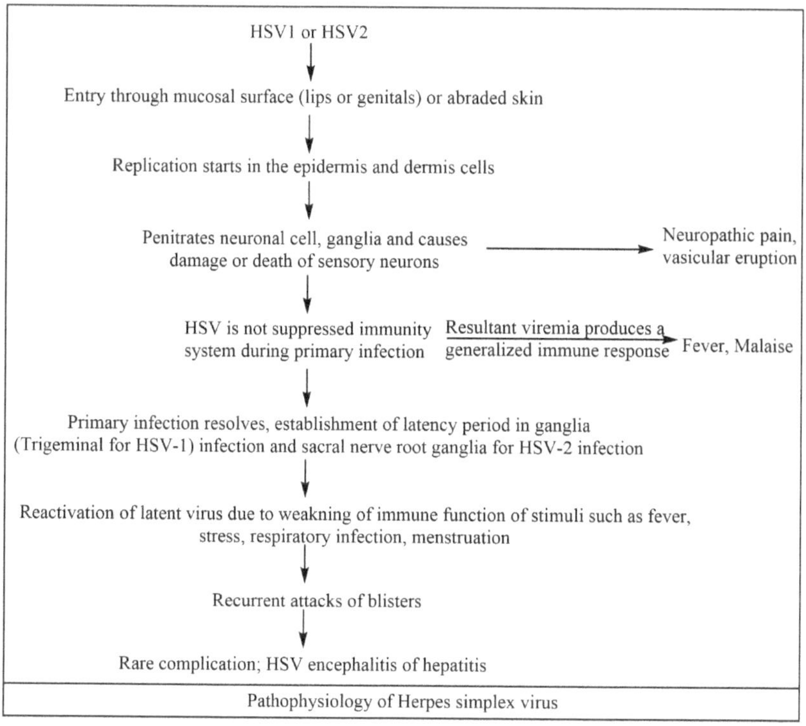

FIGURE 20.2 Pathophysiology of herpes simplex virus.

Antiherpes drugs

Acyclovir and valacyclovir

Mechanism of action: Acyclovir, a prototype, is a deoxiguanosine analog, which undergoes three phosphorylation steps to get converted into its active metabolite. First step involves its conversion to acyclovir monophosphate by viral thymidine kinase, so acyclovir selectively attacks infected cells only. Then cellular kinase of host cell converts monophosphate to diphosphate and finally to active acyclovir triphosphate. Acyclovir triphosphate acts by competitively inhibiting the viral DNA polymerase and stopping the elongation of viral DNA strand by getting incorporated into it. This terminated DNA template attaches the DNA polymerase and inhibits its action irreversibly. Affinity for viral DNA polymerase is 10–30 times more than the host cell DNA polymerase.

Acyclovir resistance develops due to the mutation of viral thymidine kinase, which decreases thymidine kinase activity or altered substrate specificity and DNA polymerase resistance to acyclovir activity.[83,84]

Valacyclovir is an ester (L-valine) prodrug of acyclovir with improved bioavailability. After oral administration, it gets converted to acyclovir during first-pass metabolism through the liver and kidney.

Both drugs are highly effective against initial herpes infections than recurrent HSV infections. These drugs are effectively used in immunosuppressed patients because they are more vulnerable to both severe HSV and varicella zoster virus (VZV) infections. Higher doses of acyclovir are used for treating VZV infection because they are less susceptible than HSV. Currently valacyclovir is used in VZV infection and recurrent genital herpes as the resultant acyclovir after oral valacyclovir has a comparable bioavailability to that of IV acyclovir. Acyclovir is therapeutically ineffective against established cytomegalovirus (CMV) and Epstein–Barr virus (EBV).[85,86]

Penciclovir and famciclovir

Penciclovir is a guanine nucleoside analog and configurationally similar to acyclovir. Famciclovir is the diacetyl ester prodrug of penciclovir.

Penciclovir inhibits viral DNA synthesis in the same mechanism as antiviral drug acyclovir, although it is less potent than acyclovir. Famciclovir is active against HSV and herpes zoster but is resistant to acyclovir-resistant strains.[87]

Idoxuridine

Idoxuridine is an iodinated deoxyuridine that acts as thymidine analog. It competitively inhibits replication of viral DNA by replacing thymidine and itself getting incorporated into the viral DNA strand. However, idoxuridine lacks selectivity and gets incorporated into DNA of uninfected cells which causes toxicity. Its use is limited to topical ophthalmic treatment of HSV virus keratitis.[1–3]

Trifluridine

Trifluridine is a fluorinated thymidine analog that is effective against both types of HSV, CMV, and other related viruses. Trifluridine blocks viral DNA polymerase enzyme and thus inhibits DNA synthesis and is effective against acyclovir-resistant HSV strains. It also inhibits host cell DNA synthesis and therefore exhibits cytotoxicity.[1–3]

Foscarnet

The inorganic pyrophosphate analog, foscarnet, prevents replication of herpesvirus, including cytomegalovirus and HIV.

Mechanism of action: Foscarnet interacts with the viral DNA polymerase enzyme or HIV RT and thereby inhibits the viral nucleic acid synthesis. Foscarnet inhibits the pyrophosphate region of the herpetic DNA polymerase, stopping cleavage of the pyrophosphate from newly attached nucleotide and thus inhibits the viral chain elongation. It is 100 times more selective for viral DNA polymerase.[87]

Docosanol

Docosanol is a saturated long alcohol chain, which is allowed in some countries as over the counter 10% ointment for herpes orolabialis. Docosanol prevents the replication of lipid-enveloped viruses such as HSV strains, CMV, and some RNA virus, including influenza virus. It prevents the viral entry into host cell by blocking the fusion between host cell membrane and viral envelope. Viral resistance is minimal as it does not affect viral replication process.[88]

Influenza virus

Influenza viruses are most prevalent as a seasonal infection and are most common cause of respiratory tract infection. It has become most significant in developing countries because they possess high death rate in immune-distressed patients, elderly individuals, and infants. Influenza virus contains single-stranded RNA as its genetic material and belongs to Orthomyxoviridae family.

There are three distinct types of influenza virus: A, B, and C; out of these, influenza A and B are highly contagious to humans. Influenza A virus is further subdivided into a number of subtypes on the basis of antigenic properties of envelop proteins, namely, hemagglutinin (H) and neuraminidase (N); 16 distinct HA subtypes and 9 subtypes of N have been discovered so far.[89]

Pathophysiology: Human respiratory epithelium is the main site of influenza virus replication where surface protein *Haemagglutinin* is cleaved effectively thereby generating new virions.

Viral transmission takes place through contaminated nasal and respiratory droplets. Influenza A is the prevailing viral cause of acute respiratory distress syndrome and pneumonia.

The viral infection of respiratory epithelium generates immune response to combat viral spreading resulting in lung inflammation. This inflammation can rigorously spread and cause multiple organ failures.

Host and viral mechanism of influenza-associated pathogenesis:

Virus-induced pathology includes:

- epithelial necrosis involving shrinkage and vacuolization followed by shedding of these cells,
- deterioration of alveolar structure,

- obstruction of airways resulting inadequate gas exchange, and
- structural changes appear due to degradation of extracellular matrix.[90]

Antiinfluenza drugs

Baloxavir marboxil

Baloxavir marboxil is a prodrug of bolaxavir acid, in which phenolic hydroxyl group is added to increase oral absorption. Influenza A and B viruses are composed of basic polymerase 1 (PB1) and 2 (PB2) as well as polymerase acidic protein (PA). Baloxavir inhibits viral replication by targeting endonuclease a protein required for viral transcription by cleaving capped mRNA which is bound to PB2. Resistance may develop due to mutation in PA subunit of influenza viruses, therefore interfering in cap-dependent endonuclease inhibition by baloxavir.[91]

Favipiravir: Favipiravir is a nucleotide precursor, undergoes phosphorylation by host cell enzymes into favipiravir-ribofuranosyl-5′-triphosphate (F-RTP), an active form. It is active against viral RNA-dependent RNA polymerase. The antiviral spectrum includes all subtypes and strains of influenza viruses, also comprising those resistant to neuraminidase and M2 inhibitors. F-RTP has high affinity for viral replication than host cell transcription and, therefore, has high selective index. Mutation facilitates the development of resistance against the drug.[92]

Oseltamivir and zanamivir

1. *Oseltamivir*: Oseltamivir is a sialic acid analog, effective against wide spectrum viral activity covering amantadine and rimantadine sensitive as well as resistant, some zanamivir-resistant and influenza A virus. Oseltamivir is hydrolyzed during absorption by hepatic enzymes to an activated form—oseltamivir carboxylate. The antiviral activity and potency of oseltamivir carboxylate are similar to zanamivir.
2. Mechanism of action: It inhibits the influenza virus neuraminidase enzyme which is important for liberation of progeny virions from infected cells. Thus, blockage of neuraminidase activity causes viral accumulation at cell surface and check viral spread. Resistance can be developed by mutation of viral neuraminidase enzyme.[38,87]
3. *Zanamivir*: Zanamivir is also a neuraminidase inhibitor that acts against influenza A and influenza B viruses and other resistant variants of amantadine and rimantadine drugs. The mode of action, potency, and clinical use is similar to that of oseltamivir. Oral bioavailability is very low so it is administered by inhalation.[38,87]
4. *Peramivir*: Peramivir is a new FDA-approved neuraminidase inhibitor, indicated in serious condition of hospitalized patients with H1N1

influenza infection. Peramivir is used as IV because its oral bioavailability is very poor.
5. *Laninamivir*: Laninamivir is a new neuraminidase inhibitor, active against oseltamivir-resistant influenza strains. It is administered as inhaler.[1,2]

Amantadine and rimantadine

Amantadine and rimantadine (x-methyl analog of amantadine) are synthetic tricyclic amines with similar pharmacological profile. Both drugs are effective for treating influenza A virus but ineffective against influenza B virus and mumps virus.

They inhibit initial step of viral replication by preventing uncoating of viral RNA as well as the later step, that is, viral assembly. The M2 protein, present within the membrane of influenza A virus, acts as primary sight of action and, thus inhibiting, M2 protein prevents H^+-mediated dissociation of ribonucleotide complex, which is an important step in viral replication. M2 inhibition potentiates acidic pH-induced conformational alteration of hemagglutinin and hence blocks viral assembly. Resistance for amantadine and rimantadine develops due to mutation in M2 protien.[87]

Hepatitis virus

Hepatitis viruses infect liver causing inflammation and necrosis. It is one of the main causes of illness and death globally. Hepatitis virus includes hepatitis A, B, C, D, and E viruses. Hepatitis A does not cause chronic infection whereas hepatitis B, C, and D cause cirrhosis, liver failure, and hepatocellular carcinoma (Fig. 20.3).[92]

Antihepatitis B drugs

1. *Adefovir dipivoxil*: Adefovir is an acyclic analog of adenosine monophosphate. Adefovir dipivoxil is deesterified to adefovir that undergoes phosphorylation to activated diphosphate by cellular enzymes. It competitively blocks DNA polymerase of hepatitis B virus and causes chain termination. It may cause nephrotoxicity if the treatment continues for 1 year.[1–3,96]
2. Telbivudine: Telbivudine, synthetic analog of thymidine, that is, is phosphorylated to triphosphate form by cellular kinase enzyme that inhibits HBV DNA polymerase and prevents chain elongation. It is used to treat chronic hepatitis B infection.[97]
3. *Entecavir*: Entecavir is guanosine analog that undergoes phosphorylation to form active triphosphate intracellularly. It competitively blocks all functions of HBV polymerase (RT) and hence prevents viral replication.[87]
4. *Besifovir*: Besifovir is a new acyclic nucleotide phosphonate that inhibits viral DNA polymerase. The active triphosphate form gets incorporated into viral DNA and inhibits DNA synthesis.[87]

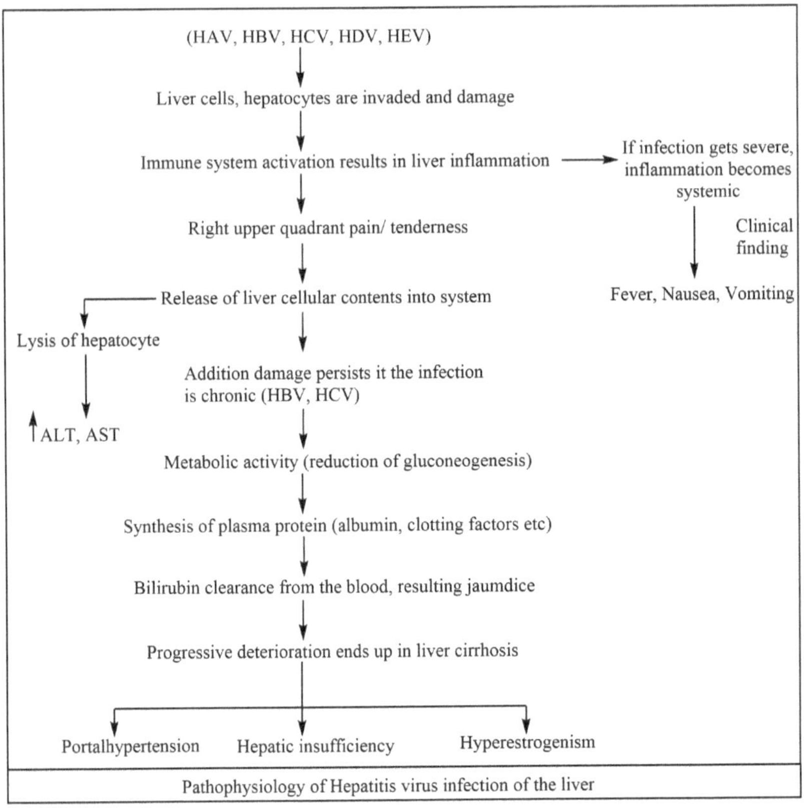

FIGURE 20.3 Pathophysiology of Hepatitis virus infection of the liver.[93–95]

5. *TAF*: TAF (prodrug) is a phosphonate derivative of TFV. It inhibits RT of HBV and HIV-1 virus. TAF is deesterified in liver and phosphorylated to TFV diphosphate, which blocks RT competitively, thus preventing chain elongation.[1,2]
6. TDF: TDF, a prodrug of TFV, is an inhibitor of RT, which is effective against HIV and hepatitis B virus.

Antihepatitis C drugs

1. *Glecaprevir/pibrentasvir*: Glecaprevir is a novel hepatitis C NS3/4A protease inhibitor. It is effective against all genotypes 1–6 of HCV. It is also effective against HCV protease from genotype 3 that is very difficult to treat. It is used in a combination with NS5A inhibitor pibrentasvir. Pibrentasvir is a novel NS5A inhibitor, which is active against all

common resistance-associated variants. Glecaprevir and pibrentasvir are coformulated as fixed-dose combination tablet.[98]

2. *Grazoprevir/elbasvir*: Grazoprevir an HCV NS3/4A protease inhibitor and is developed as single fixed-dose combination tablet with elbasvir, NS5A inhibitor. Grazoprevir inhibits HCV NS3/4A protease that is responsible for the proteolytic breakdown of viral replication and viral-encoded polyprotein and prevents the formation of viral RNA. Food and drug administration (FDA) has approved the combination for treating HCV genotype 1 or 4 infection.[99]
3. *Paritaprevir/ombitasvir/dasabuvir/ritonavir*: Paritaprevir is NS3 protease inhibitor and ombitasvir is NS5A phosphoprotein inhibitor. Dasabuvir inhibits the active sight of NS5B polymerase resulting in conformational change in NS5B. Ritonavir is CYP3A inhibitor and not effective against HCV, and it is used to decrease the frequency of dosing.[2]
4. *Simeprevir*: Simeprevir is a macrocyclic HCV NS3 protease inhibitor that prevents protease's cleavage of viral polyprotein thus checks viral replication in infected cells.[100]
5. *Vaniprevir* and *danoprevir* are direct-acting antivirals that act against HCV NS3/4A protease and exhibit advancement in treatment of chronic HCV infection.[101]
6. *Velpatasvir*: Velpatasvir is NS5A protein inhibitor. This protein plays an essential role in HCV replication and is also involved in cell signaling. Velpatasvir is combined with sofosbuvir which after getting metabolized incorporates into viral RNA and terminates chain elongation process; therefore it acts as NS5B RNA-dependent RNA polymerase inhibitor. The combination is effective for treating different genotypes 1–6 of hepatitis C.
7. *Daclatasvir*: Daclatasvir is effective against both viral RNA replication and virion aggregation by binding to the N-terminus of NS5A. It is coformulated with sofosbuvir for treating HCV genotype-3 infection. In Japan a combination of daclatasvir with NS3/4A protease inhibitor is approved.[102]
8. *Ledipasvir*: Ledipasvir inhibits NS5A phosphoprotein and is manufactured as fixed-dose combination tablet with sofosbuvir.[1,2]
9. *Sofosbuvir*: Sofosbuvir is a uridine nucleotide analog that undergoes phosphorylation within the cells to produce its action. The metabolism takes place in liver cells; therefore the active compound formed is called GS-461203. This analog then competitively blocks the NS5B polymerase, thus preventing HCV-RNA synthesis by terminating RNA chain elongation.[103]

Varicella zoster virus

Varicella zoster belongs to alpha herpesvirus family with double-stranded DNA genome.[104–107] VZV being highly communicable directly infects human through direct contact with skin lesions or air borne route. Its main target sites are T-lymphocytes, epithelial cells, and ganglia.

Primary infection causes chickenpox (varicella) in adults mainly in immunocompromised individuals, which often goes severe. It is characterized by fever, rashes on skin, headache, malaise, and loss of appetite.

Zoster (shingles) generally develops after the reactivation from latent period which resides in neurons of cranial nerve ganglia, dorsal root ganglia, and enteric and autonomic ganglia.

The early symptoms are pain, itching, numbness or tingling, sensitivity to touch, a later maculopapular rash appears which develop into vesicles. Furthermore, other complications included are myelitis, cranial nerve, palsies, meningitis, and vasculopathy (Fig. 20.4).

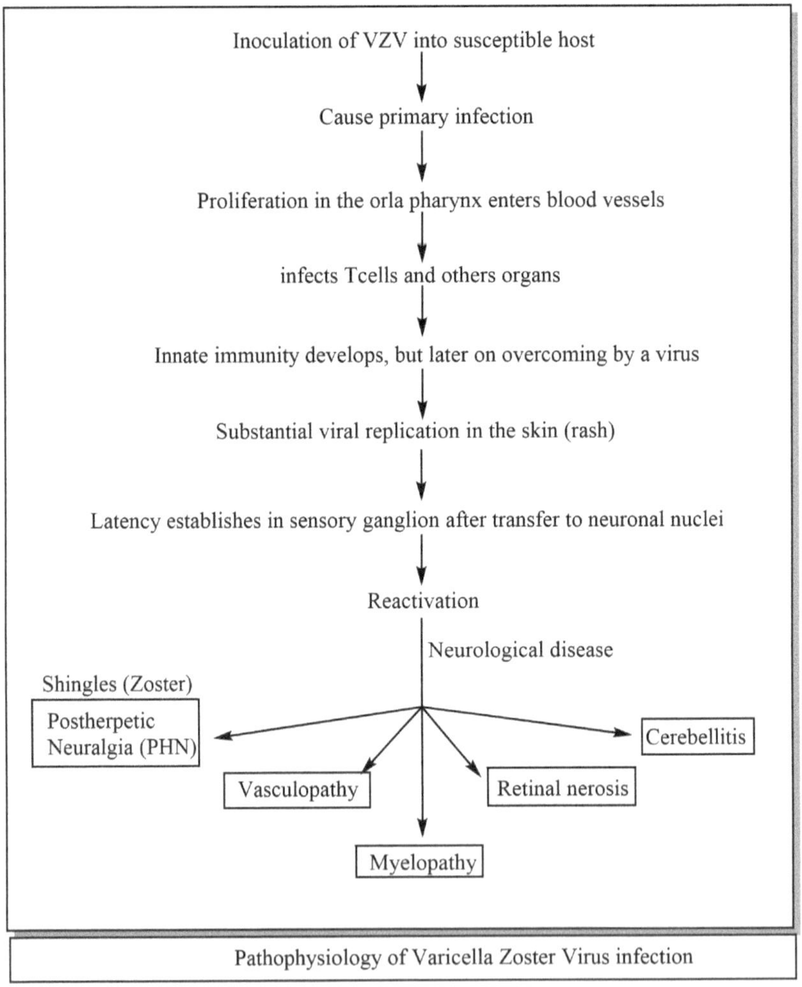

FIGURE 20.4 Pathophysiology of varicella zoster virus infection.

Antivaricella zoster virus drugs

1. *Brivudine*: Brivudine, a thymidine analog, has similar mechanism of action as acyclovir. Brivudine undergoes phosphorylation by viral thymidine kinase to an active compound which blocks viral DNA polymerase and thus prevents viral DNA synthesis. Brivudine is effective against HSV1, VZV, and EBV, but ineffective against other herpesviruses and cytomegalovirus. It is more effective against VZV compared to acyclovir and has got approval in Europe for treating herpes zoster and HSV keratitis.[82]
2. *Vidarabine*: Vidarabine is a nucleoside analog of adenine obtained from bacteria *Streptomyces antibioticus*.[2] It has an inhibitory effect on viral DNA synthesis. Like acyclovir, it blocks DNA polymerase and terminates DNA chain elongation. Selectivity of viral DNA polymerase is more compared to the host DNA polymerase. Vidarabine resistance develops due to mutation in DNA polymerase[108]

Mechanism of action of acyclovir, famciclovir, valaciclovir is discussed in antiherpes drugs.

Cytomegalovirus

Cytomegalovirus, the largest virus among herpesvirus, is double-stranded DNA virus of beta-herpesvirus subfamily.

CMV infection generally occurs during childhood, through subjection to bodily secretion (such as tears, saliva, urine, and semen) from infected person. Transmission can also occur via fomites or via organ tissue transplantation and blood transfusion.

CMV infection in healthy host is usually asymptomatic, although sometimes it may be characterized by fever, lymphadenopathy, and lymphocytosis.

After initial infection, CMV establishes latency in endothelial cell, epithelial cell, smooth-muscle cells, and fibroblasts where virus multiplies and reaches different parts of body. The initial infection produces CMV-specific immunoglobulins, IgM and IgG, that prevent and control viral replication on reactivation of viral in healthy immunocompetent host. On contrary, in immunocompromised host such as in HIV infection, patients of organ transplantation or hematopoietic stem-cell transplant suffer low CMV-specific T cells, therefore unchecked viral replication, leading to subsequent clinical diseases.[109,110]

Anticytomegalovirus drugs

Cidofovir: Cidofovir is a nucleotide analog of cytidine that gets phosphorylated to cidofovir diphosphate that inhibits viral DNA polymerase.[111] Oral bioavailability of cidofovir is very poor. It is given intravenously or applied topically. Cidofovir is active against acyclovir, ganciclovir, foscarnet-resistant CMV strains.

Ganciclovir and valganciclovir

Ganciclovir is a nucleoside analog of acyclovir. It is active against all herpesvirus and mostly against CMV.

1. *Mechanism of action*: Ganciclovir after conversion to active metabolite, that is, ganciclovir triphosphate, intracellularly by viral thymidine kinase preferentially, inhibits viral DNA polymerase and, thereby, terminates its replication. Ganciclovir triphosphate exhibits much higher concentration in CMV-infected cells.
2. *Valganciclovir* is a prodrug (L-valine ester) of ganciclovir. It is metabolized to ganciclovir after being absorbed in GIT and has higher bioavailability, about 60%.

Resistance to ganciclovir develops in a similar manner as developed in acyclovir: mutation of the protein kinase gene owing to reduced intracellular ganciclovir phosphorylation and mutation of DNA polymerase.

Antirespiratory syncytial virus drugs

Palivizumab: Palivizumab is a humanized monoclonal antibody, effective against the RSV F (RSV surface glycoprotein, helps virus to fuse with cell and form syncytia). It neutralizes RSV and prevents viral fusion with respiratory endothelial, thereby preventimg replication. It is used to treat RSV infection in children and infants.[112]

Severe acute respiratory syndrome coronavirus 2

Coronavirus is an enveloped and unsegmented virus, composing capped (+) single-stranded RNA. Coronavirus belongs to family Coronaviridae.[113,114] It transmits through respiratory droplets and aerosols. The virus attaches itself to host receptor and enters through fusion or endocytosis. The virus is made of four proteins, named, the spike (S), membrane (M), envelop (E), and nucleocapsid (N) proteins. The spike protein helps in the attachment and penetration. This protein contains two subunits (S1 and S2); S1 helps in binding and S2 subunit helps in fusion of virus and host cellular membranes (Fig. 20.5).

Anti-Covid drugs

Remdesivir: Remdesivir is a nucleoside analog, which blocks the viral RNA-dependent RNA polymerase (RdRp), interfering the viral genome replication

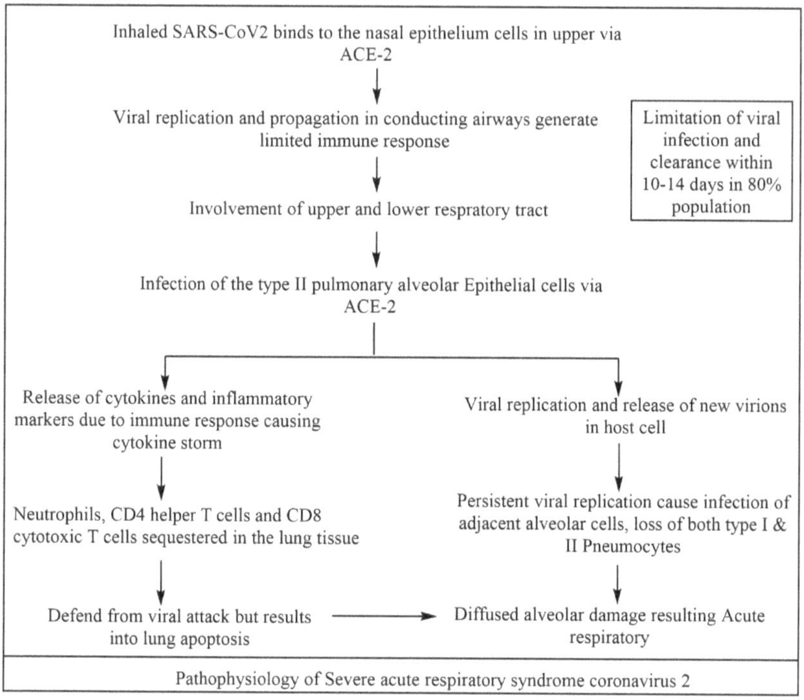

FIGURE 20.5 Pathophysiology of severe acute respiratory syndrome coronavirus 2.

process. Nucleoside analogs are required to undergo phosphorylation to easily permeate the cell wall. The phosphorylated compound formed is nucleoside triphosphate which resembles adenosine triphosphate (ATP) and plays a role in genome replication. The phosphorylated remdesivir competes with ATP and gets integrated by the RdRp enzymes or complex and thereby terminates RNA synthesis and viral replication.[115]

Conclusion

The emergence of newer antivirals has changed the landscape of antiviral therapies but still there is a lacuna in the prevention of emerging and reemerging viral infections. To fight a pandemic situation like recently, we encountered one, that is, Covid-19 infection; broad spectrum antivirus should be explored. For identification of lead compounds to target host proteins, potential natural bioactives should be looked into. This chapter is a small contribution in the path of development of novel antivirals for targeting emerging and reemerging viral infection.

References

1. Sharma HL, Sharma KK. *Sharma & Sharma's Principles of Pharmacology*. 3rd ed. Paras Medical Publisher; 2017.
2. Brunton L, Knollman B, Hilal-Dandan R. *Goodman and Gilman's The Pharmacological Basis of Therapeutics*. 13th ed. McGraw Hill Professional; 2017.
3. Thripathi KD. *Essentials of Medical Pharmacology*. 13th ed. Jaypee Brothers Medical Publishers; 2018.
4. Fields BN, Knipe DM, Howley PM. *Fields Virology*. 6th ed. Lippincott Williams & Wilkins; 2013.
5. Enquist LW. Virology in the 21st century. *J Virol*. 2009;83:5296–5308.
6. Cann AJ. *Replication of Viruses*. Leicester: Elsevier; 2008.
7. Mayo MA, Pringle CR. Virus taxonomy-1997. *J Gen Virol*. 1998;79:649–657.
8. De Clercq E, et al. A novel selective broad-spectrum anti-DNA virus agent. *Nature*. 1986;323:464–467.
9. Lou Z, Sun Y, Rao Z. Current progress in antiviral strategies. *Trends Pharmacol Sci*. 2014;35:86–102.
10. Yu F, Lu L, Du L, et al. Approaches for identification of HIV-1 entry inhibitors targeting gp41 pocket. *Viruses*. 2013;5:127–149.
11. McDonald CK, Kuritzkes DR. Human immunodeficiency virus type 1 protease inhibitors. *Arch Intern Med*. 1997;157:951.
12. Kiser JJ, Flexner C. Direct-acting antiviral agents for hepatitis C virus infection. *Annu Rev Pharmacol Toxicol*. 2013;53:427–449.
13. Kiser JJ, Flexner C. Direct-acting antiviral agents for hepatitis C virus infection. *Annu Rev Pharmacol Toxicol*. 2013;53:427–449.
14. Buttinelli G, Donati V, Fiore S, et al. Nucleotide variation in Sabin type 2 poliovirus from an immunodeficient patient with poliomyelitis. *J Gen Virol*. 2003;84:1215–1221.
15. Akaike T. Role of free radicals in viral pathogenesis and mutation. *Rev Med Virol*. 2001;11:87–101.
16. Kumari R, et al. Pretective effect of *Basella alba* leaf against diabetic nephropathy in rats. *Adv Tradit Med*. 2021;21:111–119.
17. Armogida M, Nisticò R, Mercuri NB. Therapeutic potential of targeting hydrogen peroxide metabolism in the treatment of brain ischaemia. *Br J Pharmacol*. 2012;166:1211–1224.
18. Ratnam DV, Ankola DD, Bhardwaj V, et al. Role of antioxidants in prophylaxis and therapy: a pharmaceutical perspective. *J Control Release*. 2006;113:189–207.
19. Li G, et al. *Antiviral classification*. 4th ed. *Encyclopedia of Virology*. Vol. 5. Elsevier; 2021.
20. De Clerq E. Fifty years in search of selective antiviral drugs. *J Med Chem*. 2019;2019 (62):7322–7339.
21. Arts EJ, Hazuda JD. HIV-1 antiretroviral drug therapy. *Cold Spring Harb Perspect Med*. 2012;2012(2):a007161.
22. German Advisory Committee Blood (Arbeitskreis Blut), Subgroup 'Assessment of Pathogens Transmissible by Blood'. Human immunodeficiency virus (HIV). *Transfus Med Hemother*. 2016;43(3):203–222.
23. Freed OE. HIV-1 replication. *Somatic Cell Mol Genet*. 2001;26(1/6). Nov 2001 (©2002).
24. Walker MC, et al. CD8 + lymphocytes can control HIV infection in vitro by suppressing virus replication. *Science*. 1986;234:1563–1566. Available from: http://science.sciencemag.org/. on April 25, 2017.

25. Levy AJ. Pathogenesis of human immunodeficiency virus infection. *Microbiol Rev.* 1993;1993:183–289.
26. Kreuzer KA, Rockstroh J. Pathogenesis and pathophysiology of anemia in HIV infection. *Ann Hematol.* 1997;75:179–187.
27. John Palios NPE. The pathophysiology of HIV-/HAART-related metabolic syndrome leading to cardiovascular disorders: the emerging role of adipokines. *J Diabetes Res.* 2012;2012. Kadoglou, Stylianos Lampropoulos, Article ID 103063, 7 pages.
28. Rothman MS, Bessesen MT. HIV infection and osteoporosis: pathophysiology, diagnosis, and treatment options. *Curr Osteoporos Rep.* 2012;10:270–277.
29. Nou E, Lo J, Hadigan C, Grinspoon SK. Pathophysiology and management of cardiovascular disease in patients with HIV. *Lancet Diab Endocrinol.* 2016;4(7):598–610.
30. Budka H, Costanzi G, Cristina S, et al. Brain pathology induced by infection with the human immunodeficiency virus (HIV). *Acta Neuropathol.* 1987;75:185–198.
31. Furman PA, Fyfe JA, St Clair MH, et al. Phosphorylation of 3′-azido-3′-deoxythymidine and selective interaction of the 5′-triphosphate with human immunodeficiency virus reverse transcriptase. *Proc Natl Acad Sci USA.* 1986;83(21):8333–8337.
32. Mitsuya H, Weinhold KJ, Furman PA, et al. 3′-Azido-3′-deoxythymidine (BW A509U): an antiviral agent that inhibits the infectivity and cytopathic effect of human T-lymphotropic virus type III/lymphadenopathy-associated virus in vitro. *Proc Natl Acad Sci USA.* 1985;82 (20):7096–7100.
33. Taggart AK, Kero J, Gan X, et al. (D)-beta-Hydroxybutyrate inhibits adipocyte lipolysis via the nicotinic acid receptor PUMA-G. *J Biol Chem.* 2005;280(29):26649–26652.
34. Sluis-Cremer N, Arion D, Parniak M. Molecular mechanisms of HIV-1 resistance to nucleoside reverse transcriptase inhibitors (NRTIs). *Cell Mol Life Sci.* 2000;57:1408–1422.
35. Sperling R. Zidovudine. *Infect Dis Obstet Gynecol.* 1998;6(5):197–203.
36. Anderson P.L., Rower J.E. Zidovudine and lamivudine for HIV infection. Clin Med Rev Ther. 2010;2:a2004. PMID: 20953318; PMCID: PMC2954111.
37. Piscitelli SC, Polis MA. An update on drug interactions with zidovudine. *AIDS Patient Care STDs.* 1998;12(9):687–690.
38. De Clercq E. Antiviral drugs in current clinical use. *J Clin Virol.* 2004;30(2):115–133. Available from: https://doi.org/10.1016/j.jcv.2004.02.009.
39. Mirmehrabi M, Rohani S, Jennings MC. Stavudine. *Acta Crystallogr C.* 2005;61(Pt 12): o695–o698. Available from: https://doi.org/10.1107/S0108270105034591. Epub 2005 Nov 19.
40. Hurst M, Noble S. Stavudine: an update of its use in the treatment of HIV infection. *Drugs.* 1999;58(5):919–949.
41. Menéndez-Arias L, Álvarez M, Pacheco B. Nucleoside/nucleotide analog inhibitors of hepatitis B virus polymerase: mechanism of action and resistance. *Curr Opin Virol.* 2014;8:2–3.
42. Melroy J, Nair V. The antiviral activity, mechanism of action, clinical significance and resistance of abacavir in the treatment of pediatric AIDS. *Curr Pharm Des.* 2005;11:3847–3852.
43. Kearney BP, Flaherty JF, Shah J. Tenofovir disoproxil fumarate: clinical pharmacology and pharmacokinetics. *Clin Pharmacokinet.* 2004;43(9):595–612.
44. Kaufman B, Zehtabchi S. Tenofovir for prevention of HIV infection. *Am Fam Physician.* 2017;96(1). Online.
45. Wang Y, De Clercq E;, Li G. Current and emerging non-nucleoside reverse transcriptase inhibitors (NNRTIs) for HIV-1 treatment. *Expert Opin Drug Metab Toxicol.* 2019;. *17425255.2019.1673367.*

46. Agbowuro AA, Huston WM, Gamble AB, Tyndall JDA. Proteases and protease inhibitors in infectious diseases. *Med Res Rev*. 2018;38(4):1295–1331.
47. Cvetkovic RS, Goa KL. Lopinavir/ritonavir: a review of its use in the management of HIV infection. *Drugs*. 2003;63(8):769–802.
48. Rock BM, Hengel SM, Rock DA, Wienkers LC, Kunze KL. Characterization of ritonavir-mediated inactivation of cytochrome P450 3A4. *Mol Pharmacol*. 2014;86(6):665–674.
49. Vella S, Floridia MS. Clinical pharmacology and efficacy. *Clin Pharmacokinet*. 1998;34(3):189–201.
50. la Porte CJ. Saquinavir, the pioneer antiretroviral protease inhibitor. *Expert Opin Drug Metab Toxicol*. 2009;5(10):1313–1322.
51. Pollak EB, Parmar M. *Indinavir. StatPearls*. Treasure Island, FL: StatPearls Publishing; 2020. 2021 Jan.
52. Plosker GL, Noble S. Indinavir: a review of its use in the management of HIV infection. *Drugs*. 1999;58(6):1165–1203.
53. Gupta A.K., Li B., Cerniglia G.J., Ahmed M.S., Hahn S.M., Maity A. The HIV protease inhibitor nelfinavir downregulates Akt phosphorylation by inhibiting proteasomal activity and inducing the unfolded protein response. Neoplasia. 2007;9(4):271–278. https://doi.org/10.1593/neo.07124. 17460771.
54. Flexner C. HIV-protease inhibitors. *N Engl J Med*. 1998;338:1281–1293.
55. Chandwani A, Shuter J. Lopinavir/ritonavir in the treatment of HIV-1 infection: a review. *Ther Clin Risk Manag*. 2008;4(5):1023–1033.
56. Havlir D.V., O'Marro S.D. Atazanavir: New option for treatment of HIV infection. Clin Infect Dis. 2004;38(11):1599–1604. https://doi.org/10.1086/420932.
57. Pennings PS. HIV drug resistance: problems and perspectives. *Infect Dis Rep*. 2013;5(suppl).
58. Croom KF, Dhillon S, Keam SJ. Atazanavir: a review of its use in the management of HIV-1 infection. *Drugs*. 2009;69(8):1107–1140.
59. Chapman TM, Plosker GL, Perry CM. Fosamprenavir: a review of its use in the management of antiretroviral therapy-naive patients with HIV infection. *Drugs*. 2004;64(18):2101–2124.
60. Wire MB, Shelton MJ, Studenberg S. Fosamprenavir: clinical pharmacokinetics and drug interactions of the amprenavir prodrug. *Clin Pharmacokinet*. 2006;45(2):137–168.
61. [No authors listed]. 2012. Fosamprenavir *LiverTox: Clinical and Research Information on Drug-Induced Liver Injury*. Bethesda, MD: National Institute of Diabetes and Digestive and Kidney Diseases; 2017.
62. Plosker GL, Figgitt DP. Tipranavir. *Drugs*. 2003;63(15):1611–1618.
63. King JR, Acosta EP. Tipranavir: a novel nonpeptidic protease inhibitor of HIV. *Clin Pharmacokinet*. 2006;45(7):665–682.
64. Davis DA, Soule EE, Davidoff KS, Daniels SI, Naiman NE, Yarchoan R. Activity of human immunodeficiency virus type 1 protease inhibitors against the initial autocleavage in Gag-Pol polyprotein processing. *Antimicrob Agents Chemother*. 2012;56(7):3620–3628.
65. Purohit R, Sethumadhavan R. Structural basis for the resilience of darunavir (TMC114) resistance major flap mutations of HIV-1 protease. *Interdiscip Sci*. 2009;1(4):320–328.
66. Eckhardt BJ. *Drugs for HIV infection. Infectious Diseases (Fourth Edition)*. 2. Elsevier; 2017:1293–1308.e2.
67. Rathbun RC, Lockhart SM, Miller MM, Liedtke MD. Dolutegravir, a second-generation integrase inhibitor for the treatment of HIV-1 infection. *Ann Pharmacother*. 2013;48(3):395–403.

68. Chapman T, McGavin J, Noble S. Tenofovir disoproxil fumarate. *Drugs*. 2003;63 (15):1597–1608.
69. Antela A, Aguiar C, et al. The role of tenofovir alafenamide in future HIV management. *HIV Med*. 2016;17(suppl 2):4–16.
70. Pham HT, Mesplède T. Bictegravir in a fixed-dose tablet with emtricitabine and tenofovir alafenamide for the treatment of HIV infection: pharmacology and clinical implications. *Expert Opin Pharmacother*. 2019;1–13.
71. Al-Majed AA, Bakheit AHH, Al-Qahtani BM, Al-Kahtani HM, Abdelhameed AS. Emtricitabine. *Profiles Drug Subst Excip Relat Methodol*. 2019;45(2020):55–91.
72. Mostashari Rad T, Saghaie L, Fassihi A. HIV-1 entry inhibitors: a review of experimental and computational studies. *Chem Biodivers*. 2018;15(10):e1800159.
73. Fung HB, Guo Y. Enfuvirtide: a fusion inhibitor for the treatment of HIV infection. *Clin Ther*. 2004;26(3):352–378.
74. Oldfield V, Keating GM, Plosker G. Enfuvirtide: a review of its use in the management of HIV infection. *Drugs*. 2005;65(8):1139–1160.
75. Chen RY, Kilby JM, Saag MS. Enfuvirtide. *Expert Opin Investig Drugs*. 2002;11 (12):1837–1843.
76. Zhang H, Jin R, Yao C, et al. Combination of long-acting HIV fusion inhibitor albuvirtide and LPV/r showed potent efficacy in HIV-1 patients. *AIDS Res Ther*. 2016;13:8.
77. Su B, Yao C, Zhao QX, et al. Efficacy and safety of the long-acting fusion inhibitor albuvirtide in antiretroviral-experienced adults with human immunodeficiency virus-1: interim analysis of the randomized, controlled, phase 3, non-inferiority TALENT study. *Chin Med J (Engl)*. 2020;133(24):2919–2927.
78. Markham A. Fostemsavir: first approval. *Drugs*. 2020;80(14):1485–1490.
79. Sayana S, Khanlou H. Maraviroc: a new CCR5 antagonist. *Expert Rev Anti Infect Ther*. 2008;7(1):9–19.
80. Bradshaw MJ, Venkatesan A. Herpes simplex virus-1 encephalitis in adults: pathophysiology, diagnosis, and management. *Neurotherapeutics*. 2016;13(3):493–508.
81. Mustafa M, Illzam EM, Muniandy RK, Sharifah AM, Nang MK, Ramesh B. Herpes simplex virus infections, pathophysiology and management. *IOSR J Dent Med Sci (IOSR-JDMS)*. 2016;15(7):85–91. *e-ISSN: 2279-0853, p-ISSN: 2279-0861. Ver. III (July 2016)*.
82. De SK, Hart JC, Breuer J. Herpes simplex virus and varicella zoster virus: recent advances in therapy. *Curr Opin Infect Dis*. 2015;28(6):589–595.
83. O'Brien JJ, Campoli-Richards DM. Acyclovir. An updated review of its antiviral activity, pharmacokinetic properties and therapeutic efficacy. *Drugs*. 1989;37(3):233–309.
84. Richards DM, Carmine AA, Brogden RN, Heel RC, Speight TM, Avery GS. Acyclovir. A review of its pharmacodynamic properties and therapeutic efficacy. *Drugs*. 1983;26 (5):378–438.
85. Cunha BA, Baron J. The pharmacokinetic basis of oral valacyclovir treatment of herpes simplex virus (HSV) or varicella zoster virus (VZV) meningitis, meningoencephalitis or encephalitis in adults. *J Chemother*. 2017;29(2):122–125.
86. Brantley JS, Hicks L, Sra K, Tyring SK. Valacyclovir for the treatment of genital herpes. *Expert Rev Anti Infect Ther*. 2006;4(3):367–376.
87. Razonable RR. Antiviral drugs for viruses other than human immunodeficiency virus. *Mayo Clin Proc*. 2011;86(10):1009–1026.
88. Leung DT, Sacks SL. Docosanol: a topical antiviral for herpes labialis. *Expert Opin Pharmacother*. 2004;5(12):2567–2571.
89. Luo M. Influenza virus entry. *Adv Exp Med Biol*. 2012;726:201–221.

90. Taubenberger JK, Morens DM. The pathology of influenza virus infections. *Annu Rev Pathol.* 2008;3:499–522.
91. O'Hanlon R, Shaw ML. Baloxavir marboxil: the new influenza drug on the market. *Curr Opin Virol.* 2019;35:14–18.
92. Goldhill DH, Te Velthuis AJW, Fletcher RA, et al. The mechanism of resistance to favipiravir in influenza. *Proc Natl Acad Sci USA.* 2018;115(45):11613–11618.
93. Lanini S, Ustianowski A, Pisapia R, Zumla A, Ippolito G. Viral hepatitis: etiology, epidemiology, transmission, diagnostics, treatment, and prevention. *Infect Dis Clin North Am.* 2019;33(4):1045–1062.
94. Menéndez-Arias L, Álvarez M, Pacheco B. Nucleoside/nucleotide analog inhibitors of hepatitis B virus polymerase: mechanism of action and resistance. *Curr Opin Virol.* 2014;8:1–9.
95. Nainan OV, Xia G, Vaughan G, Margolis HS. Diagnosis of hepatitis a virus infection: a molecular approach. *Clin Microbiol Rev.* 2006;19(1):63–79.
96. Oakes K. Hepatitis B: prevalence and pathophysiology. *Nurs Times.* 2014;110(7):12–16.
97. Dando T, Plosker G. Adefovir dipivoxil: a review of its use in chronic hepatitis B. *Drugs.* 2003;63(20):2215–2234.
98. [No authors listed]. 2012. Telbivudine *LiverTox: Clinical and Research Information on Drug-Induced Liver Injury.* Bethesda, MD: National Institute of Diabetes and Digestive and Kidney Diseases; 2020.
99. Carrion AF, Martin P. Glecaprevir + pibrentasvir for treatment of hepatitis C. *Expert Opin Pharmacother.* 2018;19(4):413–419.
100. Keating GM. Elbasvir/grazoprevir: first global approval. *Drugs.* 2016;76(5):617–624.
101. Chopp S, Vanderwall R, Hult A, Klepser M. Simeprevir and sofosbuvir for treatment of hepatitis C infection. *Am J Health Syst Pharm.* 2015;72(17):1445–1455.
102. Xue W, Ban Y, Liu H, Yao X. Computational study on the drug resistance mechanism against HCV NS3/4A protease inhibitors vaniprevir and MK-5172 by the combination use of molecular dynamics simulation, residue interaction network, and substrate envelope analysis. *J Chem Inf Model.* 2014;54(2):621–633.
103. Keating GM. Daclatasvir: a review in chronic hepatitis C. *Drugs.* 2016;76 (14):1381–1391.
104. [No authors listed]. Sofosbuvir with velpatasvir. *Aust Prescr.* 2017;40(5):200–201.
105. Zerboni L, Sen N, Oliver SL, Arvin AM. Molecular mechanisms of varicella zoster virus pathogenesis. *Nat Rev Microbiol.* 2014;12(3):197–210.
106. Mueller NH, Gilden DH, Cohrs RJ, Mahalingam R, Nagel MA. Varicella zoster virus infection: clinical features, molecular pathogenesis of disease, and latency. *Neurol Clin.* 2008;26(3):675–697. viii.
107. Dayan RR, Peleg R. Herpes zoster – typical and atypical presentations. *Postgrad Med.* 2017;129(6)):567–571. 6.
108. Seifert R. Vidarabine is neither a potent nor a selective AC5 inhibitor. *Biochem Pharmacol.* 2014;87(4):543–546.
109. Griffiths P, Baraniak I, Reeves M. The pathogenesis of human cytomegalovirus. *J Pathol.* 2015;235(2):288–297.
110. Sinnott 4th JT, Cancio MR. Cytomegalovirus. *Infect Control.* 1987;8(2):79–82.
111. Biron KK. Antiviral drugs for cytomegalovirus diseases. *Antivir Res.* 2006;71 (2–3):154–163.
112. Groothuis JR, Nishida H. Prevention of respiratory syncytial virus infections in high-risk infants by monoclonal antibody (palivizumab). *Pediatr Int.* 2002;44(3):235–241.

113. Yuki K, Fujiogi M, Koutsogiannaki S. COVID-19 pathophysiology: a review. *Clin Immunol*. 2020;215:108427.
114. Parasher A. COVID-19: current understanding of its Pathophysiology, clinical presentation and treatment. *Postgrad Med J*. 2021;97(1147):312–320.
115. Eastman RT, Roth JS, Brimacombe KR, et al. Remdesivir: a review of its discovery and development leading to emergency use authorization for treatment of COVID-19. *ACS Cent Sci*. 2020;6(5):672–683.

Chapter 21

Insight into the molecular mechanism of action of anticancer drugs

Monalisha Sengupta[1], Arijit Guha[2], Rudranil Bhowmik[3], Imran Kazmi[4], Salman Bakr I. Hosawi[4], Fahad Al-Abbasi[4] and Mohammed Kaleem[4]

[1]Narayana Superspeciality Hospital, Howrah, West Bengal, India, [2]Bagda Rural Hospital, Mohanpur, West Bengal, India, [3]Bioeuivalence Study Centre, Department of Pharmaceutical Technology, Jadavpur University, Kolkata, West Bengal, India, [4]Department of Biochemistry, Faculty of Science, King Abdulaziz University, Jeddah, Saudi Arabia

Introduction

Cancer comprises a collection of diseases by excessive proliferation of cells in the body that cannot be effectively regulated and the cancerous cells also conquer and destroy normal cells.[1] This disease is also categorized as an epigenetic disease due to its genetic and cytogenetic character.[2]

Every year, millions of cases of cancers are identified, which ultimately leading to end of life. Most cancer, including chronic leukemia, cannot be permanently cured. As per the information from American Cancer Society, it is estimated that cancer encounters 2%–3% of the total annual deaths recorded worldwide.[3] Therapeutic approaches for cancer involve surgery, radiotherapy, chemotherapy, and immunotherapy.

Generally, the clinical or medical conditions of the patients are categorized, based on the severity of the disease, into the following stages: Stage 1, Stage II, Stage III, and Stage IV.

Surgical treatment removes solid tumor quickly. However, it is effective, for early tumors. Those who have not benefitted from surgical treatment undergo radiation therapy. Radiation therapy is long term and expensive. Chemotherapy categorizes as systemic therapy that involves the introduction of antineoplastic agents in the body. Side effects are high as they kill cancer cells with the normal cells.

How Synthetic Drugs Work. DOI: https://doi.org/10.1016/B978-0-323-99855-0.00021-X

Immunotherapy modulates patient's own immune system to produce an antitumor effect, normally prescribed to those who are in the last stage of the disease involved critical organs.

Anticancer drugs may be at different sites—cancer cells, endothelium, extracellular matrix (ECM), the immune system or host cells. More precisely tumor cells can be targeted at the DNA, RNA, or protein level. Most classical antineoplastic agents interact with tumor DNA, whereas monoclonal antibody and other small molecules target protein.

Recently, a new drug classification based on target is prepared by Espinosa et al. Target may be located at the DNA/protein or RNA level of tumor, endothelium, ECM, etc.

Pathophysiology

In molecular level, it is discovered that in human tumors, there is a drastic change in DNA methylation and histone modifications are found. It is mostly witnessed in epigenetic alteration of human tumors that there is huge alteration done by DNA methylation particularly silencing of tumor-suppressor genes.[4] Another approach, the aberrant pattern of histone modifications, is also an important route under the epigenetic route. The basic mechanisms of gene expression involve nucleosomes, which plays a key role. These nucleosomes are consisting of 146 DNA base pairs which are wrapped around 8 histone subunits which are pairs of H2A, H2B, H3, and H4 each. The important modifications like acetylation, methylation, phosphorylation, and ubiquitination are done by the most valuable amino acid, that is, lysine, which is found in large amount in these proteins. The reading of these posttranslational modifications by different proteins and complexes, which are involved in chromatin remodeling and transcriptional activation or repression, ultimately leads to the formation of required "histone code."[2,3] An involvement of the enzymes like HATs (histone acetyltransferase) and HDACs (histone deacetylases) is to control the histone modifications, like reversible acetylation of some lysine residues of histones H3 and H4. The relevance of the acetylation is the association of acetylated lysine with less condensed chromatin and a transcriptionally active gene; otherwise association of deacetylated ones with heterochromatin and transcriptional gene silencing will be experienced.[5–7] Not only the epigenetics is one of the major causes of unnatural gene expression of cancer cells, but also the genetic and cytogenetic pathways which involve gene mutations, homozygous deletions, loss of heterozygosity, monosomies, trisomies, homogenous staining regions, etc. are also important.[5] Dense hypermethylation of the CpG islands and histone hypoacetylation caused by targeting the HDACs to the gene promoter are the two methods of epigenetic gene silencing.

Due to involvement of many tumor-suppressor genes, such as $p16^{INK4a}$, BRCA1, hMLH1, MGMT, VHL, and E-cadherin, the first mechanism became most popular for cancer therapeutics.[4] This is approached by restoring the utility of $p14^{ARF}$ and hMLH1 silent genes with the use of DNA-demethylating agents.[8–10] Though having toxicity in a significant amount, these drugs can be used to restore the expression of tumor-suppressor gene by reducing their dose and due to having synergistic effects, they are used in combination with HDAC inhibitors,[8,11] whereas individual HDACs are unable to do the same.

Similarly, the involvement of promoter hypoacetylation of histones by recruitment of HDACs for gene silencing is less studied. For an example, the archetypical gene, which is cyclin-dependent kinase inhibitor $p21^{WAF1}$, in human cancer is silenced in this manner[12–14] Though the epigenetic reactivation of this archetypical gene ($p21^{WAF1}$) with the interference of the HDAC inhibitors in cancer cell lines has been observed,[12,13] and the restoration of the same is aligned with the enhancement of hyperacetylated histones at the $p21^{WAF1}$ promoter.[14]

$p21^{WAF1}$: $p21^{WAF1}$, an original tumor-suppressor gene, proves this ability in $p21^{WAF1}$ knockout mice by developing tumors.[13] Though this gene expression is always not found in broad spectrum types of tumors[14,15] but overexpressed $p21^{WAF1}$ shows its growth arrest properties particularly in deficient cancer cells.[12]

United States Food and Drug Administration

Due to a huge number of deaths in account of advanced solid tumor, there is a need for new effective drugs or therapies. To fulfill this demand, researcher is continuously working globally on development of new effective antitumor or anticancer agents which appear in the interval of every few months under the supervision of regulatory authority, that is, the United States Food and Drug Administration (USFDA).

The USFDA, a famous federal agency of the Department of Health and Human Services, is responsible for taking care of public health by commanding on food safety, prescription, and over-the-counter pharmaceutical drugs (medications), vaccines, biopharmaceuticals, cosmetics,[15] and veterinary products. It has also the power to control the marketing of new or existing molecules or drugs by following the proper safety profile. The global acceptance of USFDA-approved drugs proves the importance of USFDA. The Centre for Drug Evaluation and Research (CDER), a division of USFDA, mainly looks after the matter regarding the availability of the safe and effective drugs to improve the health of welfare. Considering the role of USFDA in providing approval to newer cancer and blood therapies, 2019 established a strong milestone by sanctioning new therapies for prostate, bladder, breast, and lung cancers.[16]

Newer United States Food and Drug Administration–approved drugs

The most unique cancer therapy, which is based on the presence of specific genetic marker in any types of tumors, was approved by the CDER in this year. This approach differs from the traditional treatment because the treatment involves specific characteristic of a tumor instead of its site of origin. Along with this, approvals to many newer therapies have been accomplished which includes two new bone marrow cancer therapies, one new drug for patients with diffuse large B-cell lymphoma, therapy for patients with mantle cell lymphoma, a new treatment for a certain type of myelofibrosis, patients with acute hepatic porphyria, a first-in-class drug for patients requiring red blood cell transfusions, therapy for adult patients with chronic lymphocytic leukemia or small lymphocytic lymphoma. Additionally, CDER also approved the first FDA-approved therapy for the treatment with acquired thrombotic thrombocytopenic purpura, a disorder that may lead to brain damage or death in 2019. Some of the FDA-approved drugs[17] within the last five decades are enlisted in Table 21.1.

TABLE 21.1 List of anti-cancer drugs with their therapeutic application, target gene and year of approval by USFDA.

Major class	Drug	Therapeutic area	Target gene	Approval year
Cytotoxic	Radium 223 dichloride	Prostate cancer	Unknown	2013
	Omacetaxine mepesuccinate	Leukemia	RPL3	2012
	Asparaginase erwinia chrysanthemi	Leukemia	Biological	2011
	Eribulin mesylate	Breast cancer	TUBA4A; TUBB1	2010
	Pralatrexate	Lymphoma	DHFR; TYMS	2009
	Ixabepilone	Breast cancer	TUBB3	2007
	Nelarabine	Leukemia; lymphoma	DNA synthesis	2005
	Oxaliplatin	Colorectal cancer	DNA synthesis	2002
	Daunorubicin hydrochloride	Leukemia	DNA synthesis; TOP2A; TOP2B	1998
	Topotecan hydrochloride	Ovarian cancer; lung cancer; cervical cancer	TOP1; TOP1MT	1996
	Gemcitabine	Ovarian cancer; pancreatic cancer; lung cancer; breast cancer	DNA synthesis; RRM1; TYMS	1996

(Continued)

TABLE 21.1 (Continued)

Major class	Drug	Therapeutic area	Target gene	Approval year
	Docetaxel	Prostate cancer; breast cancer; head and neck cancer; stomach cancer; lung cancer; brain cancer	TUBA4A; TUBB1	1996
	Thiotepa	Breast cancer; ovarian cancer; bladder cancer	DNA synthesis	1994
	Paclitaxel	Breast cancer; lung cancer; pancreatic cancer; ovarian cancer; sarcoma	TUBA4A; TUBB1	1992
	Carboplatin	Ovarian cancer	DNA synthesis	1989
	Ifosfamide	Testicular cancer	DNA synthesis	1988
	Etoposide	Testicular cancer; lung cancer	TOP2A; TOP2B	1983
	Cisplatin	Testicular cancer; ovarian cancer; bladder cancer	DNA synthesis	1978
	Carmustine	Brain cancer; lymphoma; Multiple myeloma	DNA synthesis	1977
	Doxorubicin hydrochloride	Leukemia; breast cancer; stomach cancer; Lymphoma; ovarian cancer; lung cancer; sarcoma; thyroid cancer; bladder cancer; kidney cancer; brain cancer	TOP2A; DNA synthesis	1974
	Bleomycin	Head and neck cancer; lymphoma; penile cancer; cervical cancer; vulvar cancer; testicular cancer	DNA synthesis	1973

(Continued)

TABLE 21.1 (Continued)

Major class	Drug	Therapeutic area	Target gene	Approval year
	Fluorouracil	Breast cancer; colorectal cancer; stomach cancer; pancreatic cancer	DNA synthesis	1970
	Vinblastine sulfate	Lymphoma; testicular cancer; choriocarcinoma; breast cancer	TUBA1A; TUBB; TUBD1; TUBE1; TUBG1	1965
	Cyclophosphamide	Lymphoma; multiple myeloma; leukemia; brain cancer; ovarian cancer; retinoblastoma; breast cancer	DNA synthesis	1959
	Mercaptopurine	Leukemia	HPRT1	1953
	Methotrexate	Leukemia; breast cancer; head and neck cancer; lung cancer; lymphoma; bone cancer; gestational trophoblastic disease	DHFR	1953
Targeted	Nivolumab	Melanoma	PDCD1	2014
	Obinutuzumab	Leukemia	Ms4A1	2013
	Cabozantinib	Thyroid cancer	KDR; MET; RET	2012
	Ipilimumab	Melanoma	CTLA4	2011
	Denosumab	Bone cancer	TNFSF11	2010
	Ofatumumab	Leukemia	Ms4A1	2009
	Degarelix	Prostate cancer	GNRHR	2008
	Temsirolimus	Kidney cancer	MTOR	2007
	Panitumumab	Colorectal cancer	EGFR	2006
	Lenalidomide	Multiple myeloma; lymphoma	CRBN	2005

(Continued)

TABLE 21.1 (Continued)

Major class	Drug	Therapeutic area	Target gene	Approval year
	Cetuximab	Head and neck cancer; colorectal cancer	EGFR	2004
	Trastuzumab	Breast cancer; stomach cancer	ERBB2	1998
	Thalidomide	Multiple myeloma	CRBN	1998
	Rituximab	Lymphoma; leukemia	Ms4A1	1997
	Interferon Alfa-2b, recombinant	Sarcoma; leukemia; melanoma; lymphoma	IFNAR1; IFNAR2	1986
	Tamoxifen citrate	Breast cancer	ESR1; ESR2	1977
	Fluoxymesterone	Breast cancer	AR; ESR1; NR3C1; PRLR	1956

Classification of anticancer drugs/therapies

As mentioned, the last one to two decades have witnessed an appearance of a great number of anticancer drugs, among which many of them will not fit into the simple traditional classification and may require to establish new classification.[18] Generally, a drug classification is done to achieve the objectives mainly for a comprehensive view of the available drugs and the design of combination therapy. The objective also is to remember the drugs and their mechanism of action and also for teaching purposes.[18]

As the focus of newer therapies is started to move from site of origin or organ-to-genetic- based target-oriented therapies, likewise newer approach of drug classification will follow the same trends from therapy based on specific target organ which was established by *Espinosa* et al.[18] It can include drugs targeting endothelium and ECM, and the immune system elements involved in carcinogenesis, potential host cells, etc. which can be located at the DNA, RNA or protein level.[18] Though the proper mechanism of action of every new drug is not possible to explain in detail due to uncertainty of mechanisms and some limitations at various phases of clinical trial.[18]

The classical and modern classifications of anticancer drugs are depicted briefly in Table 21.2.

TABLE 21.2 Classification of anticancer drugs.[18,19]

Therapy	Class of drugs	Name of drugs
Chemotherapy (cytotoxic drugs)	*Alkylating agents*	
	Nitrogen mustards	Mechlorethamine, cyclophosphamide
	Ethyleneamine	Thiotepa
	Alkyl sulfonate	Busulfan
	Nitrosourea	Carmustine
	Triazine	Dacarbazine
	Antimetabolites	
	Folate antagonist	Methotrexate (Mtx)
	Purine Antagonist	6-Mercaptopurine (6-MP)
	Pyrimidine Antagonist	5-Fluorouracil (5-FU)
	Vinca alkaloids	Vincristine, vinblastine
	Taxanes	Paclitaxel
	Epipodophyllotoxin	Etoposide
	Camptothecin analogs	Topotecan
	Antibiotics	Actinomycin D
	Miscellaneous	Hydroxyurea, procarbazine
Hormonal therapy (drugs altering the hormonal milieu)	*Glucocorticoids*	Prednisolone
	Estrogens	Fosfestrol
	Selective estrogen receptor modulators	Tamoxifen
	Selective estrogen receptor down regulators	Fulvestrant
	Aromatase inhibitors	Letrozole
	Antiandrogen	Flutamide
	5-α-Reductase inhibitor	Finasteride
	GnRH analogs	Triptorelin
	Progestins	Hydroxyprogesterone
Immunotherapy (drugs acting on immune system)	*Interferon*	
	Interleukin 2	
	Vaccines	

(*Continued*)

TABLE 21.2 (Continued)

Therapy	Class of drugs	Name of drugs
Modern classification of anticancer drugs[18]		
Target organ	**Location**	**Name of drugs/treatment**
Endothelium	*DNA*	Combretastatin
	Proteins	Monoclonal antibodies
		Small molecules
Extracellular matrix	*MMPs*	MMPs inhibitors
	Other elements	Monoclonal antibodies (mab) and small molecules
Host cells	*Bone cells*	Bisphosphonates, osteoprotogerin
Immune system	*Lymphocytes and macrophages*	Interferons, interleukin 2
Tumor	*DNA (nonspecific)*	
	DNA break:	Chemotherapy
	DNA-related proteins:	Chemotherapy
	DNA (specific)	
		Hormonal therapy, retinoids
		Interferon α, gene therapy
	RNA	Antisense oligonucleotides
	Proteins	
	Membrane receptors	
	Extracellular domain:	Monoclonal antibodies (mab)
	Intracellular domain:	Small molecules
	Cytoplasm	
	Intracellular pathways	Small molecules
	Tubulin	Chemotherapy

MMPs, Matrix metalloproteinases.

Considering Table 21.2, we can come to the decision that the modern classification of anticancer drugs is more acceptable than the classical classification as it covers both the ancient and newer approved drugs in such a way which follows modern treatments. So, here we will discuss about the mechanisms of anticancer drugs as per the modern classification.[18]

Mechanism of action

Drugs acting on endothelium

Drugs that show activities against the endothelium act either as endothelial growth factor inhibitor or the inhibitor of receptors of such factors due to antiangiogenic effects.

DNA

The target of anticancer therapies is on how to induce stress-mediated apoptosis in tumor cells and tumor-associated endothelium in response to DNA damage.[20] Chemoresistance can be promoted by suppressing apoptotic mechanisms of growth factors like basic fibroblast growth factor (bFGF) and vascular endothelial cell growth factor (VEGF) in tumor cells.[21] These growth factors are inhibited by thalidomide,[22,23] carboxyamidotriazole[24,25] whereas interferon α reduces VEGF synthesis in tumor cells.[26–28]

Growth factors

Generally, bFGF and VEGF are growth factors in the microenvironment, where VEGF is highly specific for endothelial cells (ECs), and bFGF act in a broader way. These growth factors are controlling both physiologic and tumor angiogenesis functions.[29]

In a molecular level, it is found that bFGF or VEGF activates Raf-1 for the protection of EC from the apoptotic stimuli.[30,31] Normally, bFGF is responsible for translocation of Raf-1 to the mitochondria along with protection of ECs from the stress-mediated apoptosis, whereas remarkable protection from death ligand-induced apoptosis is done by VEGF making small effect on stress-mediated death. These findings prove the fact that activation of common pathways of cell proliferation, which leads to angiogenesis, is done by angiogenic growth factors.[21]

Combretastatin

In the context of drugs acting on endothelium, combretastatin shows its high potency as an antimitotic agent by inhibiting the mitotic spindle in the endothelium which ultimately leads to apoptosis[32,33] due to its simple structure. This apoptotic cell death is stimulated by the disruption of microtubules which is followed by arresting the cell cycle during metaphase to anaphase

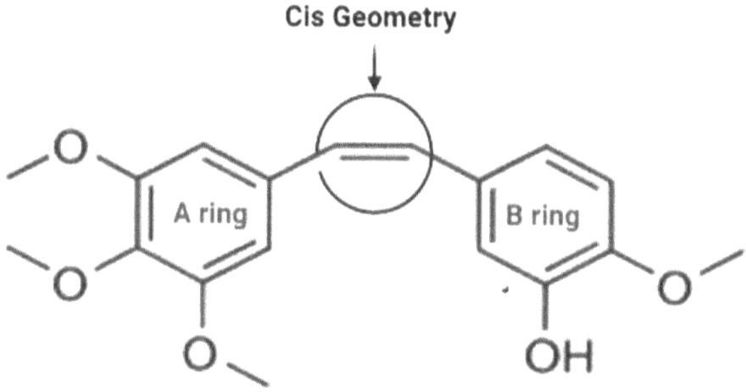

FIGURE 21.1 Structure of combretastatin.

transition where combretastatin binds particularly to the subunit of tubulin at the colchicine binding site.[34,35]

Chemistry: Combretastatin is a naturally obtained oxygenated stilbene derivative, isolated from the bark of African willow tree *Combretum caffrum* in the year 1982 by Pettit and coworkers.[36] An ethylene bridge, for connecting two phenyl rings (Rings A and B) and maintenance of cis-geometry across the central double bond, was found in the structure of combretastatin (Fig. 21.1).[37]

MOA

In general, it is established that combretastatin with 0.53–3.0 μM IC_{50}[35] is able to inhibit polymerization of tubulin by binding with it to colchicine binding site, which ultimately causes disruption of dynamic equilibrium. α- and β-tubulin heterodimers are leading to the formation of microtubules followed by the formation of abnormal mitotic spindles with the help of disruption of dynamic equilibrium. As a consequence, the cell cycle is arrested at the M-phase and finally causes targeted apoptotic cell death.[35] Mitotic catastrophe which is characterized by formation of giant, multinucleated cells by activation of caspase 9 (cysteine protease), is another approach to cell death by combretastatin.[35]

In case of neovasculature, to maintain the cell shape, the role of cellular microtubule network is very crucial. In contrast, combretastatin shows a strong antivascular effect as it is related to its antitubulin effect and causes rapid depolymerization of microtubules. The depolymerization results round-up of elongated ECs, disruption of blood vessels surrounding EC layer, etc. which leads to blood vessel congestion. Then necrosis of tumor cells is done due to less blood flow, oxygen flow and nutrient supply to tumor cells.[35]

The prodrug of combretastatin, 2, sodium phosphate is rapidly metabolized into combretastatin after administration by endogenous nonspecific phosphatases and is under clinical trials.[38]

Protein

Monoclonal antibodies

It has been shown that the monoclonal antibodies (mab) have a great role in medical research, by involving in diagnostics and clinical applications derives, due to their high affinity to bind with same type of two antigens and for their in vitro and in vivo elevated stability. mAbs also show higher specificity and lesser chance to be contaminated by pathogens due to their polyclonal counterparts in the structure which are obtained by immunization of animal serum.[39] FDA and other international regulatory agencies have approved murine, chimeric, and human antibodies as a therapy of several ailments which also include autoimmune diseases and cancer[39–41] Recent approved few mAbs within last 5 years in cancer treatment by FDA are enlisted in Table 21.3.[16]

TABLE 21.3 Lists of Food and Drug Administration–approved recent mAbs for cancer therapy.[16]

Name	Antigen	Format unconjugated antibodies	Indications	Year of approval
Isatuximab	CD38	Chimeric IgG1	Multiple Myeloma	2020
Sacituzumab govitecan	TROP2	Humanized ADC	Triple-negative breast cancer	2020
Enfortumab vedotin	Nectin-4	Human ADC	Bladder cancer	2019
Polatuzumab vedotin	CD79B	Humanized ADC	B-Cell Lymphoma	2019
Trastuzumab deruxtecan	HER-2	Humanized ADC	Breast cancer	2019
Atezolizumab	PD-L1	Humanized IgG1	Non–small cell lung cancer	2019
Atezolizumab	PD-L1	Humanized IgG1	Triple-negative breast cancers	2019
Moxetumomab pasudotox	CD22	Mouse ADC	Hairy-cell leukemia	2018
Bevacizumab	VEGF	Humanized IgG1	Ovarian Cancers	2018
Cemiplimab	PD-1	Human IgG4	Cutaneous squamous-cell carcinoma	2018

(*Continued*)

TABLE 21.3 (Continued)

Name	Antigen	Format unconjugated antibodies	Indications	Year of approval
Ipilimumab	CTLA4	Human IgG1	Renal cell carcinoma	2018
Nivolumab	PD-1	Human IgG4	Renal cell carcinoma	2018
Avelumab	PD-L1	Human IgG1	Urothelial carcinoma	2017
Avelumab	PD-L1	Human IgG1	Merkel cell carcinoma	2017
Durvalumab	PD-L1	Human IgG1	Bladder cancer	2017
Inotuzumab ozogamicin	CD22	Humanized ADC	Acute lymphoblastic leukemia	2017
Olaratumab	PDGFRα	Human IgG1	Sarcoma	2016
Daratumumab	CD38	Human IgG1	Multiple myeloma	2015
Dinutuximab	GD2	Chimeric IgG1	Neuroblastoma	2015
Elotuzumab	SLAMF7	Humanized IgG1	Multiple myeloma	2015

Muromonab, a murine, is the first ever mAb which got approval to use in humans in the treatment of transplant rejection,[42] whereas infliximab, a recent chimeric, an anti-TNFα mAb, is recommended for rheumatoid arthritis and Crohn's disease[43,44] and ofatumumab, an anti-CD20 mAb which is derived entirely from human, is used for the chronic lymphocytic leukemia treatment.[45] The antibody format of the international nonproprietary names of mAbs can be easily denoted by the suffix, which is summarized in Table 21.4.[46]

The bevacizumab is demonstrated as a humanized anti-VEGF monoclonal antibody and shows improved survival rates in combination with chemotherapy, particularly in those patients who are previously untreated with metastatic colorectal cancer in comparison to chemotherapy alone. As a result, it serves angiogenic properties and received FDA approval for first time.[47] In context to binding with VEGF receptors, the bevacizumab shows its activity with all the receptors.[18,24,48,49]

TABLE 21.4 List of international suffixes for mAbs.

Suffix	Antibody format
-omab	Mouse IgG2
-ximab	Chimeric IgG1
-zumab	Humanized IgG1
-umab	Human antibody from phage display/transgenic mice technology
-axomab	Trifunctional (bispecific) mouse–rat hybrid mAb
-cept	Fc (constant fragment) fusion protein
-stim	Fc (constant fragment) fusion peptide

Bevacizumab

Bevacizumab (Avastin), a humanized IgG1 mAb with size of 149 kDa, shows the activities of selective binding and inhibition of VEGF. Generally, the VEGF is responsible for the activation of angiogenesis and metastasis of tumors. Overexpressed VEGF has been led to a worsened prognosis in patients.[50] In 2004 bevacizumab received its first approval to be used in combination with 5-fluorouracil-based chemotherapy for the treatment of metastatic colon and rectal cancer, in the United States. In Europe, bevacizumab is authorized since 2005 for a combination therapy with various chemotherapeutic agents, particularly in the treatment of renal cell carcinoma, non–small cell lung carcinoma (NSCLC), ovarian neoplasms, breast neoplasms, and colorectal neoplasms. Recently in the United States, bevacizumab is indicated as a second-line monotherapy for the treatment of glioblastoma only.[51]

Small molecules

SU-5416, SU-6668 are categorized as small molecules that act as an anticancer agent by binding with the receptors of different growth factors. SU-5416 is binding to the tyrosine kinase of both VEGFR-1 and VEGFR-2,[24,52] along with platelet-derived growth factor receptor (PDGFR) and c-kit. Clinically SU-5416 is more potent small molecule which leads to the initiation of clinical trials with SU-5416 in hematological malignancies and colorectal cancer patients. Similarly, SU-6668 also shows its activities to bind with VEGFR, bFGFR, and PDGFR.[18,53,54]

Drugs acting on extracellular matrix

It has been observed that most drugs acting in the ECM inhibit matrix metalloproteinases (MMPs). They all have antiangiogenic effects

Matrix metalloproteinases

MMP which is also known as matrixin is a main cause for degradation of collagen (structural component of connective tissue) and other protein in ECM.[55] This MMPs plays a crucial role in several physiological and pathological activities like tumor growth, invasion, and metastasis. Since last three to four decades MMPs have been considered promising targets for cancer therapy, which ultimately leads to the development of a number of different synthetic and natural MMP inhibitors as cytostatic and antiangiogenic agents.[56] Numerical biological functions are depicted by MMPs in the development of cancer from metastatic initiation to outgrowth followed by apoptosis and angiogenesis.[55] Not only that, MMPs are also responsible for stimulating the release of VEGF, bFGF, and insulin growth factor.[18]

A number of MMP inhibitors are currently under extensive clinical examination as potential anticancer drugs.[57] They are mainly divided into synthetic inhibitors of the enzyme activity which includes marimastat,[58–60] prinomastat or BAY 12–956657, and natural inhibitors which include isoflavonoids and shark cartilage.[55]

Marimastat

Marimastat is the most common synthetic MMP inhibitors with a broad-spectrum activity. It is an orally bioavailable drug with mild-to-severe dose-dependent side effects on joint and muscle pain, has lower molecular weight.[61] Different phases of clinical trials reveal many facts about this drug. In Phase III, though it was not showing any significant advantage over conventional first-line treatment, but an improved survival rate was reported in inoperable colorectal hepatic metastases patients.[62] This outcome is followed by further clinical trials of Marimastat only in patients with cancer of the gastrointestinal tract, where survival benefit was modest,[63] and showing most prominent effect in postchemotherapeutic patients with advanced gastric cancer.[56,58]

Drugs acting on Host Cell

This section is less cultivated in comparison to other segments. Currently, it deals with only in those compounds which can inhibit or interfere with the function and microenvironment of bone cells. This includes only bisphosphonates,[64,65] osteoprotogerin,[66] and PTHRP antibodies. But there will be a great scope in the future, to develop more drugs which will target other organs at risk of metastasis.[18]

Drugs acting on immune system

One of the latest and great breakthroughs, particularly in cancer, is immunotherapy especially due to the checkpoint inhibitors[67] and chimeric antigen receptor (CAR) T cells.[68,69] Generally, the progression of cancer is done due to chronic inflammation in tumor sites. The tumor-derived factors or signals are downregulating the antitumor function of various immune effector cells, which are employed at the tumor site. To overcome this situation, reprogramming of the tumor-associated macrophages are required specially to inhibit the functions of lymphocyte. It is achieved by releasing the inhibitory cytokines such as interleukin 2, interleukin 10, prostaglandins, or reactive oxygen species.[70–72]

Drugs directed against tumor DNA

Most antineoplastic drugs act on DNA by breaking the helix. They also interfere with DNA related proteins or modify specific genes.[73]

DNA helix

Alkylating agents prevent cell division primarily by cross-linking of DNA particularly at the N-7 position. Replication of DNA and transcription of RNA are prevented by cross-links. As a result, imbalance of other cell constituents including RNA and protein and the cell dies. Activity of anticancer drugs doesn't not depend on DNA synthesis of target cells except cyclophosphamide which inhibits DNA synthesis.[74,75]

Alkylating agents are small molecules that can covalently bind an alkyl group to electron-rich nucleophilic moieties to form adduct and exert cytotoxic effect on cancer cells by binding to DNA molecules. Alkylators belong to one of several families[76]:

1. nitrogen mustard
2. triazenes
3. nitrosoureas
4. platinum compounds
5. antibiotics

Some proper alkylating agents are cisplatin, oxaliplatin, carboplatin, etc. Bleomycin and mitomycin-C are alkylator antibiotic.

DNA-related proteins

Topoisomerases are enzymes that regulate DNA topology and are essential for the integrity of the genetic material during transcription, replication, and recombination processes. It cuts and reseals DNA strands. During replication/transcription a significant amount of torsional strain is placed on DNA helix. This strain is relieved during breaking of DNA strands which is created by enzyme topoisomerase I (for single-stranded DNA) and topoisomerase II (for double-stranded DNA). Topoisomerases reseal the break after tension has been relieved.[77–79]

Topoisomerase inhibitors block the resealing step leading to large amount of fragmented DNA. This leads to destabilize the cell leading to cell death. Inhibitors of these enzymes are topotecan, irinotecan, rubitecan, lurtotecan, exatecan, etc.[80]

In addition, antimetabolites act as anticancer agents by exerting their cytotoxic effects by interfering with DNA or RNA synthesis. They are structurally resembled with normal substrate but differ enough to interfere with the metabolism.

Antimetabolites are categorized into two groups.

1. structural analog of immediate in the biosynthesis of nucleotides such as purine analog (mercaptopurine, thioguanine) and pyrimidine analog (cytarabine, gemcitabine)
2. structural analogs of vital cofactors in the synthesis of nucleotides such as folic acid analog methotrexate.

Specific genes

Several antineoplastic agents act by modifying expression of specific genes, for example, steroids, antihormones, and retinoids. They bind to receptor protein to activate regulatory sequences in DNA. For instance, antiestrogen blocks estrogenic receptor which is a ligand regulated transcription factor.[81,82]

Gene therapies also target specific genes. But its mode of action as it is introduced in vector to either repair or block specific DNA sequences.

Drugs targeted against tumor RNA

Some anticancer drugs interfere with RNA synthesis. Antisense oligonucleotides include in this group. These molecules act against specific mRNAs of bcl2, myb, P53, Her-2, etc.[83]

Drugs directed against proteins in the tumor cells. Monoclonal antibodies are included in this class. Some small molecules also act through this mechanism. Large molecules, that is, monoclonal antibody, block extracellular domain of receptor where the small molecules inhibit intracellular domain.[84] Rituximab was the first anticancer antibody.[85–87]

Passive immunotherapy refers to the preparation of antitumor antibodies or cells in vitro and then injected into the body for treatment. VEGF and antihuman EGFR-2 (HER-2) are commonly used in passive immunotherapy.[88,89]

Drugs directed against proteins in tumor cell

More than the last 10 years have been contributed to this group by providing a great number of compounds, such as monoclonal antibodies (mab) and small molecules. Their functions are all target specific by binding to the membrane receptors or cytoplasmic proteins and the effect is specialized into cytostatic rather than cytotoxic. For these reasons, this group is growing by joining more and more new potent compounds.[18]

Receptor in the tumor membrane

Both the monoclonal antibodies (mab) and small molecules have shown their activities on receptor in the tumor membrane in an absolutely distinguish ways. Normally, the performance of mAbs depends on the blockage of the extracellular domain of the receptor, whereas the small molecules depend on the inhibition of the intracellular domain, mainly a tyrosin kinase by crossing the tumor membrane easily due to its size.[18] Though the term "'small molecule'" may be a cause of misleading, due to use of small-sized classical chemotherapeutic compounds, but there will be a distinction always with mAbs.[18]

Monoclonal antibodies (mab): The lymphoid antigens like CD20 and CD52 are the most responsible elements behind the story of the development of first antitumor antibodies. Among them some combine the antibody with an isotope for more effectiveness.[90–94] As a result, the possibilities of treatment in patients with refractory lymphomas have highly expanded by these highly active compounds and followed by evaluation of the compounds as in first-line therapy. Currently many new antibodies like anti-CD33 gemtuzumab and the anti-CD22 epratuzumab are under the clinical investigation to strengthen the group.[95,96]

There are many more antibodies available in the market after getting the FDA approval (Table 21.3) for one or more indications. Trastuzumab[97,98] and cetuximab[99,100] are also those FDA-approved antibodies that have shown their great activities against carcinoma. Normally, Her-2 positive breast tumors are treated with either trastuzumab alone or in combination with chemotherapy. Along with this indication, new possible indications are also being studied. Similarly, the use of antibody like an anti-MUC antibody as a vaccine in the future for the patients with carcinomas is also being studied.[101]

Small molecules: The function of these molecules only expressed after binding with the epidermal growth factor receptor (EGFR) family. Small molecules like PKI-166 inhibit the activities of both Her-1 and Her-2[102] whereas gefitinib (ZD-1839)[103,104] and OSI-774[105] are showing their specific activities only toward the Her-1, which are representative of EGFR group. On the other hand, CI-1033 shows its irreversible inhibition activity toward all the EGFR.[106] Among the many small molecules only gefitinib went through different phases of clinical trials so far, which followed up by recognition of it as a single agent for NSCLC and head and neck tumors.

Intracellular pathways in tumor cells

The distinct intracellular pathways are playing a key role in the matter of growth, because the signal for the proliferation is conveyed to the nucleus by several metabolic pathways, which are interrelated to each other. Generally, growth factors are there to influence these pathways and some specific drugs make them as their target. The foremost drug in this specific group of drugs is imatinib which shows major effects in chronic myeloid leukemia and in gastrointestinal stromal tumors. It mainly acts by inhibiting the tyrosine kinase of bcr/abl and c-kit.[107,108] Others, such as lonafarnib, R115,777, BAY 43-9006, CI-1040, CCI-779, bryostatin, and PKC-412, are targeting the ras pathway or the phosphatidylinositol pathway, along with the proteasome and the cyclin-dependent kinases. Normally, the farnesyltransferase enzyme is responsible for activation of raw protein, which is followed by the activation of raf and MEK which is shown in the Fig. 21.2. Lonafarnib and R115,777 are farnesyltransferase inhibitors, which act as a false metabolite of this enzyme,[109,110] whereas BAY 43-9006 and CI-1040 are acted on raf and MEK respectively.[111,112] Currently, most of these agents are in the first steps of clinical development.[18]

Just like ras–raf pathway, the serin threonine PI-3K helps to initiate the phosphatidylinositol pathway. This pathway is connected with mechanistic target of rapamycin (mTOR) with the help of PKB/Akt. The MTOR gene in human is responsible for regulating the rate of apoptosis as well as for maintenance of the balance between cellular catabolism and anabolism. CCI-779, a rapamycin derivative, exhibits its specific function in this pathway by blocking mTOR.[113] Similarly, the activation of the transcription factor NF-kB is done by the association of PI-3K with protein kinase C,[18] where this protein kinase C becomes target of bryostatin[114,115] and PKC-412[116] to show their inhibitory functions.

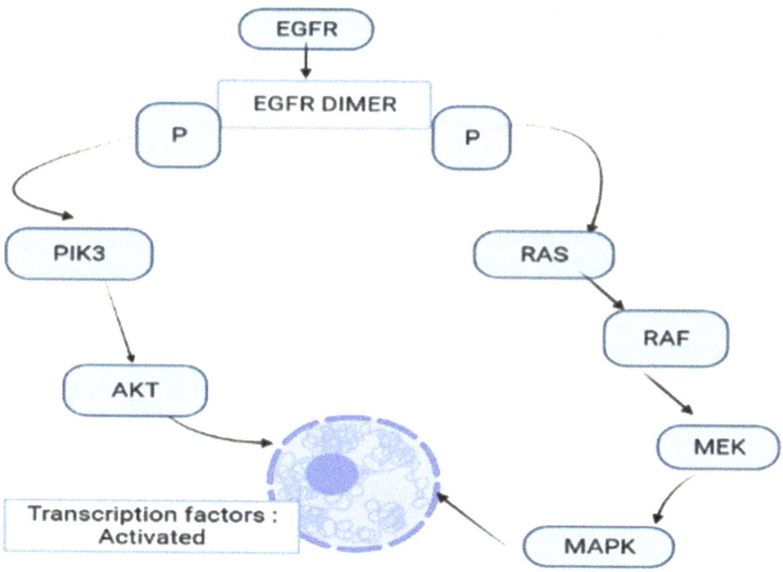

FIGURE 21.2 Schematic diagram of Ras/Raf pathway.

Tubulin

To maintain the cell shape, intracellular transport and cell mitosis tubulin play an important role. Drugs interfering with tubulin include vinca alkaloids which are used to bind at specific sites of tubulin followed by prevention of tubulin polymerization and disruption of the microtubule's formation.[18] Similarly, taxanes have also shown binding activities and stabilizing activities at distinct sites of microtubules, which ultimately cause to inhibit the normal reorganization of the microtubule network.[18] By utilizing this unique character, oral formulations of taxanes are prepared to improve the convenience when the potency of the formulation is matched with the potency of parent drugs.[117] Epothilones are another group of tubulin-stabilizing agents, which have shown promising activities in preclinical studies which followed to phase II and III clinical trials.[118,119]

Conclusion

Every year a number of anticancer drugs are introduced to the market where FDA plays a significant role in the development of novel anticancer drugs. Though the many anticancer agents are still at a developmental stage, approved newer drugs have shown different aspects of mechanisms which replace the traditional classification as well as provide a new era of cancer therapy. The target of these drugs is mostly situated in the tumor cells or in other elements which interact with the different elements of tumor cells such as endothelium, ECM, immune system, host cells. It can be expected that the new classification will be able to address new drugs coming up in the coming years and strengthen the anticancer therapies.

References

1. Shah U, Shah R, Acharya S, Acharya N. Novel anticancer agents from plant sources. *Chin J Nat Med*. 2013;11(1):16–23.
2. Villar-Garea A, Esteller M. Histone deacetylase inhibitors: understanding a new wave of anticancer agents. *Int J Cancer*. 2004;112(2):171–178.
3. Schwartsmann G, da Rocha AB, Berlinck RG, Jimeno J. Marine organisms as a source of new anticancer agents. *Lancet Oncol*. 2001;2(4):221–225.
4. Esteller M. CpG island hypermethylation and tumor suppressor genes: a booming present, a brighter future. *Oncogene*. 2002;21(35):5427–5440.
5. Jenuwein T, Allis CD. Translating the histone code. *Science*. 2001;293(5532):1074–1080.
6. Iizuka M, Smith MM. Functional consequences of histone modifications. *Curr Opin Genet Dev*. 2003;13:154–160.
7. Johnstone RW. Histone-deacetylase inhibitors: novel drugs for the treatment of cancer. *Nat Rev Drug Discov*. 2002;1:287–299.
8. Villar-Garea A, Esteller M. DNA demethylating agents and chromatin-remodelling drugs: which, how and why? *Curr Drug Metab*. 2003;4:11–31.

9. Esteller M, Cordon-Cardo C, Corn PG, et al. p14ARF silencing by promoter hypermethylation mediates abnormal intracellular localization of MDM2. *Cancer Res*. 2001;61:2816–2821.
10. Herman JG, Umar A, Polyak K, et al. Incidence and functional consequences of hMLH1 promoter hypermethylation in colorectal carcinoma. *Proc Natl Acad Sci USA*. 1998;95:6870–6875.
11. Cameron EE, Bachman KE, Myohanen S, Herman JG, Baylin SB. Synergy of demethylation and histone deacetylase inhibition in the re-expression of genes silenced in cancer. *Nat Genet*. 1999;21:103–107.
12. Archer SY, Meng S, Shei A, Hodin RA. p21WAF1 is required for butyrate-mediated growth inhibition of human colon cancer cells. *Proc Natl Acad Sci USA*. 1998;95:6791–6796.
13. Blagosklonny MV, Robey R, Sackett DL, et al. Histone deacetylase inhibitors all induce p21 but differentially cause tubulin acetylation, mitotic arrest, and cytotoxicity. *Mol Cancer Ther*. 2002;1:937–941.
14. Gui CY, Ngo L, Xu WS, Richon VM, Marks PA. Histone deacetylase (HDAC) inhibitor activation of p21WAF1 involves changes in promoter-associated proteins, including HDAC1. *Proc Natl Acad Sci USA*. 2004;101:1241–1246.
15. Hargadon KM, Johnson CE, Williams CJ. Immune checkpoint blockade therapy for cancer: an overview of FDA-approved immune checkpoint inhibitors. *Int Immunopharmacol*. 2018;62:29–39.
16. FDA. *Indications and Year of First Approval for Each Antibody Were Accessed Using the FDA Drug Database*. <https://www.accessdata.fda.gov/scripts/cder/daf/>.
17. Sun J, Wei Q, Zhou Y, Wang J, Liu Q, Xu H. A systematic analysis of FDA-approved anticancer drugs. *BMC Syst Biol*. 2017;11(5):1–7.
18. Espinosa E, Zamora P, Feliu J, Barón MG. Classification of anticancer drugs—a new system based on therapeutic targets. *Cancer Treat Rev*. 2003;29(6):515–523.
19. Tripathi KD. *Essentials of Medical Pharmacology*. JP Medical Ltd; 2013.
20. Clayton F, Tessnow KA, Fang JC, Holden JA, Moore JG. Circadian variation of topoisomerase II-α in human rectal crypt epithelium: implications for reduction of toxicity of chemotherapy. *Modern Pathol*. 2002;15(11):1191–1196.
21. Alavi AS, Acevedo L, Min W, Cheresh DA. Chemoresistance of endothelial cells induced by basic fibroblast growth factor depends on Raf-1–mediated inhibition of the proapoptotic kinase, ASK1. *Cancer Res*. 2007;67(6):2766–2772.
22. Neben K, Moehler T, Egerer G, et al. High plasma basic fibroblast growth factor concentration is associated with response to thalidomide in progressive multiple myeloma. *Clin Cancer Res*. 2001;7(9):2675–2681.
23. Raje N, Anderson KC. Thalidomide and immunomodulatory drugs as cancer therapy. *Curr Opin Oncol*. 2002;14(6):635–640.
24. Figg WD, Kruger EA, Price DK, Kim S, Dahut WD. Inhibition of angiogenesis: treatment options for patients with metastatic prostate cancer. *Invest New Drugs*. 2002;20(2):183–194.
25. Waselenko JK, Shinn CA, Willis CR, Flinn IW, Grever MR, Byrd JC. Carboxyamido-triazole (CAI)—a novel "static" signal transduction inhibitor induces apoptosis in human B-cell chronic lymphocytic leukemia cells. *Leuk Lymphoma*. 2001;42(5):1049–1053.
26. Dreau D, Foster M, Hogg M, Swiggett J, Holder WD, White RL. Angiogenic and immune parameters during recombinant interferon-a2b adjuvant treatment in patients with melanoma. *Oncol Res*. 2000;12(5):241–251.

27. Kawano Y, Matsui N, Kamihigashi S, Narahara H, Miyakawa I. Effects of interferon-gamma on secretion of vascular endothelial growth factor by endometrial stromal cells. *Am J Reprod Immunol.* 2000;43(1):47–52.
28. Jonasch E, Haluska FG. Interferon in oncological practice: review of interferon biology, clinical applications, and toxicities. *Oncologist.* 2001;6(1):34–55.
29. Ferrara N. Vascular endothelial growth factor as a target for anticancer therapy. *Oncologist.* 2004;9:2–10.
30. Alavi A, Hood JD, Frausto R, Stupack DG, Cheresh DA. Role of Raf in vascular protection from distinct apoptotic stimuli. *Science.* 2003;301:94–96.
31. Hood JD, Bednarski M, Frausto R, et al. Tumor regression by targeted gene delivery to the neovasculature. *Science.* 2002;296:2404–2407.
32. Dowlati A, Robertson K, Cooney M, et al. A phase I pharmacokinetic and translational study of the novel vascular targeting agent combretastatin A-4 phosphate on a single-dose intravenous schedule in patients with advanced cancer. *Cancer Res.* 2002;62 (12):3408–3416.
33. Ohno T, Kawano K, Sasaki A, et al. Antitumor and antivascular effects of AC-7700, a combretastatin A-4 derivative, against rat liver cancer. *Int J Clin Oncol.* 2002;7 (3):171–176.
34. Cushman M, Nagarathnam D, Gopal D, He HM, Lin CM, Hamel E. Synthesis and evaluation of analogues of (*Z*)-1-(4-methoxyphenyl)-2-(3, 4, 5-trimethoxyphenyl) ethene as potential cytotoxic and antimitotic agents. *J Med Chem.* 1992;35(12):2293–2306.
35. Chaudhary A, Pandeya S, Kumar P, et al. Combretastatin A-4 analogues as anticancer agents. *Mini-Rev Med Chem.* 2007;7(12):1186–1205.
36. Pettit GR, Cragg GM, Herald DL, Schmidt JM, Lohavanijaya P. Isolation and structure of combretastatin. *Can J Chem.* 1982;60(11):1374–1376.
37. Gill RK, Kaur R, Kaur G, et al. A comprehensive review on combretastatin analogues as tubulin binding agents. *Curr Org Chem.* 2014;18(19):2462–2512.
38. Pettit GR, Lippert JW. Antineoplastic agents 429. Syntheses of the combretastatin A-1 and combretastatin B-1 prodrugs. *Anticancer Drug Design.* 2000;15(3):203–216.
39. Van Epps HL. How Heidelberger and Avery sweetened immunology. *J Exp Med.* 2005;202 (10):1306.
40. Nossal GJ, Lederberg J. Antibody production by single cells. *Nature.* 1958;181 (4620):1419–1420.
41. Zahavi D, Weiner L. Monoclonal antibodies in cancer therapy. *Antibodies.* 2020;9(3):34.
42. Ortho Multicenter Transplant Study Group. A randomized clinical trial of OKT3 monoclonal antibody for acute rejection of cadaveric renal transplants. *N Engl J Med.* 1985;313 (6):337–342.
43. Lipsky PE, van der Heijde DM, St Clair EW, et al.Anti-Tumor Necrosis Factor Trial in Rheumatoid Arthritis With Concomitant Therapy Study Group Infliximab and methotrexate in the treatment of rheumatoid arthritis. Anti-Tumor Necrosis Factor Trial in Rheumatoid Arthritis With Concomitant Therapy Study Group. *N Engl J Med.* 2000;343 (22):1594–1602. Available from: https://doi.org/10.1056/NEJM200011303432202, PMID:. Available from: 11096166.
44. Present DH, Rutgeerts P, Targan S, et al. Infliximab for the treatment of fistulas in patients with Crohn's disease. *N Engl J Med.* 1999;340:1398–1405.
45. Keating MJ, Dritselis A, Yasothan U, Kirkpatrick P. Ofatumumab. *Nat Rev Drug Discov.* 2010;9(2).

46. Galluzzi L, Vacchelli E, Fridman WH, et al. Trial watch: monoclonal antibodies in cancer therapy. *Oncoimmunology*. 2012;1(1):28–37.
47. Ferrara N, Hillan KJ, Novotny W. Bevacizumab (Avastin), a humanized anti-VEGF monoclonal antibody for cancer therapy. *Biochem Biophys Res Commun*. 2005;333(2):328–335.
48. Garcia J, Hurwitz HI, Sandler AB, Miles D, Coleman RL, Deurloo R, Chinot OL. Bevacizumab (Avastin®) in cancer treatment: A review of 15 years of clinical experience and future outlook. *Cancer treatment reviews*. 2020;86:102017. Available from: https://doi.org/10.1016/j.ctrv.2020.102017.
49. Chen HX, Gore-Langton RE, Cheson BD. Clinical trials referral resource: current clinical trials of the anti-VEGF monoclonal antibody bevacizumab. *Oncology (Williston Park)*. 2001;15(8):1017. 1020, 1023–1026.
50. Ferrara N, Gerber HP, LeCouter J. The biology of VEGF and its receptors. *Nat Med*. 2003;9(6):669–676.
51. Ebbers HC, van Meer PJ, Moors EH, Mantel-Teeuwisse AK, Leufkens HG, Schellekens H. Measures of biosimilarity in monoclonal antibodies in oncology: the case of bevacizumab. *Drug Discov Today*. 2013;18(17–18):872–879.
52. Stopeck A, Sheldon M, Vahedian M, Cropp G, Gosalia R, Hannah A. Results of a Phase I dose-escalating study of the antiangiogenic agent, SU5416, in patients with advanced malignancies. *Clin Cancer Res*. 2002;8(9):2798–2805.
53. Fabbro D, Manley P. Su-6668. SUGEN. *Curr Opin Investig Drugs*. 2001;2:1142–1148.
54. Hoekman K. SU6668, a multitargeted angiogenesis inhibitor. *Cancer J*. 2001;7(suppl 3): S134–S138.
55. Jabłońska-Trypuć A, Matejczyk M, Rosochacki S. Matrix metalloproteinases (MMPs), the main extracellular matrix (ECM) enzymes in collagen degradation, as a target for anticancer drugs. *J Enzyme Inhib Med Chem*. 2016;31(suppl 1):177–183.
56. Mannello F, Tonti G, Papa S. Matrix metalloproteinase inhibitors as anticancer therapeutics. *Curr Cancer Drug Targets*. 2005;5(4):285–298.
57. Hoekstra R, Eskens FA, Verweij J. Matrix metalloproteinase inhibitors: current developments and future perspectives. *Oncologist*. 2001;6(5):415–427.
58. Bramhall SR, Hallissey MT, Whiting J, et al. Marimastat as maintenance therapy for patients with advanced gastric cancer: a randomised trial. *Br J Cancer*. 2002;86(12):1864–1870.
59. Bramhall SR, Schulz J, Nemunaitis J, Brown PD, Baillet M, Buckels JA. A double-blind placebo-controlled, randomised study comparing gemcitabine and marimastat with gemcitabine and placebo as first line therapy in patients with advanced pancreatic cancer. *Br J Cancer*. 2002;87(2):161–167.
60. Groves MD, Puduvalli VK, Hess KR, et al. Phase II trial of temozolomide plus the matrix metalloproteinase inhibitor, marimastat, in recurrent and progressive glioblastoma multiforme. *J Clin Oncol*. 2002;20(5):1383–1388.
61. Vihinen P, Kähäri VM. Matrix metalloproteinases in cancer: prognostic markers and therapeutic targets. *Int J Cancer*. 2002;99(2):157–166.
62. King J, Zhao J, Clingan P, Morris D. Randomised double blind placebo control study of adjuvant treatment with the metalloproteinase inhibitor Marimastat in patients with inoperable colorectal hepatic metastases: significant survival advantage in patients with musculoskeletal side-effects. *Anticancer Res*. 2003;23:639–645.
63. Ramnath N, Creaven PJ. Matrix metalloproteinase inhibitors. *Curr Oncol Rep*. 2004;6:96–102.
64. Coleman RE. Treatment of skeletal complications of cancer with zoledronic acid. *Semin Oncol*. 2002;29(suppl 21):1–49.

65. Body JJ, Mancini I. Bisphosphonates for cancer patients: why, how, and when? *Support Care Cancer*. 2002;10:399–407.
66. Body JJ, Greip P, Coleman RE, et al. A phase I study of AMGN-0007, a recombinant osteoprotegerin construct, in patients with multiple myeloma or breast carcinoma related bone metastases. *Cancer*. 2003;97(suppl 3):887–892.
67. Ribas A, Wolchok JD. Cancer immunotherapy using checkpoint blockade. *Science*. 2018;359(6382):1350–1355.
68. June CH, Sadelain M. Chimeric antigen receptor T cells. *N Engl J Med*. 2018;379:64–73.
69. Guedan S, Ruella M, June CH. Emerging cellular therapies for cancer. *Annu Rev Immunol*. 2019;37:145–171.
70. Mantovani A, Sozzani S, Locati M, Allavena P, Sica A. Macrophage polarization: tumor-associated macrophages as a paradigm for polarized M2 mononuclear phagocytes. *Trends Immunol*. 2002;23(11):549–555.
71. Martinez FO, Sica A, Mantovani A, Locati M. Macrophage activation and polarization. *Front Biosci*. 2008;13:453–461.
72. Sato T, Terai M, Tamura Y, Alexeev V, Mastrangelo MJ, Selvan SR. Interleukin 10 in the tumor microenvironment: a target for anticancer immunotherapy. *Immunol Res*. 2011;51(2):170–182.
73. Fong CW. Platinum anti-cancer drugs: free radical mechanism of Pt-DNA adduct formation and anti-neoplastic effect. *Free Radic Biol Med*. 2016;95:216–229.
74. McCann JJ, Lo TM, Webster DA. Cross-linking of DNA by alkylating agents and effects on DNA function in the chick embryo. *Cancer Res*. 1971;31(11):1573–1579.
75. Ralhan R, Kaur J. Alkylating agents and cancer therapy. *Expert Opin Ther Pat*. 2007;17(9):1061–1075.
76. Oronsky BT, Reid T, Knox SJ, Scicinski JJ. The scarlet letter of alkylation: a mini review of selective alkylating agents. *Transl Oncol*. 2012;5(4):226–229.
77. Liu LF, Rowe TC, Yang L, Tewey KM, Chen GL. Cleavage of DNA by mammalian DNA topoisomerase II. *J Biol Chem*. 1983;258(24):15365–15370.
78. Hiasa H, Yousef DO, Marians KJ. DNA strand cleavage is required for replication fork arrest by a frozen topoisomerase-quinolone-DNA ternary complex. *J Biol Chem*. 1996;271(42):26424–26429.
79. Nelson EM, Tewey KM, Liu LF. Mechanism of antitumor drug action: poisoning of mammalian DNA topoisomerase II on DNA by 4′-(9-acridinylamino)-methanesulfon-*m*-anisidide. *Proc Natl Acad Sci USA*. 1984;81(5):1361–1365.
80. Ulukan H, Swaan PW. Camptothecins. *Drugs*. 2002;62(14):2039–2057.
81. Dauvois S, White R, Parker MG. The antiestrogen ICI 182780 disrupts estrogen receptor nucleocytoplasmic shuttling. *J Cell Sci*. 1993;106(4):1377–1388.
82. Halachmi S, Marden E, Martin G, MacKay H, Abbondanza C, Brown M. Estrogen receptor-associated proteins: possible mediators of hormone-induced transcription. *Science*. 1994;264(5164):1455–1458.
83. Shen L, Li J, Xu L, et al. miR-497 induces apoptosis of breast cancer cells by targeting Bcl-w. *Exp Ther Med*. 2012;3(3):475–480.
84. Ritter CA, Arteaga CL. *The epidermal growth factor receptor–tyrosine kinase: a promising therapeutic target in solid tumors. Seminars in Oncology*. 30. WB Saunders; 2003:3–11.
85. Plosker GL, Figgitt DP. Rituximab. *Drugs*. 2003;63(8):803–843.
86. Weiner GJ. *Rituximab: mechanism of action. Seminars in Hematology*. 47. WB Saunders; 2010:115–123.

87. Onrust SV, Lamb HM, Balfour JA. Rituximab. *Drugs*. 1999;58(1):79–88.
88. Jotereau F, Labarrière N, Gervois N, Pandolfino MC, Dreno B. Passive immunotherapy of melanoma. *Bull Cancer*. 2003;90(7):583–586.
89. Foy KC, Liu Z, Phillips G, Miller M, Kaumaya PT. Combination treatment with HER-2 and VEGF peptide mimics induces potent anti-tumor and anti-angiogenic responses in vitro and in vivo. *J Biol Chem*. 2011;286(15):13626–13637.
90. Davis TA, Grillo-Lopez AJ, White CA, et al. Rituximab anti-CD20 monoclonal antibody therapy in non-Hodgkin's lymphoma: safety and efficacy of re-treatment. *J Clin Oncol*. 2000;18(17):3135–3143.
91. Vose JM, Wahl RL, Saleh M, et al. Multicenter phase II study of iodine-131 tositumomab for chemotherapy-relapsed/refractory low-grade and transformed low-grade B-cell non-Hodgkin's lymphomas. *J Clin Oncol*. 2000;18(6):1316–1323.
92. Gibson A, Jain VK, Zelenetz A, Leonard J. Iodine-131 tositumomab (Bexxar) in relapsed/refractory non-Hodgkin's lymphoma: update from the 2001 American Society of Hematology Meeting. *Clin Lymphoma*. 2002;2(4):209–211.
93. Rai KR, Freter CE, Mercier RJ, et al. Alemtuzumab in previously treated chronic lymphocytic leukemia patients who also had received fludarabine. *J Clin Oncol*. 2002;20(18):3891–3897.
94. Lundin J, Kimby E, Bjorkholm M, et al. Phase II trial of subcutaneous anti-CD52 monoclonal antibody alemtuzumab (Campath-1H) as first-line treatment for patients with B-cell chronic lymphocytic leukemia (B-CLL). *Blood*. 2002;100(3):768–773.
95. Roboz GJ, Knovich MA, Bayer RL, et al. Efficacy and safety of gemtuzumab ozogamicin in patients with poor-prognosis acute myeloid leukemia. *Leuk Lymphoma*. 2002;43(10):1951–1955.
96. Larson RA, Boogaerts M, Estey E, et al. Antibody-targeted chemotherapy of older patients with acute myeloid leukemia in first relapse using Mylotarg (gemtuzumab ozogamicin). *Leukemia*. 2002;16(9):1627–1636.
97. Ligibel JA, Winer EP. Trastuzumab/chemotherapy combinations in metastatic breast cancer. *Semin Oncol*. 2002;29(3 suppl 11):38–43.
98. McKeage K, Perry CM. Trastuzumab: a review of its use in the treatment of metastatic breast cancer overexpressing HER2. *Drugs*. 2002;62(1):209–243.
99. Baselga J. The EGFR as a target for anticancer therapy—focus on cetuximab. *Eur J Cancer*. 2001;37(suppl 4):S16–S22.
100. Robert F, Ezekiel MP, Spencer SA, et al. Phase I study of anti-epidermal growth factor receptor antibody cetuximab in combination with radiation therapy in patients with advanced head and neck cancer. *J Clin Oncol*. 2001;19(13):3234–3243.
101. Reddish M, MacLean GD, Koganty RR, et al. Anti-MUC1 class I restricted CTLs in metastatic breast cancer patients immunized with a synthetic MUC1 peptide. *Int J Cancer*. 1998;76(6):817–823.
102. Baker CH, Kedar D, McCarty MF, et al. Blockade of epidermal growth factor receptor signaling on tumor cells and tumor-associated endothelial cells for therapy of human carcinomas. *Am J Pathol*. 2002;161(3):929–938.
103. Herbst RS, Kies MS. ZD1839 (Iressa) in non-small cell lung cancer. *Oncologist*. 2002;7(suppl 4):9–15.
104. Ranson M. ZD1839 (Iressa): for more than just non-small cell lung cancer. *Oncologist*. 2002;7(suppl 4):16–24.
105. Hidalgo M, Siu LL, Nemunaitis J, et al. Phase I and pharmacologic study of OSI-774, an epidermal growth factor receptor tyrosine kinase inhibitor, in patients with advanced solid malignancies. *J Clin Oncol*. 2001;19(13):3267–3279.

106. Allen LF, Lenehan PF, Eiseman IA, Elliott WL, Fry DW. Potential benefits of the irreversible pan-erbB inhibitor, CI-1033, in the treatment of breast cancer. *Semin Oncol.* 2002;29(3 suppl 11):11–21.
107. Cohen MH, Moses ML, Pazdur R. Gleevec for the treatment of chronic myelogenous leukemia: U.S. Food and Drug Administration regulatory mechanisms, accelerated approval, and orphan drug status. *Oncologist.* 2002;7(5):390–392.
108. Joensuu H, Fletcher C, Dimitrijevic S, Silberman S, Roberts P, Demetri G. Management of malignant gastrointestinal stromal tumours. *Lancet Oncol.* 2002;3(11):655–664.
109. Hoover RR, Mahon FX, Melo JV, Daley GQ. Overcoming STI571 resistance with the farnesyl transferase inhibitor SCH66336. *Blood.* 2002;100(3):1068–1071.
110. Karp JE, Kaufmann SH, Adjei AA, Lancet JE, Wright JJ, End DW. Current status of clinical trials of farnesyltransferase inhibitors. *Curr Opin Oncol.* 2001;13(6):470–476.
111. Hotte SJ, Hirte HW. BAY 43-9006: early clinical data in patients with advanced solid malignancies. *Curr Pharm Des.* 2002;8(25):2249–2253.
112. Dancey JE. Agents targeting ras signaling pathway. *Curr Pharm Des.* 2002;8(25):2259–2267.
113. Elit L. CCI-779 Wyeth. *Curr Opin Investig Drugs.* 2002;3(8):1249–1253.
114. Brockstein B, Samuels B, Humerickhouse R, et al. Phase II studies of bryostatin-1 in patients with advanced sarcoma and advanced head and neck cancer. *Invest New Drugs.* 2001;19(3):249–254.
115. Pfister DG, McCaffrey J, Zahalsky AJ, et al. A phase II trial of bryostatin-1 in patients with metastatic or recurrent squamous cell carcinoma of the head and neck. *Invest New Drugs.* 2002;20(1):123–127.
116. Virchis A, Ganeshaguru K, Hart S, et al. A novel treatment approach for low grade lymphoproliferative disorders using PKC412 (CGP41251), an inhibitor of protein kinase C. *Hematol J.* 2002;3(3):131–136.
117. Rose WC, Long BH, Fairchild CR, Lee FY, Kadow JF. Preclinical pharmacology of BMS-275183, an orally active taxane. *Clin Cancer Res.* 2001;7(7):2016–2021.
118. Lee FY, Borzilleri R, Fairchild CR, et al. BMS-247550: a novel epothilone analog with a mode of action similar to paclitaxel but possessing superior antitumor efficacy. *Clin Cancer Res.* 2001;7(5):1429–1437.
119. Stachel SJ, Biswas K, Danishefsky SJ. The epothilones, eleutherobins, and related types of molecules. *Curr Pharm Des.* 2001;7(13):1277–1290.

Chapter 22

An insight into the agents used for immunomodulation and their mechanism of action

Avishek Mandal[1], Priti Das[2], Rudranil Bhowmik[1], Hindol Mazumdar[1], Md. Adil Shaharyar[1], Reshma Kumari[1], Sandipan Jana[1], Susmita Patra[3], Pallab Kanti Haldar[1] and Sanmoy Karmakar[1]

[1]Bioeuivalence Study Centre, Department of Pharmaceutical Technology, Jadavpur University, Kolkata, West Bengal, India, [2]TCG Life Sciences Pvt Ltd (formerly "Chembiotek Research International"), Kolkata – R&D Centre, Chemistry, Kolkata, West Bengal, India, [3]Department of Pharmaceutical Technology, Adamas University, Barasat, Kolkata, West Bengal, India

Introduction

In our body, the immune system consists of the tissue and various types of cells like white blood cells derived from the thymus gland, lymph nodes, and lymph vessels which protect from viruses, bacteria, parasites, and fungus.[1] The outer parts of our body, like hair, nails, the skin, complex construction that covers our body, protect the deeper tissues, and its cellular composition works in harmony to prevent infection.[1] Several types of exogenous and endogenous agents contribute to the ability and function of the immune system that leads to immunosuppression or immunostimulant.[1] The host immunity abnormal progression can lead to various types of infectious disease and cancer. There are several types of antiinflammatory and immunosuppressive drugs like a vaccine, therapeutic antibodies [(monoclonal antibodies and polyclonal antibodies (pAbs)], and Toll-like receptor agonists among the immune system modulators allowed by the US Foods and Drug Administration (FDA).[2] Oral infections such as mucosal infections that spread via cell or physiological reactions persistently focused toward epithelial or connective structures recurring series represent a large category of oral mucosal diseases.[3] Our bodies can fight against all kinds of pathogens and poisons that might harm our tissues or organs. Immunity is a term used to describe persons' ability to defend themselves. The first step to resist bacterium, virus, or toxin by our body is called innate immunity.[4] Some types of

How Synthetic Drugs Work. DOI: https://doi.org/10.1016/B978-0-323-99855-0.00022-1

viral infections are hog cholera, cattle plague, and distemper (viral infection), where a huge percentage of animals are affected, which are resistant to our body by the innate immunity.[4] Various compounds and microorganisms in the blood of innate immunity bind to foreign organisms or poisons and eliminate them. A natural killer cell is able to detect pathogens, foreign substance eliminated, and even a few virus-infected cells.[4] The specific protective system that forms an antibody and activated lymphocyte that attack and destroy the specific invading organism or toxin involves the adaptive immune system. Acquired immunity provides a significant level of protection against toxin, botulinum toxin, tetanizing toxin of tetanus, which could be protected against in doses as high as 100,000 times the amount that would be lethal without immunity.[4] Immunity leads to protect the infection. When any foreign substances stimulate the immune environment, it is called mainly antigen. Several components are involved in the immune system like humoral immunity, cellular immunity, immunoglobulin, lymph node, spleen, and thymus. Mostly two types of immunity we have identified: that is active and passive. Immunotherapies affect the immune system at various stages. As a consequence, various drugs that selectively inhibit or enhance specific classes and subgroups of immune-sensitive cells have been introduced, that is, T cell, B cell, lymphocyte, cytotoxicity, chemokine, macrophage, and antibodies. Immunotherapeutic drugs alter the immune response by raising (immunostimulatory) or decreasing (immunosuppressives) serum antibody generation.[1] Immunostimulants, often recognized as immunostimulatory, are agents (drugs and nutrients) that cause or enhance the function of most of the immune elements of the system, that is, the granulocyte-macrophage colony-stimulating factor. Immunosuppressive medications weaken the immune system and reduce the chance of foreign substances, such as implant organs, being rejected. The mechanisms of action of different types of immunosuppressive agents differentiate, that is, mammalian target of rapamycin (mTOR) inhibitor: sirolimus, steroids: prednisone. The mechanism and function of immunomodulation are described in this chapter (Fig. 22.1).[5,6]

Immunomodulators

Immunomodulators are natural or synthesized medicines that can regulate immunological disorders by altering or stabilizing immunity. In several other terms, they restore the equilibrium of immune systems by strengthening damaged immune systems or moderating overly aggressive immune systems.[1] Immunomodulators are divided into two categories: immunostimulants and immunosuppressants. Immunostimulants are drugs designed to improve the body's resilience to infections by boosting the immune system's baseline response, which is particularly important in the immune system deficient.[2] Immunosuppressants are used in treatments to inhibit the immunity function and are used to treat an organism's immunological reactions

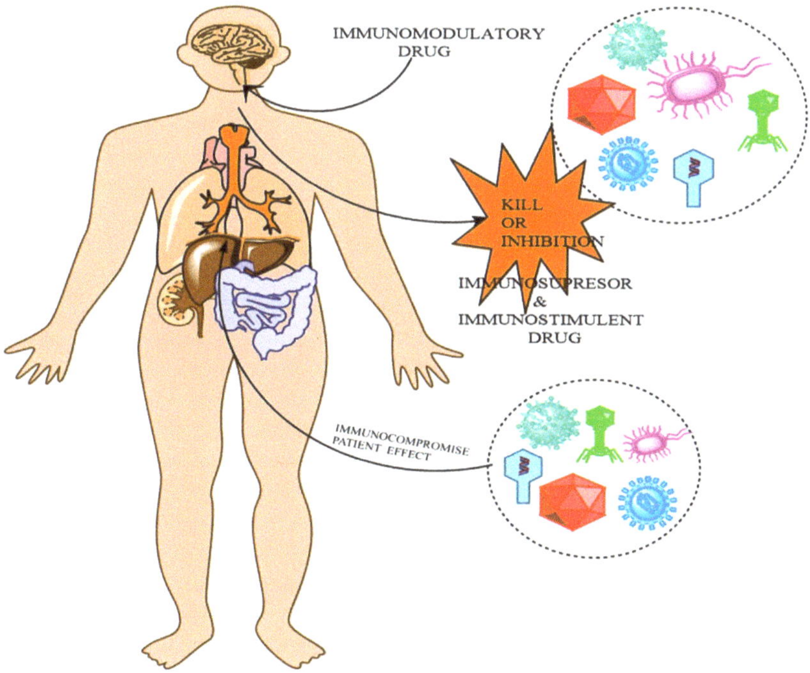

FIGURE 22.1 Immunomodulatory drug function against foreign elements.

against its own healthy cells and hypersensitivity.[7] This study would focus on immunomodulatory drug classes and their mechanisms of action given in Fig. 22.2.

Immunosuppressants

Immunosuppressants are such treatments that are used to calm down an overactive immune function that is causing harm to the host, such as in cases of autoimmune disorders or oversensitivity. Standard immune suppressant drugs, steroid-sparing medicines, and biologic drugs can all be generically categorized based on their method of action and origin.[8] These different groups' modes of operation and indications are discussed in further detail.[8]

Glucocorticoid

Glucocorticoids are a component of the immune system's mechanism which decreases inflammation and other facets of immune function. As a reason, these medications are used to treat diseases like allergies, asthma, autoimmune diseases, and sepsis, which are exacerbated by an overactive immune system. Although glucocorticoids have a spectrum of impact, including potential health

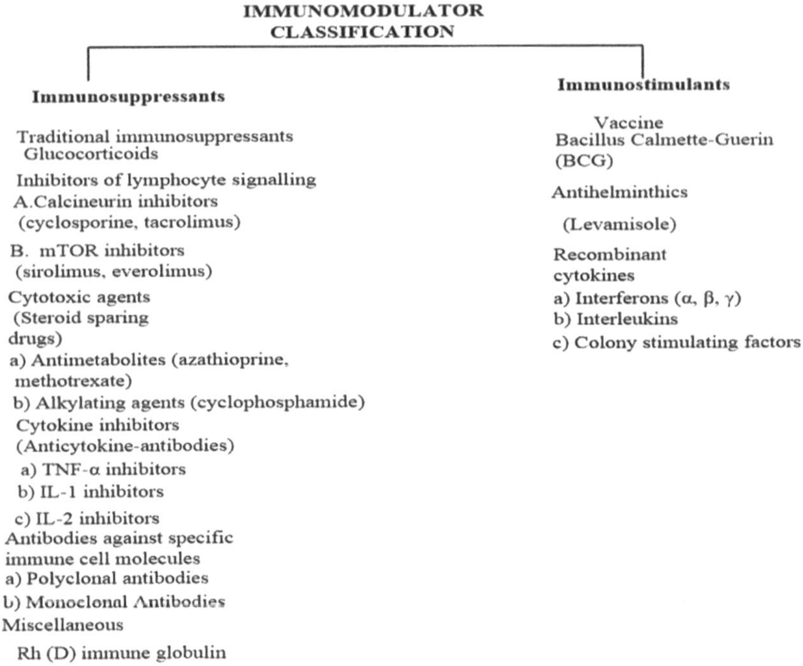

FIGURE 22.2 Immunomodulators classification.

risks, they are seldom available over-the-counter.[9] They also disrupt some of the pathological pathways of cancer cells, so they are used to cure cancer at elevated doses. This involves inhibiting lymphocyte differentiation in the treatment of lymphomas and leukemias, as well as reducing anticancer medication side effects. In particular, corticosteroids have progressed to become the standard of care for a broad range of clinical manifestations and disorders having an allergy and alter the immune condition, or inflammation.[9]

Mechanism of action of classical immunomodulatory drugs

Several cells that have been linked to inflammatory response, such as macrophages, T lymphocytes, mast cells, dendritic cells (DCs), and neutrophilic leukocytes, are inhibited by the medications.

Proinflammatory transcription factors like nuclear factor-B (NFB) and activator protein 1 regulate gene transcription changes. These proinflammatory transcription factors used the activation of transcriptional coactivator proteins and changes in chromatin modifications such as histone acetylation to turn on inflammatory genes.[10] Through inhibiting the phospholipase A2 enzyme, glucocorticoids also reduce prostaglandin activity. Several genes that signal for inflammation cytokines, chemokines, inflammatory enzymes, receptors, as well as macromolecules of binding are inhibited by the glucocorticoids, which is the most significant impact.[11,12] The mechanisms of the drugs, observation, doses, administration, and approval of FDA are presented in Table 22.1.

Prednisone

Prednisone is an immunomodulatory medicine that is a synthesized antiinflammatory glucocorticoid generated with cortisone. It was approved by the FDA for the first time on February 21, 1955. Prednisone is used to treat allergic reactions, dermatological, kidney-related infections, hematological, ophthalmological, nervous system, renal, cardiovascular, rheumatologic, viral, endocrine, or neoplastic diseases, as well as organ donation recipients.[25] Prednisone is converted to its active form, prednisolone, a glucocorticoid agonist corticosteroid, in the liver. Corticosteroids have short-term effects such as decreased vasodilation and capillary permeability, as well as reduced leukocyte migration to immune cells. Glucocorticoids suppress neutrophil apoptosis and demargination; inhibited phospholipase A2, which reduces arachidonic acid derivative development; therefore the suppression of NF-Kappa B and other inflammatory transcription factors; and they stimulate antiinflammatory genes such as IL-10 (Interleukin). This medication causes corticosteroids that have an antiinflammatory function at lower doses, but they suppress the immune system at higher doses.[26] It is clinically important that high doses of glucocorticoids cause sodium levels to rise and potassium levels to decline.[27] It is mostly found in tablet shape in the market. Clinical trials for COPD patients, progressive follicular lymphoma, IgA nephropathy, and rheumatoid arthritis have already been completed.[28]

Hydrocortamate

This drug is a synthetic glucocorticoid used to treat inflammation caused by corticosteroid-responsive dermatoses because of its antiinflammatory or immunosuppressive properties. It has a character that binds to the cortisol receptor while glucocorticoid steroid hormones are present.[29] This results in a variety of essential cardiovascular, biochemical, immunologic, and homeostatic impacts. Hydrocortamate suppresses hyperimmunity mainly. It works by blocking the cytokines IL-1, IL-2, IL-3, IL-4, IL-5, IL-6, IL-8, and tumor necrosis factor (TNF)-alpha, with IL-2 being the most prominent.[1] T-cell proliferation is limited by reduced cytokine production. The action mechanism in the cytosol, hydrocortamate, attaches to the glucocorticoid receptor.[1] In the cell the newly created receptor–ligand complex translocated the nucleus after binding the receptor, where it connects to a number of glucocorticoid reaction elements in the promoter region of the target genes. Lipocortins, phospholipase A2 inhibitory proteins that regulate the

TABLE 22.1 Mechanisms, observation, doses, and administration, Foods and Drug Administration (FDA)-approved drug.

Steroid-free drugs	Sl no	Drug	Mechanisms	Observation	Doses and administration	Approval of FDA
Calcineurin inhibitor	1	Cyclosporine	Activates genes encoding IL-3, IL-5 in basophils and mast cells	Electrolytes, blood pressure	2.5-5 mg/kg/d, oral	1983[13–15]
	2	Tacrolimus	T-cell activation and cytokine release		0.1%–0.3%, 0.3 mg/kg/d, ointment	2006[16–18]
Antibiotics	3	Dapsone (sulfone antibiotic)	Inhibits neutrophil chemotaxis by blocking myeloperoxidase	CBC, G6PD activity, LFT, and RFT	25-50 mg/d, oral	2016[1,19]
Antimetabolites	4	Azathioprine	Inhibits RNA and DNA syntheses	CBC and LFT	3-4 mg/week	1968[20]
	5	Methotrexate	RNA synthesis during S phase, interferes with transmethylation suppression	CBC, electrolytes, RFT, and LFT	15 mg/week	1953[21]
	6	Mycophenolate mofetil	Inhibits inosine monophosphate dehydrogenase	CBC, liver enzymes	0.5-1.5 g twice daily	1995[22]
Alkylating agents	7	Cyclophosphamide	Effective against B and T cells	CBC with platelets, RFT, urine	1-g IV	1959[23,24]

CBC, Complete blood count; *G6PD*, glucose-6-phosphate dehydrogenase; *LFT*, liverfunction test.

prostaglandins and leukotrienes formation by inhibiting arachidonic acid, are thought to be associated with corticosteroids' antiinflammatory effects. As DNA interacts with a basic transcription factor, gene expression rises.[30,31]

Calcineurin inhibitors

Three medications make calcineurin inhibitors (CNIs) (cyclosporine, tacrolimus, and pimecrolimus). CNIs are mainly used as immunosuppressive medications that block the main signaling phosphatase calcineurin. For this action, these medications are useful in the long-term treatment of patients with allografts. CNIs suppress the immune system and inhibit T-cell proliferation by inhibiting the phosphatase calcineurin, which is a central signaling phosphatase in the immune system.[32]

Cyclosporine

Cyclosporine is an immunomodulatory drug known as a CNI that helps resist organ transplant rejection which is used to treat inflammatory and autoimmune diseases. It was first marketed by Sandoz and the FDA accepted it for usage in 1983.[13] Allograft rejection, graft versus host disease, and inflammatory autoimmune disease are some of the severe immune-mediated reactions that prevent this drug and manage it. T-cell activation is inhibited by cyclosporine, a CNI. It binds to the cyclophilin-1 receptor; hence, it is a cyclophilin-1 receptor binder inside cells and it joins cyclosporine and cyclophilin to produce the cyclosporine–cyclophilin complex.[14] Such combination then inhibits calcineurin, which prevents nuclear factor dephosphorylation and regulation in activated T cells nuclear factor of activated T-cells (NF-AT), which is responsible for inflammatory responses. Our bodies' immune system's (NF-AT) is a transcription factor that creates cytokines mainly IL-2, IL-4, and interferon-gamma, including TNF-α, that are all active in the inflammatory process. Cyclosporine's immunosuppressive effects are suggested to be related to its inhibition of IL-2, which is needed for T-cell activation and proliferation.[14] In rodents the oral LD50 is 1480 mg/kg, while in humans, the TDLO is 12 mg/kg.[15] In the market, liquid, injection, solution, and capsule forms are available. Clinical trials for acute renal failure, heart transplantation, pterygia, dry eyes, and cataracts have also been approved.

Tacrolimus

Tacrolimus is an immunosuppressive treatment used to decrease the functions and an immunological system of the patient; therefore the threat can arise of organ rejection after an organ transplant.[16] This was approved by the FDA to be used in liver transplantation in 1994. Tacrolimus specifically attaches to the immunophilin FKBP-12 (FK506-binding protein) and creates a new inhibitory complex peptidylprolyl isomerase action. This inhibits all the T-lymphocyte signaling and IL-2 transcription. It has shown potential effects in the treatment of eczema, especially in atopic eczema, when applied topically. It functions in a similar way to steroids in terms of reducing inflammation, except it is not as powerful. Tacrolimus' mode of action in atopic dermatitis is unknown.[17] T-lymphocyte activation is inhibited by tacrolimus that attaches to a protein found inside the cell called FKBP-12. The phosphatase activity calcineurin is blocked by making a complex with tacrolimus-FKBP-12, calcium, calmodulin, and calcineurin. It prevents the nuclear factor of activated T cells (NF-AT), a nuclear portion considered to trigger gene transcript used for lymphokine production, which is being dephosphorylated and translocated. This drug prevents the transcript of the genes that encode IL-3, IL-4, IL-5, GM-CSF, and TNF-α in its initial phases of T-cell stimulation. Tacrolimus has also been demonstrated to lower the expression of FceRI on Langerhans cells and prevent the production of mast cells in the skin and basophils. It is only available in capsule form in the market. [18] There are no clinical trial accepted treatments for liver diseases, kidney transplant failure, or rejection have been established.

Mammalian target of rapamycin inhibitors

A new class of immunosuppressants is inhibitors of the mTOR. Immunosuppressants such as sirolimus and everolimus are very active found in various types of studies. They may not suppress calcineurin and, therefore, signal I of T-cell activation, unlike other macrolides, including tacrolimus and cyclosporine A. Besides binding and signaling through two protein complexes, mTORC1 and mTORC2, mTOR regulates cellular metabolism, development, and proliferation.[33]

Sirolimus

Sirolimus is an immunosuppressive drug that also has antifungal and anticancer effects. A macrolide derived from streptomyces hygroscopic inhibits cytokine synthesis by specifically inhibiting cytokine overexpression. Sirolimus drug activate different way than other immunosuppressants in inhibiting antigenic and cytokine (IL-2, IL-4, and IL-15) stimulation stimulates T lymphocyte activation.[34] Sirolimus effectively prevents the development of antibodies. In cells, sirolimus forms an immunosuppressive complex with the immunophilin FK Binding Protein-12 (FKBP-12). It connects to the mTOR, a central regulatory kinase, and inhibits its activation. This inhibition prevents T-cell proliferation triggered by cytokines from progressing the G1 to S cycle cell division. Markets are mostly fond of tablets. The clinical trials for coronary artery restenosis, coronary heart disease, rejection transplant, renal allograft recipients, transplant, and kidney therapy are almost finished.[25]

Everolimus

Everolimus is a rapamycin (sirolimus) derivative that acts as an mTOR inhibitor in the same form as rapamycin. These are most commonly used to avoid organ rejection after a transplant as an immunosuppressant. The mechanism of action mTOR inhibitor that link to the FK506 binding protein-12 (FKBP-12) with high affinity, producing a drug combination that prevents mTOR activation.[35] It causes a block in the transition of cells from G1 to S process, causing cell growth hampered and apoptosis. Cell proliferation, angiogenesis, and glucose absorption are all reduced as mTOR is inhibited by everolimus.[35] It can be found on the market as a tablet.

Antimetabolite

An antimetabolite is a compound that prevents the use of a metabolite and occurs naturally in the metabolism. Although antimetabolites can also have toxic effects on cells, such as preventing cell growth and differentiation, these substances have been used as a cancer treatment.[36]

Leflunomide

The DMARD (disease-modifying antirheumatic drug) family of medicines involves leflunomide. It is also called pyrimidine synthesis inhibitor.[37] It was approved by FDA in 1999. Leflunomide is used to treat acute rheumatoid arthritis (RA) in adults. T cell is elevated in RA, which is an autoimmune condition. The inhibition of dihydroorotate dehydrogenase by leflunomide would have a significant impact on produced T cells, which depends on de novo pyrimidine synthesis and starts to the salvage pathway of pyrimidine synthesis.[38] The metabolites are mostly accountable for the drug action in vivo system. Leflunomide's mechanism of action is unknown, although it seems to mainly involve the modulation of autoimmune lymphocytes. It binds to a position near the flavin mononucleotide in the hydrophobic passage. The inhibition of dihydroorotate dehydrogenase blocks the de novo pathway from producing ribonucleotide uridine monophosphate (rUMP), resulting in lower rUMP level, G1 cell cycle delay, decreased DNA and RNA synthesis, and suppression of cell proliferation.[39] Leflunomide inhibits tyrosine kinases. Tyrosine kinases stimulate DNA repair, apoptosis, and cell proliferation through activating signaling pathways. Tyrosine kinase inhibition can facilitate the treatment of cancer by stopping tumor cells from repairing themselves.[39]

6-Mercaptopurine pathology and treatment

6 Mercaptopurine has antineoplastic, antimetabolite, and immunomodulatory properties. It inhibits purine metabolism, therefore, inhibiting nucleic acid

synthesis, and prevention in recovery management for leukemia, normally in combination with other medications.[40] The pharmacodynamics of this drug is a wide class purine analog that inhibits nucleic acid biosynthesis which is shown to be effective contradiction of human leukemia.[41] This analog is mainly based on adenine and hypoxanthine. It is unclear whether the mercaptopurine's and metabolite's biochemical is directly or indirectly important for cell death. The treatment of Crohn's disease (CD), acute lymphocytic leukemia, lymphoma, lymphoblastic leukemia, and childhood acute promyelocytic leukemia has also been reported. Mercaptopurine is transformed to thioinosinic acid by interacting with hypoxanthine and guanine for the enzyme hypoxanthine-guanine phosphoribosyl transferase (HGPRTase) (TIMP). TIMP inhibits a number of inosinic acid (IMP)-related reactions, including the change of IMP to xanthylic acid (XMP) and the alteration of IMP to adenylic acid (AMP) through adenyl succinate (SAMP).[42] TIMP changes 6-methylthioinosinate (MTIMP) after methylation, which inhibits glutamine-5 phosphoribosyl pyrophosphate aminotransferase as well as TIMP.[43] The enzyme as their unique property from the de novo link for purine ribonucleotide synthesis is glutamine-5-phosphoribosylpyrophosphate amidotransferase.[44] Mercaptopurine can be extracted from DNA and create deoxythioguanosine, as per experiments using radiolabelled mercaptopurine. Inosinate (IMP) dehydrogenase and xanthylate (XMP) aminase, which transform TIMP to thioguanylic acid, can convert some mercaptopurine to nucleotide derivatives of 6-thioguanine (6-TG) (TGMP).[45]

Alkalyting agent

Alkylating agents are divided into five categories: mustards that are high in nitrogen (e.g., bendamustine, chlorambucil, cyclophosphamide, ifosfamide, mechlorethamine, and melphalan); nitrosoureas are a kind of nitrosourea (e.g., carmustine, lomustine, and streptozocin); alkyl sulfonates are a type of alkyl sulfonate (e.g., busulfan); triazines are a form of triazine (e.g., dacarbazine and temozolomide).[46] Several cancers are treated with alkylating agents. They are, however, cytotoxic to normal cells, particularly those that differentiate regularly, such as those in the gastrointestinal tract, bone marrow, testicles, and ovaries, which can lead to infertility.[47] The majority of alkylating agents are carcinogenic as well. The use of hyperthermia to improve the effects of alkylating agents is particularly effective.

Steroid-free medications

Immunosuppressive drugs are often used in conjunction with steroid treatment to reduce the number of steroids required and thereby avoid any of the negative aspects of steroid therapy. As a result, these treatments are often referred to as "steroid-sparing" or "adjuvant" medicines. Steroid sparing therapy refers to nonsteroid immune suppressants that enable partial or complete removal of corticosteroids. Based on their mode of action, these drugs can be classified into three groups: alkylating (cyclophosphamide and chlorambucil), antimetabolite (methotrexate, mycophenolate mofetil, and azathioprine), and antibiotic/CNI (cyclosporine, tacrolimus, and sirolimus).[48] Corticosteroid medication mainly benefited (1) the potency to lower systemic corticosteroid to a normal dosage of 10 mg or less of oral prednisone; (2) clinically lower pain; (3) recovery or reduction of symptoms such as pain; and (4) patient awareness to any medication and their effects and all criteria for corticosteroid-sparing therapy performance.[49]

Oral signs and symptoms

1. SLE (systemic lupus erythematosus) and scleroderma are connective tissue diseases.[50]
2. Behcet's disease, erythema multiforme, lichen planus, pemphigus, pemphigoid, epidermolysis bullosa, RA, Sjogren's syndrome (SS), and Wegener's granulomatosis are all immune-mediated diseases. In the circumstance of graft rejection, these are whether acute or chronic.[50,51]

Cyclophosphamide

Immunosuppressive agent cyclophosphamide is activated in the liver to become active aldophosphamide. Lymphoma and leukemia have also been treated with it. Cyclophosphamide is an anticancer drug that belongs to the alkylating agent family.[23] It is used to treat a variety of cancers. They inhibit tumor development by actively attaching DNA with cross-linking guanine bases in double-helix strands. These molecules are unable to make coiling and disperse as a result of formation. The cells can no longer differentiate because this is needed for DNA replication. Alkylating agents work in three ways: (1) they attach alkyl clusters to DNA bases, causing DNA to be split by restoration enzymes as they try to change the alkylated bases, stopping DNA and RNA from the affected DNA; (2) it causes DNA harm by forming cross-links (bonds with in the DNA), averting DNA from being detached for transcription; and (3) that initiation of nucleotide mispairing, which results in genetic changes.[24] Markets also provide injection, liquid, lyophilized, solution, tablet, and capsule forms.

Definition of biologics

Any medical substance made in or derived from a biological source is referred to as biopharmaceuticals—biologics or biological agents (BA).[52] Immunocytes or their metabolites are often targeted by biologics, which target various steps in proinflammatory pathways.[53] The receptors implicated in the pathological of immune related and neoplastic diseases is to be related their function. In contrast to corticosteroids and traditional corticosteroid-sparing immunosuppressants, mediators offer a huge number of selective antiinflammatory or immunosuppressive effects. As a result, they are likely to be more selective like medication than mere palliative therapy, which has cytokines, antibodies, or fusion proteins.[52]

Biologics are divided into three groups based on their chemical composition

1. Biologics: signaling proteins that are almost equivalent to biochemical human insulin, erythropoietin, cell activator, and hormone.
2. Monoclonal antibodies (mAbs) are "customized biotechnologically designed" antibodies that inhibit a specific biological agent or target and damage a particular cell category.
3. Cell-surface forms, also known as a recombinant protein, are made by combining various genes that code for the same protein. Chimerization is the process of removing fragments of a mouse antibody that is separate from a human antibody to eliminate side effects; this is demonstrated by adding -xi- to the name.[5]

Mechanism of action of newer immunomodulators

Hormones, blood products, cytokines, growth factors, vaccines, gene and cellular treatments, fusion proteins, insulin, interferon, human (suffix "mab"), humanized (suffix "zumab"), or chimeric (mouse–human; suffix "ximab") monoclonal antibodies are examples of biologics.[5] The particular steps in proinflammatory processes, are often targeted with biologics. T lymphocytes, B cells, granulocytes, antigen-presenting cells, DCs, macrophages, and other immunocytes may function in this way by binding directly to immunocytes or immune mediators (cytokines, chemokines, growth factors, and complement components). They mainly block activity, stop them from homing to lymphoid organs and inflammatory areas, and deplete the cells' energy.[54–57]

Usage of biologics for clinical indications

1. Immune-mediated disorders with oral symptoms include pemphigus, Behcet's illness, mucous membrane pemphigoid, oral lichen planus, and recurrent aphthous ulcers. TNF-α inhibitors, including etanercept and adalimumab, help patients with refractory ulcerative lesions, RA, and inflammatory conditions.[55]
2. Orofacial granulomatosis, Melkersson–Rosenthal syndrome, and biologics (TNF-α inhibitors) may support patients with symptoms outside of

the gastrointestinal tract like Crohn's disease, including oral Crohn's disease and related disorders.[54]

3. SS: Rituximab, on the other hand, has enhanced SS symptoms (xerostomia, etc.) and improved salivary gland activity in some patients, and mucosa-associated lymphoid tissue symptoms have been inhibited. In systemic extra glandular difficulties of fatigue, cryoglobulinemia, pulmonary disease, polysynovitis, arthralgia, and peripheral neuropathy, rituximab tends to have a therapeutic advantage.[58]
4. Cancer: Antiangiogenic biologics, like VEGF antagonists (bevacizumab) and antiepidermal growth factor receptor (anti-EGFR) agents, are currently applicable for clinical application. The monoclonal antibody, like cetuximab, greatly increased the recovery of oral cancer patients.[59]

Tumor necrosis factor-alpha Inhibitor

A TNF inhibitor is a drug that inhibits the physiologic response to TNF, a component of the immune response. Antibodies mainly made in in vitro conditions from human or animal tissues are TNF inhibitors. When it comes into contact with blood, it triggers an immune system response that inhibits inflammation. TNF-α inhibitors are treated for RA, psoriatic arthritis, juvenile arthritis, Crohn's disease, ulcerative colitis, ankylosing spondylitis, and psoriasis, among other inflammatory diseases.[60]

Categorization

TNF blockers, lymphocyte modulators, IL inhibitors, and miscellaneous agents are the four major types of BAs.

1. TNF inhibitors: TNF is a primary proinflammatory cytokine that promotes enhanced leukocyte stimulation and starts to place tissue inflammation, which is vital in the pathogenesis of the immunologically induced disease. TNF causes inflammation or programmed cell death by binding to the TNF receptor (TNFR) on the plasma membrane. TNFR 1 is found in all kinds of cells, while TNFR 2 is mainly found in endothelial and immune cells. TNF causes apoptosis by attaching to TNFR 1, which causes the caspase 3–8 cascade to be activated. TNF-$\propto$ can lead to inflammation through binding to specific receptors 1 and 2 and activating several of the receptor's pathways: (1) JNK (c-Jun N-terminal kinase); (2) MAPK (mitogen-activated protein kinases) kinase cascade; and (3) NF-κB (nuclear factor-kappa).[61]
2. Lymphocyte modulators: Specify lymphocyte antigens [cluster of differentiation (CD) antigens] targeted by lymphocyte modulators. They are further subdivided into the categories: (1) T-cell modulators; (2) B-cell modulators; and (3) B-cell modulators.[62]

3. IL inhibitors: ILs include a family of cytokines (IL group) that are generated primarily with lymphocytes, monocytes, and macrophages and play a major character in immunological property. IL blockers are immunomodulatory drugs that block a variety of ILs and a wide range of applications dependent on which IL they regulate.[63]
4. Miscellaneous biologic agents: Provide a huge spectrum of biologics used with a wide range of applications, including cancer care.[64]
   a. Products that are anticoagulant and neovascularizing.
   b. anti-EGFR.
   c. Nuclear factor kappa B ligand-blocking receptor activator.[64]
   d. Antimicrobial substances.
   e. Vaccines.

The drug names, mechanisms, doses, and routes, FDA-approved newer drug are given in Table 22.2.

Etanercept

Etanercept applies for mild-to-highly effective RA in adults and frequent mild-to-heavy plaque psoriasis in people between the ages 4 and up.[65] It is used to treat ankylosing spondylitis and psoriatic symptoms. This attaches to TNF directly, modulating biochemical mechanisms that TNF induces or regulates.[65] The level of adhesion molecules produced and also serum cytokines and matrix metalloproteinases are examples of mechanisms or molecules that are affected. TNFRs are divided into two types: a 55-kilodalton protein (p55) and a 75-kilodalton protein (p75).[66] This is a soluble dimeric version of the p75 TNFR which attaches to both TNFs and remove them from distribution. Then its attaching site is situated in the cleft among subunits. Etanercept can only bind to the activated trimeric form of TNF. TNF levels are higher in RA, psoriatic arthritis, ankylosing spondylitis, and plaque psoriasis patients' tissues and fluids.[67] There has no evidence of major protein binding. Injection and solution formulations are available on the market.

Infliximab

Infliximab prevents the initiation of the proinflammatory signaling pathway. It is also used to suppress inflammatory cell penetration into inflammatory areas. Infliximab is also an IgG1 protein that attaches to both solubilizing and transmembrane forms of TNF-α with strong potential, disrupting the proinflammatory signaling cascade.[68] The antibody binds to TNF-α which inhibits it from interacting with its targets. TNF-α (lymphotoxin-α), a similar cytokine that uses similar receptors as TNF-α, is not neutralized by infliximab.[68] Downregulation of proinflammatory cytokines (i.e., IL-1 and IL-6), decrease of lymphocyte and leukocyte movement to the place of

TABLE 22.2 Drug names, mechanisms, doses and routes, Foods and Drug Administration (FDA)-approved new drugs.

Biologic agents	Sl. no.	Drug names	Mechanisms of action	Doses and route	FDA new approval
TNF-α inhibitors	1	Etaneracept	TNF receptor types—II blocks circulating TNF and lymphotoxin-A	25-50 mg, 1-2 times/week	2016[65–67]
	2	Infliximab	Blocked actions of TNF-α reduction of lymphocyte and does not neutralize TNF-β	3-5 mg/kg IV 2-6 weeks	2017[68–70]
	3	Adalimumab	Inhibits p55 and p75 cell line. Human recombinant monoclonal antibody to TNF-α	Single dose of 40 mg/0.8 mL, subcutaneously every 14–15 days	2018[1,71]
Inhibitory agents (T-cell modulators)	4	Alefacept	Inhibits T-lymphocyte production by binding to the CD2 lymphocyte antigen	15 mg intramuscularly once weekly for 12 weeks	2003[72]
Inhibitory agents (T-cell costimulators)	5	Abatacept	Costimulation modulator, like CTLA-4, inhibits T-cell (T lymphocyte) activation blocking interaction with CD28	$<$60 kg 500 mg 60–100 kg 750 mg $>$100 kg 1000 mg	2005[1,73]
Inhibitory agents (B-cell modulators)	6	Rituximab	Targets the CD20 antigen depletion of circulating B lymphocytes expressed on the surface of B lymphocytes	375 mg/m^2 Intravenous infusion once weekly for 4 weeks	2018[1,74]
Interleukin inhibitors	7	Belimumab	Monoclonal antibody targeting soluble reduces B cell–mediated immunity the autoimmune response	200 mg once a week	2011[75]

TNF, Tumor necrosis factor.

inflammation, initiation of apoptosis of TNF-α making cells (i.e., activated monocytes and T lymphocytes), amplified huge number of NFB inhibitor, and decrease of endothelial adhesion molecules are all consequences of TNF-α blocking actions.[69] Infliximab decreases synovitis and joint erosions in collagen-make arthritis and enabled eroded joints to recover, according to a transgenic mouse study that formed polyarthritis due to high levels of human TNF-α.[70] Injections, powders, and lyophilized products for solution preparation are available on the market.

Interleukin-1 inhibitors

Interleukin 1 (IL-1 and IL-II) is an essential moderator of the inflammatory response, contributing to the body's normal responses as well as the formation of acute pathological conditions that contribute to the inflammatory process and cellular damage. Even so, it remains a promising therapeutic option for a variety of autoimmune, metabolic, skin, and cardiovascular diseases.[76]

Anakinra

Anakinra is mainly a nonglycosylated recombinant human IL-1 receptor antagonist (IL-1Ra). The *Escherichia coli* speech scheme is used to create it. Anakinra is a protein that contains 153 individual amino acids.[77] The FDA gave its approval on November 14, 2001. Inflammatory triggers activate the release of IL-1, which mediates a variety of physiological responses, including inflammatory and immunological responses.[78] IL-1 levels are higher in RA patients. Anakinra mechanism mainly attaches to the IL-1 type I in a reasonable fashion, inhibiting the activity of high levels of IL-1, which can cause cartilage downturn and bone resorption.[79] Markets provide injection and solution forms.

Daclizumab

The human IL-2 receptor is bounded by a humanized IgG1 Mab (anti-Tac or anti-CD25). Older people with relapsing forms of multiple sclerosis, which is treated with daclizumab, have a therapeutic humanized monoclonal antibody.[1,80] Daclizumab is made up of 90% human antibody sequences and 10% murine antibody sequences. This is an inhibitor of the IL-2 receptor. It stops IL-2-like lymphocyte initiation, a key mechanism in the immune feedback that plays a role in allograft rejection.[81] Daclizumab prevents IL-2 binding by binding to the Tac subunit of the high-affinity IL-2 receptor complex with strong potential. On active lymphocytes the IL-2 receptor (Tac) subunit antigen is activated, though not on active lymphocytes.[82] Injection and solution are available in the market.

Polyclonal antibody

pAbs are a set of antibodies formed in the body by various B cells. They have the ability to recognize and attach to a variety of antigen epitopes. An immunogen is injected into an animal to create pAbs.[83] Following a primary immune reaction to a single antigen, on the other hand, animals are given a secondary, tertiary immunization to create top titters of antibodies to that antigen. pAbs should be extracted either with the serum or filtered from to produce an extraction that is free from other serum proteins after immunization. The B cells that clone the single parent cell produce monoclonal antibodies (mAbs).[83] Similarly monoclonal antibodies have a single affinity, meaning they only recognize the same antigen epitope (Fig. 22.3).

Antithymocyte immunoglobulin (ATG)

Thymoglobulin is a complex type of antibody proposed to bind to various cell-surface antigens. The utmost important mechanism of action is to decrease T cells specifically.[84] Antithymocyte globulin (ATG) is a highly enriched antihuman T-lymphocyte immunoglobulin originating from rabbits

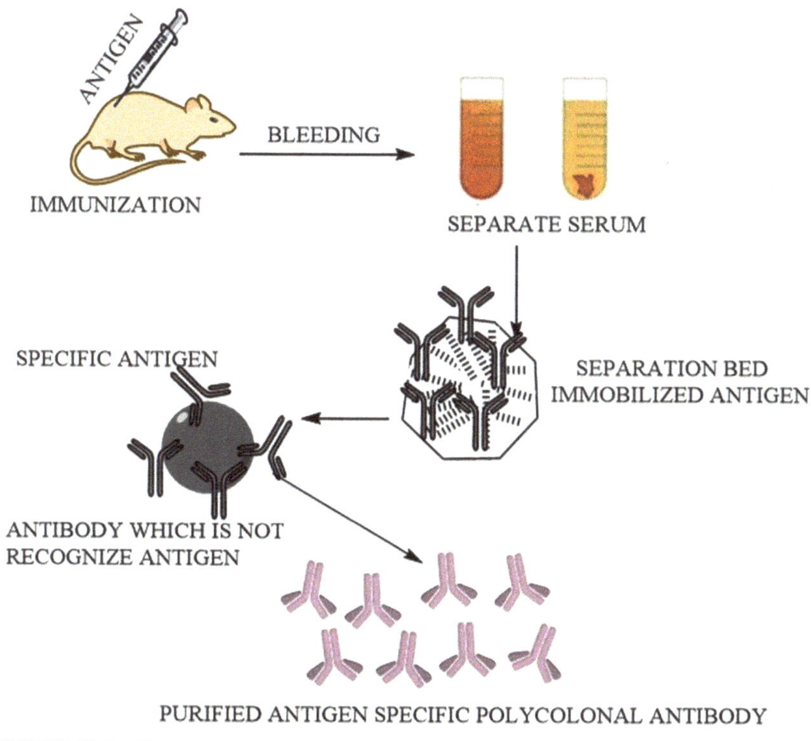

FIGURE 22.3 The polyclonal antibody generation process.

immunized with a T-lymphoblast cell line. ATG is an immunoregulatory medication used to avoid and treat acute organ rejection after transplantation. ATG suppresses the immune response to tissue transplants and organ allografts in the host.[43] It attaches to several T-cell antigens, causing complement-mediated cytotoxicity or apoptosis in T-lymphocyte cells.[85] There are injections, powders, and lyophilized solutions available for sales on the market.

Monoclonal antibodies

Monoclonal antibodies (mAb or moAb) are immunoglobulins that are similar and are developed by a single B-cell duplication. Special epitopes, or binding sites, on a single antigen are recognized by these antibodies. Monoclonal antibodies are distinguished from pAbs by their origin in a single B-cell clone and subsequent targeting of a single epitope. In biochemistry, molecular biology, and medicine, this has been a useful technique (Fig. 22.4).[86]

Alemtuzumab

An antibody of lymphocyte antigens has been humanized. It is a humanized monoclonal antibody (Campath-1H) derived from recombinant DNA against the 21–28 kD cell-surface glycoprotein CD52. Campath-1H is an IgG1 kappa antibody with a human parameter system and stable domains, as well as the complementarity-determining area of research from a murine (rat) monoclonal antibody (Campath-1G).[87] Campath is made in a culture medium of mammalian cells (Chinese hamster ovary) in a neomycin-type liquid. CD52 is a cellular protein present on almost both B and T lymphocytes, as well as the bulk of monocytes, macrophages, and granulocytes. Erythrocytes and hematopoietic stem

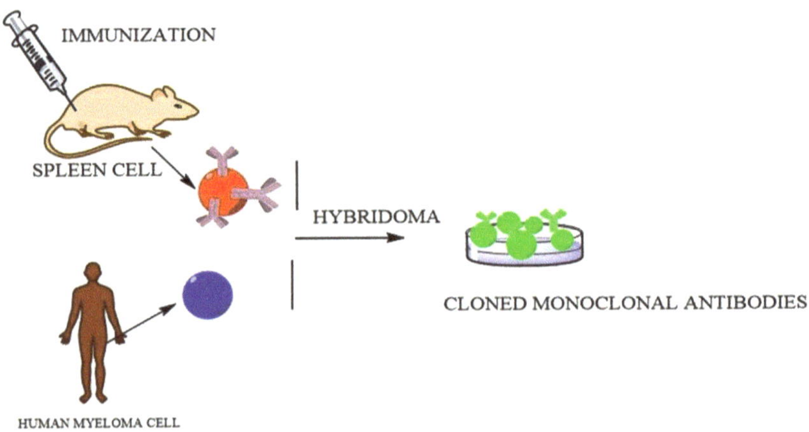

FIGURE 22.4 Monoclonal antibody process.

cells do not contain the CD52 antigen. Since B and T cells are overrepresented in leukemia, Campath allows for the particular factor of lymphocyte communities. Markets sell only injections, solutions, and concentrates.[88]

Vaccine

A vaccination is a biological substance that involved creating acquired immunity against a specific communicable disease. A vaccine usually involves an agent that looks like a disease-causing microorganism and is produced from damaged or destroyed microbes, their metabolites, or one of their surface proteins. This product activates the immune system to recognize and kill the agent as a weapon, as well as any related microorganisms it might develop in the future. Vaccines could be either therapeutics (to stop or mitigate the symptoms of potential infection by a natural or "wild" pathogen) or preventive (to treat an existing disease) (to fight a disease that has already occurred, such as cancer).[89]

Bacillus Calmette-Guérin

The vaccine type—Mycobacterium bovis, Bacillus Calmette–Guérin (BCG), is used to avoid tuberculosis as well as other mycobacterial pathogens. BCG is the only tuberculosis standard therapy. The BCG vaccine is a relatively effective vaccine that has not been linked to any serious side effects. Infection with mycobacteria, such as tuberculosis, vaccination, or natural acquisition which may protect against potential infection with mycobacteria, even tuberculosis.[90] The BCG vaccine could well be administered intradermally or intracutaneously. Since normal infection and sensitization to *Mycobacterium tuberculosis* in humans appear to occur in the respiratory system, research is currently being performed on respiratory control.[91]

Antihelminthics

Antihelmintics, also known as antihelminthics, are antiparasitic medicines that are used to remove parasitic worms (helminths) and other internal parasites from the body by stunning or destroying them without harming the organ. Infected animals are also treated with these medications.[92] Mebendazole and albendazole are the medications of choice for soil-transmitted helminths; praziquantel is the medication of choice for schistosomiasis and tapeworms.

Albendazole

A broad-spectrum benzimidazole anthelmintic that is structurally similar to mebendazole is selective against a variety of diseases. Albendazole is such an anthelmintic with a broad spectrum of action.[93] Albendazole's main mechanism of action is to prevent tubulin polymerization, which outcomes in the degradation of cytoplasmic microtubules. Albendazole induces degeneration in the worm's tegument and intestinal cells by reducing its energy generation, resulting in the parasite's immobilization and death. This functions by attaching to tubulin's colchicine-sensitive location, preventing it from polymerizing or assembling into microtubules.[94] It functions by attaching to tubulin's colchicine-sensitive site, preventing it from polymerizing or assembling in microtubules. Since cytoplasmic microtubules are necessary for glucose production in the larval and adult stages of susceptible parasites, the parasites' stored glycogen is degraded. Decreased development of adenosine triphosphate, the source of power needed for the helminth's survival, is caused by deteriorating changes in the endoplasmic reticulum, the germinal layer's mitochondria, and the resulting release of lysosomes.[95] Markets provide tablet and suspension forms.

Discussion

Immune-mediated diseases are characterized by lymphocytic invasion of a host cell and signs of an immune reaction to self-antigens attributable to either autoantibodies or immune cells. Allergies and hypersensitivity conditions of exogenous antigens, such as medications, curative products, and nutritional ingredients, cause hypersensitivity reactions. Type 1 (immediate hypersensitivity), Type 2 (antibody mediated), Type 3 (immune complex mediated), and Type 4 (cell-mediated or delayed hypersensitivity) are the different types of hypersensitivity. Immunoproliferative diseases lead to immune system cancers (multiple myeloma, lymphoma, leukemia, etc.). Immune oxidative stress characterizes immune-mediated inflammatory disorders, which result in acute or chronic inflammation and tissue death degradation. Inappropriate secretion of proinflammatory cytokines such as IL1, IL-6, and TNF-α is one of the causes of immune dysregulation. Management for these conditions should focus on treating the underlying immunity inhibitor, stopping repetition and preserving organ unity and function, in addition to relieving symptoms.

Conclusion

In the type of immunomodulatory medications and biologics, there seems to be a new variety of treatment options for steroid-tolerant or recalcitrant oral lesions. Nevertheless, several randomized control studies of these newer medications should be performed to better understand the risk–benefit relationship in the case of management.

References

1. Chambers E, Vukmanovic-Stejic M. Skin barrier immunity and ageing. *Immunology*. 2019;160(2):116–125. Available from: https://doi.org/10.1111/imm.13152.
2. Bascones-Martinez A, Mattila R, Gomez-Font R, Meurman J. Immunomodulatory drugs: oral and systemic adverse effects. *Med Oral Patol Oral Cir Bucal*. 2014;e24–e31.
3. Imanguli M, Alevizos I, Brown R, Pavletic S, Atkinson J. Oral graft-vs-host disease. *Oral Dis*. 2008;14(5):396–412.
4. Khonsary S. Guyton and hall: textbook of medical physiology. *Surg Neurol Int*. 2017; 8(1):275.
5. Konidena A, Sharma S, Patil D, Dixit A, Gupta R, Kaur M. Immunosuppressants in oral medicine: a review. *J Indian Acad Oral Med Radiol*. 2017;29(4):306.
6 Ballas Z. Immunomodulators: A brave new world. *Journal Of Allergy And Clinical Immunology*. 2008;21(2):331–333. Available from: https://doi.org/10.1016/j.jaci.2007.12.1158.
7. Nagapreeti N, Rajeshwari P. An overview of immunomodulators. *Int J Curr Pharm Clin Res*. 2014;4:108–114.
8. Marder W, McCune WJ. Advances in immunosuppressive drug therapy for use in autoimmune disease and systemic vasculitis. *Semin Respir Crit Care Med*. 2004;25(5):581–594.
9. Tripathi DK. *Corticosteroids. Essentials of Medical Pharmacology*. 5th ed. New Delhi: Jaypee Brothers Medical Publishers (P) Ltd;; 2003:254–265.
10. Funder J. Experimental and clinical pharmacology: corticosteroids – mechanisms of action. *Aust Prescr*. 1996;16(2):41–44.
11. Ito T, Ikeda U. Inflammatory cytokines and cardiovascular disease. *Curr Drug Targets Inflamm Allergy*. 2003;2(3):257–265.
12. Tamesis R, Rodriguez A, Christen W, Akova Y, Messmer E, Foster C. Systemic drug toxicity trends in immunosuppressive therapy of immune and inflammatory ocular disease. *Ophthalmology*. 1996;103(5):768–775.
13. Lichtiger S, Present DH, Kornbluth A, et al. Cyclosporine in severe ulcerative colitis refractory to steroid therapy. *N Engl J Med*. 1994;330(26):1841–1845 [PubMed: 8196726].
14. Kappers-Klunne MC, van't Veer MB. Cyclosporin A for the treatment of patients with chronic idiopathic thrombocytopenic purpura refractory to corticosteroids or splenectomy. *Br J Haematol*. 2001;114(1):121–125. Available from: https://doi.org/10.1046/j.1365-2141.2001.02893.x [PubMed: 11472356].
15. Occhiutto ML, Freitas FR, Maranhao RC, Costa VP. Breakdown of the blood-ocular barrier as a strategy for the systemic use of nanosystems. *Pharmaceutics*. 2012;4(2):252–275. Available from: https://doi.org/10.3390/pharmaceutics4020252 [PubMed: 24300231].
16. Labrande C, Velly L, Canolle B, et al. Neuroprotective effects of tacrolimus (FK506) in a model of ischemic cortical cell cultures: role of glutamate uptake and FK506 binding protein 12 kDa. *Neuroscience*. 2006;137(1):231–239. Epub 2005 Nov 10. [PubMed: 16289353].
17. Zheng H, Zeevi A, Schuetz E, et al. Tacrolimus dosing in adult lung transplant patients is related to cytochrome P4503A5 gene polymorphism. *J Clin Pharmacol*. 2004;44 (2):135–140. Available from: https://doi.org/10.1177/0091270003262108 [PubMed: 14747421].
18. Lampen A, Christians U, Guengerich FP, et al. Metabolism of the immunosuppressant tacrolimus in the small intestine: cytochrome P450, drug interactions, and interindividual variability. *Drug Metab Dispos*. 1995;23(12):1315–1324 [PubMed: 8689938].

19 Zhao, Q., Alhilali, K., Alzahrani, A., Almutairi, M., Amjad, J., Liu, H., Sun, Y., Sun, L., Zhang, H., Meng, X., Gibson, A., Ogese, M. O., Kevin Park, B., Liu, J., Ostrov, D. A., Zhang, F., & Naisbitt, D. J. *(2019). Dapsone- and nitroso dapsone-specific activation of T cells from hypersensitive patients expressing the risk allele HLA-B*13:01. Allergy, 74(8), 1533–1548.* Available from: https://doi.org/10.1111/all.13769.

20. Lampe JW, King IB, Li S, et al. Brassica vegetables increase and apiaceous vegetables decrease cytochrome P450 1A2 activity in humans: changes in caffeine metabolite ratios in response to controlled vegetable diets. *Carcinogenesis.* 2000;21(6):1157–1162 [PubMed: 10837004].

21. Breedveld P, Zelcer N, Pluim D, et al. Mechanism of the pharmacokinetic interaction between methotrexate and benzimidazoles: potential role for breast cancer resistance protein in clinical drug-drug interactions. *Cancer Res.* 2004;64(16):5804–5811 [PubMed: 15313923].

22. Sanquer S, Maison P, Tomkiewicz C, et al. Expression of inosine monophosphate dehydrogenase type I and type II after mycophenolate mofetil treatment: a 2-year follow-up in kidney transplantation. *Clin Pharmacol Ther.* 2008;83(2):328–335. Epub 2007 Aug 22. [PubMed: 17713475].

23. Harmsen S, Meijerman I, Beijnen JH, Schellens JH. Nuclear receptor mediated induction of cytochrome P450 3A4 by anticancer drugs: a key role for the pregnane X receptor. *Cancer Chemother Pharmacol.* 2009;64(1):35–43. Available from: https://doi.org/10.1007/s00280-008-0842-3. Epub 2008 Oct 7. [PubMed: 18839173].

24. Yang L, Yan C, Zhang F, et al. Effects of ketoconazole on cyclophosphamide metabolism: evaluation of CYP3A4 inhibition effect using the in vitro and in vivo models. *Exp Anim.* 2018;67(1):71–82. Available from: https://doi.org/10.1538/expanim.17-0048. Epub 2017 Nov 13. [PubMed: 29129847].

25. Nagy H, Goda K, Fenyvesi F, et al. Distinct groups of multidrug resistance modulating agents are distinguished by competition of P-glycoprotein-specific antibodies. *Biochem Biophys Res Commun.* 2004;315(4):942–949 [PubMed: 14985103].

26. Yates CR, Chang C, Kearbey JD, et al. Structural determinants of P-glycoprotein-mediated transport of glucocorticoids. *Pharm Res.* 2003;20(11):1794–1803 [PubMed: 14661924].

27. Dilger K, Schwab M, Fromm MF. Identification of budesonide and prednisone as substrates of the intestinal drug efflux pump P-glycoprotein. *Inflamm Bowel Dis.* 2004;10(5):578–583 [PubMed: 15472518].

28. Matoulkova P, Pavek P, Maly J, Vlcek J. Cytochrome P450 enzyme regulation by glucocorticoids and consequences in terms of drug interaction. *Expert Opin Drug Metab Toxicol.* 2014;10(3):425–435. Available from: https://doi.org/10.1517/17425255.2014.878703. Epub 2014 Jan 23. [PubMed: 24451000].

29. Chadfield HW. Corticosteroid therapy in current dermatological practice. *Postgrad Med J.* 1963;39:526–533. Available from: https://doi.org/10.1136/pgmj.39.455.526 [PubMed: 14046902].

30 Skov L, Bendtzen K. Biologiske laegemidler til behandling af ikkecancerrelaterede sygdomme [Biological response modifiers in the treatment of immunoinflammatory diseases]. Ugeskr Laeger. 2008 Jun 9;170(24):2120-6. Danish. PMID: 18565292.

31. *Composition and Method for Control and Treatment of Cutaneous Inflammation.*

32. Hamawy MM. Molecular actions of calcineurin inhibitors. *Drug News Perspect.* 2003;16(5):277–282 [PubMed].

33. Pópulo H, Lopes J, Soares P. The mTOR signalling pathway in human cancer. *Int J Mol Sci.* 2012;13(2):1886–1918.

34. Arceci RJ, Stieglitz K, Bierer BE. Immunosuppressants FK506 and rapamycin function as reversal agents of the multidrug resistance phenotype. *Blood*. 1992;80(6):1528–1536 [PubMed: 1381629].
35. Picard N, Levoir L, Lamoureux F, Yee SW, Giacomini KM, Marquet P. Interaction of sirolimus and everolimus with hepatic and intestinal organic anion-transporting polypeptide transporters. *Xenobiotica*. 2011;41(9):752–757. Available from: https://doi.org/10.3109/00498254.2011.573882. Epub 2011 Apr 27. [PubMed: 21524191].
36. Peters G, van der Wilt C, van Moorsel C, Kroep J, Bergman A, Ackland S. Basis for effective combination cancer chemotherapy with antimetabolites. *Pharmacol Ther*. 2000;87 (2–3):227–253.
37. Goldenberg MM. Leflunomide, a novel immunomodulator for the treatment of active rheumatoid arthritis. *Clin Ther*. 1999;21(11):1837–1852. discussion 1821. [PubMed: 10890256].
38. Herrmann ML, Schleyerbach R, Kirschbaum BJ. Leflunomide: an immunomodulatory drug for the treatment of rheumatoid arthritis and other autoimmune diseases. *Immunopharmacology*. 2000;47(2–3):273–289 [PubMed: 10878294].
39. Fukushima R, Kanamori S, Hirashiba M, et al. Teratogenicity study of the dihydroorotate-dehydrogenase inhibitor and protein tyrosine kinase inhibitor Leflunomide in mice. *Reprod Toxicol*. 2007;24(3–4):310–316. Epub 2007 May 18. [PubMed: 17604599].
40. Sahasranaman S, Howard D, Roy S. Clinical pharmacology and pharmacogenetics of thiopurines. *Eur J Clin Pharmacol*. 2008;64(8):753–767. Available from: https://doi.org/10.1007/s00228-008-0478-6. Epub 2008 May 28. [PubMed: 18506437].
41. Dubinsky MC. Azathioprine, 6-mercaptopurine in inflammatory bowel disease: pharmacology, efficacy, and safety. *Clin Gastroenterol Hepatol*. 2004;2(9):731–743 [PubMed: 15354273].
42. Gaulton A, Bellis LJ, Bento AP, et al. ChEMBL: a large-scale bioactivity database for drug discovery. *Nucleic Acids Res*. 2012;40(Database issue):D1100–D1107. Available from: https://doi.org/10.1093/nar/gkr777. Epub 2011 Sep 23. [PubMed: 21948594].
43. Chen X, Ji ZL, Chen YZ. TTD: therapeutic target database. *Nucleic Acids Res*. 2002;30 (1):412–415 [PubMed: 11752352].
44. Esses SI, Morley TP. Spinal arachnoiditis. *Can J Neurol Sci*. 1983;10(1):2–10. Available from: https://doi.org/10.1017/s0317167100044486, PMID. Available from: 6404543.
45. Coelho J, Beaugerie L, Colombel JF, et al. Pregnancy outcome in patients with inflammatory bowel disease treated with thiopurines: cohort from the CESAME Study. *Gut*. 2011;60 (2):198–203. Available from: https://doi.org/10.1136/gut.2010.222893, PMID. Available from: 21115547.
46. Wiedemann GJ, Robins HI, Gutsche S, et al. Ifosfamide, carboplatin and etoposide (ICE) combined with 41.8 degrees C whole body hyperthermia in patients with refractory sarcoma. *Eur J Cancer*. 1996;32A(5):888–892. Available from: https://doi.org/10.1016/0959-8049(95)00622-2, PMID. Available from: 9081372.
47. Takimoto CH, Calvo E. Principles of oncologic pharmacotherapy. In: Pazdur R, Wagman LD, Camphausen KA, Hoskins WJ, eds. *Cancer Management: A Multidisciplinary Approach*. 11th ed. UBM Medica; 2008.
48. Agrawal A, Daniel MJ, Srinivasan SV, Jimsha VK. Steroid sparing regimens for management of oral immune mediated diseases. *J Indian Acad Oral Med Radiol*. 2014;26:55–61.
49. Kruh J, Foster CS. Corticosteroid-sparing agents: conventional systemic immunosuppressants. *Dev Ophthalmol*. 2012;51:29–46.

50. Riano-Arguelles A, Martino Gorbea R, Iglesias Zamora ME, Garatea Crelgo J. Topic tacrolimus, alternative treatment for oral erosive lichen planus resistant to steroids: a case report. *Med Oral Patol Oral Cir Bucal*. 2006;11:E462–E466.
51. Mutasim DF. Therapy of autoimmune bullous diseases. *Ther Clin Risk Manag*. 2007;3:29–40.
52. Georgakopolou EA, Andreadis D, Arvanitidis E, Loumou P. Biologic agents and their clinical implications. *Acta Dermatovenerol Croat*. 2013;21:24–34.
53. Georgakopolou EA, Scully C. Biologics: what they are, how they affect oral health and how they can modulate oral health care. *Br Dent J*. 2015;218:671–677.
54. Wu Y, Zhou BP. TNF-alpha/NF-kappaB/Snail pathway in cancer cell migration and invasion. *Br J Cancer*. 2010;102:639–644.
55. Maxwell LJ, Singh JA. Abatacept for rheumatoid arthritis: a Cochrane systematic review. *J Rheumatol*. 2010;37:234–245.
56. Sfikakis P, Markomichelakis N, Alpsoy E, et al. Anti-TNF therapy in the management of Behçet's disease—review and basis for recommendations. *Rheumatology*. 2007;46: 736–741.
57. Leonardi CL. Efalizumab: an overview. *J Am Acad Dermatol*. 2003;49:98–104.
58. Moutsopoulos NM, Katsifis GE, Angelov N, et al. Lack of efficacy of etanercept in Sjögren syndrome correlates with failed suppression of tumour necrosis factor α and systemic immune activation. *Ann Rheum Dis*. 2008;67:1437–1443.
59. Elliott T, Campbell H, Escudier M, et al. Experience with anti-TNF-α therapy for orofacial granulomatosis. *J Oral Pathol Med*. 2011;40:14–19.
60. Zia K, Ashraf S, Jabeen A, et al. Identification of potential TNF-α inhibitors: from in silico to in vitro studies. *Sci Rep*. 2020;10(1).
61. Gonzalez-Gay MA, et al. Influence of anti-TNF-alpha infliximab therapy on adhesion molecules associated with atherogenesis in patients with rheumatoid arthritis. *Clin Exp Rheumatol*. 2006;24:373.
62. Watzl B, Bub A, Brandstetter B, Rechkemmer G. Modulation of human T-lymphocyte functions by the consumption of carotenoid-rich vegetables. *Br J Nutr*. 1999;82 (5):383–389.
63. Cavalli G, Larcher A, Tomelleri A, Dagna L. Interleukin-1 and interleukin-6 inhibition in patients with COVID-19 and hyperinflammation – authors' reply. *Lancet Rheumatol*. 2021;3(4):e248–e249.
64. Wei S, Teitelbaum S, Wang M, Ross F. Receptor activator of nuclear factor-κB ligand activates nuclear factor-κB in osteoclast precursors. *Endocrinology*. 2001;142 (3):1290–1295.
65. Zhou SY, Shu C, Korth-Bradley J, et al. Integrated population pharmacokinetics of etanercept in healthy subjects and in patients with rheumatoid arthritis and ankylosing spondylitis. *J Clin Pharmacol*. 2011;51(6):864–875. Available from: https://doi.org/10.1177/0091270010375961. Epub 2010 Sep 17. [PubMed: 20852002].
66. Banner DW, D'Arcy A, Janes W, et al. Crystal structure of the soluble human 55 kd TNF receptor-human TNF beta complex: implications for TNF receptor activation. *Cell*. 1993;73(3):431–445 [PubMed: 8387891].
67. Wong M, Ziring D, Korin Y, et al. TNFalpha blockade in human diseases: mechanisms and future directions. *Clin Immunol*. 2008;126(2):121–136. Available from: https://doi.org/10.1016/j.clim.2007.08.013. Epub 2007 Oct 3. [PubMed: 17916444].
68. Mimura T. Selection of one of the TNF blockers; infliximab and etanercept. *Nihon Rinsho*. 2007;65(7):1282–1286 [PubMed: 17642244].

69. Braun J, Baraliakos X, Listing J, Sieper J. Decreased incidence of anterior uveitis in patients with ankylosing spondylitis treated with the anti-tumor necrosis factor agents infliximab and etanercept. *Arthritis Rheum.* 2005;52(8):2447–2451 [PubMed: 16052578].
70. Tobin AM, Kirby B. TNF alpha inhibitors in the treatment of psoriasis and psoriatic arthritis. *BioDrugs.* 2005;19(1):47–57 [PubMed: 15691217].
71 Ternant D, Ducourau E, Fuzibet P, et al. Pharmacokinetics and concentration-effect relationship of adalimumab in rheumatoid arthritis. *British journal of clinical pharmacology.* 2015;79(2):286–297. Available from: https://doi.org/10.1111/bcp.12509.
72. Koo JY, Bagel J, Sweetser MT, Ticho BS. Alefacept in combination with ultraviolet B phototherapy for the treatment of chronic plaque psoriasis: results from an open-label, multicenter study. *J Drugs Dermatol.* 2006;5(7):623–628 [PubMed: 16865867].
73 Summary of opinion: Orencia,abatacept. (2019). *Case Medical Research.* Available from: https://doi.org/10.31525/cmr-a2e17a.
74 FDA approves first biosimilar for treatment of adult patients with non-Hodgkin's lymphoma. *Case Medical Research* 2018. Available from: https://doi.org/10.31525/fda2-ucm627009.htm.
75. US Food and Drug Administration (FDA). *FDA Approves Benlysta to Treat Lupus* (Press release). 2011. Archived from the original on 11 March 2011.
76. Bigby M. The use of anti–interleukin-12/23 agents and major adverse cardiovascular events. *Arch Dermatol.* 2012;148(6).
77. Tang YH, Zhang SP, Liang Y, Deng CQ. Effects of Panax notoginseng saponins on mRNA expressions of interleukin-1 beta, its correlative factors and cysteinyl-aspartate specific protease after cerebral ischemia-reperfusion in rats. *Zhong Xi Yi Jie He Xue Bao.* 2007;5(3):328–332 [PubMed: 17498496].
78. Do H, Vasilescu A, Carpentier W, et al. Exhaustive genotyping of the interleukin-1 family genes and associations with AIDS progression in a French cohort. *J Infect Dis.* 2006;194 (11):1492–1504. Epub 2006 Oct 26. [PubMed: 17083033].
79. So A, De Smedt T, Revaz S, Tschopp J. A pilot study of IL-1 inhibition by anakinra in acute gout. *Arthritis Res Ther.* 2007;9(2):R28 [PubMed: 17352828].
80 Jonsson B, Martinalbo J, Pignatti F. European Medicines Agency Perspective on Oncology Study Design for Marketing Authorization and Beyond. *Clinical Pharmacology & Therapeutics.* 2017;101(5):577–579. Available from: https://doi.org/10.1002/cpt.612.
81. Shamsi TS, Irfan M, Farzana T, et al. Allogeneic peripheral blood stem cell transplant (PBSCT) using anti-IL2 receptor antibody Daclizumab for the prevention of acute graft vs host disease in steroid refractory Diamond Blackfan anaemia: a case report. *J Pak Med Assoc.* 2005;55(10):454–455 [PubMed: 16304857].
82. Garcia CD, Bittencourt VB, Tumelero A, Antonello JS, Malheiros D, Garcia VD. Plasmapheresis for recurrent posttransplant focal segmental glomerulosclerosis. *Transplant Proc.* 2006;38(6):1904–1905 [PubMed: 16908318].
83. Ascoli C, Aggeler B. Overlooked benefits of using polyclonal antibodies. *Biotechniques.* 2018;65(3):127–136.
84. Imming P, Sinning C, Meyer A. Drugs, their targets and the nature and number of drug targets. *Nat Rev Drug Discov.* 2006;5(10):821–834 [PubMed: 17016423.
85. Monti P, Allavena P, Di Carlo V, Piemonti L. Effects of anti-lymphocytes and anti-thymocytes globulin on human dendritic cells. *Int Immunopharmacol.* 2003;3(2):189–196 [PubMed: 12586600].
86. Ansar W, Ghosh S. Monoclonal antibodies: a tool in clinical research. *Indian J Clin Med.* 2013;4. IJCM.S11968.

87. Rebello PR, Hale G, Friend PJ, Cobbold SP, Waldmann H. Anti-globulin responses to rat and humanized CAMPATH-1 monoclonal antibody used to treat transplant rejection. *Transplantation*. 1999;68(9):1417–1420 [PubMed: 10573085].

88. Hederer RA, Guntermann C, Miller N, et al. The CD45 tyrosine phosphatase regulates Campath-1H (CD52)-induced TCR-dependent signal transduction in human T cells. *Int Immunol*. 2000;12(4):505–516 [PubMed: 10744652].

89. Melief CJ, van Hall T, Arens R, Ossendorp F, van der Burg SH. Therapeutic cancer vaccines. *J Clin Invest*. 2015;125(9):3401–3412. Available from: https://doi.org/10.1172/JCI80009, PMC 4588240. PMID. Available from: 26214521.

90 WHO. Cho, T., Khatchadourian, C., Nguyen, H., Dara, Y., Jung, S., & Venketaraman, V. (2021). A review of the BCG vaccine and other approaches toward tuberculosis eradication. *Human vaccines & immunotherapeutics*, *17*(8), 2454–2470. Available from: https://doi.org/10.1080/21645515.2021.1885280. *Wkly Epidemiol Rec* 2018;93(8):73–968. hdl:10665/260307.

91. Hawgood BJ. Albert Calmette (1863-1933) and Camille Guérin (1872-1961): the C and G of BCG vaccine. *J Med Biogr*. 2007;15(3):139–146. Available from: https://doi.org/10.1258/j.jmb.2007.06-15, ISSN 0967-7720. PMID. Available from: 17641786.

92. Taylor-Robinson DC, Maayan N, Donegan S, Chaplin M, Garner P. Public health deworming programmes for soil-transmitted helminths in children living in endemic areas. *Cochrane Database Syst Rev*. 2019;9:CD000371. Available from: https://doi.org/10.1002/14651858.CD000371.pub7, ISSN 1469-493X. PMC 6737502. PMID. Available from: 31508807.

93. Molina AJ, Merino G, Prieto JG, Real R, Mendoza G, Alvarez AI. Absorption and metabolism of albendazole after intestinal ischemia/reperfusion. *Eur J Pharm Sci*. 2007;31(1):16–24. Epub 2007 Feb 6. [PubMed: 17350811].

94. *FDA Approved Drugs Products: Albendazole Oral Tablets*.

95. Ramirez T, Benitez-Bribiesca L, Ostrosky-Wegman P, Herrera LA. In vitro effects of albendazole and its metabolites on the cell proliferation kinetics and micronuclei frequency of stimulated human lymphocytes. *Arch Med Res*. 2001;32(2):119–122 [PubMed: 11343808].

Chapter 23

Mechanism of opioids action and their receptor-dependent signaling

Muhammad Zubair Saleem[1] and Muhammad Azhar Nisar[2]
[1]*Fujian Provincial Key Laboratory of Natural Medicine Pharmacology, Fujian Medical University, Fuzhou, P.R. China,* [2]*Department of Pathology and Laboratory Medicine, Tulane University School of Medicine, New Orleans, LA, United States*

Introduction

Over two centuries ago, a new analgesic pharmacology epoch was escorted with purification of morphine from the opium poppy.[1] Opioids are among the oldest therapies used to reduce severe pain at both, acute as well as chronic level.[2] Opioids can be the remedy medicines frequently referred to as anesthetics, or these are called as heroin – a so-called street drug. Several opioids are used to wedge the signals between the brain and the body and are taken to overcome severe pain. Besides, some people feel happy while taking opioids for pain relief and, therefore, these drugs can be addictive. Opioids are sometimes referred to as sedatives, but when used for a similar function like some other drugs, for example, Tylenol and aspirin, these drugs are not considered to be in the same category. The most frequently used opioids are OxyContin and Vicodin, which are categorized among prescribed opioids. Another common type is fentanyl, a synthetic opioid that is 50–100 times more potent than morphine. Heroin is an illegal drug that is also used very frequently. Therefore, despite its pivotal role in pain relief, opium has perilous obligations in its use.[3] To overcome this obligative pressure over the opium, a large number of studies have been conducted to identify ideal, safe, and less non-addictive opioid that would not have lethal effect of respiratory suppression or physical necessity. There are thousands of synthetic molecules having the same mode of action like opioids ranging from completely synthetic opioids like fentanyl to endogenous peptides like β-endorphin. The recent trend for the use of opioids to alleviate minor or major cancer pain has largely been accredited over last few decades.[4] As a

How Synthetic Drugs Work. DOI: https://doi.org/10.1016/B978-0-323-99855-0.00023-3

concern for non-cancerous pain, the United States has emerging prescriptions for using strong opioids in last 15 years, and hydrocodone was among the top prescribed prescription in the year 2011.[5]

There are different types of opioids available with different names. For example, Oxycodone is an opioid type that is available with the names like OxyContin, Oxycet, Percodan, Oxecta, Tylox, etc. Among hydrocodone family, some common types are Hyrdocodone-Ibuprofen, Hydrocodone-Clorpheniramine, Pseudoephedrine-Hydrocodone, Hydrocodone-Cpm-Pseudoephed, and Hydrocodone bitartrate. These are also available with different brand names. Morphine is another opioid available with names like Oramorph SR, Roxanol-T, Duramorph, etc. Besides their use for pain relief, opioids are also well-known for their side effects, for example, nausea/vomiting, sedation, paradoxical hyperalgesia, respiratory depression, and constipation.[6] The common side effects of opioids that are generally divided into peripheral effects, such as hives, bronchospasm, urinary retention, constipation, and central effects, such as respiratory depression, hypotension, cough suppression, miosis, nausea, and sedation (as given in Table 23.1). According to the report of CDC (Center for Disease Control),[7] the number of deaths due to the overdose of opioids exceeded that of car accidents.[7] Therefore, it is at urgency to develop novel therapies to either restrict the adverse effects of the current analgesics or replace them with newly developed techniques to discover better ways to deal with acute and chronic pain. For the purpose, it is needed to disclose the advancements in the opioid mode of actions. This chapter covers the general introduction along with the opioid mechanism of actions to describe how opioid receptors mediate diverse molecular responses.[8–12]

Opioid receptors

Underway the radio-ligand binding studies and later by cloning the individual receptor genes, identification of molecular targets for opioids have created a broader discernment in opioid pharmacology.[14,15] Although the understandings of molecular mechanism for opioid's mode of action are old enough, the studies have shown that there are three opioid receptors to which opioid analgesics interact; these are named as mu-opioid (MOPR) receptor, the delta-opioid (DOPR) receptor, and the kappa-opioid (KOPR) receptor, all of which belong to 7- transmembrane spanning G protein-coupled receptors (7TMRs) superfamily.[16] According to International Union of Basic and Clinical Pharmacology, the fourth receptor named nociception receptor (NOPR) along with some other endogenous opioid peptides act either lasciviously or selectively at each subtype, and they are not considered to be the opioid receptor but articulated to be opioid-related.[17,18] All of these receptors are encoded by their respective unique genes named *Oprm1*, *Oprd1*, *Oprk1*, *Oprl1* and share 60% of their amino acid composition.[19] After activation of

TABLE 23.1 Side effects of morphine and its substitutes in different organ systems.

System	Effect	Intensity in High/ Low (+/ −)
Central effect		
	Nausea and vomiting	+
	Respiration rate	−
	Analgesia	+
	Cough reflex	−
	Truncal stiffness leading to Stiff-person syndrome	+
	Pupil constriction (Miosis)	+
Peripheral effect		
Skin	Itching	+
	Feverish and flushing up body skin	+
Cardiovascular system	Heart rate	−
	Blood pressure	−
Renal Function	Urinary retention	+
	Renal function depression	+
Reproductive system changes	Uterine tone	−
Gastrointestinal function	Gastric motility, digestion	−
	Constipation	+
	Peristaltic movement in colon	−
	Esophagus reflex	+
Immune function	Natural killer cells activity	−
	Rosettes formation by lymphocytes	−

*These effects enlisted in the table are summarized on the base of all opioids used clinically.[13]

opioid receptors, a series occurs including adenylyl cyclase inhibition, K + channels activation, and Ca^{2+} channel inhibition. These events subsequently inhibit the release of presynaptic neurotransmitter, decrease excitability of neurons, and induce postsynaptic hyperpolarization. Opioid receptors, upon activation, trigger Gi/o heterotrimeric G proteins, and the Gα and Gβγ subunits detach, engage a variety of effectors, and subsequently participate in various intracellular signaling cascades that characteristically dampen the neural functionality.[13] Fig. 23.1 shows the basal and comparative opioid action on neurotransmission and signal transduction.

All of the three receptor types play a vital role in antinociception; however, the most common clinically available opioid analgesics are MOPR agonists that further support the traditional idea about the analogous positive and negative impact of MOPR agonist simultaneously. Recent studies have evaluated that targeting the DOPR and KOPR receptors may avoid side effects and improve the outcomes of using opioid analgesics rather using MOPR receptor agonists.[20] Comparatively, DOPR agonists showed the promising results in preclinical trials but lacked efficacy in phase 2 clinical trials for acute as well as chronic pain.[21] Besides, KOPR receptor agonists were found potent analgesics but with dysphoria and other central nervous system (CNS) side effects.[22] The diversification in receptor-binding molecules provides insight to probably have an ideal opioid analgesic devoid of lethality and being addicted to it.

The simultaneous agonism of NOPR and opioid receptor has been auspicious to incite less lethal analgesia.[23–25] Meanwhile, homomers and heteromers have established new stands to develop novel opioid analgesics. Besides, some proteins are activated because of opioids activity, among which β-arrestin1 is well-known. Change in as β-arrestin1 (β-arr1) and β-arrestin2 (β-arr2) modulates downstream signaling related to the adverse impact of opioids. β-arr1 and β-arr2 are widely expressed and vary in different brain regions of rodents, that is, high expression in CNS synapses and

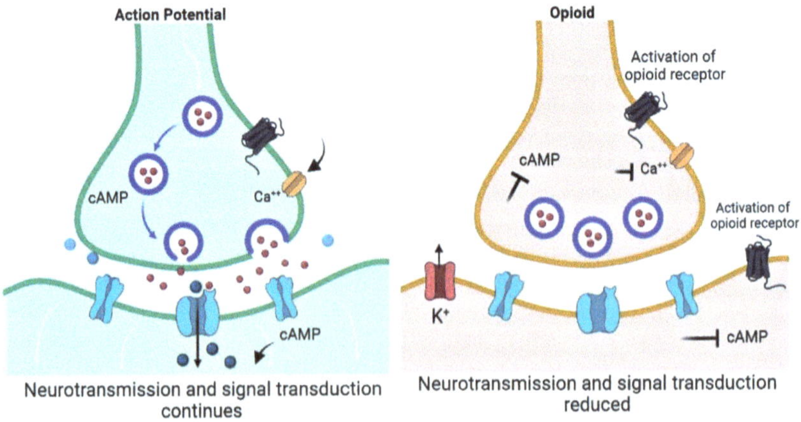

FIGURE 23.1 A comparative basal and opioid action over neurotransmission and signal transduction. Created with BioRender.com.

low in other body tissues.[26,27] Owing to the interactive properties of β-arr1with KOPR, DOPR, or NOPR, the signaling and further mechanistic approach should be evaluated further. However, recently, it was discovered that β-arr1 interferes in case of DOPR and KOPR with G-protein coupling but not in case of MOPR, which brings a variation in interference of β-arr1 in contrast to the interference of β-arr2 (i.e., with MOPR more prominently).[27–30] Moreover, the in vivo experiments have justified that antinociception of morphine is increased in the absence of β-arr2.[31,32] Some other investigations have confirmed that the mode of action of the different ligands and the subsequent cellar mechanisms prevailed are distinct.[33] The lack of direct evidence in this regard opens new explorative aspects of the role of opioid signaling in the context of β-arr1 and β-arr2.

Opioid ligands

β-endorphins, enkephalins, dynorphins, and nociceptin/orphanin are the four families of opioid ligands that are widely expressed in pain-related pathways and neuraxis. These are endogenous opioid ligands. The stored form of opioid peptides is transported to the axon terminal as in disparity to the monoamine neurotransmitters. The prepropeptides are spliced by the enzymatic activity where peptide transmitters are formed, which are specified to their receptors. For instance, proopiomelanocortin is a parental molecule from which β-endorphin is cleaved.[34] Some others include α-melanocyte-stimulating hormone (α-MSH), and corticotropin-releasing hormone (CRH). β-endorphin generally acts on MOPR, while α-MSH and CRH act on melanocortin receptors and corticotropin receptors, respectively. β-endorphin further cleaves into metenkephalin, which shows affinity to DOPR and MOPR. In a similar way, Preproenkephalin forms leu-enkephalin or met-enkephalin on its cleavage, while prodynorphin forms dynorphin-A,[4,13,16,21,31–43] dynorphin-B,[13,16,21,31–40] and α-neoendorphin on its cleavage.[39] The diversification of its cleavage into various transmitters makes it a potential agonist for the receptors. The last family of opioid ligands named nociceptin also originates from the prepronociceptin and exhibits higher affinity to the NOPR compared to that of others.[44]

Molecular recognition of opioids

About hundred years earlier to the sighting of receptors for opioids, the structure of morphine was projected, while the structural modifications led to a variety of analgesic activity of several compounds. In this regard, the key features of interactive anionic site holding positive charge, a flat surface for aromatic ring and a channel to accommodate amino group were included in a common set of rules proposed earlier.[35–37] The proteins, representative of opioid receptors, are amazingly dynamic, and thus, covalent antagonists with high affinity were used for the stabilization of the inactive conformation of receptors. X-ray crystallography along with other advancements brought the primary understandings about the structure of the four opioid receptors.[45–48] On the basis of these structural outlines, opioids were documented for their standard receptors (MOPR, DOPR, KOPR). As predicted earlier, there is an anionic aspartic acid residue at the binding site that bridges to the amino group of opioid ligands. The aliphatic elements over the amino group are lodged by a deep cavity. Synthetic opioid and co-crystallized morphinans have the phenol group that participates in a network of hydrogen bonding between conserved histidine residue and two water molecules in transmembrane helix 6 (TM6) similar to that found in H-2‘,6‘-dimethyltyrosine-Tic-Phe-Phe-NH_2 (DIPP-NH2) bound to the δOR, a bifunctional μOR agonist/δOR antagonist.[49,50] It has also been revealed that several cations (e.g., sodium) upsurge the affinity for antagonists, while magnesium, a divalent cation, increases agonist affinity, which further shows the existence of multiple conformations of opioid receptors. The details of inhibiting opioid receptors by opioid drugs and peptides are provided in Table 23.2.

TABLE 23.2 Natural opioid drugs and peptide along with their selectivity and potency to their receptors.

Opioid Drugs	MOPR (effectiveness)	DOPR (effectiveness)	KOPR (effectiveness)
Morphine	Moderate	Weak	weak
Fentanyl	Partial agonist	-	-
Codeine	Strong	Weak	-
Pethidine	Weak	Weak	Partial agonist
Pentazocine (Partial/ mixed Agonist)	Strong	Moderate	Moderate
Opioid Peptides			
b endorphin	Strong	Strong	Strong
Leu-enkephalin	Weak	Strong	-
Met-enkephalin	Intermediate	Strong	-
Dynorphin	Intermediate	Weak	Strong

The table shows effectiveness of opioid drugs and peptide to their receptors on the base of their selectivity.[51]

Classic mechanism

Primary afferent neurons, spinal cord, midbrain, and thalamus are the different regions of the nervous system where opioid receptors are present for the transmission of pain signals. These pain signals are interrupted by analgesics at the different points of transmission more often by the inhibiting the release of neurotransmitters in spinal cord from primary afferent terminals that further lead toward the inhibitory control at the midbrain. The nociceptor pathways and their ongoing activity bring changes into the levels of neurotransmitters. The reduced opioid sensitivity generally correlates to the neuropathic pain and it is because of the alterations in the neurotransmitters caused by the activated nociceptive pathways. The additional factor is the glutamate N-methyl-D-aspartate receptor, which has the ability to bring changes in the sensitivity of the pain on its activation.

Ion channels

Modulation in ion channels is the most obvious and conserved pathway that opioid receptors use to bring changes in the function of neuron. In general, the depolarization of nerve terminal and Ca^{2+} entry through channels carries the normal release of neurotransmitters from neurons. Opioids may target the Ca^{2+} channels for inhibiting the entry of Ca^{2+} or promoting the K^{+} exit outward to reduce the repolarization time and action potential due to the direct coupling of opioid receptors to voltage sensitive Ca^{2+} and K^{+} channels via G-proteins. In case of depolarization of neuron, the voltage-gated channels are activated. There are three types of Ca^{2+} channels known, namely, L-type with large conductance, T-type with small conductance, and N-type with intermediate conductance. N-, P/Q-, and L-type voltage-gated calcium channels are inhibited by modulating the channel flux.[52] Opioids usually inhibit this N-type of Ca^{2+} channel with intermediate conductance to restrict the release of neurotransmitters. However, it is not only the mechanism followed for the inhibition of neurotransmitter release.

Similar to the Ca^{2+} voltage-sensitive channels, there are several voltage-sensitive K^{+} channels known. These channels are opened by opioids for the outward flow of K^{+}, which represents the postsynaptic hyperpolarization and subsequent inhibition of neuron activity by opioids. Opioids activate G-protein gated inwardly rectifying potassium channels in a postsynaptic manner, which is mediated via $G\beta\gamma$.[53] To exhibit the value of G-protein conductance of potassium, in vivo experiments were performed. The results showed that the dysfunctional channels or their complete absence in mutant mice model led to the decreased nociception of opioids.[54,55]

In between the primary afferent nociceptors and second-order spinal cord neurons, long-term potentiation (LTP) of synaptic transmission can be provoked by withdrawing the exogeneous opioid supplementation.[56] This type of mechanism involving LTP may also contribute to the analgesic tolerance (discussed in the next section of the chapter), though the underlying mechanism is not fully understood. Some of the events required for the opioid-induced hyperalgesia are the activation of toll-like receptors, P2X4, and some other molecules like pannexin 1. Moreover, microglial activation and presynaptic MOPR also contribute to the mechanism of tolerance as well as opioid-induced hyperalgesia.[43,57,58]

Adenylate cyclase

Inhibition of adenylate cyclase is another strategy that is followed to understand the mechanism of action by opioids over neuronal signal transmission. Adenylate cyclase is an enzyme responsible for the conversion and breakdown of adenosine triphosphate to cyclic adenosine monophosphate (cAMP). Opioid receptor activity inhibits the adenylate cyclase and thus reduces cAMP production.[59] The opioid receptors are coupled to the adenylate cyclase, while its inhibition may cause the restriction of neurotransmitter release.[60]

Mitogen-activated protein kinase signaling

GPCR-regulated kinases (GRKs), for example, mitogen-activated protein kinase (MAPK) cascade, act to desensitize the activated opioid receptors that subsequently lead to the phosphorylation of receptors and β-arrestins. Three major proteins among MAPK are c-Jun N-terminal kinases (JNK), that is, 1, 2, 3, and p38, while others are extracellular signal-regulated kinases (ERK), which include ERK ½. These proteins play pivotal role in regulation of neuro-transport, ion channels, and transcription factors, while some other irrelative roles of these proteins are in apoptosis, proliferation, differentiation, and protein scaffolding.[61] These proteins are activated via their phosphorylation by almost all sub-types of opioid receptors.[13,41,62–64] However, activation of JNK is reported to engage arrestin-independent signaling.[65] Phosphatidylinositol-3-Kinase/AKT (PI3K/AKT) activation-dependent JNK phosphorylation is usually initiated by DOPR, while in others, this activity is independent of PI3K activation.[66,67] Comparatively, JNK activation is found independent of PI3K in KOPR. Researchers have also found the activation of JNK in pertussis toxin-sensitive way, while among immune cell types, this mechanism is dependent of GTPase Rac and focal adhesion kinase activity. In recent studies, it is investigated that protein kinase C (PKC) activity also plays a pivotal role in activation of JNK in case of MOPR.[68]

Another important MAPK signaling module, namely, p38 phosphorylation is verified primarily in MOPR and KOPR systems. For the activation of p38 mediated by KOPR, arrestin 3 recruitment and ser369 phosphorylation by GRK-3 are found obligatory.[40,41] Moreover, p38 activation is also required for the MOPR cross regulation of α2A-adrenergic receptors.[69] ERK ½ is considered to be the most frequent signaling observed that is induced by the opioids. Among astrocyte cultures and some transfected cell lines, activation of ERK has been found by stimulating MOPR and KOPR.[38] MOPR and KOPR can induce ERK activation within 5–10 minutes. In case of MOPR mediation, ERK activation requires protein kinase C (PKCε) activity, while GRK-3 and arrestin are required for this activity in MOPR-dependent condition.[70] These events afterward induce larger outcomes. Fig. 23.2 shows the illustrative presentation of the opioid receptor signaling.

One important phenomenon is the distinction of the expression pattern of each and every receptor across the whole nervous system.[71,72] Moreover, the crystal structures of these receptors, identified earlier, provide insights up to atomic level to uncover the binding pockets for opioids. For instance, on the basis of the structure of active MOPR, novel opioids were determined that promoted unique conformations of the active sites and initiated subsequent signaling pathways.[73] For this, molecular docking and drug designing techniques were used. A similar study for NOPR indicated that there is a missing salt bridge, present in others but not in NOPR, resulted in complete conformational changes and shift in fifth and sixth helices that might be linked to the development of receptor-specific drugs. Not only by the activation of the receptor modification via its phosphorylation and some intracellular signaling but also the opioid receptors interact with alternate GPCRs, sets of membrane proteins, and even with each other. The detailed signaling cascade in opioid pharmacology with special reference to MAPK signaling is enlisted in Table 23.3. This protein–protein interaction is an important aspect in opioid

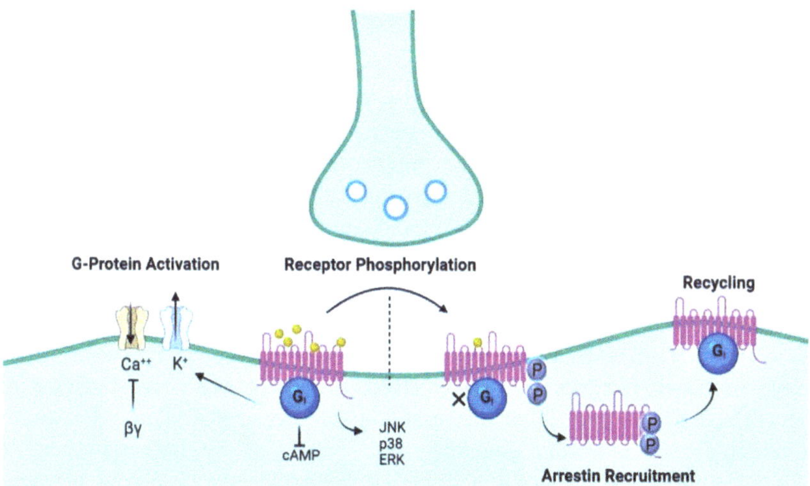

FIGURE 23.2 Illustration of the opioid receptor signaling. Arrows refer to activation steps; T lines refer to blockade or inhibition of function. Created with BioRender.com.

TABLE 23.3 Cascade/ Signaling pathways involved in different opioid receptors.

Receptor Type	Signaling Description	References
MOPR	(i) At chronic, ERK expression is decreased (ii) In arrestin-dependent pathway, ERK1/2 is activated. (iii) JNK2 is activated. (iv) STAT3 is activated via phosphorylation.	Macey et al.[64,68,69,74,75]
KOPR	(i) ERK1/2 is activated (ii) p38 MAPK is activated (iii) JNK1 is activated (iv) JAK2 and STAT3 are activated	Melief et al.[42,68,76,77]
DOPR	(i) ERK1/2 is activated (ii) PI3K/AKT is activated (iii) (iii) GSK-3β is decreased.	Shahabi et al.[67,78–80]
ORL1	(i) ERK1/2 is activated (ii) p38 MAPK is activated (iii) JNK is activated	Zhang et al.[81–83]

pharmacology that would help to explore the functional role of all the receptors at a broader level. The probable involvement of alternate signaling needs further investigations more importantly in vivo to solve the controversies in opioid-induced hyperalgesia and tolerance.

Tolerance

The chronic exposure of morphine and some other opioids induces tolerance and dependence. The term tolerance states the higher dosages of opioids to yield effects, and the background behind tolerance in case of opioids is the functional uncoupling of receptors to the G proteins consequential to the desensitization, which is not fully elucidated so far. Dependence and tolerance are two distinct phenomena, which nevertheless convoy each other generally. Endocytosis is considered to play a protective role by regulating the opioid receptors and subsequently stop developing the tolerance.[84,85] Following endocytosis, the response of the cell toward agonist is desensitized. However, receptors are re-sensitized to the agonist being recycled to the surface of the cell. This phenomenon has been proved in vivo where development of morphine tolerance was prevented by the assistance of MOPR endocytosis.[84] Once the drug has been stopped or opioid receptor antagonist, that is, naloxone has been given, the opioid drug is removed from its receptor and hence leads to unveil dependence. Afterward, self-denial or a pull-out response occurs. Dependence is a frequent mechanism compared to the tolerance.

Conclusion

The major phenomenon behind the opioids' effect in clinics is considered to be the inhibition of neurotransmitter release. Despite, the major contribution and extensive investigative studies on the cellular action of opioids and the mechanism of action of morphine and other opioids are still not fully uncovered, especially regarding the dependence and tolerance mechanisms involved in opioid usage. It is not less than a surprise that most of the applicative and powerful effects of these interesting drugs still need to be verified with the broader and refined techniques in drug development. The adverse effects of the current opioids and less selective effects affect the quality of patient's life and the utilization of these agents in clinical trials. Furthermore, the less-refined techniques have brought this topic waited for further investigations where investigators would fetch more precise outcomes in the field of opioid pharmacology with minimum or no side effects.

References

1. Manglik A. Molecular basis of opioid action: from structures to new leads. *Biol psychiatry*. 2020;87(1):6–14. Available from: https://doi.org/10.1016/j.biopsych.2019.08.028.
2. Puig S, Gutstein HB. Opioids: keeping the good, eliminating the bad. *Nat Med*. 2017;23 (3):272–273. Available from: https://doi.org/10.1038/nm.4277.
3. Rosenblum A, Marsch LA, Joseph H, Portenoy RK. Opioids and the treatment of chronic pain: controversies, current status, and future directions. *Exp Clin Psychopharmacol*. 2008;16(5):405–416. Available from: https://doi.org/10.1037/a0013628.
4. Bruera E, Paice JA. Cancer pain management: safe and effective use of opioids. *Am Soc Clin Oncol Educ Book*. 2015;e593–e599. Available from: https://doi.org/10.14694/EdBook_AM.2015.35.e593.
5. Manchikanti L, Helm S, Fellows B, et al. Opioid epidemic in the United States. *Pain physician*. 2012;15(3 Suppl). ES9-38.
6. Streicher JM, Bilsky EJ. Peripherally acting μ-opioid receptor antagonists for the treatment of opioid-related side effects: mechanism of action and clinical implications. *J Pharm Pract*. 2018;31(6):658–669. Available from: https://doi.org/10.1177/0897190017732263.
7. CDC (2013). "Vital signs: overdoses of prescription opioid pain relievers and other drugs among women–United States, 1999–2010.", in: *MMWR Morb. Mortal. Wkly. Rep*.
8. Mani Senthil Kumar KT, Gorain B, Roy DK, et al. Anti-inflammatory activity of Acanthus ilicifolius. *J Ethnopharmacol*. 2008;120(1):7–12. Available from: https://doi.org/10.1016/j.jep.2008.07.024. 18703126.
9. Nag Chaudhuri AK, Karmakar S, Roy D, Pal S, Pal M, Sen T. Anti-inflammatory activity of Indian black tea (Sikkim variety). *Pharmacol Res*. 2005;51(2):169–175. Available from: https://doi.org/10.1016/j.phrs.2004.07.008. 15629264.

10. Barik R, Sarkar R, Biswas P, et al. 5,7-dihydroxy-2-(3-hydroxy-4, 5-dimethoxy-phenyl)-chromen-4-one-a flavone from Bruguiera gymnorrhiza displaying anti-inflammatory properties. *Indian J Pharmacol*. 2016;48(3):304–311. Available from: https://doi.org/10.4103/0253-7613.182890. 27298502.
11. Barik R, Sarkar R, Biswas P, et al. Inhibition of arachidonic acid metabolism and pro-inflammatory cytokine production by Bruguiera gymnorrhiza leaf. *Orient Pharm Exp Med*. 2013;13. Available from: https://doi.org/10.1007/s13596-013-0103-9.
12. Sarkar R, Barik R, Biswas P, Sharma A, Karmakar S, Sen T. Pharmacological Studies on Bruguiera Gymnorrhiza-A Focus on Dual Inhibition of Cox and 5-Lox. *Indian J Pharmacol*. 2013;45.
13. Al-Hasani R, Bruchas MR. Molecular mechanisms of opioid receptor-dependent signaling and behavior. *Anesthesiology*. 2011;115(6):1363–1381. Available from: https://doi.org/10.1097/ALN.0b013e318238bba6.
14. Pert CB, Pasternak G, Snyder SH. Opiate agonists and antagonists discriminated by receptor binding in brain. *Science*. 1973;182(4119):1359–1361. Available from: https://doi.org/10.1126/science.182.4119.1359.
15. Wolozin BL, Pasternak GW. Classification of multiple morphine and enkephalin binding sites in the central nervous system. *Proc Natl Acad Sci U S A*. 1981;78(10):6181–6185. Available from: https://doi.org/10.1073/pnas.78.10.6181.
16. Benarroch EE. Endogenous opioid systems: current concepts and clinical correlations. *Neurology*. 2012;79(8):807–814. Available from: https://doi.org/10.1212/WNL.0b013e3182662098.
17. Imam MZ, Kuo A, Ghassabian S, Smith MT. Progress in understanding mechanisms of opioid-induced gastrointestinal adverse effects and respiratory depression. *Neuropharmacology*. 2018;131:238–255. Available from: https://doi.org/10.1016/j.neuropharm.2017.12.032.
18. Pasternak GW, Pan Y-X. Mu opioids and their receptors: evolution of a concept. *Pharmacol Rev*. 2013;65(4):1257–1317. Available from: https://doi.org/10.1124/pr.112.007138.
19. Toll L, Bruchas MR, Calo G, Cox BM, Zaveri NT. Nociceptin/orphanin FQ receptor structure, signaling, ligands, functions, and interactions with opioid systems. *Pharmacol Rev*. 2016;68(2):419–457. Available from: https://doi.org/10.1124/pr.114.009209.
20. Stein C. Opioid receptors. *Annu Rev Med*. 2016;67(1):433–451. Available from: https://doi.org/10.1146/annurev-med-062613-093100.
21. Abdallah K, Gendron L. The delta opioid receptor in pain control. In: Jutkiewicz EM, ed. *Delta Opioid Receptor Pharmacology and Therapeutic Applications*. Cham: Springer International Publishing; 2018:147–177.
22. Helal MA, Habib ES, Chittiboyina AG. Selective kappa opioid antagonists for treatment of addiction, are we there yet? *Eur J Medicinal Chem*. 2017;141:632–647. Available from: https://doi.org/10.1016/j.ejmech.2017.10.012.
23. Dahan A, Boom M, Sarton E, et al. Respiratory effects of the nociceptin/orphanin FQ peptide and opioid receptor agonist, cebranopadol, in healthy human volunteers. *Anesthesiology*. 2017;126(4):697–707. Available from: https://doi.org/10.1097/aln.0000000000001529.
24. Tzschentke TM, Kögel BY, Frosch S, Linz K. Limited potential of cebranopadol to produce opioid-type physical dependence in rodents. *Addiction Biol*. 2018;23(5):1010–1019. Available from: https://doi.org/10.1111/adb.12550.
25. Tzschentke TM, Linz K, Frosch S, Christoph T. Antihyperalgesic, antiallodynic, and antinociceptive effects of cebranopadol, a novel potent nociceptin/orphanin FQ and opioid receptor agonist, after peripheral and central administration in rodent models of neuropathic pain. *Pain Pract*. 2017;17(8):1032–1041. Available from: https://doi.org/10.1111/papr.12558.

26. Jiang T, Yu JT, Tan MS, Zhu XC, Tan L. β-Arrestins as potential therapeutic targets for Alzheimer's disease. *Mol Neurobiol.* 2013;48(3):812–818. Available from: https://doi.org/10.1007/s12035-013-8469-8.
27. Zuo Z. The role of opioid receptor internalization and β-arrestins in the development of opioid tolerance. *Anesthesia & Analgesia.* 2005;101(3).
28. Cheng ZJ, Yu QM, Wu YL, Ma L, Pei G. Selective interference of beta-arrestin 1 with kappa and delta but not mu opioid receptor/G protein coupling. *J Biol Chem.* 1998;273(38):24328–24333. Available from: https://doi.org/10.1074/jbc.273.38.24328.
29. Mittal N, Roberts K, Pal K, et al. Select G-protein-coupled receptors modulate agonist-induced signaling via a ROCK, LIMK, and β-arrestin 1 pathway. *Cell Rep.* 2013;5(4):1010–1021. Available from: https://doi.org/10.1016/j.celrep.2013.10.015.
30. Pierce KL, Lefkowitz RJ. Classical and new roles of β-arrestins in the regulation of G-protein-coupled receptors. *Nat Rev Neurosci.* 2001;2(10):727–733. Available from: https://doi.org/10.1038/35094577.
31. Bohn LM, Gainetdinov RR, Sotnikova TD, et al. Enhanced rewarding properties of morphine, but not cocaine, in beta(arrestin)-2 knock-out mice. *J Neurosci: Off J Soc Neurosci.* 2003;23(32):10265–10273. Available from: https://doi.org/10.1523/JNEUROSCI.23-32-10265.2003.
32. Bohn LM, Lefkowitz RJ, Gainetdinov RR, Peppel K, Caron MG, Lin FT. Enhanced morphine analgesia in mice lacking beta-arrestin 2. *Science.* 1999;286(5449):2495–2498. Available from: https://doi.org/10.1126/science.286.5449.2495.
33. Bahouth SW, Nooh MM. Barcoding of GPCR trafficking and signaling through the various trafficking roadmaps by compartmentalized signaling networks. *Cell Signal.* 2017;36:42–55. Available from: https://doi.org/10.1016/j.cellsig.2017.04.015.
34. Bloom FE, Rossier J, Battenberg EL, et al. Beta-endorphin: cellular localization, electrophysiological and behavioral effects. *Adv Biochem Psychopharmacol.* 1978;18:89–109.
35. Beckett A, Casy A, Harper NJ, Phillips P. Analgesics and their antagonists: some steric and chemical considerations. *J Pharm Pharmacology.* 1956;8.
36. Beckett AH, Casy AF. Synthetic analgesics: stereochemical considerations. *J Pharm Pharmacology.* 1954;6(1):986–1001. Available from: https://doi.org/10.1111/j.2042-7158.1954.tb11033.x.
37. Beckett AH, Casy AF. Analgesics and their antagonists: biochemical aspects and structure-activity relationships. *Prog Med Chem.* 1965;4:171–218. Available from: https://doi.org/10.1016/s0079-6468(08)70169-3.
38. Belcheva MM, Vogel Z, Ignatova E, et al. Opioid modulation of extracellular signal-regulated protein kinase activity is ras-dependent and involves Gbetagamma subunits. *J Neurochem.* 1998;70(2):635–645. Available from: https://doi.org/10.1046/j.1471-4159.1998.70020635.x.
39. Bower JD, Guest KP, Morgan BA. Enkephalin. Synthesis of two pentapeptides isolated from porcine brain with receptor-mediated opiate agonist activity. *J Chem Soc Perkin.* 1976;1(23):2488–2492.
40. Bruchas MR, Land BB, Aita M, et al. Stress-induced p38 mitogen-activated protein kinase activation mediates kappa-opioid-dependent dysphoria. *J Neurosci.* 2007;27(43):11614–11623. Available from: https://doi.org/10.1523/jneurosci.3769-07.2007.
41. Bruchas MR, Macey TA, Lowe JD, Chavkin C. Kappa opioid receptor activation of p38 MAPK is GRK3- and arrestin-dependent in neurons and astrocytes. *J Biol Chem.* 2006;281(26):18081–18089. Available from: https://doi.org/10.1074/jbc.M513640200.

42. Bruchas MR, Schindler AG, Shankar H, et al. Selective p38α MAPK deletion in serotonergic neurons produces stress resilience in models of depression and addiction. *Neuron*. 2011;71(3):498–511.
43. Burma NE, Bonin RP, Leduc-Pessah H, et al. Blocking microglial pannexin-1 channels alleviates morphine withdrawal in rodents. *Nat Med*. 2017;23(3):355–360. Available from: https://doi.org/10.1038/nm.4281.
44. Meunier J-C, Mollereau C, Toll L, et al. Isolation and structure of the endogenous agonist of opioid receptor-like ORL1 receptor. *Nature*. 1995;377(6549):532–535. Available from: https://doi.org/10.1038/377532a0.
45. Granier S, Manglik A, Kruse AC, et al. Structure of the δ-opioid receptor bound to naltrindole. *Nature*. 2012;485(7398):400–404. Available from: https://doi.org/10.1038/nature11111.
46. Manglik A, Kruse AC, Kobilka TS, et al. Crystal structure of the μ-opioid receptor bound to a morphinan antagonist. *Nature*. 2012;485(7398):321–326. Available from: https://doi.org/10.1038/nature10954.
47. Thompson AA, Liu W, Chun E, et al. Structure of the nociceptin/orphanin FQ receptor in complex with a peptide mimetic. *Nature*. 2012;485(7398):395–399. Available from: https://doi.org/10.1038/nature11085.
48. Wu H, Wacker D, Mileni M, et al. Structure of the human κ-opioid receptor in complex with JDTic. *Nature*. 2012;485(7398):327–332. Available from: https://doi.org/10.1038/nature10939.
49. Fenalti G, Zatsepin NA, Betti C, et al. Structural basis for bifunctional peptide recognition at human δ-opioid receptor. *Nat Struct & Mol Biol*. 2015;22(3):265–268. Available from: https://doi.org/10.1038/nsmb.2965.
50. Koehl A, Hu H, Maeda S, et al. Structure of the μ-opioid receptor-G(i) protein complex. *Nature*. 2018;558(7711):547–552. Available from: https://doi.org/10.1038/s41586-018-0219-7.
51. Chahl, L.A. (1996). Opioids-mechanisms of action.
52. Rusin KI, Giovannucci DR, Stuenkel EL, Moises HC. κ-Opioid receptor activation modulates ca2 + currents and secretion in isolated neuroendocrine nerve terminals. *J Neurosci*. 1997;17(17):6565–6574. Available from: https://doi.org/10.1523/jneurosci.17-17-06565.1997.
53. Torrecilla M, Marker CL, Cintora SC, Stoffel M, Williams JT, Wickman K. G-protein-gated potassium channels containing kir3.2 and kir3.3 subunits mediate the acute inhibitory effects of opioids on locus ceruleus neurons. *J Neurosci*. 2002;22(11):4328–4334. Available from: https://doi.org/10.1523/jneurosci.22-11-04328.2002.
54. Luján R, Marron Fernandez de Velasco E, Aguado C, Wickman K. New insights into the therapeutic potential of Girk channels. *Trends Neurosci*. 2014;37(1):20–29. Available from: https://doi.org/10.1016/j.tins.2013.10.006.
55. Nagi K, Pineyro G. Kir3 channel signaling complexes: focus on opioid receptor signaling. *Front Cell Neurosci [Online]*. 2014;8. Available from: http://europepmc.org/abstract/MED/25071446;https://www.ncbi.nlm.nih.gov/pmc/articles/pmid/25071446/pdf/?tool = EBI; https://www.ncbi.nlm.nih.gov/pmc/articles/pmid/25071446/?tool = EBI;https://doi.org/10.3389/fncel.2014.00186;https://europepmc.org/articles/PMC4085882;https://europepmc.org/articles/PMC4085882?pdf = render [Accessed 2014].
56. Zhou HY, Chen SR, Chen H, Pan HL. Opioid-induced long-term potentiation in the spinal cord is a presynaptic event. *J Neurosci*. 2010;30(12):4460–4466. Available from: https://doi.org/10.1523/jneurosci.5857-09.2010.
57. Corder G, Tawfik VL, Wang D, et al. Loss of μ opioid receptor signaling in nociceptors, but not microglia, abrogates morphine tolerance without disrupting analgesia. *Nat Med*. 2017;23(2):164–173. Available from: https://doi.org/10.1038/nm.4262.

58. Trang T, Al-Hasani R, Salvemini D, Salter MW, Gutstein H, Cahill CM. Pain and poppies: the good, the bad, and the ugly of opioid analgesics. *J Neurosci.* 2015;35(41):13879–13888. Available from: https://doi.org/10.1523/jneurosci.2711-15.2015.
59. Minneman KP, Iversen IL. Enkephalin and opiate narcotics increase cyclic GMP accumulation in slices of rat neostriatum. *Nature.* 1976;262(5566):313–314. Available from: https://doi.org/10.1038/262313a0.
60. Corder G, Castro DC, Bruchas MR, Scherrer G. Endogenous and Exogenous Opioids in Pain. *Annu Rev Neurosci.* 2018;41:453–473. Available from: https://doi.org/10.1146/annurev-neuro-080317-061522.
61. Raman M, Chen W, Cobb MH. Differential regulation and properties of MAPKs. *Oncogene.* 2007;26(22):3100–3112. Available from: https://doi.org/10.1038/sj.onc.1210392.
62. Chen L-Y, Huang J-X, Yu L-C. Involvement of ORL1 receptor and ERK kinase in the orphanin FQ-induced nociception in the nucleus accumbens of rats. *Regulatory Peptides.* 2008;151(1):43–47. Available from: https://doi.org/10.1016/j.regpep.2008.06.001.
63. Eisinger DA, Ammer H. Delta-opioid receptors activate ERK/MAP kinase via integrin-stimulated receptor tyrosine kinases. *Cell Signal.* 2008;20(12):2324–2331. Available from: https://doi.org/10.1016/j.cellsig.2008.09.002.
64. Macey TA, Lowe JD, Chavkin C. Mu opioid receptor activation of ERK1/2 is GRK3 and arrestin dependent in striatal neurons. *J Biol Chem.* 2006;281(45):34515–34524. Available from: https://doi.org/10.1074/jbc.M604278200.
65. Schattauer SS, Land BB, Reichard KL, et al. Peroxiredoxin 6 mediates Gαi protein-coupled receptor inactivation by cJun kinase. *Nat Commun.* 2017;8(1):743. Available from: https://doi.org/10.1038/s41467-017-00791-2.
66. Kam AY, Chan AS, Wong YH. Phosphatidylinositol-3 kinase is distinctively required for mu-, but not kappa-opioid receptor-induced activation of c-Jun N-terminal kinase. *J Neurochem.* 2004;89(2):391–402. Available from: https://doi.org/10.1111/j.1471-4159.2004.02338.x.
67. Shahabi NA, McAllen K, Sharp BM. δ Opioid receptors stimulate akt-dependent phosphorylation of c-jun in T cells. *J Pharmacology Exp Therapeutics.* 2006;316(2):933–939. Available from: https://doi.org/10.1124/jpet.105.091447.
68. Melief EJ, Miyatake M, Bruchas MR, Chavkin C. Ligand-directed c-Jun N-terminal kinase activation disrupts opioid receptor signaling. *Proc Natl Acad Sci.* 2010;107(25):11608–11613. Available from: https://doi.org/10.1073/pnas.1000751107.
69. Tan M, Walwyn WM, Evans CJ, Xie CW. p38 MAPK and beta-arrestin 2 mediate functional interactions between endogenous micro-opioid and alpha2A-adrenergic receptors in neurons. *J Biol Chem.* 2009;284(10):6270–6281. Available from: https://doi.org/10.1074/jbc.M806742200.
70. Groer CE, Tidgewell K, Moyer RA, et al. An opioid agonist that does not induce mu-opioid receptor--arrestin interactions or receptor internalization. *Mol Pharmacol.* 2007;71(2):549–557. Available from: https://doi.org/10.1124/mol.106.028258.
71. Mansour A, Fox CA, Burke S, et al. Mu, delta, and kappa opioid receptor mRNA expression in the rat CNS: An in situ hybridization study. *J Comp Neurol.* 1994;350(3):412–438. Available from: https://doi.org/10.1002/cne.903500307.
72. Neal Jr CR, Mansour A, Reinscheid R, et al. Opioid receptor-like (ORL1) receptor distribution in the rat central nervous system: Comparison of ORL1 receptor mRNA expression with 125I-[14Tyr]-orphanin FQ binding. *J Comp Neurol.* 1999;412(4):563–605.
73. Manglik A, Lin H, Aryal DK, et al. Structure-based discovery of opioid analgesics with reduced side effects. *Nature.* 2016;537(7619):185–190.

74. Ikeda H, Miyatake M, Koshikawa N, et al. Morphine modulation of thrombospondin levels in astrocytes and its implications for neurite outgrowth and synapse formation. *J Biol Chem*. 2010;285(49):38415–38427.
75. Miyatake M, Rubinstein TJ, McLennan GP, Belcheva MM, Coscia CJ. Inhibition of EGF-induced ERK/MAP kinase-mediated astrocyte proliferation by μ opioids: integration of G protein and β-arrestin 2-dependent pathways. *J Neurochemistry*. 2009;110(2):662–674.
76. Finley MJ, Steele A, Cornwell WD, Rogers TJ. Transcriptional regulation of the major HIV-1 coreceptor, CXCR4, by the κ opioid receptor. *J Leukoc Biol*. 2011;90(1):111–121.
77. Potter DN, Damez-Werno D, Carlezon Jr WA, Cohen BM, Chartoff EH. Repeated exposure to the κ-opioid receptor agonist salvinorin A modulates extracellular signal-regulated kinase and reward sensitivity. *Biol Psychiatry*. 2011;70(8):744–753.
78. Eisinger DA, Ammer H. Down-regulation of c-Cbl by morphine accounts for persistent ERK1/2 signaling in δ-opioid receptor-expressing HEK293 cells. *J Biol Chem*. 2009;284(50): 34819–34828.
79. Olianas MC, Dedoni S, Onali P. Regulation of PI3K/Akt signaling by N-desmethylclozapine through activation of δ-opioid receptor. *Eur J Pharmacol*. 2011;660(2-3):341–350.
80. Olianas MC, Dedoni S, Onali P. Signaling pathways mediating phosphorylation and inactivation of glycogen synthase kinase-3β by the recombinant human δ-opioid receptor stably expressed in Chinese hamster ovary cells. *Neuropharmacol*. 2011;60(7-8):1326–1336.
81. Harrison RS, Ruiz-Gomez G, Hill TA, et al. Novel helix-constrained nociceptin derivatives are potent agonists and antagonists of ERK phosphorylation and thermal analgesia in mice. *J Medicinal Chem*. 2010;53(23):8400–8408.
82. Ross J, Armstead WM. NOC/oFQ activates ERK and JNK but not p38 MAPK to impair prostaglandin cerebrovasodilation after brain injury. *Brain Res*. 2005;1054(1):95–102.
83. Zhang Z, Xin SM, Wu GX, Zhang WB, Ma L, Pei G. Endogenous δ-opioid and ORL1 receptors couple to phosphorylation and activation of p38 MAPK in NG108-15 cells and this is regulated by protein kinase A and protein kinase C. *J neurochemistry*. 1999;73(4): 1502–1509.
84. He L, Fong J, Von Zastrow M, Whistler JL. Regulation of opioid receptor trafficking and morphine tolerance by receptor oligomerization. *Cell*. 2002;108(2):271–282.
85. Whistler JL, Chuang H-h, Chu P, Jan LY, Von Zastrow M. Functional dissociation of μ opioid receptor signaling and endocytosis: implications for the biology of opiate tolerance and addiction. *Neuron*. 1999;23(4):737–746.

Chapter 24

Application of molecular pharmacology in research techniques and drug development

Mainak Chakraborty[1], Nilanjan Sarkar[1], Amrita Kumari[2], Kalyan Roy[3], Gauthaman Karunakaran[3], Priti Das[4], Jafar Abdulla Mohamed Usman[5] and Samit Karmakar[6]

[1]Department of Pharmaceutical Technology, NSHM Knowledge campus Kolkata, Group of Institutions, Kolkata, West Bengal, India, [2]Usha College of Pharmacy, Dhatkidih, Jamshedpur, Jharkhand, India, [3]Government Pharmacy College, Gangtok, Sikkim, India, [4]TCG Life Sciences Pvt Ltd (formerly "Chembiotek Research International"), Kolkata – R&D Centre, Chemistry, Kolkata, West Bengal, India, [5]Prosthetic dentistry, Faculty of dentistry, MAHSA University, Jln SP2 Selangor, Malaysia, [6]Medical College Kolkata, Kolkata, West Bengal, India

Introduction

As per today's consequences, the treatment and discovery of a new molecule are more target-oriented and more specific as compared to traditional drug discovery. Nowadays, importance is focused on the individual patient-related problems aimed to provide beneficial effects of drugs to minimize the symptoms, disabilities, and survival to balance the target-oriented and target-specific treatment or development to achieve the maximum benefits and minimum adverse effects. To achieve the goal, the treatment-oriented drug development process is more focused on a cellular and molecular level.

Few approaches of molecular pharmacology based on the knowledge of the structure and function of targets like receptors, enzymes, transport molecules, and ion channels provide the experimental techniques to analyze or screen the novel substances in the process of drug discovery.

In the last few decades, biological sciences showed more advancement in cellular target-based discovery and knowledge in the development of OMICS providing the molecular data at the genomic level.

How Synthetic Drugs Work. DOI: https://doi.org/10.1016/B978-0-323-99855-0.00024-5

The identification of genes and proteins provides a data bank of individual molecular components leading to the discovery of newer drug molecules based upon several targets related to diseases.

Target-oriented drug discovery is based upon the study of the structure of biological molecules to understand how they are assembled, what their behavior is in a complex system, and what changes will make their dynamic behavior alter. As a result, today's era of drug discovery is focused on a cellular and molecular level to identify the disease and lead compounds along with its mechanism-based drug development.[1]

It is very difficult to understand in the case of a complex disease like cancer, diabetes, and obesity where either multiple genes or a single gene is involved in gene abnormality disease problems. But OMICS data help in identifying the target and useful tools in the field of new drug development process.[2]

Additionally, the drug development process also fails in some cases due to the poor understanding of cellular and molecular pharmacological pathways, that is why it is very crucial to gain proper knowledge in molecular components to minimize the failure in the drug development process.[3]

Considering the cellular and molecular level of diseases or drug targets, which provides new opportunities to address the process of discovery on the basis of molecular targets or molecular pathways that helps to discover a new candidate from preclinical to clinical stages resulting in the development of novel biomarkers and therapies.[4]

Overall understanding of the cellular and molecular consequents and pathways that are involved in the disease-related target progression upon drug discovery processes have various applied methods and techniques that are used as a tool in the modern era.[4]

Molecular pharmacology methods and their application in drug discovery approaches

Molecular and cellular pharmacology mainly targets the phenotype and their characteristics in the biological system individually on a molecular basis.[5]

The main feature of molecular biology or pharmacology study is the characteristic feature of individual molecules. Molecular pharmacology approaches also use computational methods to generate or predict some features that can be evaluated experimentally.

In the process of drug discovery, molecular pharmacology tools or methods evaluate the multiple cellular and molecular components that allow one to measure the targets in various ways.

The application of computational methods that are based on the hypothesis data can be validated experimentally, after that the acquired data can be recapitulated to a cellular and molecular target of interest.

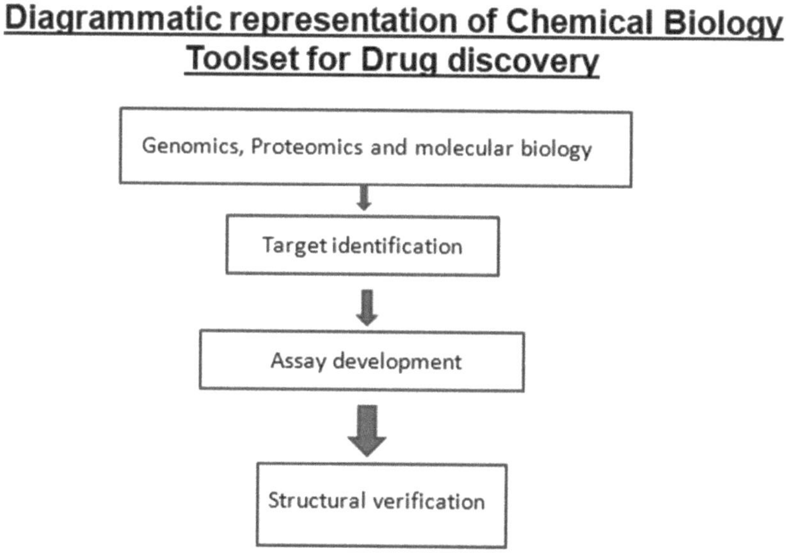

FIGURE 24.1 A diagrammatic representation showing chemical biology toolset used in drug discovery and development.

Top-down and bottom-up modeling systems are generally incorporated in cellular and molecular biological study.[6]

The data gathered on a large scale are subsequently used in OMICS or Data Bank using statistical models. Network modeling is one of the main approaches which highlights the target interaction with thousands of cellular and molecular components.

Drug discovery based on hypothesis basically characterizes the relation between molecular and cellular components, leading to the emergent behaviors of the target. The choice of application is usually based on the nature of compounds and target molecules (Fig. 24.1).[6]

Molecular approaches based on network

Collecting all data and linking them together in a biological system is like a network where a system at the cellular and molecular level established a connection that will help the scientific investigators get the appropriate knowledge to identify the target in the process of drug discovery.[7]

A biological system network is a representation of molecular and cellular components like genes, proteins, metabolites, ion channels, even a disease or its phenotypes.

The cellular and molecular network mainly represents the interaction between ligand and target, signaling pathways, regulatory genes, as well as diseased genes. Understanding these molecular networks, scientists can develop or discover many new drug candidates.[8,9]

In the drug discovery process, the cellular and molecular network provides a great insight into the developmental processes. The complex illustration of a biological system represented by a network provides strong concept of target-oriented lead identification.

Advancement in the cellular and molecular network nowadays is of significant help. They can get the total information about the properties like topology and motifs from here.[2,8] Several properties like activation or the deactivation of certain kinds of proteins, genes, enzymes, ion channels, etc. established some mechanisms at the molecular level.[8]

Studying about the degree of protein or proteomics represents the interaction property as well as network-based molecular approaches, providing information regarding target–ligand interaction, degree and extent of distribution, as well as the architecture of the target molecules, which ultimately acts as a useful part in drug discovery process.[8]

Molecular-level network-basis target illustration is very important because they are associated with biological function.[9]

The network hub and their biological role involves them into an intramodule and coexpressed manner with their interacting molecules that are prefer able to function inside the modules like cell cycle and DNA damage, gene mutation.[2,10]

Mechanism-based approach in drug discovery

By illustrating some molecular pathways, a mathematical model can be established.[11] In establishing a mechanistic equation, a large number of molecular data that are related to physiochemical theory, biomolecular processes, kinetic parameters, etc. can be evaluated.[5,12]

Thus researchers involved in mechanistic modeling get an idea from the prior knowledge like—how to make target-specific predictions—and work best with pathways where components and connectivity are relatively well established.

The utilization of mechanistic modeling is of great benefit as it provides a powerful tool to analyze the target and lead at the cellular and molecular levels.

The development of the mechanistic model is based on four steps:

1. Model design: One of the initial stages is to specify the model scope and establish the reaction scheme of all of the molecular components of interest.[12]
2. Model construction: According to the physicochemical theory, the connectivity diagram must be converted to appropriate biochemical reactions, which are mathematically represented by differential equations.[13]

3. Model calibration, also known as model regression, is one of the processes by which unknown kinetic parameter values in a model are estimated in such a manner so as to match model performance to experimental measurements. The parameter estimation is generally based on data-fitting techniques which involves an iterative process of adjusting kinetic parameter values to minimize the difference between the model-predicted value and the corresponding experimental data.[14]
4. To evaluate the goodness of a calibrated model, Model validation is used that includes making predictions which can be subjected to experimental tests. If the simulation results of a dynamic model recapitulates experimentally defined input–output relations, the model can be considered to be accurate. The input–output relations may be time–course and dose–response experimental data in the presence or absence of additional perturbations.[13]

Molecular biology method in human disease and drug discovery

As compared to the application of the traditional approach, modern molecular pharmacology tries to elucidate a complex disease by understanding the genetic level and cellular and molecular pathways. The tools that are used to study the target and lead at the ground level are provided by molecular networking, which includes the studies of (1) global relationships between human disease and associated genes, (2) predictions of treatment response, (3) investigations of the underlying mechanism of diseases, and (4) predictions of new disease-associated genes. These are monumental contributors to the drug discovery process.[8]

Human disease networks and molecular pharmacology

Previously the drug discovery process contained the studying of one gene–one disease concept, whereas development in the field of molecular pharmacology, that is, elucidation of network-based technique supported the better understanding of multiple genes that are associated with the diseases.[15] Such systematic approaches have provided a foundation for a genome-scale network analysis of complex diseases, such as cancer,[16] neurodegenerative diseases,[17] inflammatory diseases,[18] and also pathogen causing responses.[19]

Molecular pharmacology in treatment response prediction

Molecular biology is such an important area where the discovery of biomarkers provides a great insight into disease-specific drug development processes. Genomics and proteomics tools provide many of the disease profiles with system-wide maps of the pathways to identify biomarkers that are able to diagnose disease severity and predict disease outcomes. A network-based

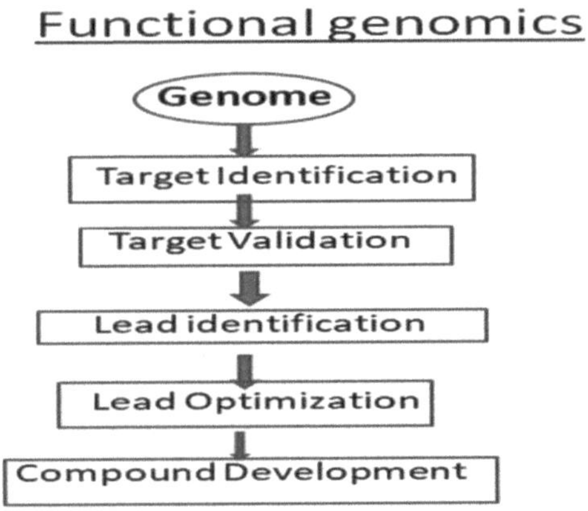

FIGURE 24.2 Flowchart representation showing functional genomics leading to drug discovery.

molecular approach that identifies subnetworks with coherent expression patterns can also be used to identify novel markers for disease purpose.[20] Network-based molecular pharmacology is also a useful analytical tool for OMICS to predict the relative risk for disease progression and patient survivability.[21–24] In all the cases the goal is to identify biomarkers not as lists of individual genes or proteins but as functionally related groups of genes or proteins where their aggregated properties account for the phenotypic differences between the different populations of patient.[25] Unlike traditional diagnostic markers based on individual genes, network-based diagnostic markers should be inherently more reliable as they are useful to biological interpretation for the association between the subnetwork biomarker and the particular type of disease (Fig. 24.2).[26]

Investigation of disease mechanisms by molecular pharmacology

The application of molecular biology as large-scale molecular profiling is possible nowadays, providing an insight into the physiological regulation and pathological consequences in a disease condition.[26,27]

Recent observations have shown that the wiring of biological networks can change from healthy to diseased states.[28] Their network-based integrative analysis not only highlights the strong association between immune pathways and pathophysiology of the disease but also identified the key network regulators that may serve as an effective target for therapeutic intervention. Another thrust in system biology involves combining dynamical modeling of regulatory pathways with molecular and cellular experiments so as to understand the precise regulatory mechanisms of networks that are altered in diseases.[29–31]

Gene regulation and disease state

The quest for disease-causing genes is a long-standing goal of biomedical research. Molecular pharmacology is playing an interesting role in this field through the computational integration of multiple genome-scale measurements. The application of network-based molecular pharmacology is able to predict the unidentified human disease–associated genes. Similar network-based computational frameworks have been proposed to reliably predict disease-associated genes.[32,33] Overall, the molecular pharmacology approaches at the network level provide the highly efficient method for addressing the problems of identifications of genes, thus playing a pivotal role in human disease.

Molecular pharmacology approaches in drug discovery

The molecular biology technique has long been used in the field of drug discovery to understand the mechanism of action as well as the effectiveness of selected compounds.

Utilizing the molecular biology technique and computational approach in a combined form exposes the researchers to the introduction of systemic pharmacology, which mainly[34] describes a field of research that provides us with a comprehensive view of drug action rooted in molecular interactions between drugs and their targets in a human cellular context.

Advancement with the molecular pharmacology tools gives us long-term benefit in the discovery of a new drug candidate more specific and target-oriented manner, which ultimately helps us in patient care management.

Several methods of approaches and tools of molecular pharmacology make a significant contribution in the process of drug discovery; some important techniques that could be considered major targets are (1) drug–target networks, (2) predictions of drug–target interactions, (3) investigations of the adverse effects of drugs, (4) drug repositioning, and (5) predictions of drug combination.

Drug–target networks and molecular pharmacology

Molecular pharmacology approaches allow us to study the ligand versus target interaction and polypharmacology.[35,36] Topological analyses of the molecular network provide the identification of target proteins. Many proteins are targeted by more than one drug containing distinct chemical structures. This new appreciation of the role of polypharmacology has significant implications in the drug development process. Although the single-target approach remains the main strategy presently, some remarkable efforts are being put into the development of "promiscuous" drugs (also called "dirty drugs") that can bind to multiple targets.

Integrating systems biology and polypharmacology hold the promise of expanding the current opportunities to improve clinical efficacy and decrease side effects and toxicity. Advances in these areas are creating the foundation of the next paradigm in drug discovery, that is, "network pharmacology."[37]

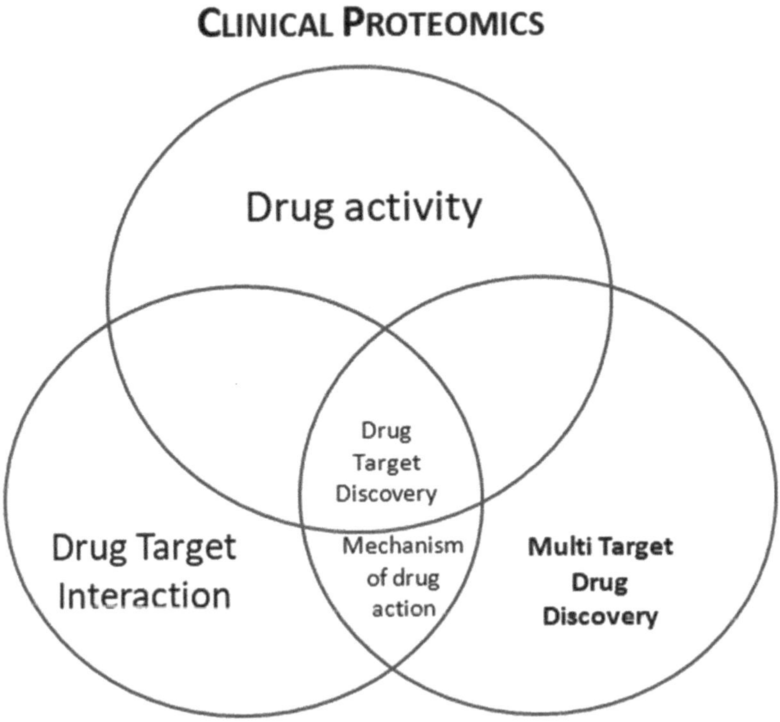

FIGURE 24.3 A diagrammatic representation showing the role of clinical proteomics in drug discovery and development.

Predictions of drug–target interactions

Polypharmacology study mainly focuses on multidirectional target identification and target validation. To understand the mechanism of action, polypharmacology study is more relevant.[38] Unlike the traditional conventional approaches based on sequence or structural similarity between targets, the "similarity ensemble approach" defines each target by its set of known ligands, searches for drugs with a chemical structure similar to the known ligands, and then predicts new drug–target associations (Fig. 24.3).[39]

Investigations of drug adverse effects by molecular pharmacology approaches

The safety and toxicity profile of a drug or drug component is very much crucial in the drug discovery process. By integrating the biological data and molecular pharmacology, there are many techniques that could change the concept of the drug discovery process.[40] Approximately half of their predictions were confirmed by experimental assays. An association metric was developed to prioritize new off-targets that explained side effects better than any known target of a given drug, creating a drug–target–adverse drug reaction network.[41] By investigating the associations between drug and off-targets, their research has explored the molecular basis of several adverse events. Other studies that integrate systems biology with structural or chemoinformatics analysis have also been conducted to successfully predict drug adverse effects.[42,43]

Drug repositioning and molecular pharmacology

It is the process of exploring the potential therapeutic application of the existing drug. The main advantage of drug repositioning is that it drastically reduces the risk of drug development and facilitates repositioned drugs to enter clinical phases more rapidly.[44] By understanding the network pharmacology and molecular pathways, the lead can be modified or targeted on different other diseases, the OMICS data also support the repositioning theory.[45] This new method is based on the premise that drugs indicated for etiologically or pathologically similar type of diseases based on their chemical/structural similarity, may be effectively deployed for the prediction of novel indications of existing drugs. Furthermore, numerous approaches based on gene expression data for in-silico drug repositioning have been published.[46,47]

Predictions of drug combination and molecular pharmacology approaches

To achieve great therapeutic benefits, output of the combination approaches are being explored nowadays. As the diseases involve complex molecular pathways and multiple genes or proteins, combination oriented approaches are very much beneficial as compared to the single drug concept.[48] Molecular biology methods have been applied to explain and predict potential drug combinations.[49] Computational approaches that utilize dynamic modeling have already been used to simulate the effects of drug combinations and generate experimentally demonstrable interventions.[38,50]

Conclusion

In the current scientific scenario, molecular pharmacology is dramatically advancing. The understanding of disease (target) through cellular and molecular pathways provides a great insight into the process of lead identification and lead optimization. Traditional techniques are sufficient to explore the whole process of the gene causing diseases and drug–target relations in the context of biological systems. This comprehensive chapter gives an insight into the role of molecular pharmacology in the drug discovery processes.

References

1. British Pharmacological Society, Pharmacology Skill for Drug Discovery, <http://www.rsb.org.uk%2Fimages%2FPharmacology_Skills_for_Drug_Discovery.pdf&clen = 37255&chunk = true>. Accessed 23.10.21.
2. Barabási A-L, Gulbahce N, Loscalzo J. Network medicine: a network-based approach to human disease. *Nat. Rev. Genet.* 2011;12(1):56–68.
3. Araujo RP, Liotta LA, Petricoin EF. Proteins, drug targets and the mechanisms they control: the simple truth about complex networks. *Nat. Rev. Drug Discov.* 2007;6(11):871–880.
4. Pujol A, Mosca R, Farrés J, Aloy P. Unveiling the role of network and systems biology in drug discovery. *Trends Pharmacol. Sci.* 2010;31(3):115–123.
5. Sobie EA, Lee Y-S, Jenkins SL, Iyengar R. Systems biology—biomedical modeling. *Sci. Signal.* 2011;4(190). article tr2.
6. Faratian D, Clyde RG, Crawford JW, Harrison DJ. Systems pathology—taking molecular pathology into a new dimension. *Nat. Rev. Clin. Oncol.* 2009;6(8):455–464.
7. Schenone M, Dančík V, Wagner BK, Clemons PA. Target identification and mechanism of action in chemical biology and drug discovery. *Nature chemical biology.* 2013;9(4):232–240. Available from: https://doi.org/10.1038/nchembio.1199.
8. Ma'ayan A. Introduction to network analysis in systems biology. *Sci. Signal.* 2011;4(190). article tr5.
9. Vidal M, Cusick ME, Barabási A-L. Interactome networks and human disease. *Cell.* 2011;144(6):986–998.
10. Chang X, Xu T, Li Y, Wang K. Dynamic modular architecture of protein-protein interaction networks beyond the dichotomy of "date" and "party" hubs. *Sci Rep.* 2013;3. article 1691.
11. Aldridge BB, Burke JM, Lauffenburger DA, Sorger PK. Physicochemical modelling of cell signalling pathways. *Nat. Cell Biol.* 2006;8(11):1195–1203.
12. Neves SR. Developing models in virtual cell. *Sci. Signal.* 2011;4(192). article tr12.
13. Neves SR. Obtaining and estimating kinetic parameters from the literature. *Sci Signal.* 2011;4(191). article tr8.
14. Costa KD, Kleinstein SH, Hershberg U. Biomedical model fitting and error analysis. *Sci. Signal.* 2011;4(192). article tr9.
15. Goh K-I, Cusick ME, Valle D, Childs B, Vidal M, Barabási A-L. The human disease network. *Proc. Nat. Acad. Sci. USA.* 2007;104(21):8685–8690.
16. Wu G, Feng X, Stein L. A human functional protein interaction network and its application to cancer data analysis. *Genome Biol.* 2010;11(5). article R53.
17. Hwang D, Lee IY, Yoo H, et al. A systems approach to prion disease. *Mol. Syst. Biol.* 2009;5. article 252.
18. Yosef N, Shalek AK, Gaublomme JT, et al. Dynamic regulatory network controlling TH17 cell differentiation. *Nature.* 2013;496(7446):461–468.
19. Arnit I, Garber M, Chevrier N, et al. Unbiased reconstruction of a mammalian transcriptional network mediating pathogen responses. *Science.* 2009;326(5950):257–263.
20. Chuang H-Y, Lee E, Liu Y-T, Lee D, Ideker T. Network-based classification of breast cancer metastasis. *Mol. Syst. Biol.* 2007;3. article 140.
21. Taylor IW, Linding R, Warde-Farley D, et al. Dynamic modularity in protein interaction networks predicts breast cancer outcome. *Nat Biotechnol.* 2009;27(2):199–204.
22. Breitkreutz D, Hlatky L, Rietman E, Tuszynski JA. Molecular signaling network complexity is correlated with cancer patient survivability. *Proc. Nat. Acad. Sci.* 2012;109(23):9209–9212.

23. Chuang HY, Rassenti L, Salcedo M, et al. Subnetwork-based analysis of chronic lymphocytic leukemia identifies pathways that associate with disease progression. *Blood*. 2012;120 (13):2639–2649.
24. Huang T, Wang J, Cai Y-D, Yu H, Chou K-C. Hepatitis c virus network based classification of hepatocellular cirrhosis and carcinoma. *PLoS ONE*. 2012;7(4). Article ID e34460.
25. Andersen JN, Sathyanarayanan S, Di Bacco A, et al. Pathway-based identification of biomarkers for targeted therapeutics: personalized oncology with PI3K pathway inhibitors. *Sci. Transl. Med*. 2010;2(43):43ra55.
26. Carro MS, Lim WK, Alvarez MJ, et al. The transcriptional network for mesenchymal transformation of brain tumours. *Nature*. 2010;463(7279):318–325.
27. Bromberg KD, Ma'ayan A, Neves SR, Iyengar R. Design logic of a cannabinoid receptor signaling network that triggers neurite outgrowth. *Science*. 2008;320(5878):903–909.
28. Saez-Rodriguez J, Alexopoulos LG, Zhang MS, Morris MK, Lauffenburger DA, Sorger PK. Comparing signaling networks between normal and transformed hepatocytes using discrete logical models. *Cancer Res*. 2011;71(16):5400–5411.
29. Stites EC, Trampont PC, Ma Z, Ravichandran KS. Network analysis of oncogenic Ras activation in cancer. *Science*. 2007;318(5849):463–467.
30. Klinke II DJ. Signal transduction networks in cancer: quantitative parameters influence network topology. *Cancer Res*. 2010;70(5):1773–1782.
31. Liu B, Zhang J, Tan PY, et al. A computational and experimental study of the regulatory mechanisms of the complement system. *PLoS Computational Biol*. 2011;7(1). Article ID e1001059.
32. Wu X, Jiang R, Zhang MQ, Li S. Network-based global inference of human disease genes. *Mol Syst Biol*. 2008;4. article 189.
33. Vanunu O, Magger O, Ruppin E, Shlomi T, Sharan R. Associating genes and protein complexes with disease via network propagation. *PLoS Computational Biol*. 2010;6(1). Article ID 1000641.
34. Zhao S, Iyengar R. Systems pharmacology: network analysis to identify multiscale mechanisms of drug action. *Annu Rev Pharmacology Toxicol*. 2012;52:505–521.
35. Yıldırım MA, Goh K-I, Cusick ME, Barabási A-L, Vidal M. Drug-target network. *Nat Biotechnol*. 2007;25(10):1119–1126.
36. Paolini GV, Shapland RHB, Van Hoorn WP, Mason JS, Hopkins AL. Global mapping of pharmacological space. *Nat Biotechnol*. 2006;24(7):805–815.
37. Hopkins AL. Network pharmacology: the next paradigm in drug discovery. *Nat Chem Biol*. 2008;4(11):682–690.
38. Zou J, Luo S-D, Wei Y-Q, Yang S-Y. Integrated computational model of cell cycle and checkpoint reveals different essential roles of Aurora-A and Plk1 in mitotic entry. *Mol Biosyst*. 2011;7(1):169–179.
39. Campillos M, Kuhn M, Gavin A-C, Jensen LJ, Bork P. Drug target identification using side-effect similarity. *Science*. 2008;321(5886):263–266.
40. Lounkine E, Keiser MJ, Whitebread S, et al. Large-scale prediction and testing of drug activity on side-effect targets. *Nature*. 2012;486(7403):361–367.
41. Kuhn M, Al Banchaabouchi M, Campillos M, et al. Systematic identification of proteins that elicit drug side effects. *Mol. Syst. Biol*. 2013;9:663.
42. Chang RL, Xie L, Xie L, Bourne PE, Palsson BØ. Drug off-target effects predicted using structural analysis in the context of a metabolic network model. *PLoS Computational Biol*. 2010;6(9). Article ID e1000938.
43. Chen L, Lu J, Zhang J, Feng K-R, Zheng M-Y, Cai Y-D. Predicting chemical toxicity effects based on chemical-chemical interactions. *PLoS One*. 2013;8(2). Article ID e56517.

44. Iorio F, Bosotti R, Scacheri E, et al. Discovery of drug mode of action and drug repositioning from transcriptional responses. *Proc. Natl. Acad. Sci. USA*. 2010;107(33):14621–14626.
45. Gottlieb A, Stein GY, Ruppin E, Sharan R. PREDICT: a method for inferring novel drug indications with application to personalized medicine. *Mol. Syst. Biol*. 2011;7. article 496.
46. Sirota M, Dudley JT, Kim J, et al. Discovery and preclinical validation of drug indications using compendia of public gene expression data. *Sci. Transl. Med*. 2011;3(96):96ra77.
47. Jin G, Fu C, Zhao H, Cui K, Chang J, Wong STC. A novel method of transcriptional response analysis to facilitate drug repositioning for cancer therapy. *Cancer Res*. 2012;72(1):33–44.
48. Jia J, Zhu F, Ma X, Cao ZW, Li YX, Chen YZ. Mechanisms of drug combinations: interaction and network perspectives. *Nat. Rev. Drug Discov*. 2009;8(2):111–128.
49. Fitzgerald JB, Schoeberl B, Nielsen UB, Sorger PK. Systems biology and combination therapy in the quest for clinical efficacy. *Nat. Chem. Biol*. 2006;2(9):458–466.
50. Iadevaia S, Lu Y, Morales FC, Mills GB, Ram PT. Identification of optimal drug combinations targeting cellular networks: integrating phospho-proteomics and computational network analysis. *Cancer Res*. 2010;70(17):6704–6714.

Index

Note: Page numbers followed by "*f*" and "*t*" refer to figures and tables, respectively.

A

Abacavir, 454
$\alpha_{1\beta}$ – adrenergic receptors, 57
Abnormal impulse conduction, 304
Aborted sudden cardiac death, 292–293
Absorption, 6
Aceclofenac, 79–80
Acetazolamide, 373
Acetylcholine, 393
  biochemistry of, 29–30
Acetylcholinesterase inhibitors, 12
Acetyl coenzyme A (acetyl-COA), 95–96
Acid, peripheral regulation of, 392–393
Activator protein 1, 506–507
Active transport, 5
Acyclovir, 459–460
Adefovir dipivoxil, 463
Adenosine, 319, 371
Adenosine receptor antagonist, 371–373
Adenylate cyclase, 536
Adenylyl cyclase, inhibition of, 34–43
  anticholinergic drugs, 35–43, 40*t*
  anticholinesterases, 35, 38*t*
  cholinergic agonists, 35
Adrenaline, 48
Adrenergic drugs, 48–49, 48*f*
  adrenergic nerve receptors, 49–58, 50*t*
  nervous system, 47–48, 48*f*
  pharmacological actions, 49
Adrenergic nerve receptors, 49–58, 50*t*
  α and β receptors, 52–58
    abstinent heroin addicts, dug-related memory reconsolidation in, 53
    α_1-adrenergic drugs, 54
    attention deficit hyperactivity disorder, animal model of, 55
    β_1-adrenergic receptor, agonist activation, 54
    β_2 – adrenergic receptor discovery of agonists, 58
    β – adrenergic receptor-ROS signaling, 57
    $\alpha_{1\beta}$ – adrenergic receptors, 57
    β-adrenergic receptors, molecular docking and drug discovery in, 57
    chronic obstructive pulmonary disease, 58
    diadenosine tetraphosphate, 56
    Down syndrome, formoterol, a long-acting 2-adrenergic agonist, 56
    endothelial progenitor cells dysfunction, 53
  G-protein, 51–52
  G protein-coupled receptor, molecular structure of, 51
Afterdepolarizations, 302–303
Agonists, 12
Albendazole, 521–522
Albiglutide, 117
Albuvirtide, 458
Aldosterone, 84
Aldosterone-induced proteins (AIPs), 356
Aldosterone-producing adenomas, 86
Aldosterone receptor antagonist, 383
Alemtuzumab, 520–521
Aliphatic antipsychotics, 233*t*
Aliskiren, 361
Alkalyting agent, 492, 512
Allergic rhinitis, 69
α and β receptors, 52–58
α-glucosidase inhibitors, 108–110
α_1-Adrenergic drugs, 54
Aluminum-containing antacids, 397
Amantadine, 463
Amiloride, 383–384
Amiodarone, 317
Amlodipine, 359
AMP-dependent protein kinase (AMPK), 105–107
Amphotericin B, 438–441
Amylin analog, 117

Anabolic-androgenic steroids (AAS), 148–153
Anakinra, 518
Andamide (AEA), 169
Andpropargylamines, 207
Androgen
biosynthesis of, 123–127, 124*f*
characteristics of, 125*t*
hormonal imbalance
in females, 127–129
in males, 129–130
hormonal therapy, 132–133
mechanism of action of, 127
Andropause, 129
AngII receptor antagonist (ARBs), 355, 360–361
Angina pectoris, 329–332, 343
consequences of, 329–332, 332*f*
pathophysiology of, 329–332, 331*f*
Angiogenesis, 339
Angiotensin-converting enzyme (ACE) inhibitors, 283, 355, 359–360
Angiotensin-II blockers, 283
Aniline derivatives, nonsteroidal anti-inflammatory drugs, 81, 82*t*
Antacids, 396–398
classification, 397
contraindication, 398
side effects, 397–398
Antagonism, 356
Antagonist, 12
Antianginal
antianginal drugs, USFDA classification of, 332–333
beta-blockers, mechanism of action of, 335–337, 337*f*
dipyridamole, 339
fasudil, 341–342, 342*f*
ivabradine, 342–343, 343*f*
nitrates, mechanism of action, 333–335
pathophysiology associated with angina pectoris, 329–332
potassium channel opener, mechanism of action of, 338–339
ranolazine, 340–341, 342*f*
trimetazidine, 340, 341*f*
Antianginal drugs, USFDA classification of, 332–333
Antianxiety medications, 161, 164–170, 165*t*
Antiarrhythmic drugs
antiarrhythmic therapy, new developments in, 320
cardiac arrhythmia, 290–293, 305–311
approach, 290
atrioventricular nodal tachycardias, 308–309
bradycardia, 305–306
genetics of, 293–294, 295*t*
palpitations, 290–291
physical findings, 293
sudden cardiac arrest and aborted sudden cardiac death, 292–293
supraventricular tachyarrhythmia, 306–308
syncope and presyncope, 291–292, 292*t*
ventricular tachyarrhythmia, 309–311
channelopathies, 299–300
catecholaminergic polymorphic ventricular tachycardia, 299–300
class I antiarrhythmic drugs, 311–312
classification of, 311, 312*t*
class II antiarrhythmic drugs, 315–316
class IV antiarrhythmic drugs, 318–319
electrophysiology, principles of, 300–304
cardiac arrhythmias, mechanisms of, 302–304, 303*t*
descriptive physiology, 300–302, 301*f*
QT-opathies, 294–299
drug-induced torsade de pointes, 297–299
long-QT syndrome, 294–299
short-QT syndrome, 297
specific class IA drugs, 313–314
specific class IB drugs, 314
specific class IC drugs, 314–315
Antiarrhythmic therapy, new developments in, 320
Antibacterial agents
β-lactams, classification of, 421–422
carbapenems, 422
cell wall biosynthesis inhibitors, 422
cephalosporins, 422–423
50S and 30S ribosomal subunits, protein synthesis inhibitors, 423–425, 423*f*
ATP synthase inhibitors, 425
membrane function inhibitors, 424
nucleic acid synthesis, inhibitors of, 424–425
Antibiotics, for *Helicobacter pylori* infection, 400–401, 402*t*, 403*t*
Antibodies to citrullinated protein antigens (ACPAs), 66–67
Anticancer drugs
classification of, 483–486, 484*t*
Newer United States Food and Drug Administration, 479–486, 484*t*

Anticancer drugs, 478
  bevacizumab, 490
  combretastatin, 486–487, 487*f*
  DNA, 486
  DNA helix, 492
  DNA-related proteins, 492–493
  drugs targeted against tumor RNA, 493
  marimastat, 491
  matrix metalloproteinases, 491
  mechanism of action, 486–496
  MOA, 487
  Newer United States Food and Drug Administration, 479–486
  pathophysiology, 478–479
  protein, 488–489
  small molecules, 490
  specific genes, 493
  tumor cell, drugs directed against proteins in, 493–496
  United States Food and Drug Administration, 479
Anticholinergics, 35–43, 40*t*, 407
Anticholinesterases, 35, 38*t*
Anti-covid drugs, 468–469
Anticytomegalovirus drugs, 467–468
Antidepressants
  adverse effect and interaction of, 266–267
  depression pathophysiology, assimilation of hypotheses on, 260–261
  dysbiosis/gut/brain axis hypotheses, 259
  fundamental pharmacology of, 261–264
    5-hydroxytryptamine receptor modulators, 263–264
    monoamine oxidase inhibitors, 264
    selective serotonin reuptake inhibitors, 261–262
    serotonin-norepinephrine reuptake inhibitors, 262–263
  glutamate hypotheses, 260, 261*f*
  glutamate signaling antagonist, 265, 266*t*
  major depression, pathophysiology of, 255–256
  monoamines and neurotransmitters hypotheses, 256–257, 257*f*
  neurotrophic hypotheses, 257–258, 258*f*
  stress-responsive/HPA axis hypotheses, 258–259
Antidiabetic drugs
  adipose cells, amaryl in, 105
  albiglutide, 117
  biguanides, 105–107
  classification, sulfonylureas, 103–104
  diabetes mellitus. *See* Diabetes mellitus
  GLP-1 agonist, 115–116
  glucose-lowering agents, 117
    pramlintide, 117, 118*f*
  K_{ATP} channel modulators, 108–117
    bromocriptine, 115
    dipeptidyl peptidase-4 inhibitors, 110
    α-glucosidase inhibitors, 108–110
    gut, dipeptidyl peptidase-4 inhibition, 110–112
    mechanism of action, 110, 112–114
    repaglinide, 108
    thiazolidinediones, 112
  liraglutide, 116–117
  metformin, 107
  metformin and organic cation transporters, 107–108
  Na^+-glucose transporter-2 inhibitors, 115
Antidiarrheal agents, 410
Antidiuretic hormone receptor (vasopressin) antagonist, 384–385
Antiemetics, 401–409
  classification of, 404–407, 406*t*
  D_2 receptors antagonists/neuroleptics, 405–406
  5-hydroxytryptamine 3 receptor antagonist, 404–405
  prochlorperazine, 406
  stimulants for vomiting, 404, 405*t*
  vomiting, 401–403, 403*f*, 404*f*
Antiepileptic drugs
  bromide, 183
  epilepsy, pathophysiology and pathogenesis of, 178–180
  GABA, role of, 180
  general treatment, 182–185
  glutamate, role of, 180–182, 181*f*
  mechanism of action
    benzodiazepines, 184
    brivaracetam, 186
    carbamazepine, 184
    eslicarbazepine acetate, 186
    ethosuximide, 184–185
    gabapentin, 185
    lacosamide, 186–187
    levetiracetam, 186
    phenobarbital, 183
    phenytoin, 183–184
    valproic acid, 185
Antifungal agents
  black fungus and COVID-19, 441
  classification of, 436–437

Antifungal agents (*Continued*)
fungal infections, 432
mechanism of, 437–440
pathophysiology, 432–436
source, 441
sudden development, reasons for, 441–442
symptoms, 442
treatments, 442
Antihelminthics, 521
Antihepatitis B drugs, 463–464
Antihepatitis C drugs, 464–465
Antiherpes drugs, 459–460
Antihistamines, 407
Antihuman immunodeficiency virus drugs, 453
Antiinfluenza drugs, 462
Antimanic drugs, 252*t*
Antimetabolites, 493, 511
Anti-Parkinson's disease drugs, 202–203
dopamine agonists, 203
levo-DOPA, 202–203
Antipsychotics, 215–216
environmental factors, 228–230
pollution, 228–230
intracellular calcium, regulation of, 246–253
carbamazepine, 246–247, 252
glycogen synthase kinase, 246, 247*f*
lamotrigine, 253
lithium carbonate, 247
mechanism, 247–249
olanzapine, 249
risperidone, 249–251
sodium valproate, 252–253
valproic acid, 247
mechanism of action of, 239
lithium, 239
psychological disorder
behaviors represented by, 217
cannabis use, 223, 224*t*
causes, 219
complications of, 221
definition of, 217–223
familial clustering, 223
gene involvement, 229*t*
genetic changes, 223–228
genetic factors, 221
genome-wide association study data and major histocompatibility complex locus, 227–228
neurotransmitters, 222
non-MHC loci, significance of, 228
physical symptoms of, 219
pregnancy and birth complications, 222
risk factors, 219
schizophrenia, etiology of, 221
schizophrenia, genetics of, 223
season of birth, 222
serious symptoms, 219
symptoms of, 218
treatment of, 220
ways to improvement, 220
psychological disorders at glance, 216–217
psychotic disease, pathophysiology of, 230–239
Antirespiratory syncytial virus drugs, 468
Antithymocyte immunoglobulin (ATG), 519–520
Antivaricella zoster virus drugs, 467
Antiviral drugs
viral targets, classification of, 448–450, 451*t*
viruses, pathophysiology of, 450–469
abacavir, 454
adhesion inhibitor, 458
amantadine and rimantadine, 463
anti-covid drugs, 468–469
anticytomegalovirus drugs, 467–468
antihepatitis B drugs, 463–464
antihepatitis C drugs, 464–465
antiherpes drugs, 459–460
antihuman immunodeficiency virus drugs, 453
antiinfluenza drugs, 462
antirespiratory syncytial virus drugs, 468
antivaricella zoster virus drugs, 467
atazanavir, 456
CCR5 receptor inhibitor, 458
cytomegalovirus, 467
darunavir, 457
docosanol, 461
fosamprenavir, 456
foscarnet, 460–461
fusion peptide inhibitor, 457–458
ganciclovir and valganciclovir, 468
hepatitis virus, 463, 464*f*
herpesvirus, 458, 459*f*
human immunodeficiency virus, 450–453
idoxuridine, 460
indinavir, 456
influenza virus, 461–462
integrase inhibitors, 457
lamivudine and emtricitabine, 453

lopinavir, 456
nelfinavir, 456
nucleotide reverse transcriptase inhibitors, 454–455
oseltamivir and zanamivir, 462–463
penciclovir and famciclovir, 460
protease inhibitors, 455
ritonavir, 455
saquinavir, 455–456
stavudine, 453
tipranavir, 456
trifluridine, 460
varicella zoster virus, 465–466
zidovudine, 453
virus life cycle and pathogenesis, 447–448, 449*f*
Anxiety, 164–170, 165*t*, 231
Anxiolytics, novel molecules with diverse pharmacological targets
endocannabinoid system, 169
GABA system, 170
glutamate system, 168
systems containing monoamines, 164–167
Apo-B monomers, 101
Apomorphine, 409
2-Arachidonoylglycerol (2-AG), 169
Aripiprazole, 251
Aspergillosis, 432–433
Aspirin, 75–76, 529–530
Asthma, 67
AT1 antagonists, 283
Atazanavir, 456
ATP synthase inhibitors, 425
Atrial fibrillation, 307
Atrial flutter, 307
Atrial premature complexes (APCs), 306
Atrial tachycardias, 307–308
Atrianatriuretic peptide, 385
Atrioventricular conduction block, 305–306
Atrioventricular junctional tachycardias, 308
Atrioventricular nodal reentrant tachycardia, 308
Atrioventricular nodal tachycardias, 308–309
Attention deficit hyperactivity disorder (ADHD), 55
Automaticity, 302
Autonomic nervous system (ANS), 27
Autonomic neurotransmitters, chemistry of, 29
Avastin, 490
AVN-101, 167
Azole antifungal, 437

B

Bacillus Calmette-Guerin (BCG), 521
Baloxavir marboxil, 462
Barbiturates, 171
Bedaquiline, 425
Benperidol, 238
Benzhexol, 238–239
Benzodiazepines, 170–171
mechanism of action, 184
Besifovir, 463
β – adrenergic receptor-ROS signaling, 57
β-adrenergic receptors, molecular docking and drug discovery in, 57
Beta-blockers, 283–284, 316
of antianginal and vasodilating agent, 335–337, 337*f*
β-cell demise and dysfunction, 102
β-lactams, classification of, 421–422
Bevacizumab, 489–490
Bictegravir, 457
Biguanides, 105–107
Biological system network, 547
Biologics, 514
definition of, 513–514
usage of, 514–515
Birth complications, pregnancy and, 222
Black fungus, antifungal agents, 441
Blastomycosis, 433
Blood perfusion, 6
Blood pressure (BP), 349
Blood pressure, normal regulation of, 350–354, 351*f*
renin and prorenin receptor, 353–354
renin secretion, control of, 352–353, 353*f*
Bottom-up modeling systems, 547
Bowman's capsule, 371
Bradycardia, 305–306
Brain axis hypotheses, 259
Brain-derived neurotrophic factor (BDNF), 227
Brain natriuretic peptide, 385
Brexpiprazole, 167
Brivaracetam, 186
Brivudine, 467
Bromide, 183
Bromocriptine, 115
Brugada syndrome, 299–300
Buformin, 105–107
Bumetanide, 376

C

Ca^{2+} channel blockers, 355, 358–359
Caffeine, 371–373

Calcineurin inhibitors, 509
Calcium channel blockers (CCBs), 284, 284*f*, 311
Canagliflozin, 373–376
Cancer, 477, 515
estrogen, progesterone and androgen, 130–132
Candesartan, 360–361
Candidal vaginitis, 433
Candidiasis, 433
Cannabidiol, 187
Cannabinoids, 408
Carbamazepine, 246–247, 252
mechanism of action, 184
Carbapenems, 422
Carbonic anhydrase inhibitors, 373
Cardiac arrhythmia
genetics of, 293–294, 295*t*
mechanisms of, 302–304, 303*t*
abnormal impulse conduction, 304
impulse initiation, alterations in, 302
triggered automaticity and afterdepolarizations, 302–303
signs and symptoms of, 290–293
approach, 290
palpitations, 290–291
physical findings, 293
sudden cardiac arrest and aborted sudden cardiac death, 292–293
syncope and presyncope, 291–292, 292*t*
types of, 305–311
atrioventricular nodal tachycardias, 308–309
bradycardia, 305–306
supraventricular tachyarrhythmia, 306–308
ventricular tachyarrhythmia, 309–311
Cardiac electrophysiology, 289
Cardiovascular lesions, 452
Carrier transport, 5–6
Carvedilol, 357
Cascade/signaling pathways, 538*t*
Catecholaminergic polymorphic ventricular tachycardia, 299–300
Brugada syndrome, 299–300
clinical description and manifestations, 299
sick sinus syndrome, 300
Catechol-o-methyltransferase, 203–204, 205*t*
Catechol-o-methyltransferase inhibitors, 203–204
Cathartics, 409–410, 411*t*
CCR5 receptor inhibitor, 458
Celecoxib, 80–81
Cell adhesion molecules (CAM), 64–65
Cell-surface forms, 514
Cell wall biosynthesis inhibitors, 422
Central nervous system (CNS), 27
lesions, 452
Cephalosporins, 422–423
Chloral hydrate, 171
Chloramphenicol, 424
Chlorothiazide, 378–382
Chlorpromazine, 232–239, 237*f*
benperidol, 238
benzhexol, 238–239
droperidol, 238
fluphenazine, 232
haloperidol, 238
mesoridazine, 237–238
penfluridole, 238
pimozide, 232–237
trifluoperazine, 232
Chlorthalidone, 378–382
Cholesterol, 84
Cholinergic agonists, 35, 36*t*
Cholinergic drugs
acetylcholine, biochemistry of, 29–30
autonomic neurotransmitters, chemistry of, 29
muscarinic receptors, 32–43, 33*t*
adenylyl cyclase, inhibition of, 34–43
nicotinic receptor, 31–32
signal transduction mechanisms, 30–31
Chronic obstructive pulmonary disease (COPD), 58, 67–68
Cidofovir, 467–468
Circulatory system, 64–65
c-Jun N-terminal kinases (JNK), 536
Class I antiarrhythmic drugs, 311–312
Class II antiarrhythmic drugs, 315–316
Class III antiarrhythmic drugs, 316–318
Class IV antiarrhythmic drugs, 318–319
Classic angina, pathology of, 331–332
Clevidipine, 359
Clonidine, 358
Clozapine, 250
Coccidioidomycosis, 433–434
Cognitive disorders, 231
Combretastatin, 486–487, 487*f*
COMT, 227
Conivaptan, 384–385
Conjugated equine estrogen (CEE), 138
Coronary arteries, 329–332
Corticosteroid-binding globulin (CBG), 127

Corticosteroids
  anti-inflammatory mechanism, 69, 82–86
  classification of, 73–74
    glucocorticoids, 74
    mineralocorticoids, 74
  contraindications of, 86
Corticosteroid sparing medication, 512–513
Cortico-striato-cerebello-thalamocortical (CSPTC) loops, 199–201
COVID-19
  antifungal agents, 441
COX-2 inhibitor, 73, 80–81
C-reactive protein (CRP), 66–67
Crohn's disease (CD), 511–512
Cryptococcosis, 434
C-type natriuretic peptide, 385
Cutaneous candidiasis, 433
Cyclobenzaprine VLD (TNX-102), 167
Cyclophosphamide, 513
Cyclopropylamines, 207
Cyclosporine, 509
Cytomegalovirus, 467
Cytosine permease, 438

D

Daclatasvir, 465
Daclizumab, 518
Danazol, 154–156
Danoprevir, 465
Dapagliflozin, 373–376
Darunavir, 457
Dasabuvir, 465
Delta-opioid (DOPR) receptor, 532
Dementia, rapid disease progression without, 197
Depression, 11, 231, 255
  pathophysiology, assimilation of hypotheses on, 260–261
Diabetes mellitus, 95
  biochemical background of, 95–96
  classification, 96
    type 1, 96
    type 2, 96–97
  drug/chemical-induced, 98
  endocrinopathies, 97–98
  etiology, 99–102
    genetic component, 99–102
  exocrinepancreas, diseases of, 97–98
  gestational diabetes mellitus, 99
  immune-mediated diabetes, uncommon forms of, 99
  infections, 99
  insulin action, genetic defects in, 97
Diadenosine tetraphosphate, 56
Diclofenac, 79–80
Dienogest, 147–148
5α-Dihydrotestosterone (DHT), 154
Digoxin, 282
  atrioventricular node inhibition, 282
  positive ionotropic, 282
Diltiazem, 318
Dimorphic fungi, 432
Dipeptidyl peptidase-4 inhibitors, 110–112
Dipyridamole, 339
Direct renin inhibitor, 355, 361
Disease-modifying antirheumatic drug (DMARD), 511
Disoproxil fumarate (TDF), 464
Disopyramide, 314
Disrupted in schizophrenia 1 (DISC1), 227
Distal convoluted tubule (DCT), 377–382
Diuretic and anti-diuretic drugs, 281–282, 354–356, 369
  classification of, 370–371
  distal convoluted tubule, 378–382
  glomerulus, 371–373
    adenosine receptor antagonist, 371–373
  hypocalcaemia and hypomagnesemia, mechanism of, 376
  hypokalemia and metabolic alkalosis, mechanism of, 377–378
  nephron, anatomy and physiology of, 369–370, 370*f*
  nephron and related diuretics, physiology, 371
  osmotic diuretics, 385–386
  proximal convoluted tubule, 373–376
    carbonic anhydrase inhibitors, 373
    sodium-glucose cotransporter 2 inhibitors, 373–376
  thick ascending limb, 376
  tubule system, 383–385
    aldosterone receptor antagonist/mineralocorticoid receptor antagonist, 383
    antidiuretic hormone receptor (vasopressin) antagonist, 384–385
    nonspecific cation channel inhibitor, 385
    renal epithelial Na^+ channel, inhibitors of, 383–384
DJ-1 gene mutation, 199
DNA helix, 492
DNA-related proteins, 492–493

DNA virus, 448, 449*f*
Docosanol, 461
Dofetilide, 317–318
Dolutegravir, 457
Donepezil, 35
Dopamine, 48
Dopamine agonists, 203
Doravirine, 455
Dorzolamide, 373
Down syndrome, 56
Doxazosin, 357
D1 receptor agonist, 362
D_2 receptors antagonists/neuroleptics, 405–406
Dronedarone, 317
Droperidol, 238
Drospirenone, 147–148
Drug/chemical-induced diabetes mellitus, 98
Drug discovery, 547
  mechanism-based approach in, 548–549
  molecular biology method in, 549
  molecular pharmacology, 551
    methods and application, 546–547
Drug discovery process, 548
Drug distribution, 7
Drug excretion, 9–10
Drug-induced torsade de pointes, 297–299
Drug metabolism, 8
Drug repositioning, and molecular pharmacology, 553
Drugs, 1
Drugs, used in hypertension
  AngII receptor antagonist, 360–361
  angiotensin-converting enzyme inhibitors, 359–360
  blood pressure, normal regulation of, 350–354, 351*f*
    renin and prorenin receptor, 353–354
    renin secretion, control of, 352–353, 353*f*
  Ca^{2+} channel blockers, 358–359
  classification of, 354–355
  direct renin inhibitor, 361
  diuretics, 355–356
  D1 receptor agonist, 362
  hypertension, etiology of, 350
  sympatholytic agents, 356–358
  vasodilators, 361
Drug-target interactions, predictions of, 552
Drug-target networks, and molecular pharmacology, 551
Dysbindin (DTNBP1), 227
Dysbiosis, 259

E

Earlier disease onset (EDO), 197
eCB system, targets for, 169
Echinocandins, 438
Edrophonium, 35
Efavirenz (EFV), 454
Elbasvir, 465
Electrolytes, 243–244
Electrophysiology, principles of, 300–304
Elsulfavirine, 455
Elvitegravir, 457
Emetics, 401–409
Empagliflozin, 373–376
Emtricitabine, 453, 457
Enalapril, 360
Endocannabinoid system, 77, 169
  eCB system, targets for, 169
  fatty acid amide hydrolase, inhibitors of, 169
Endocrine lesions, 453
Endocrinopathies, 98
Endocytosis, 538–539
Endogenous antioxidants, 448
Endogenous catecholamines, 48*f*
Endogenous steroid sex hormones, 127
Endothelial progenitor cells (EPC) dysfunction, 53
Endothelium, 486–490
Enfuvirtide, 457–458
Enolic acid, 77–79
Entecavir, 463
Enzymatic receptors, 17–19
  JAK/STAT pathway, 19
  RAS/RAF pathway, 18
Epicardial vessels, 329–332
Epilepsy, pathophysiology and pathogenesis of, 178–180
Eplerenone, 383
Epothilones, 496
Eprosartan, 360–361
Erythromycin, 423–424
Esketamine, 265
Eslicarbazepine acetate, 186
Estradiol, 133–137
Estradiol esters, 138–139
Estrogen(s)
  biosynthesis of, 123–127, 124*f*
  cancer, 130–132
  characteristics of, 125*t*
  hormonal imbalance
    in females, 127–129
    in males, 129–130

hormonal therapy, 132–133
mechanism of action of, 127, 133–139, 134t, 139f
Estrogen carcinogenesis, 130–131
Estrogen receptors (ERs), 130–131
Estrogen response elements (ERE), 133–137
Estrone sulfate, 138
Etanercept, 516
Ethacrynic acid, 376
Ethinyl estradiol (EE), 137–138
Ethosuximide, 184–185
Ethoxzolamide, 373
Etodolac, 79–80
Etomidate, 173
Etoricoxib, 80–81
Etravirine, 455
Everolimus, 511
Excitatory postsynaptic potential (EPSP), 180
Exenatide, 116
Exercise therapy, 275–276
Exocrinepancreas, diseases of, 97–98
Extracellular fluid, 7
Extracellular matrix, 490–491

F

Facilitated diffusion, 6
Famciclovir, 460
Familial clustering, 223
Fasudil, 341–342, 342f
Fatty acid amide hydrolase, inhibitors of, 169
Fatty acid steal phenomenon, 113
Favipiravir, 462
Felodipine, 359
Fenamate, 76
Fenoldopam, 362
Fertility, 127–128
50S and 30S ribosomal subunits, protein synthesis inhibitors, 423–425, 423f
ATP synthase inhibitors, 425
membrane function inhibitors, 424
nucleic acid synthesis, inhibitors of, 424–425
Filtration, 5
First-generation progestins, 147
First-order kinetics, 8
Flucytosine, 438
Fluoxymesterone, 154–156
Fluphenazine, 232
Flurbiprofen, 77
Focal atrial tachycardias (FATs), 308
Formoterol, 56
Fosamprenavir, 456
Foscarnet, 460–461
Fostemsavir, 458
Fourth-generation progestins, 147–148
Free fatty acid (FFA), 100–101
Functional disorders, 231
Fungal infections, 432
Furosemide, 376
Fusion peptide inhibitor, 457–458
Fusion proteins, 29–30

G

Gabapentin, 185
γ-aminobutyric acid (GABA), 170, 180
Ganciclovir, 468
Gastric mucosa, 392–393
Gastrin, 393, 394t
Gastroesophageal reflex disease (GERD), 398
Gastrointestinal acid regulation, 392–393
gastrin, 393, 394t
peripheral regulation of acid, 392–393
Gastrointestinal diseases
anticholinergics, 407
antidiarrheal agents, 410
antiemetics and emetics, 401–409
classification of, 404–407, 406t
stimulants for vomiting, 404, 405t
vomiting, 401–403, 403f, 404f
antihistamines, 407
cannabinoids, 408
emetics, 409
gastrointestinal acid regulation, 392–393
gastrin, 393, 394t
peripheral regulation of acid, 392–393
gastrointestinal tract, neuronal and hormonal control over, 392
glucocorticoids, 408
laxatives, purgatives, and cathartics, 409–410, 411t
neutralizing and inhibiting acid release, drugs used for, 396–399
antacids, 396–398
H^+/K^+ ATPase inhibitor/ proton pump inhibitor (PPIs), 399–401
histamine receptor antagonist, 398–399
oral rehydration supplements, 410–414, 415t
peptic ulcer, 394–396, 395t
causes of, 395–396, 396f
vitamin B6, 409
Gastrointestinal tract (GIT), 391–392
neuronal and hormonal control over, 392
G-cells, 393

Gene regulation, 551
Genetic defects, in insulin action, 97
Gestagen, 140
Gestational diabetes mellitus, 99
Gestogen, 140
G72(DAOA)/G30, 227
GI lesions, 452
Glecaprevir/pibrentasvir, 464–465
Glomerulus, 371
GLP-1 agonist, 115–116
Glucocorticoid, 505–506
Glucocorticoid-inducedleucine zipper (GILZ), 83
Glucocorticoid receptors (GRs), 83–84
Glucocorticoids, 74, 84, 408
Glutamate, 168, 180–182, 181*f*
  ketamine, 168
  xenon gas, 168
Glutamate hypotheses, 260, 261*f*
Glycerol, 385–386
Glyceryl trinitrate (GTN), 334
Glycogen synthase kinase, 246
Gonadotropin-releasing hormone (GnRH), 133–137
GPCR-regulated kinases (GRKs), 536
G protein-coupled receptor, 13–16, 14*f*
  cAMP pathway, 14–15
  IP3/DAG pathway, 15
  linked to ion channels, 16
  molecular structure of, 51
G-proteins, 51–52
Grazoprevir, 465
Griseofulvin, 438
Growth factors, 486
Guanabenz, 358
Guanadrel, 358
Guanfacine, 358
Gut, 259
  dipeptidyl peptidase-4 inhibition, 110–112

H

Haemagglutinin, 461
Haloperidol, 238
H_2 blocker drugs, 398–399
Heart failure (HF), 275
  angiotensin-converting enzyme inhibitors, 283
  angiotensin-II blockers, 283
  beta-blockers, 283–284
  calcium channel blockers, 284, 284*f*
  classification of, 275–277
  digoxin, 282
  diuretics, 281–282
  etiology, 277
  management of, 281, 281*t*
  newer agents, 284–285
  pathophysiology, 277–280
    cell, changes in, 279–280
    hemodynamics, changes in, 277–278, 278*f*
    neurohormones, changes of, 279, 280*f*
  vasodilators, 282
Helicobacter pylori infection, antibiotics for, 400–401, 402*t*, 403*t*
Hemodynamics, changes in, 277–278, 278*f*
Hepatitis virus, 463, 464*f*
Herpesvirus, 458, 459*f*
Histamine, 393
Histamine receptor antagonist, 398–399
Histone code, 478
Histoplasmosis, 434
Hormonal imbalance, 127–129
Hormonal therapy, 132–133
Human disease, molecular biology method in, 549
Human disease networks, 549
Human immunodeficiency virus (HIV), 450–453
  HIV RT, 454
Hydralazine, 361
Hydrazines, 207
Hydrochlorothiazide, 378–382
Hydrocortamate, 507–509
5-Hydroxytryptamine 3 receptor antagonist, 404–405
5-Hydroxytryptamine receptor modulators, 263–264
Hyoscine, 171
Hypertension, 85, 350
Hypnotics, 161
  administered intravenously, 173
  benzodiazepines, 170–171
  selection of hypnotic agent, 171–172
Hypocalcaemia, 376
Hypokalemia, mechanism of, 377–378
Hypomagnesemia, 376
Hypothalamic–pituitary–ovary (HPO) axis, 128–129
Hysterical dramatic symptoms, 232

I

Ibuprofen, 77
Ibutilide, 317–318
Idiopathic diabetes, 96
Idoxuridine, 460

IKr channel blockers, 298–299
Immune-mediated diabetes, uncommon forms of, 99
Immune-mediated disorders, 514
Immune system, anticancer drugs, 491–492
Immunity, 503–504
Immunoglobulin (IgE) mucosal response, 67
Immunomodulators, 504–505
  albendazole, 521–522
  alemtuzumab, 520–521
  alkalyting agent, 512
  anakinra, 518
  antihelminthics, 521
  antimetabolite, 511
  antithymocyte immunoglobulin, 519–520
  Bacillus Calmette-Guerin, 521
  biologics, 514
    definition of, 513–514
    usage of, 514–515
  calcineurin inhibitors, 509
  categorization, 515–516
  classification, 506*f*
  cyclophosphamide, 513
  cyclosporine, 509
  daclizumab, 518
  etanercept, 516
  everolimus, 511
  glucocorticoid, 505–506
  hydrocortamate, 507–509
  immunosuppressants, 505
  infliximab, 516–518
  interleukin-1 inhibitors, 518
  leflunomide, 511
  mammalian target of rapamycin inhibitors, 510
  mechanism of action of classical immunomodulatory drugs, 506–507, 508*t*
  mechanism of action of newer immunomodulators, 514
  6 mercaptopurine pathology and treatment, 511–512
  monoclonal antibodies, 520, 520*f*
  oral signs and symptoms, 513
  polyclonal antibody, 519, 519*f*
  prednisone, 507
  sirolimus, 510
  steroid-free medications, 512–513
  tacrolimus, 509–510
  tumor necrosis factor-alpha Inhibitor, 515
  vaccine, 521
Immunostimulants, 503–504
Immunosuppressive drugs, 505, 512–513
Immunotherapy, 477–478
Impulse initiation, 302
Indapamide, 378–382
Indinavir, 456
Indomethacin, 75
Inflammation, 61–65
  effective and controlled provocative reaction, 62–63
  inflammation and inflammatory pathway, pathophysiology of, 63–65
  inflammatory diseases, 65–69
    allergic rhinitis, 69
    asthma, 67
    chronic obstructive pulmonary disease, 67–68
    inflammatory bowel disease, 68
    multiple sclerosis, 69
    rheumatoid arthritis, 65–69
    treatment, 69, 70*t*
  inflammatory mediators, 65, 66*t*
Inflammatory mediators, 65, 66*t*
Infliximab, 516–518
Influenza virus, 461–462
Inhaled aspergillosis, 432–433
Inhibitory postsynaptic potential (IPSP), 180
Inositol tris-phosphate (IP3), 244–245
Insulin resistance, 100–101
Integrase inhibitors, 457
Interleukin inhibitors, 516
Interleukin-1 inhibitors, 518
Interleukins (ILs), 279
Intracellular calcium, regulation of, 246–253
  carbamazepine, 246–247, 252
  glycogen synthase kinase, 246, 247*f*
  lamotrigine, 253
  lithium carbonate, 247
  mechanism, 247–249
  olanzapine, 249
  risperidone, 249–251
  sodium valproate, 252–253
  valproic acid, 247
Intramuscular route, 3–4
Intra-myocardial arteries, 329–332
Intravenous propofol, 171
Intravenous route, 3
Intrinsic ion channels, receptors with
  mitogen activated protein kinases, 17
  Rho/Rho kinase, 17
Inverse agonist, 12
Ion channels, 301–302
  opioids, 535–536

Ipecacuanha, 409
Irbesartan, 360–361
Irritation, 11
Isosorbide, 385–386
Isosorbide dinitrate, 334
Isotonic hydrochloric acid, 393
Isradipine, 359
Ivabradine, 342–343, 343*f*

J

Janus kinases (JAK)/Signal Transducer and Activator of Transcription (STAT) pathway, 19
Junctional premature complexes (JPCs), 306
Juxtaglomerular apparatus, 352

K

Kappa-opioid (KOPR) receptor, 532
K_{ATP} channel modulators, 108–117
  bromocriptine, 115
  dipeptidyl peptidase-4 inhibitors, 110
  α-glucosidase inhibitors, 108–110
  gut, dipeptidyl peptidase-4 inhibition, 110–112
  mechanism of action, 110, 112–114
  repaglinide, 108
  thiazolidinediones, 112
K-channel openers(KCO), 103–104
Ketamine, 168, 173, 265
Ketoprofen, 77
Ketorolac, 75

L

Labetalol, 357
Lacosamide, 186–187
Lamivudine, 453
Lamotrigine, 253
Laninamivir, 463
Laxatives, 409–410, 411*t*
Lazabemide, 207, 209*t*
Ledipasvir, 465
Leflunomide, 511
Leucine-rich repeat kinase-2 (LRRK-2) mutation, 198–199
Leukemia, 513
Levetiracetam, 186
Levo-DOPA, 202–203
Lidocaine, 314, 315*f*
Ligand, 13
Ligand-gated ion channels, 16
Lincosamides, 423–424
Liraglutide, 116–117
Lisinopril, 360
Lithium, 239
  mechanisms of action, 239–245
    electrolytes, membrane transport, membrane potential, 243–244
    monoaminergic signaling, 243–244
    second messenger system, 244–245
    transcription factors, 245
Lithium carbonate, 247
LKB1-AMPK-dependent pathway, 107
Long-acting 2-adrenergic agonist, 56
Long-chain 3-ketoacylcoenzyme A thiolase (LC 3-KAT), 340
Long-QT syndrome, 294–299, 310–311
  clinical description and manifestations, 294
  genetic basis, 294–296
  phenotypic correlates, 296–297
Long-term potentiation (LTP), 535–536
Loop diuretics, 376
Loop of Henle, 374–376
Lopinavir, 456
Loxapine, 250
Lymphocyte modulators, 515
Lymphoma, 513
Lysergic acid (LSD), 263–264

M

Macrolides, 423–424
Madurella mycetomatis, 435
Magnesium, 319
Major depression, pathophysiology of, 255–256
Major depressive disorder (MDD), 255
Mammalian target of rapamycin inhibitors, 510
Mannitol, 385–386
MAP kinases, 17
Maraviroc, 458
Marimastat, 491
Matrixin, 491
Matrix metalloproteinases (MMP), 491
Mechanism-based approach, in drug discovery, 548–549
Meglitinides, 108–117
Melkersson-Rosenthal syndrome, 514–515
Meloxicam, 78–80
Membrane function inhibitors, 424
Membrane potential, 243–244
Membrane transport, 243–244

Menstruation, 127–128
Mental disorders, 215
Mephenemic acid, 76
6 Mercaptopurine, pathology and treatment, 511–512
Mescaline, 263–264
Mesoridazine, 237–238
Metabolic alkalosis, mechanism of, 377–378
Metabolic syndrome (MetS), 102
Metamizole, 81
Metformin, 107
  and organic cation transporters, 107–108
Methazolamide, 373
Methyldopa, 357–358
Metolazone, 378–382
Metoprolol, 356–357
Mexiletine, 314, 315*f*
Mineralocorticoid receptor antagonist, 383
Mineralocorticoids, 74
Minoxidil, 361
Mitogen-activated protein kinase signaling, opioids, 536–538
Moclobemide, 264
Model regression, 549
Molds, 432
Molecular biology, 549–550
Molecular pharmacology
  disease mechanisms, investigation of, 550
  drug adverse effects, investigations of, 552–553
  drug combination, predictions of, 553
  in drug discovery, 551
  drug discovery approaches, molecular pharmacology methods and application, 546–547
  drug discovery, mechanism-based approach in, 548–549
  drug repositioning and, 553
  drug-target interactions, predictions of, 552
  drug-target networks and, 551
  gene regulation and disease state, 551
  human disease and drug discovery, molecular biology method in, 549
  human disease networks and, 549
  methods and application, 546–547
  network, molecular approaches based on, 547–548
  in treatment response prediction, 549–550
Monoamine oxidase (MAO), 206
Monoamine oxidase-A, 206–207
Monoamine oxidase-B, 206–207
Monoamine oxidase-B inhibitor, 207
Monoamine oxidase inhibitors, 264
Monoaminergic signaling, 244
Monoamines, 256–257, 257*f*
Monoclonal antibodies (mab), 487–489, 488*t*, 490*t*, 494, 514
  immunomodulators, 520, 520*f*
Morphine, side effects of, 530, 531*t*
mPGES-1, 78–79
Mucocutaneous lesions, 452
Mucormycosis, 435
Multifocal atrial tachycardia (MAT), 307
Multiple sclerosis, 69
Muromonab, 489
Muscarinic receptors, 32–43, 33*t*
Musculoskeletal lesions, 452
Mycetoma, 435
Mycoses, 432
Myosin light chain kinase (MLCK), 333–334

N

Na^+-glucose transporter-2 inhibitors, 115
Nandrolone, 156–157
Naproxen, 77
Natural opioid drugs, 533–534, 534*t*
Nebumetone, 75
Nefazodone, 263–264
Nefopam, 81
Nelfinavir, 456
Neosporin, 424
Neostigmine, 35
Nephron, anatomy and physiology of, 369–370, 370*f*
Nephron and related diuretics, physiology, 371
Nervous system, 47–48, 48*f*
Network, molecular approaches, 547–548
Neurohormones, changes of, 279, 280*f*
Neuroleptic drugs, 215–216
Neurotransmitters, 222
Neurotransmitters hypotheses, 256–257, 257*f*
Neurotrophic hypotheses, 257–258, 258*f*
Neutrophils, 64–65
Nevirapine (NVP), 455
Newer United States Food and Drug Administration, anticancer drugs, 479–486
Nicotinic receptor, 31–32
Nimesulide, 79–80
Nisoldipine, 359
Nitrates, 333–335
Nitroprusside, 361

Nonabsorbable antacids, 397
Non-NRTIs (NNRTIs), 454
Nonselective COX inhibitor, 73–79
  nonsteroidalanti-inflammatory drugs, 74–79
Nonspecific cation channel inhibitor, 385
Nonsteroidal anti-inflammatory drugs (NSAIDs), 72–73
  contraindications of, 86
  molecular mechanism of action, 74–81
    aniline derivatives, 81, 82*t*
    nonselective COX inhibitors, 74–79
    preferential COX II inhibitors, 79–80
    selective COX-2 inhibitors, 80–81
  newly approved NSAID drugs, 73
  nonselective COX inhibitor, 73
  preferential cyclooxygenase II inhibitor, 73
  selective COX-2 inhibitor, 73
Nonsulfonyl ureas, 108–117
Nonsustained ventricular tachycardia, 309
Non tremor dominant (TD), 197
Noradrenaline, 28–29, 48
Norgestimate, 147
Norgestrel, 147
NRG1, 223–226
Nuclear factor-B (NFB), 506–507
Nuclear receptors, 19–20
Nucleic acid synthesis, inhibitors of, 424–425
Nucleoside reverse transcriptase inhibitors (NRTIs), 453
Nucleotide-binding folds (NBF), 103–104
Nucleotide reverse transcriptase inhibitors, 454–455

O

Obesity, 100
Obsessive compulsive disorder (OCD), 231
Olanzapine, 249, 251
Ombitasvir, 465
Opioid(s), 529–530
  adenylate cyclase, 536
  classic mechanism, 535
  ion channels, 535–536
  mitogen-activated protein kinase signaling, 536–538
  molecular recognition of, 533–534
  opioid receptors, 530–533
  tolerance, 538–539
Opioid receptors, 530–533
Oral rehydration supplements, 410–414, 415*t*
Oral route, 2
Oral thrush, 433
Organic cation transporters, metformin and, 107–108
Organic nitrates, 333
Orofacial granulomatosis, 514–515
Oseltamivir, 462–463
Osmotic diuretics, 385–386
Oxicams, 77–78
Oxidative stress, in diabetes mellitus, 101
  pathophysiology of, 101–102, 102*t*
Oxycodone, 530
OxyContin, 529–530

P

Pain, 529–530
Paliperidone, 251
Palivizumab, 468
Palpitations, 290–291
Paracetamol, 81
Parecoxib, 80–81
Paritaprevir, 465
Parkinson's disease (PD), 195–196
  anti-Parkinson's disease drugs, 202–203
    dopamine agonists, 203
    levo-DOPA, 202–203
  catechol-o-methyltransferase, 203 204, 205*t*
  catechol-O-methyltransferase inhibitors and, 203–204
  epidemiology and risk factors for, 198–199, 198*t*
  inhibitors of monoamine oxidase-A and monoamine oxidase-B, 207
  monoamine oxidase, 206
  monoamine oxidase-A and monoamine oxidase-B, 206–207
  monoamine oxidase-B inhibitor lazabemide and, 207, 209*t*
  monoamine oxidase-B inhibitor selegiline and, 207, 208*f*
  pathophysiology and pathoanatomy of, 201, 202*f*
  substantia nigra and association with neuronal components, 199–201
  symptoms and subtypes, 196–197, 197*t*
PARK-2 mutation, 199
Pars compacta, 199–201
Pars reticulata, 199–201
Partial agonist, 12
Passive diffusion, 4–5
Penciclovir, 460
Penfluridole, 238
Penicillium chrysogenum, 422
Penicillium notatum, 422
Peptic ulcer, 394–396, 395*t*
  causes of, 395–396, 396*f*
Peramivir, 462–463

Perampanel, 186
Peripheral nervous system, 47–48
Peroxisomal proliferator-activated receptor gamma (PPAR)γ, 112–113
Persistent generalized lymphadenopathy, 452
Pharmacological therapy, 289–290
Pharmacology, 1
  absorption, 6
  absorption of drugs, factors affecting, 6
  distribution, apparent volume of, 8
  drug administration, local routes of, 4
  drug distribution, 7
  drug excretion, 9–10
  drug metabolism, 8
  history of, 1–2
  kinetics of metabolism, 8–9
    phase II reactions, 9
    phase I reactions, 9
  mechanism of drug actions
    chemical action, 12
    physical action, 11
    through enzymes, 12
    through receptors, 12
  nature of receptors, 13
  pharmacodynamics, 10–11
    drug action, principles of, 10–11
  pharmacokinetic and pharmacodynamic steps, 2, 2*f*
  pharmacokinetics, 4–5
    filtration, 5
    passive diffusion, 4–5
  pinocytosis, 6
  plasma protein binding of drugs, 8
  routes of drug administration, 2–4, 3*f*
    enteral routes, 2–3
    parenteral routes of drug administration, 3–4
  specialized transport, 5–6
    active transport, 5
    carrier transport, 5–6
    facilitated diffusion, 6
  transducer mechanisms, 13–20
    enzymatic receptors, 17–19
    G protein–coupled receptors, 13–16, 14*f*
    nuclear receptors, 19–20
    receptors with intrinsic ion channels, 16–17
  water compartments, 7
    extracellular fluid, 7
    plasma compartment, 7
    total body water, 7
Phase I reactions, 9
Phase II reactions, 9
Phenformin, 105–107
Phenobarbitone, 183
Phenothiazine, 216, 222
Phenylbutazone, 74
Phenytoin, 183–184
Phobic states, 231
Phosphodiesterase 7B (PDE7B), 156–157
Physostigmine, 35
Pibrentasvir, 464–465
Pimozide, 232–237
Pinocytosis, 6
Piroxicam, 77–79
Plasma compartment, 7
Pollution, 228–230
  environmental damages, 229–230
  toxicology of, 229
Polyclonal antibody, 519, 519*f*
Polycystic ovary syndrome (PCOS), 128–129
Polyene antibiotic, 438–441
Posttraumatic stress disorders, 232
Postural baroreflex, 351–352
Potassium bromide, 183
Potassium channel opener, 338–339
PPAR-responsive elements (PPRE), 113
Pramlintide, 117, 118*f*
Prazosin, 357
Prednisone, 507
Preferential COX II inhibitors, nonsteroidal anti-inflammatory drugs, 79–80
Preferential cyclooxygenase II inhibitor, 73
Preganglionic parasympathetic neurons, 29
Pregnancy, and birth complications, 222
Premature ventricular complexes (PVCs), 309
Presyncope, 291–292
Procainamide, 314
Prochlorperazine, 406
Prodrugs, 156–157
Profens, 77
Progestagen, 140
Progesterone
  biosynthesis of, 123–127, 124*f*
  carcinogenesis, 131
  characteristics of, 125*t*
  mechanism of action of, 127
Progestin(s)
  hormonal imbalance
    in females, 127–129
    in males, 129–130
  hormonal therapy, 132–133
  mechanism of action, 140–148, 141*t*, 146*f*
Progestin generations, 140

Progestogen, 140
Proinflammatory transcription factors, 506–507
Prokinetic drugs, 406–407
Propiphenazone, 81
Propofol, 173
Propranolol, 356–357
Prorenin receptor, 353–354
Prostaglandins, 67–68
Protease inhibitors, 455
Protein, anticancer drugs, 488–489
Protein synthesis inhibitors, 422–423
  50S and 30S ribosomal subunits, 423–425, 423*f*
    ATP synthase inhibitors, 425
    membrane function inhibitors, 424
    nucleic acid synthesis, inhibitors of, 424–425
Proximal convoluted tubule, 371–376
  carbonic anhydrase inhibitors, 373
  sodium-glucose cotransporter 2 inhibitors, 373–376
Psychological disorder, 215–217
  behaviors represented by, 217
  cannabis use, 223, 224*t*
  causes, 219
  complications of, 221
  definition of, 217–223
  familial clustering, 223
  gene involvement, 229*t*
  genetic changes, 223–228
  genetic factors, 221
  genome-wide association study data and major histocompatibility complex locus, 227–228
  neurotransmitters, 222
  non-MHC loci, significance of, 228
  physical symptoms of, 219
  pregnancy and birth complications, 222
  risk factors, 219
  schizophrenia, etiology of, 221
  schizophrenia, genetics of, 223
  season of birth, 222
  serious symptoms, 219
  symptoms of, 218
  treatment of, 220
  ways to improvement, 220
Psychosis, 215, 230–231
Psychotherapy, 220
Psychotic disease, pathophysiology of, 230–239
  chlorpromazine, 232–239, 237*f*
  psychoses, 230–231
  schizophrenia, 231–232, 233*t*
Pulmonary aspergillosis, 432
Pulmonary diseases, 434
Pulmonary lesions, 452
Purgatives, 409–410, 411*t*
P2X4, 535–536
Pyrazolone derivative-oxyphenylbutazone, 74
Pyridostigmine, 35

Q

QT-opathies, 294–299
  drug-induced torsade de pointes, 297–299
  long-QT syndrome, 294–299
  short-QT syndrome, 297
Quetiapine, 250
Quinidine, 313–314

R

Raltegravir, 457
Ranolazine, 340–341, 342*f*
Ras/Raf pathway, 195, 495*f*
Rat Sarcoma (RAS)/Rapidly Accelerated Fibrosarcoma (RAF) pathway, 18
Rauwolfia serpentina, 358
Rectal route, 3
Reentry, 304
Remdesivir, 468–469
Renal epithelial Na^+ channel, inhibitors of, 383–384
Renal lesions, 452
Renin, 353–354
Renin secretion, control of, 352–353, 353*f*
Repaglinide, 108
Repolarization reserve, 298–299
Rheumatoid arthritis (RA), 66–67
Rho/Rho kinase, 17
Rilpivirine (RPV), 454
Rimantadine, 463
Risperidone, 249–251
  aripiprazole, 251
  clozapine, 250
  loxapine, 250
  olanzapine, 251
  paliperidone, 251
  quetiapine, 250
  risperidone, 250–251
  thioridazine, 249–250
  triflupromazine, 250
  zotepine, 251
Ritonavir, 455, 465

Rituximab, 515
Rivastigmine, 35
RNA virus, 448, 449*f*

S

Salicylates, 66–67, 75–76
Saquinavir, 455–456
Schizophrenia, 231–232, 233*t*
  etiology of, 221
  genetics of, 223
Schizophrenia-like disorders, 215
Second-generation progestins, 147
Second messenger system, 244–245
Sedatives, 161, 170–173
  administered intravenously, 173
  anxiety and antianxiety medications, 164–170
  benzodiazepines, 170–171
  generalized mode of action, 161–164, 163*f*
  novel molecules with diverse pharmacological targets
    endocannabinoid system, 169
    GABA system, 170
    glutamate system, 168
    systems containing monoamines, 164–167
Seizure, 182
Selective serotonin reuptake inhibitors (SSRIs), 261–262
Selegiline, 207, 208*f*
Septic shock, 62–63
Serotonin-norepinephrine reuptake inhibitors (SNRIs), 262–263
Serotonin reuptake transporter (SERT), 261–262
17α-alkylated AAS, 154–156
Severe acute respiratory syndrome coronavirus 2, 468
Sevoflurane, 171
Sex hormone, 127
Sex hormone–binding globulin (SHBG), 127
Short-QT syndrome, 297
  clinical description and manifestations, 297
  genetic basis, 297
  genotype-phenotype correlates, 297, 298*f*
Sick sinus syndrome (SSS), 300
Signal transduction mechanisms, 30–31
Simeprevir, 465
Sinoatrial node dysfunction (SND), 305
Sinus tachycardia, 306
Sirolimus, 510
Small molecules, 490, 494
Sodium bromide, 183
Sodium channel binding, 311–312
Sodium-glucose cotransporter 2 inhibitors, 373–376
Sodium valproate, 252–253
Sofosbuvir, 465
Sotalol, 316, 318
Sphingosine 1-phosphate stimulation, 57
Spironolactone, 383
Spontaneous (fourth phase) diastolic depolarization, 302
Spontaneously hypertensive rat (SHR), 55–56
Sporotrichosis, 435–436
Stavudine, 453
Steroid-free medications, 512–513
Steroid hormones, 123
Steroid receptors, 19–20
Stimulation, 11
Stiripentol, 187
Street drug, 529–530
Stress-responsive/HPA axis hypotheses, 258–259
Stroke, 320
Subcutaneous route, 4
Sublingual/buccal, 3
Substantia nigra, and association with neuronal components, 199–201
Sudden cardiac arrest (SCA), 290, 292–293
Sulfonylurea receptor (SUR), 103–104
Sulfonylureas, 103–104
Supraventricular tachyarrhythmia, 306–308
  atrial fibrillation, 307
  atrial flutter, 307
  atrial premature complexes (APCs), 306
  junctional premature complexes (JPCs), 306
  sinus tachycardia, 306
Surface area
  for absorption, 6
  retention time at, 6
Susceptibility loci, 100–102
  β-cell demise and dysfunction, 102
  insulin resistance, 100–101
  obesity and physical inactivity, 100
  oxidative stress, in diabetes mellitus
    pathophysiology of, 101–102, 102*t*
Sustained ventricular tachycardia, 310
Sympathetic nervous system (SNS), 28–29
Sympatholytic agents, 354–358
Synapses, 178
Synapsin-I, 103–104
Synaptosomal nerve-associated proteins (SNAPs), 29–30

Syncope, 291–292, 292*t*
Synthetic androgens, 148–157, 149*t*, 155*f*
Synthetic estrogens, 133–139, 134*t*, 139*f*
Synthetic progestins, 140–148, 141*t*, 146*f*
Systemic candidiasis, 433
Systems containing monoamines, 164–167
  AVN-101, 167
  brexpiprazole, 167
  cyclobenzaprine VLD (TNX-102), 167
  vilazodone, 167

T

Tachycardias, with accessory atrioventricular pathways, 308–309
Tacrine, 35
Tacrolimus, 509–510
Target-oriented drug discovery, 546
Taxanes, 496
Telbivudine, 463
Telmisartan, 360–361
Tenofovir, 454–455
Tenofovir alafenamide (TAF), 464
Tenoxicam, 77–79
Terbinafine, 437–438
Testosterone deficiency syndrome, 129
Testosterone, esters of, 154
Theobromine, 371–373
Theophylline, 371–373
Thiazide diuretics, 378–382
Thiazolidinediones, 112
Thick ascending limb (TAL), 375–376
Thiopentone, 173
Thioridazine, 249–250
Thioxanthene, 216
Third-generation progestins, 147
Thyroid dysregulation, 259
Thyroid hormone receptors
Tipranavir, 456
Tissue degeneration, 64–65
TNF inhibitors, 515
Tolvaptan, 384–385
Top-down modeling systems, 547
Topoisomerases, 492
Torsades de pointes, 310
Torsemide, 376
Total body water, 7
Toxoplasma gondii, 69
Transmembranedomains (TMD), 103–104
Transmembrane helix 6 (TM6), 533–534
Trazodone, 263–264
Tremor dominant (TD), 197
Triamterene, 383–384
Triazines, 512
Triclofos, 171
Tricyclic antidepressants (TCAs), 261–263
Trifluoperazine, 232
Triflupromazine, 250
Trifluridine, 460
Triggered automaticity, 302–303
Trimetazidine, 340, 341*f*
Tubule system, 380–385, 381*f*, 382*f*
  aldosterone receptor antagonist/ mineralocorticoid receptor antagonist, 383
  antidiuretic hormone receptor (vasopressin) antagonist, 384–385
  nonspecific cation channel inhibitor, 385
  renal epithelial Na^+ channel, inhibitors of, 383–384
Tubulin, 496
Tumor cell
  drugs directed against proteins in, 493–496
  intracellular pathways in, 494–495
Tumor DNA, anticancer drugs, 492–496
Tumor membrane, receptor in, 494
Tumor necrosis factor (TNF), 279
Tumor necrosis factor-alpha Inhibitor, 515
Tumor-suppressor genes, 478–479
Tylenol, 529–530
Type 1 diabetes (T1DM), 95–96
  pathophysiology of, 96–97
Type 2 diabetes, 95–97
  pathophysiology of, 97

U

United States Food and Drug Administration (USFDA), anticancer drugs, 479
Urea, 385–386
Urodilatin, 385
Use-dependent blockage, 312

V

Vaccine, 521
Valacyclovir, 459–460
Valganciclovir, 468
Valproic acid, 185, 247
Valsartan, 360–361
Vaniprevir, 465
Variant angina, pathology of, 332
Varicella zoster virus, 465–466

Vasodilating agent
antianginal drugs, USFDA classification of, 332–333
beta-blockers, mechanism of action of, 335–337, 337*f*
dipyridamole, 339
fasudil, 341–342, 342*f*
ivabradine, 342–343, 343*f*
nitrates, mechanism of action, 333–335
pathophysiology associated with angina pectoris, 329–332
potassium channel opener, mechanism of action of, 338–339
ranolazine, 340–341, 342*f*
trimetazidine, 340, 341*f*
Vasodilators, 282, 355, 361
Vasospastic angina, 332
Velpatasvir, 465
Venlafaxine, 262–263
Ventricular flutter, 310
Ventricular tachyarrhythmia, 309–311
long-QT syndrome, 310–311
premature ventricular complexes, 309
ventricular flutter, 310
ventricular tachycardia, 309–310
Ventricular tachycardia, 309–310
Verapamil, 318
Vernakalant, 320
Vesicle-associated membrane proteins (VAMPs), 29–30
Vesicular acetylcholine transporter (VAChT), 29–30
Vicodin, 529–530
Vidarabine, 467
Vilazodone, 167
Viruses, 447, 450–469
abacavir, 454
adhesion inhibitor, 458
amantadine and rimantadine, 463
anti-covid drugs, 468–469
anticytomegalovirus drugs, 467–468
antihepatitis B drugs, 463–464
antihepatitis C drugs, 464–465
antiherpes drugs, 459–460
antihuman immunodeficiency virus drugs, 453
antiinfluenza drugs, 462
antirespiratory syncytial virus drugs, 468
antivaricella zoster virus drugs, 467
atazanavir, 456
CCR5 receptor inhibitor, 458
cytomegalovirus, 467
darunavir, 457
docosanol, 461
fosamprenavir, 456
foscarnet, 460–461
fusion peptide inhibitor, 457–458
ganciclovir and valganciclovir, 468
hepatitis virus, 463, 464*f*
herpesvirus, 458, 459*f*
human immunodeficiency virus, 450–453
idoxuridine, 460
indinavir, 456
influenza virus, 461–462
integrase inhibitors, 457
lamivudine and emtricitabine, 453
lopinavir, 456
nelfinavir, 456
nucleotide reverse transcriptase inhibitors, 454–455
oseltamivir and zanamivir, 462–463
penciclovir and famciclovir, 460
protease inhibitors, 455
ritonavir, 455
saquinavir, 455–456
stavudine, 453
tipranavir, 456
trifluridine, 460
varicella zoster virus, 465–466
zidovudine, 453
Vitamin B6, 409
Voltage-gated ion channels, 302
Vomiting, 401–403, 403*f*, 404*f*
stimulants for, 404, 405*t*

W

Wasting syndrome, 452
White blood cells, 64–65

X

Xenon gas, 168

Y

Yeast-*Cryptococcus neoformans*, 432
Yeast-like fungi, 432

Z

Zanamivir, 462–463
Zero-order kinetics, 9
Zidovudine, 453
Zotepine, 251

FSC
www.fsc.org
MIX
Papier | Fördert
gute Waldnutzung
FSC® C083411

Kolibri 360 GmbH
Ferdinand-Jühlke-Straße 7
99095 Erfurt, Deutschland
produktsicherheit@kolibri360.de